Evidence Based
Clinical Gynecology

Evidence Based Clinical Gynecology

Editors

Devender Kumar MD (OG)
Professor
Department of Obstetrics and Gynecology
Maulana Azad Medical College and Lok Nayak Hospital
New Delhi, India

Nilanchali Singh MS (OG)
Assistant Professor
Department of Obstetrics and Gynecology
Maulana Azad Medical College and Lok Nayak Hospital
New Delhi, India

Anjali Tempe MD (OG)
Director-Professor and Head
Department of Obstetrics and Gynecology
Maulana Azad Medical College and Lok Nayak Hospital
New Delhi, India

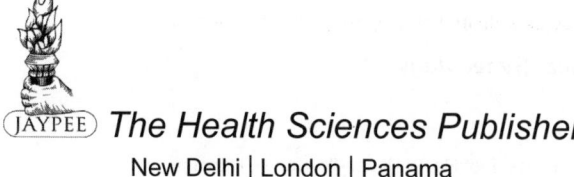

The Health Sciences Publisher
New Delhi | London | Panama

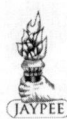
Jaypee Brothers Medical Publishers (P) Ltd.

Headquarters
Jaypee Brothers Medical Publishers (P) Ltd.
4838/24, Ansari Road, Daryaganj
New Delhi 110 002, India
Phone: +91-11-43574357
Fax: +91-11-43574314
E-mail: jaypee@jaypeebrothers.com

Overseas Offices

J.P. Medical Ltd.
83, Victoria Street, London
SW1H 0HW (UK)
Phone: +44-20 3170 8910
Fax: +44(0) 20 3008 6180
E-mail: info@jpmedpub.com

Jaypee-Highlights Medical Publishers Inc.
City of Knowledge, Bld. 235, 2nd Floor, Clayton
Panama City, Panama
Phone: +1 507-301-0496
Fax: +1 507-301-0499
E-mail: cservice@jphmedical.com

Jaypee Brothers Medical Publishers (P) Ltd.
17/1-B, Babar Road, Block-B, Shaymali
Mohammadpur, Dhaka-1207
Bangladesh
Mobile: +08801912003485
E-mail: jaypeedhaka@gmail.com

Jaypee Brothers Medical Publishers (P) Ltd.
Bhotahity, Kathmandu, Nepal
Phone: +977-9741283608
E-mail: kathmandu@jaypeebrothers.com

Website: www.jaypeebrothers.com
Website: www.jaypeedigital.com

© 2017, Jaypee Brothers Medical Publishers

The views and opinions expressed in this book are solely those of the original contributor(s)/author(s) and do not necessarily represent those of editor(s) of the book.

All rights reserved. No part of this publication may be reproduced, stored or transmitted in any form or by any means, electronic, mechanical, photocopying, recording or otherwise, without the prior permission in writing of the publishers.

All brand names and product names used in this book are trade names, service marks, trademarks or registered trademarks of their respective owners. The publisher is not associated with any product or vendor mentioned in this book.

Medical knowledge and practice change constantly. This book is designed to provide accurate, authoritative information about the subject matter in question. However, readers are advised to check the most current information available on procedures included and check information from the manufacturer of each product to be administered, to verify the recommended dose, formula, method and duration of administration, adverse effects and contraindications. It is the responsibility of the practitioner to take all appropriate safety precautions. Neither the publisher nor the author(s)/editor(s) assume any liability for any injury and/or damage to persons or property arising from or related to use of material in this book.

This book is sold on the understanding that the publisher is not engaged in providing professional medical services. If such advice or services are required, the services of a competent medical professional should be sought.

Every effort has been made where necessary to contact holders of copyright to obtain permission to reproduce copyright material. If any has been inadvertently overlooked, the publisher will be pleased to make the necessary arrangements at the first opportunity.

Inquiries for bulk sales may be solicited at: jaypee@jaypeebrothers.com

Evidence Based Clinical Gynecology

First Edition: **2017**
ISBN: 978-93-86261-78-6
Printed at Rajkamal Electric Press, Plot No. 2, Phase-IV, Kundli, Haryana.

Dedicated to

Humanities in medical education and all learners.

Contributors

Akanksha Sharma
Senior Resident
Department of Obstetrics and Gynecology
Maulana Azad Medical College and
Lok Nayak Hospital
New Delhi, India

Akansha Shrivastava
Senior Resident
Department of Obstetrics and Gynecology
Maulana Azad Medical College and
Lok Nayak Hospital
New Delhi, India

Anjali Tempe
Director-Professor and Head
Department of Obstetrics and Gynecology
Maulana Azad Medical College and
Lok Nayak Hospital
New Delhi, India

Anoosha K Ravi
Resident
Department of Obstetrics and Gynecology
Maulana Azad Medical College and
Lok Nayak Hospital
New Delhi, India

Arun Kumar Rathi
Professor
Department of Radiotherapy
Maulana Azad Medical College and
Lok Nayak Hospital
New Delhi, India

Ashok Kumar
Director-Professor
Department of Obstetrics and Gynecology
Maulana Azad Medical College and
Lok Nayak Hospital
New Delhi, India

Asmita M Rathore
Director-Professor
Department of Obstetrics and Gynecology
Maulana Azad Medical College and
Lok Nayak Hospital
New Delhi, India

Asmita Patil
Assistant Professor
Department of Physiology
All India Institute of Medical Sciences (AIIMS)
New Delhi, India

Bhavya Sareen
Resident
Department of Obstetrics and Gynecology
Maulana Azad Medical College and
Lok Nayak Hospital
New Delhi, India

Bhoomika Tantuway
Senior Resident
Department of Obstetrics and Gynecology
Maulana Azad Medical College and
Lok Nayak Hospital
New Delhi, India

Bidhisha Singha
Specialist
Department of Obstetrics and Gynecology
Maulana Azad Medical College and
Lok Nayak Hospital
New Delhi, India

Chetna Arvind Sethi
Specialist
Department of Obstetrics and Gynecology
Maulana Azad Medical College and
Lok Nayak Hospital
New Delhi, India

Deepali Dhingra
Senior Resident
Department of Obstetrics and Gynecology
Maulana Azad Medical College and
Lok Nayak Hospital
New Delhi, India

Deepti Goswami
Director-Professor
Department of Obstetrics and Gynecology
Maulana Azad Medical College and
Lok Nayak Hospital
New Delhi, India

Devender Kumar
Professor
Department of Obstetrics and Gynecology
Maulana Azad Medical College and
Lok Nayak Hospital
New Delhi, India

Divya Arora
Resident
Department of Obstetrics and Gynecology
Maulana Azad Medical College and
Lok Nayak Hospital
New Delhi, India

Gauri Gandhi
Director-Professor
Department of Obstetrics and Gynecology
Maulana Azad Medical College and
Lok Nayak Hospital
New Delhi, India

Gunjan Bhatnagar
Senior Resident
Department of Obstetrics and Gynecology
Maulana Azad Medical College and
Lok Nayak Hospital
New Delhi, India

Karishma Bhatia
Resident
Department of Obstetrics and Gynecology
Maulana Azad Medical College and
Lok Nayak Hospital
New Delhi, India

Kishore Singh
Head and Director-Professor
Department of Radiotherapy
Maulana Azad Medical College and Lok Nayak
Hospital, New Delhi, India

Komal Rastogi
Senior Resident
Department of Obstetrics and Gynecology
Maulana Azad Medical College and
Lok Nayak Hospital
New Delhi, India

Krishna Agarwal
Professor
Department of Obstetrics and Gynecology
Maulana Azad Medical College and
Lok Nayak Hospital
New Delhi, India

Latika Sahu
Professor
Department of Obstetrics and Gynecology
Maulana Azad Medical College and
Lok Nayak Hospital
New Delhi, India

Leena Wadhwa
Professor
Department of Obstetrics and Gynecology
ESI-Postgraduate Institute of Medical Sciences
and Research
Basai Darapur, New Delhi, India

Madhavi M Gupta
Professor
Department of Obstetrics and Gynecology
Maulana Azad Medical College and
Lok Nayak Hospital
New Delhi, India

Meenoo S
Resident
Department of Obstetrics and Gynecology
Maulana Azad Medical College and
Lok Nayak Hospital
New Delhi, India

Neelam Yadav
Senior Resident
Department of Obstetrics and Gynecology
Maulana Azad Medical College and
Lok Nayak Hospital
New Delhi, India

Niharika Dhiman
Assistant Professor
Department of Obstetrics and Gynecology
Maulana Azad Medical College and
Lok Nayak Hospital
New Delhi, India

Nikhil Khattar
Professor
Department of Urology
Postgraduate Institute of Medical Education and
Research and Dr Ram Manohar Lohia Hospital
New Delhi, India

Nilanchali Singh
Assistant Professor
Department of Obstetrics and Gynecology
Maulana Azad Medical College and
Lok Nayak Hospital
New Delhi, India

Nupur Ahuja
Senior Resident
Department of Obstetrics and Gynecology
Maulana Azad Medical College and
Lok Nayak Hospital
New Delhi, India

Pooja Rani
Resident
Department of Obstetrics and Gynecology
ESI-Postgraduate Institute of Medical Sciences
and Research
Basai Darapur, New Delhi, India

Poonam Kashyap
Specialist
Department of Obstetrics and Gynecology
Maulana Azad Medical College and
Lok Nayak Hospital
New Delhi, India

Poonam Sachdeva
Senior Specialist
Department of Obstetrics and Gynecology
Maulana Azad Medical College and
Lok Nayak Hospital
New Delhi, India

Preeti Singh
Assistant Professor
Department of Obstetrics and Gynecology
Maulana Azad Medical College and
Lok Nayak Hospital
New Delhi, India

Pushpa Mishra
Senior Medical Officer
Department of Obstetrics and Gynecology
Maulana Azad Medical College and
Lok Nayak Hospital
New Delhi, India

Rachna Sharma
Senior Specialist
Department of Obstetrics and Gynecology
Maulana Azad Medical College and
Lok Nayak Hospital
New Delhi, India

Reena Rani
Senior Resident
Department of Obstetrics and Gynecology
Maulana Azad Medical College and
Lok Nayak Hospital
New Delhi, India

Renu Tanwar
Professor
Department of Obstetrics and Gynecology
Maulana Azad Medical College and
Lok Nayak Hospital
New Delhi, India

Reva Tripathi
Director-Professor
Department of Obstetrics and Gynecology
Maulana Azad Medical College and
Lok Nayak Hospital
New Delhi, India

Rini Pachori
Resident
Department of Obstetrics and Gynecology
Maulana Azad Medical College and
Lok Nayak Hospital
New Delhi, India

Ritesh Kumar Singh
Senior Resident
Department of Urology
Postgraduate Institute of Medical Education and
Research and Dr Ram Manohar Lohia Hospital
New Delhi, India

Sangeeta Bhasin
Chief Medical Officer (NFSG)
Department of Obstetrics and Gynecology
Maulana Azad Medical College and
Lok Nayak Hospital
New Delhi, India

Sangeeta Gupta
Professor
Department of Obstetrics and Gynecology
Maulana Azad Medical College and
Lok Nayak Hospital
New Delhi, India

Savita Arora
Assistant Professor
Department of Radiotherapy
Maulana Azad Medical College and
Lok Nayak Hospital
New Delhi, India

Shakun Tyagi
Assistant Professor
Department of Obstetrics and Gynecology
Maulana Azad Medical College and
Lok Nayak Hospital
New Delhi, India

Shipra Chandra
Senior Resident
Department of Physiology
All India Institute of Medical Sciences (AIIMS)
New Delhi, India

Shristi
Resident
Department of Obstetrics and Gynecology
Maulana Azad Medical College and
Lok Nayak Hospital
New Delhi, India

Shubhi Yadav
Senior Resident
Department of Obstetrics and Gynecology
ESI-Postgraduate Institute of Medical Sciences
and Research
Basai Darapur, New Delhi, India

Siddhidatri Mishra
Senior Resident
Department of Obstetrics and Gynecology
Maulana Azad Medical College and
Lok Nayak Hospital
New Delhi, India

Snigdha Pathak
Resident
Department of Obstetrics and Gynecology
Maulana Azad Medical College and
Lok Nayak Hospital
New Delhi, India

Yedla Manikya Mala
Director-Professor
Department of Obstetrics and Gynecology
Maulana Azad Medical College and
Lok Nayak Hospital
New Delhi, India

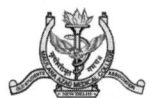

Dr Deepak K Tempe
(MD FRCA FAMS)
DEAN

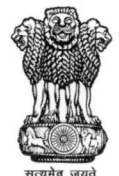

सत्यमेव जयते

**Maulana Azad Medical College &
Associated GB Pant, LNH & GNEC Hospitals**
Bahadur Shah Zafar Marg
New Delhi - 110002 (India)
Ph. : 91-11-23231478, 23231438
Fax: 91-11-23235574 Ext.: 101-102
Email : deanmamc.2012@gmail.com

Foreword

Maulana Azad Medical College (MAMC) has a rich tradition of academic excellence and the credit goes to its mentors, faculty and the students. It is said that the buildings do not make an institution, it is the individuals who make it. Therefore, the contribution by the faculty, residents, nursing and other support staff is paramount. In particular, ethical practice, innovations, and upbringing of talents deserve a special mention.

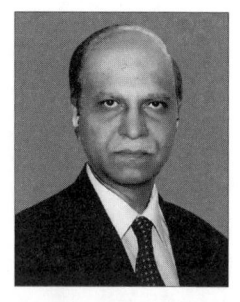

Every department has a role to play in this endeavor, and the department of obstetrics and gynecology is one of the major departments that strive to provide quality patient care. Postgraduate practical course is one of the many initiatives that the department has undertaken in this direction. The main objective of this course is to impart the knowledge, clinical skills, and nontechnical skills (cognitive, social and personal resource skills) to the students in order to provide the comprehensive training to them, so that they transform into clinicians, who maintain ethical standards while providing quality care to the patients.

The postgraduate practical course and CME are spread over three days, consisting of case discussions of almost all types of commonly encountered conditions. These cases usually form a part of the assessment process of the postgraduates during the examination. So this unique practical course provides much-needed skills to the students regarding how to approach a long case and handle the discussions regarding various clinical aspects. The tradition of publishing a book during this course has brought out pearls of wisdom on the subject. The present publication *Evidence Based Clinical Gynecology* is one of them. This year, the faculty from the All India Institute of Medical Sciences, Employees' State Insurance-Postgraduate Institute of Medical Education and Research, and Department of Radiotherapy (MAMC), have also contributed. This has merged the basics with recent advances in gynecology to provide crisp but concrete skills in clinical gynecology. The topics are relevant to the subject and the contents are lucid and well supported with the evidences. A lucid account of the clinical skills and how to reach the diagnosis with relevant investigations, is the hallmark of the book. This book will certainly help all the postgraduates in this subject and is a must for all the clinicians.

I extend my best wishes to the editorial team and the authors for providing a happy learning.

(Deepak K Tempe)

Preface

Clinical gynecology is next to obstetrics care to improve the health of women in our country. The treatment modalities have changed significantly in recent years due to improvement in diagnostic techniques, still women keep on suffering with gynecological problems and unable to alleviate their problems. The reason is evident, the inability of the treating physician to collect proper information from the patients and recognize their concerns. Recent advances for preventive measures and early diagnosis should reach all healthcare providers in a simple and understandable format, towards that this book is a small attempt.

Healthcare providers must improve their communication skills and justify the need of investigations to support their clinical diagnosis. Ethical practices forbid unnecessary investigations. *Evidence Based Clinical Gynecology* is one step towards reaching that goal. Rationalization of investigations and treatment options is the need of time. Awareness of all investigations is knowledge, but the appropriate use of those tools is wisdom.

Since long, we felt a need that we must disseminate what we practice, and provide evidence why we do so. Our authors and mentors have decades of clinical experience, which is beyond what could be available in a single textbook. Relevance of the content and clinical approach is the hallmark of this publication. Some parts of the chapters are new concepts that are unlikely to have been defined at one place anywhere else. Basic concepts in the subject are nurtured diligently, and enhanced with clinical experience in this book.

The General Gynecology section of this book precisely defines the most used skills in gynecology. Clinical aspect of menstruation, menopause, ultrasonography, minor procedures, recent advances in contraceptions and endoscopies are must for any gynecologist. The other two sections on Benign and Malignant Gynecological Diseases are also conceptualized to provide clinically relevant information of common diseases like infections, infertility, abnormal uterine bleeding, genital prolapse, stress urinary incontinence and malignancies seen routinely in gynecology OPD.

We convey our deepest regards and gratitude to all authors in this publication from the Department of Obstetrics and Gynecology, Maulana Azad Medical College, and look forward to feedback on the content from the readers.

Devender Kumar
Nilanchali Singh
Anjali Tempe

Contents

SECTION 1: General Gynecology

1. Endocrinology of Menstruation — 3
Akansha Shrivastava, Shipra Chandra, Asmita Patil

Organs Involved *3* • Regulation of Menstruation *12*

2. Ultrasonography in Gynecology — 17
Niharika Dhiman

Consent *17* • Technique *18* • Uterus *18* • Endometrium *18*
The Postmenopausal Endometrium *19*
Ultrasonographic Features of Benign Ovarian Cyst *22*
Safety Profile of Ultrasonography *25*

3. Endoscopies in Gynecology: Principles and Equipment — 26
Leena Wadhwa, Shubhi Yadav, Pooja Rani

Indications of Laparoscopy *26* • Surgical Technique of Laparoscopy *27*
Left Upper Quadrant (Palmer's Point) *27* • Pneumoperitoneum *27*
Direct Trocar Insertion *28* • Open Laparoscopy (Hasson Technique) *29*
Laparoscopic Instruments *29* • Disposable Shielded Trocars *30*
Single Incision Laparoscopic Surgery *32* • Complications *33*
Contraindications *34* • Hysteroscopy *34*
Hysteroscopy and its Role in Cancers *37*

4. Minor Procedures in Gynecology — 39
Bidhisha Singha

Conventional Pap Test *39* • Colposcopy *41*
Cervical Biopsy (Punch Biopsy) *42* • Dilatation of Cervix *43*
Dilatation and Curettage *44* • Endometrial Biopsy *44*
Office Hysteroscopy *45* • Hysterosalpingogram *46*
Intrauterine Insemination *46*

5. Recent Advances in Contraceptions — 49
Rachna Sharma, Siddhidatri Mishra

Vaginal Rings *49* • Transdermal Contraception *50* • Implants *51*
Hormonal Injectable Contraceptives *52* • Intrauterine Contraceptive Devices *53*
Chewable Low Dose Oral Contraceptive Pills *54*
Recent Methods of Female Sterilization *54* • Newer Emergency Contraceptives *55*
Postpartum Intrauterine Contraceptive Device *55* • Newer Male Contraceptive *55*

6. Menopause — 57
Poonam Kashyap

Hormonal Changes 58 • Clinical Presentation 58 • Management 60
Vasomotor Symptoms 61 • Bone Loss (Osteoporosis) and Fracture Risk 62
Postmenopausal Vulvovaginal Atrophy 64 • Cardiovascular Disease 66
Differential Diagnosis 67 • Monitoring or Follow-up 67

SECTION 2: Benign Gynecological Diseases

7. Vaginal Discharge — 73
Sangeeta Gupta, Bhavya Sareen

Diagnostic Approach to Vaginal Discharge 73 • Investigations 73
Treatment 75 • Leukorrhea 78

8. Pelvic Inflammatory Disease — 80
Ashok Kumar, Gunjan Bhatnagar

Clinical Presentation 81
Difference between Acute and Chronic Pelvic Inflammatory Disorders 81
Differential Diagnosis 82 • Treatment 82 • Follow-up 84
Pelvic Inflammatory Disease Prevention 84

9. Genital Tuberculosis — 86
Pushpa Mishra, Nupur Ahuja, Deepali Dhingra

Pathogenesis 86 • Mode of Spread 86 • Clinical Presentation 87
Diagnosis 88 • Indirect Tests 88 • Direct Tests 88
Management 90 • Fertility Prognosis 90

10. Viral Infections in Gynecology — 92
Shakun Tyagi

Herpes Simplex Virus 92 • Genital Warts 94
Molluscum Contagiosum 97 • Human Immunodeficiency Virus 97

11. Abnormal Uterine Bleeding — 101
Krishna Agarwal

Causes and Classifications of Abnormal Uterine Bleeding in
a Reproductive Age Woman 101
Treatment of Abnormal Uterine Bleeding in Adolescents 106

12. Fibroid Uterus — 108
Chetna Arvind Sethi, Divya Arora

Clinical Presentation 108 • Risk Factors 109 • Differential Diagnosis 109
Types of Fibroids 110 • Diagnosis 110 • Examination 110
Investigations 110 • Treatment 111 • Expectant Management 112

Medical Management *112* • Surgical Therapies *112*
Minimally Invasive Techniques *117* • General Treatment Plan *119*

13. Endometriosis and Adenomyosis — 123
Nilanchali Singh, Deepali Dhingra, Nupur Ahuja

Endometriosis *123* • Adenomyosis *132*

14. Chronic Pelvic Pain — 138
Preeti Singh, Neelam Yadav, Rini Pachori

Pathophysiology *138* • Etiology *139* • Gynecological Causes *140*
Urological Causes *142* • Gastrointestinal Causes *143*
Musculoskeletal Problems *143* • Psychological Factors *144*
History *144* • Examination *145* • Investigations *145*
Treatment *146* • Follow-up *148* • Recommendations *148*

15. Ectopic Pregnancy — 151
Sangeeta Bhasin, Reena Rani

Classification *151* • Risk Factors *152* • Sequelae of Ectopic Pregnancy *152*
Diagnosis *152* • Investigations *152* • Management *154*
Expectant Management *155* • Medical Management *155*
Surgical Management *157* • Nontubal Ectopic Pregnancy *158*
Ovarian Pregnancy *159* • Cervical Pregnancy *160*
Abdominal Pregnancy *160* • Previous Scar Pregnancy *161*

16. Amenorrhea — 163
Deepti Goswami

Primary Amenorrhea *163* • Secondary Amenorrhea *167*

17. Polycystic Ovary Syndrome — 172
Madhavi M Gupta

Pathophysiology *173* • Clinical Features *173*
Diagnosis *173* • Management *174*

18. Hirsutism — 177
Madhavi M Gupta

Androgen Biosynthesis, Transport and Metabolism in Women *177*
Causes of Hirsutism *178* • Investigations *179* • Treatment Options *179*

19. Female Infertility — 182
Renu Tanwar, Shristi

Causes of Infertility *182* • Clinical Presentations *183*
Diagnosis *183* • Investigations *184*

20. Ovarian Stimulation Protocols in *In Vitro* Fertilization and Ovarian Hyperstimulation Syndrome 187
Anjali Tempe, Komal Rastogi, Deepali Dhingra

GnRH Agonist Down-regulation and Gonadotropin Stimulation:
The 'Long' Protocol *187*
GnRH Agonist 'Flare' and Gonadotropin Stimulation Protocol *188*
GnRH Antagonist and Gonadotropin Stimulation Protocol *189*
Minimal Stimulation Protocol *190* • Management Options for High Responders *190*
Management Options for Poor Responders *190*
Ovarian Hyperstimulation Syndrome *191*

21. Pelvic Organ Prolapse 196
Anoosha K Ravi, Devender Kumar

Pelvic Floor Anatomy *196* • Pathophysiology of Pelvic Organ Prolapse *198*
Clinical Evaluation of Pelvic Organ Dysfunction *200* • Local Genital Examination *200*
Classifications for Pelvic Organ Prolapse *200* • Evaluation of Bladder Function *205*
Mapping of Tears *205* • Surgeries for Pelvic Organ Prolapse *206*

22. Urodynamics in Stress Urinary Incontinence 208
Nikhil Khattar, Ritesh Kumar Singh

What to Look for in Urodynamics? *209*
Evidence for and against Urodynamics *213*

23. Benign Adnexal Masses 216
Akansha Shrivastava, Asmita M Rathore

Evaluation of Adnexal Masses *216* • Prepubertal Age Group *219*
Reproductive Age *221* • Postmenopausal Age Group *225*
Complications of Adnexal Masses *227*

SECTION 3: Malignant Gynecological Diseases

24. Premalignant Lesions of Female Lower Genital Tract 233
Poonam Sachdeva, Akanksha Sharma

Cervical Intraepithelial Neoplasia *233* • Colposcopic-Directed Biopsy *239*
Vaginal Intraepithelial Neoplasia *249* • Vulvar Intraepithelial Neoplasia *251*

25. Gestational Trophoblastic Neoplasia 254
Reva Tripathi, Meenoo S

Follow-up after Molar Evacuation *254* • Clinical Presentation *255*
Investigations *255* • Persistent Gestational Trophoblastic Neoplasia *256*
Invasive Mole *257* • Choriocarcinoma *257*
Placental Site Trophoblastic Tumor *257* • Epithelioid Trophoblastic Tumor *258*
Metastatic Gestational Trophoblastic Neoplasia *258*
Management of Gestational Trophoblastic Neoplasia *258*

Treatment of Low-risk Gestational Trophoblastic Nonmetastatic Neoplasia *258*
Management of High-risk Metastatic GTN *259* • Prophylactic Chemotherapy *260*
Indications of Hysterectomy *260* • Emergency Situations *260*
Management of Metastases at Various Sites *261*
Newer Options in Patients with EMACO Resistance *261*
Follow-up and Surveillance *261* • Contraception *261*
Advice on Future Pregnancy *261* • Quiescent Gestational Trophoblastic Disease *262*

26. Vulval Cancer — 265
Gauri Gandhi, Snigdha Pathak

Pathology of Vulvar Cancer—Histological Types *265*
Etiology and Risk Factors *265* • Clinical Presentation *266*
Confirmation of Diagnosis *266* • Routes of Spread *267*
Treatment of Primary Disease *268* • Surgical Management *268*
Postoperative Complications *272* • Role of Radiation *272*
Role of Chemotherapy *272* • Follow-up *273* • Recurrence *273*

27. Vaginal Cancer — 275
Gauri Gandhi, Snigdha Pathak

Vaginal Cancer *275*

28. Carcinoma Cervix — 278
Pushpa Mishra

Epidemiology *278* • Risk Factors *278* • Classification *279*
Clinical Presentation *279* • Diagnosis *280* • Management *281*
Treatment Modalities *281* • Special Scenarios *285*

29. Endometrial Carcinoma — 289
Yedla Manikya Mala, Bhoomika Tantuway, Karishma Bhatia

Clinical Presentation *289* • Investigations *291*
Staging of Endometrial Cancer *291* • Management *292*
Adjuvant Therapy *294* • Fertility Sparing Options *294*

30. Ovarian Cancer — 297
Latika Sahu

Risk Factors *297* • Clinical Presentation *297* • Epithelial Ovarian
Cancer Screening *298* • FIGO Ovarian Cancer Staging *299*
Newer Therapy Trials *304* • Germ Cell Cancer *304*
Sex Cord Stromal Tumor *305*

31. Borderline Ovarian Tumors — 309
Devender Kumar, Savita Arora

Incidence *309* • Classification of Ovarian Tumors *309*
Clinical Presentation *309* • Malignancy Index Score *310*
Histology of Borderline Ovarian Tumors *310* • Follow-up *311*

32. Introduction to Radiotherapy and Chemotherapy 313
Kishore Singh, Savita Arora, Arun Kumar Rathi

Radiotherapy *313* • Intracavitary Radiotherapy *314*
Chemotherapy *314* • Principles of Chemotherapy *314*

33. Chemotherapy in Gestational Trophoblastic Neoplasia 316
Kishore Singh, Savita Arora, Arun Kumar Rathi

Low-risk *316* • Duration of Chemotherapy and Follow-up *317*
High Risk Gestational Trophoblastic Neoplasia *317*
Duration of Chemotherapy and Follow-up *317*
Role of Surgery/Radiotherapy *317* • Recurrent/Residual Lesion *318*

34. Chemoradiotherapy in Carcinoma Vulva 319
Kishore Singh, Savita Arora, Arun Kumar Rathi

Role of Surgery *319* • Role of Radiation Therapy *320*
Locally Advanced Vulvar Cancer *321* • Definitive Chemoradiotherapy *322*

35. Chemoradiotherapy in Carcinoma Vagina 325
Kishore Singh, Savita Arora, Arun Kumar Rathi

Treatment Options Overview *325*
Stagewise Treatment Approach *326*
Recurrent Vaginal Cancer *327*

36. Chemoradiotherapy in Carcinoma Cervix 329
Kishore Singh, Savita Arora, Arun Kumar Rathi

Diagnosis and Workup *329* • Primary Management *329*
Concurrent Chemoradiotherapy *333* • Dose of Radiotherapy *333*
Recent Advances *334*

37. Chemoradiotherapy in Carcinoma Endometrium 336
Kishore Singh, Savita Arora, Arun Kumar Rathi

Risk Factors *336* • Prognostic Variables in Endometrial Carcinoma *336*
Primary Treatment *336* • Systemic Therapy in Endometrial Carcinoma *337*
Hormonal Therapy *338* • Recent Advances *338*

38. Chemotherapy in Ovarian Cancer 339
Kishore Singh, Savita Arora, Arun Kumar Rathi

Diagnostic Workup *339* • Treatment of Epithelial Ovarian Tumors *339*
Postoperative Management *340* • Radiotherapy *342*
Germ Cell Tumors *343*

Index   *345*

PLATE 1

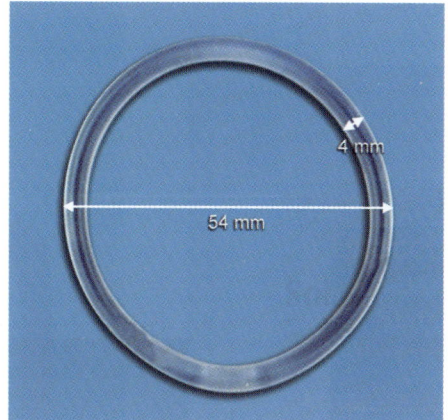

Fig. 5.1 NuvaRing

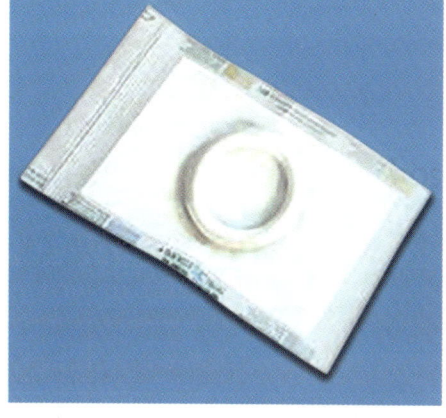

Fig. 5.2 Progesterone vaginal ring

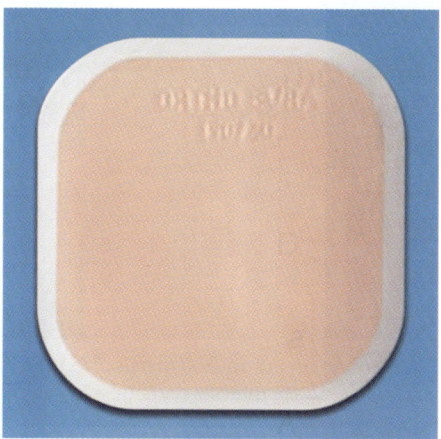

Fig. 5.3 Ortho Evra

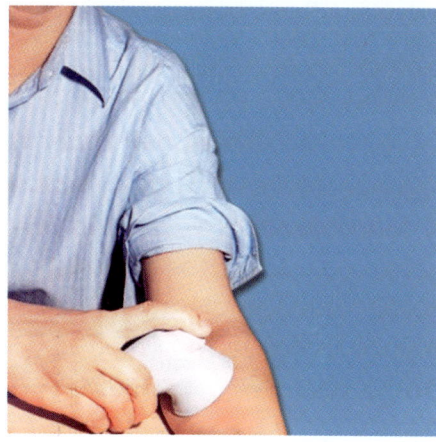

Fig. 5.4 Spray on contraceptive

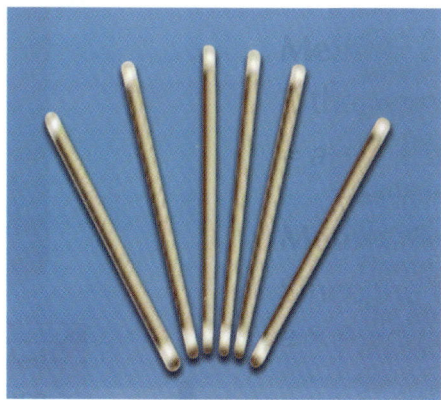

Fig. 5.5 Norplant

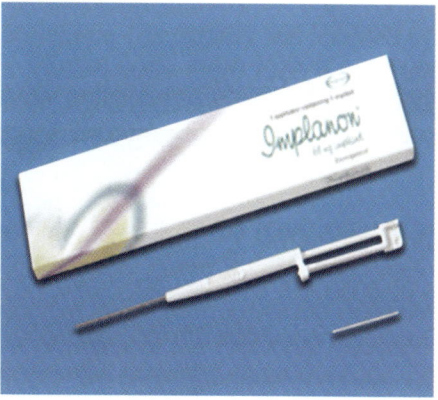

Fig. 5.6 Implanon

PLATE 2

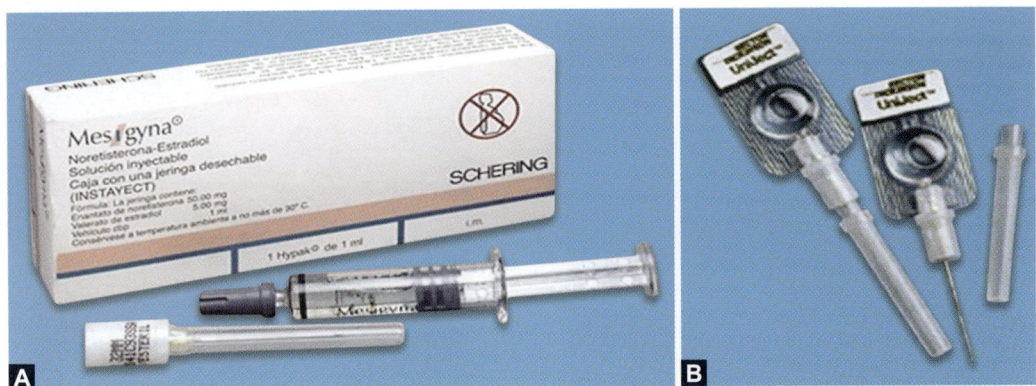

Figs 5.7A and B Subcutaneous DMPA

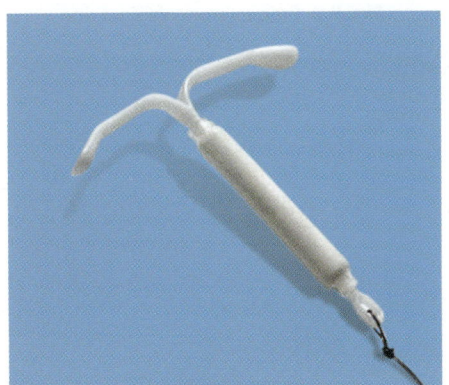

Fig. 5.8 Mirena

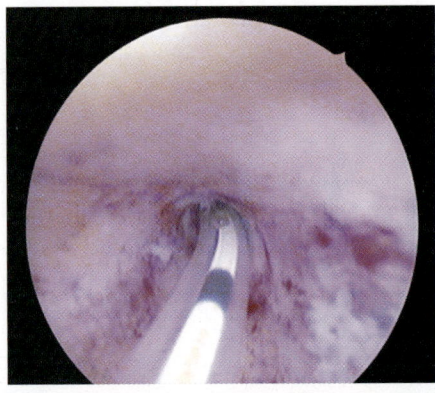

Fig. 5.10 Adian introduced in fallopian tube to cause thermal damage

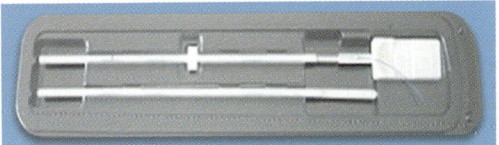

Fig. 5.9 Frameless IUCD

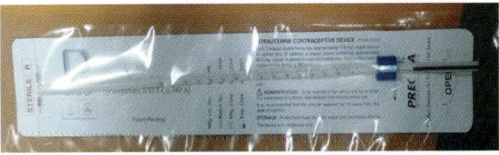

Fig. 5.12 PPIUCD inserter

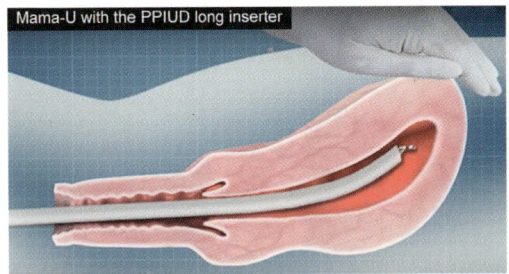

Fig. 5.13 Mama-U (PPIUCD) from Pregna international company

PLATE 3

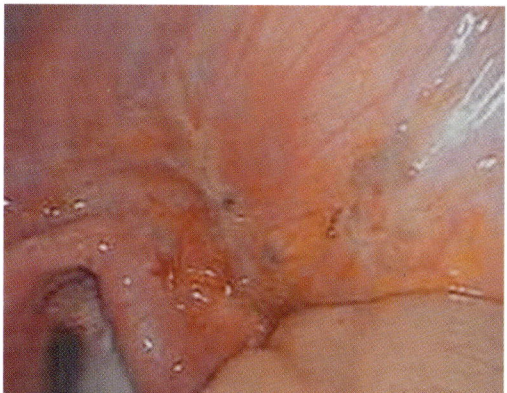

Fig. 13.1 Bluish puckered lesions and small vesicles surrounded by some fibrosis (typical lesion)

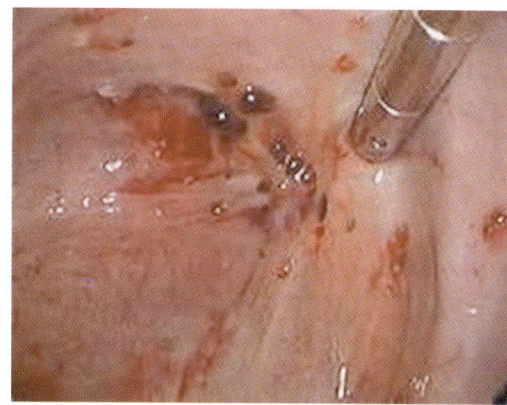

Fig. 13.2 Red implants with petechiae and vesicles (atypical lesion)

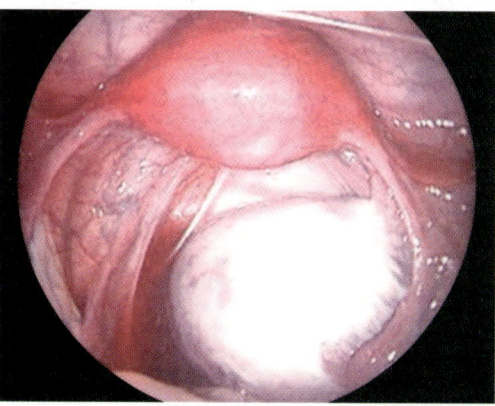

Fig. 13.3 Large endometrioma arising from right ovary

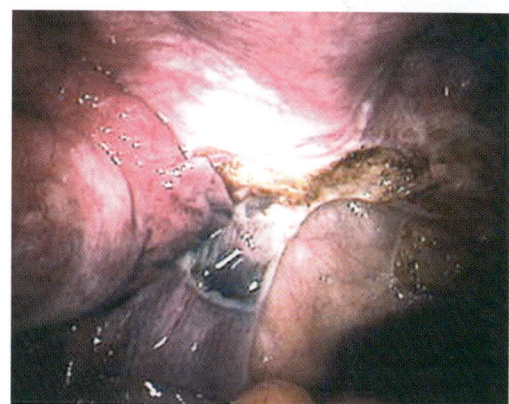

Fig. 13.4 Infiltrative lesion of the uterosacral ligament obliterating the pouch of Douglas

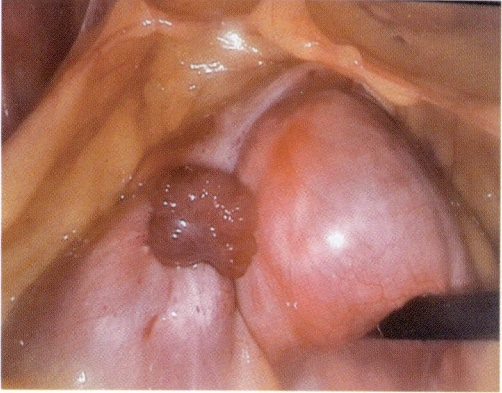

Fig. 13.5 Dense adhesions due to endometriosis leading to tubo-ovarian mass formation, suggestive of moderate-to-severe disease

PLATE 4

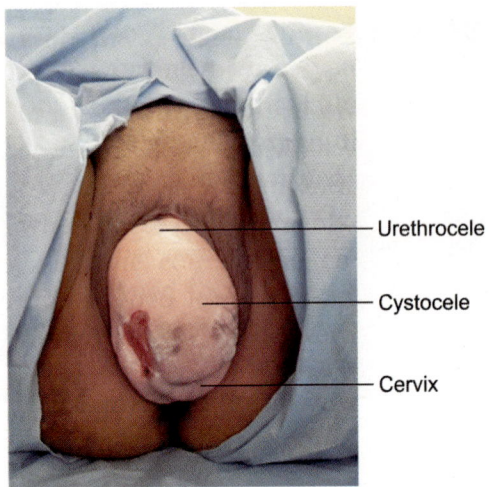

Fig. 21.7 Example of prolapse with all three compartment defects. According to Shaw's classification, it is a 3rd degree cervical descent with urethrocystocele, enterocele and rectocele with decubitus ulcer

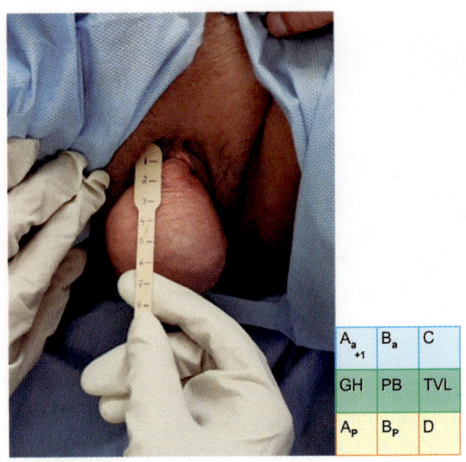

Fig. 21.10 Point A_a: fixed point 3 cm from the hymen on the anterior wall

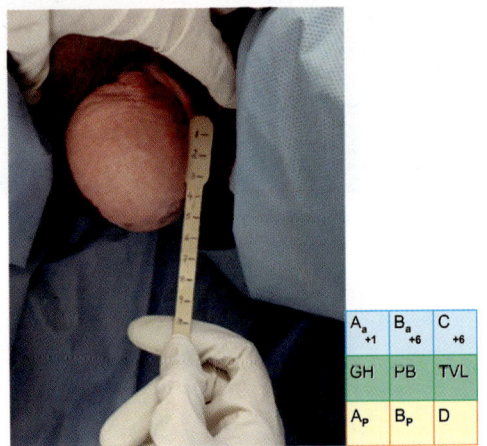

Fig. 21.11 Point B_a: most leading point on the anterior wall from point A_a to apex; Point C: most distal point on the cervix
Abbreviations: TVL, total vaginal length; PB, perineal body; GH, genital hiatus

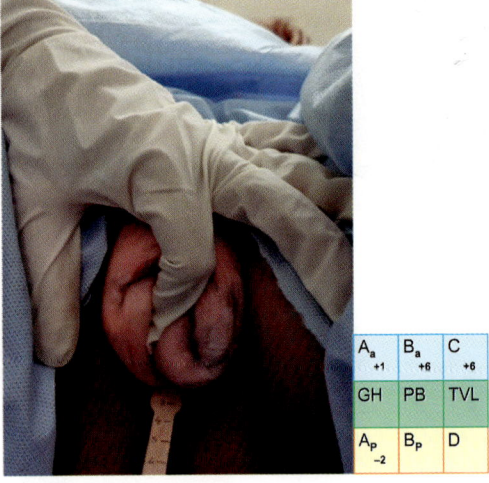

Fig. 21.12 Point A_p: fixed point 3 cm from the hymen on the posterior wall

PLATE 5

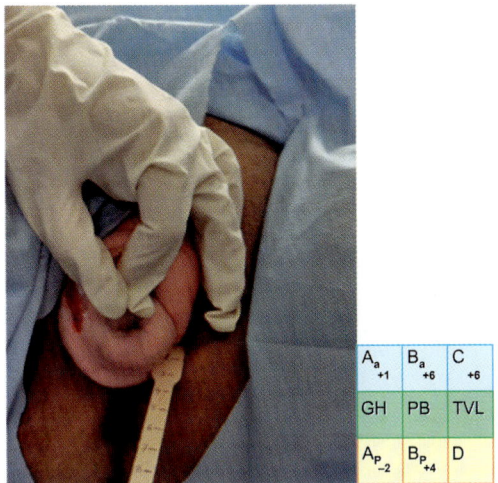

Fig. 21.13 Point B$_p$: most leading point on the posterior wall from point A$_p$ to apex

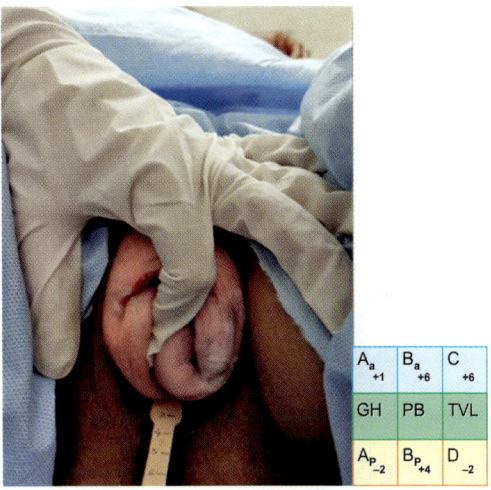

Fig. 21.14 Point D is posterior fornix

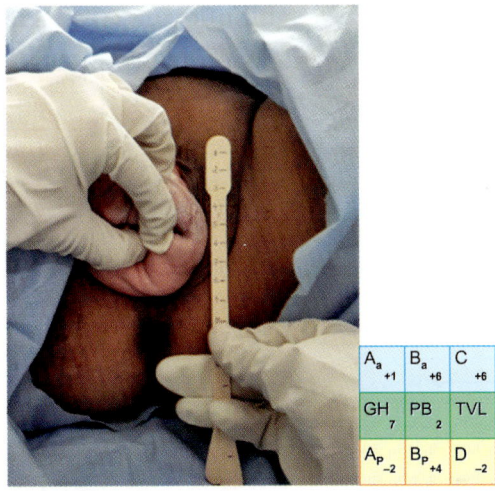

Fig. 21.15 GH measured from the middle of external urethral meatus to the inferior hymenal ring; PB measured from inferior hymenal ring to middle of anal orifice

PLATE 6

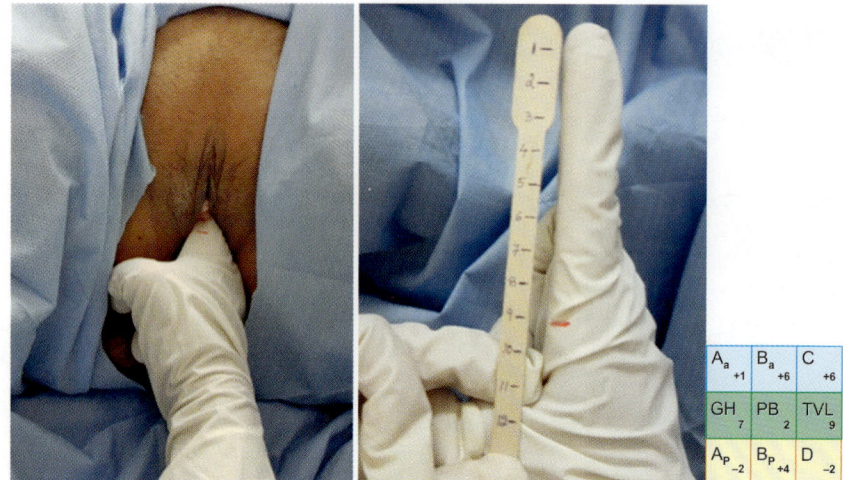

Fig. 21.16 Total vaginal length

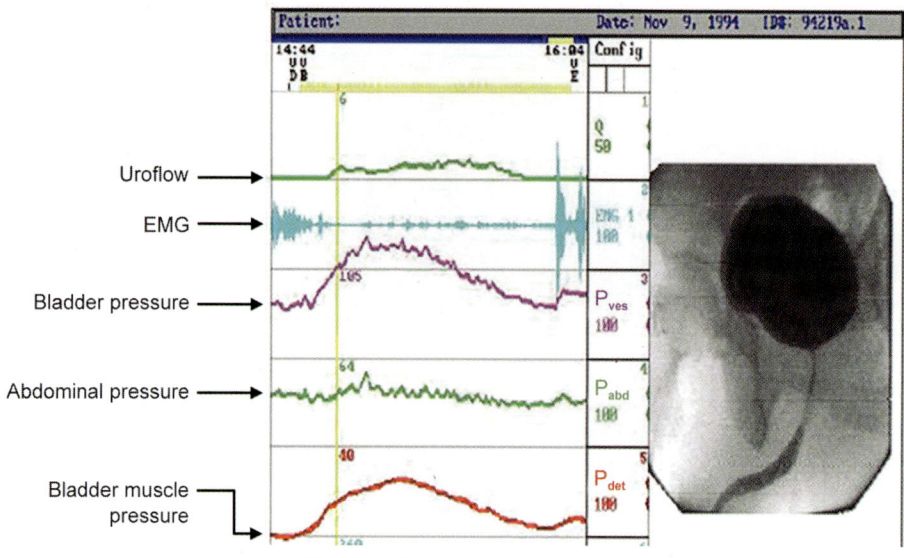

Fig. 22.5 Videourodynamics

PLATE 7

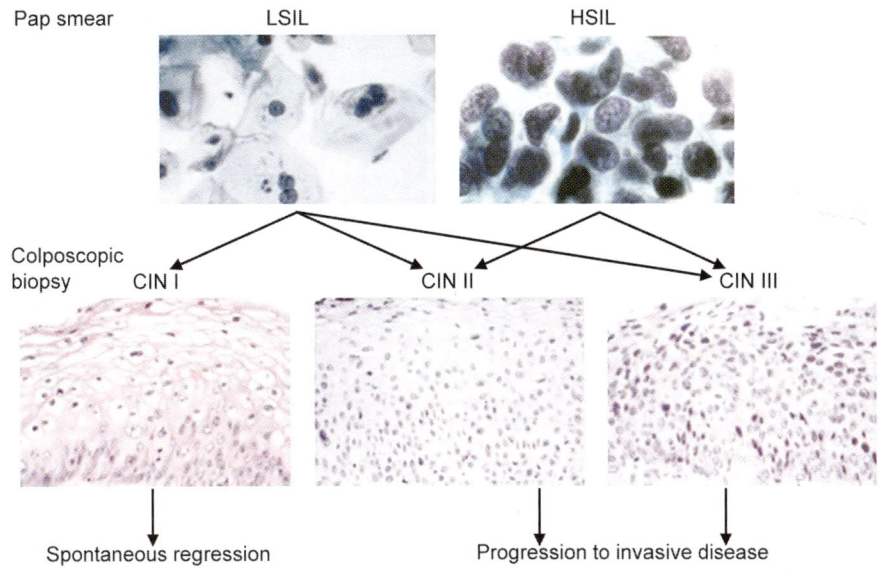

Fig. 24.1 Abnormal cytology and histopathology

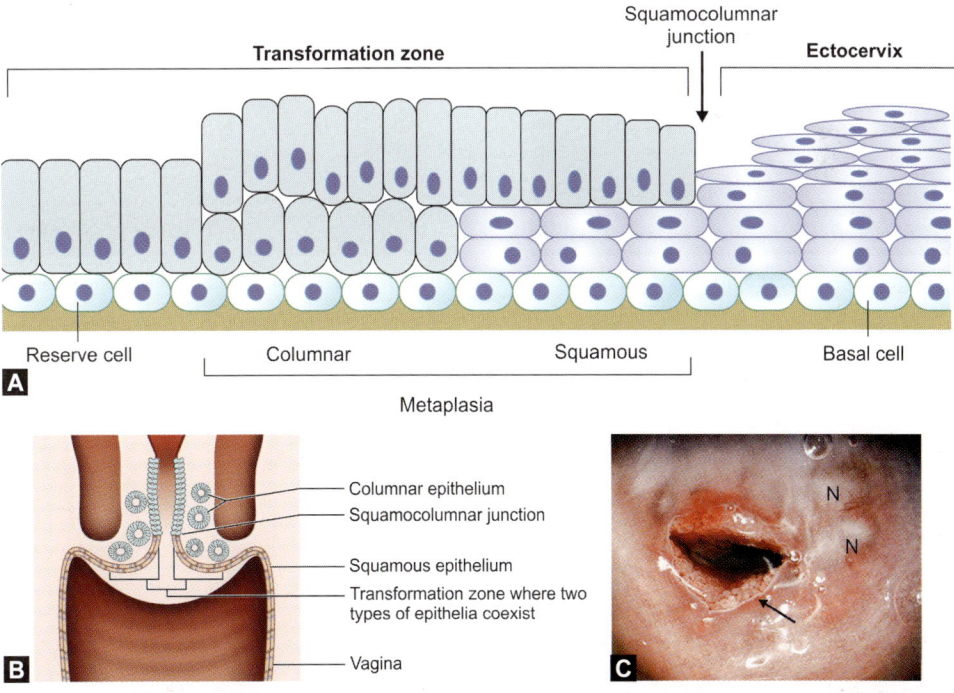

Figs 24.4A to C (A) Schematic display of histology; (B) Longilindual view to understand the location; (C) Colposcopic view of normal cervix. Normal or typical transformation zone: Tongues of metaplastic epithelium, gland openings, nabothian follicles, islands of columnar epithelium

PLATE 8

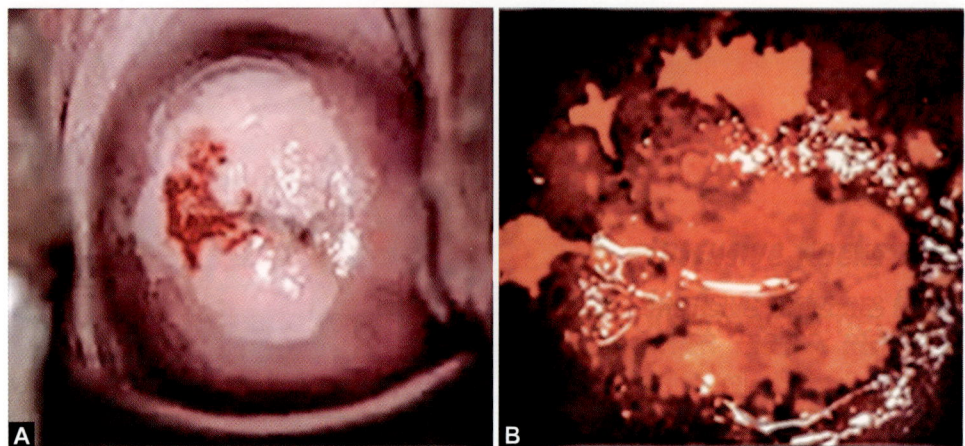

Figs 24.6A and B VIA (A) VILI (B) positive cervix

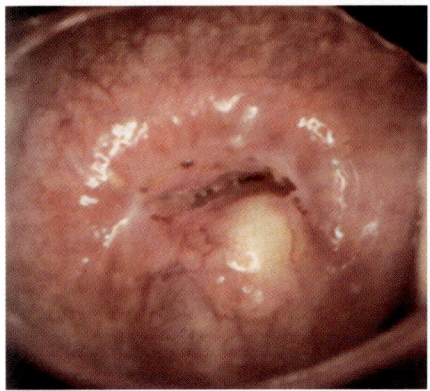

Fig. 24.7 Colposcopic of normal cervix

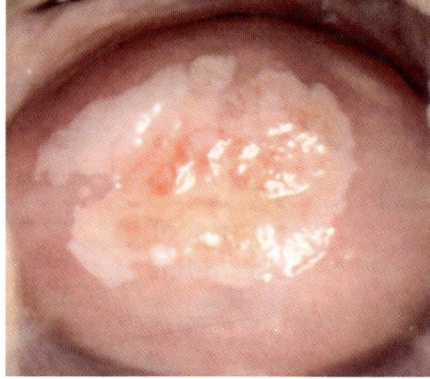

Fig. 24.8 Colposcopic of acetowhite cervix

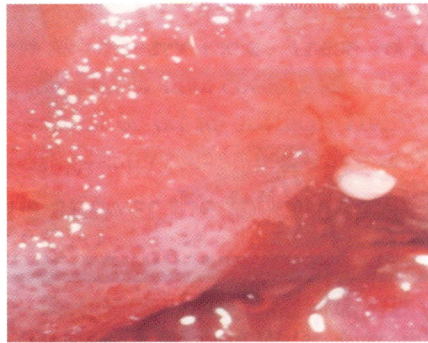

Fig. 24.9 Colposcopic showing punctations

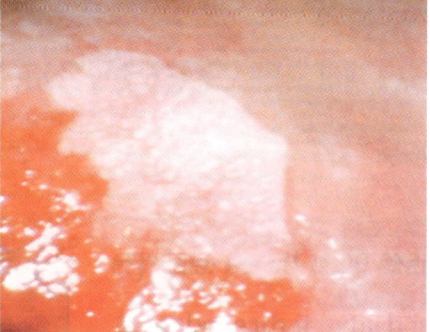

Fig. 24.10 Colposcopic picture showing coarse mosaic pattern

PLATE 9

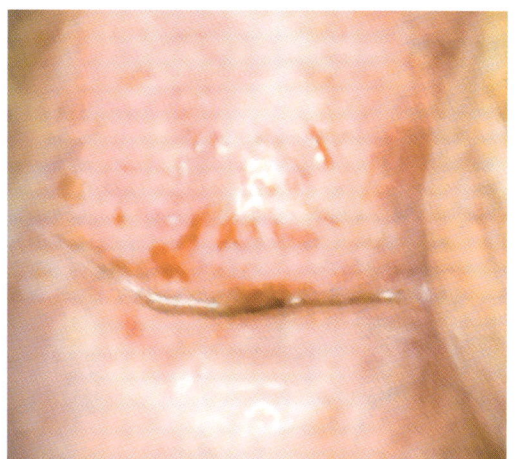

Fig. 24.11 Abnormal vessels on colposcopy of cervix

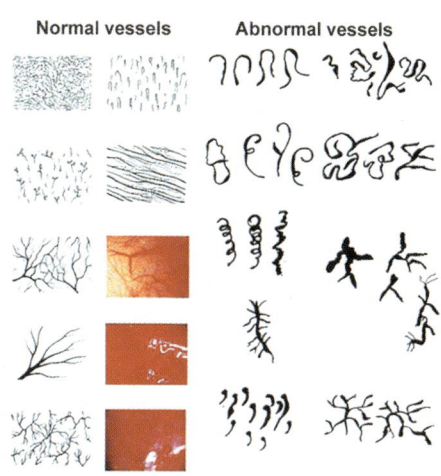

Fig. 24.12B Normal and abnormal vessel pattern on colposcopy

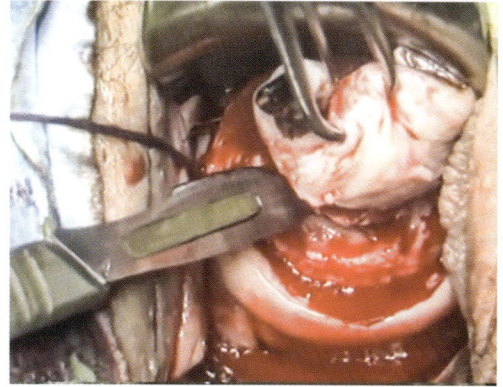

Fig. 24.13 Cone biopsy with cold knife

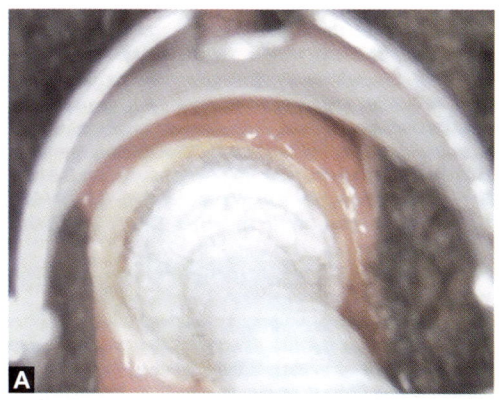
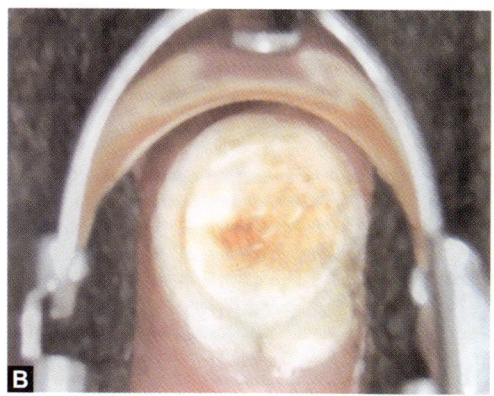

Figs 24.15A and B (A) Cryotherapy probe on cervix; (B) Frozen Cx after cryoprobe removed

PLATE 10

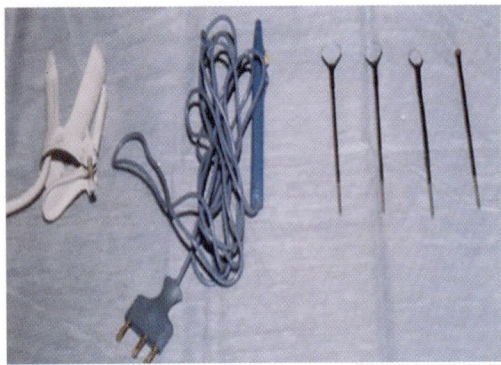

Fig. 24.16 Large loop excision of transformation zone (LLETZ) Instruments and procedure: Insulated cuscos speculum, loops in 3 sizes (Large, medium, small) and roller ball cautery

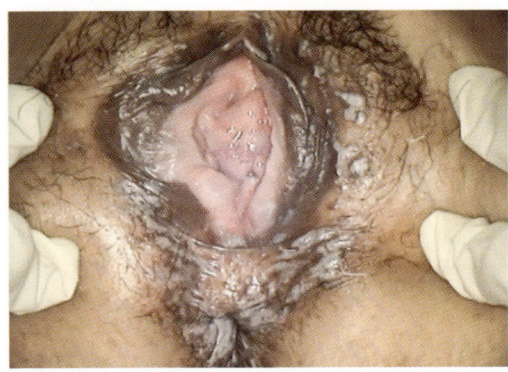

Fig. 24.18 Vulvar intraepithelial neoplasia (VIN)

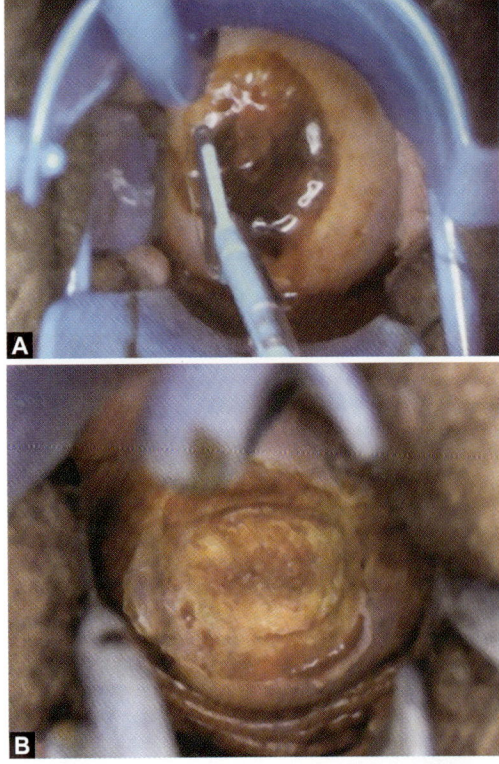

Figs 24.17A and B (A) Large loop excision of transformation zone (LLETZ); (B) Crater after Large loop excision of transformation zone (LLETZ)

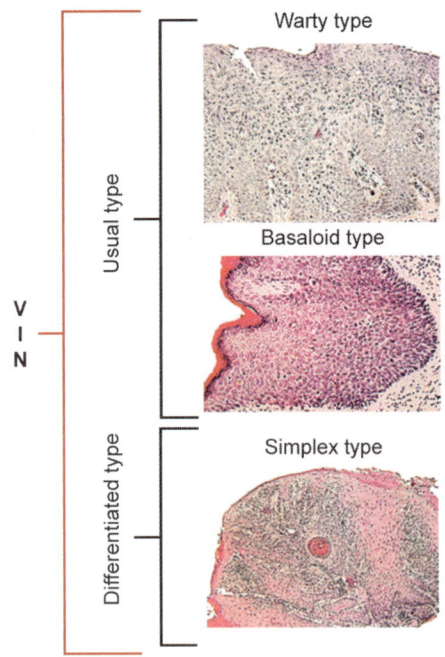

Fig. 24.19 VIN histopathology

SECTION 1

General Gynecology

Chapters

- Endocrinology of Menstruation
- Ultrasonography in Gynecology
- Endoscopies in Gynecology: Principles and Equipment
- Minor Procedures in Gynecology
- Recent Advances in Contraceptions
- Menopause

1

Endocrinology of Menstruation

Akansha Shrivastava, Shipra Chandra, Asmita Patil

The origin of the word "menstruation" relates to the Latin word mensis (month), which is further related to the Greek word mene (moon). Hence, in earlier times, women were said to be in their moon phase during menstruation. They were secluded during these times and refrained from the normal day-to-day functioning.[1,2]

Menstruation is a clinically significant phase of menstrual cycle when endometrial shedding occurs. Various factors contribute to the regulation of this process including hormones, paracrine and autocrine factors. The cyclical secretion of hypothalamic and pituitary hormones determines the ovarian cycle. The ovarian sex steroids in turn interact through different nuclear receptors and regulate the expression of local factors within the endometrium. The shedding or sustaining of endometrium is primarily due to estrogen and progesterone hormones secreted from ovary. In pregnancy, placenta takes over this function and sustains the endometrium to decidualize, in turn maintains the pregnancy.

ORGANS INVOLVED

- Hypothalamus
- Pituitary gland
- Ovaries
- Uterus.

Hypothalamus

Located below the thalamus and above the pituitary, it forms the base of the third ventricle. The median eminence of hypothalamus secretes a small peptide, gonadotropin-releasing hormone (GnRH), also known as luteinizing hormone-releasing hormone (LHRH). This decapeptide is synthesized in arcuate nucleus of the hypothalamus and is released at the nerve endings near tuber cinereum. Hypothalamus is connected to the anterior pituitary gland through special hypothalamo-hypophyseal portal system of vessels. Until puberty, these GnRH secreting cells are in dormant state under the inhibitory influence of adrenal cortex, and the higher cortical center. Gradual sensitization of these cells occurs around 8–12 years and resumes its full function by the age of 13–14 years completely establishing the hypothalamo-pituitary-ovarian axis. Near puberty leptin produced by the adipose tissue triggers GnRH release and function.

This is the basis for earlier menarche in obese girls and delayed puberty in lean individuals.

Regulation of GnRH

The factors that control GnRH pulse frequency and amplitude are not fully characterized.

Neuroendocrine factors that likely play a major role in regulating GnRH secretion include kisspeptin and leptin. Other steroids that play an important role in regulating GnRH secretion include the gonadal steroids, estradiol, progesterone, and testosterone. Neuroendocrine system works through several loops, both positive and negative.
- Long loops through estrogen and progesterone
- Short loop through anterior pituitary gland
- Ultrashort loop within the hypothalamus.

Kisspeptin
Regulation of GnRH is not directly through GnRH neuron but rather through KISS1 neurons. KISS1 neurons contain ER-alpha receptors that regulate the transcription of KISS1, the gene that encodes the peptide kisspeptin. This kisspeptin acts on GnRH neurons through KISS1 receptors and stimulates the GnRH release. There are two population KISS1 neurons, one in the Arcuate (ARC) nucleus and another in anteroventral periventricular (AVPV) nucleus of the hypothalamus. There is differential regulation and actions of ARC versus AVPV KISS1 neurons in the control of GnRH in mediating the negative- and positive-feedback effects of ovarian sex steroids on GnRH and gonadotropin secretion (Fig. 1.1). It has been found that the administration of an intravenous bolus of the C-terminal decapeptide of kisspeptin (amino acids 112-121) results in an immediate LH pulse, with an amplitude that is twice as large as LH pulses observed prior to the administration of kisspeptin. A single dose of kisspeptin stimulates LH secretion for approximately 17 minutes.[3] In humans, loss of function mutations in genes that code for GnRH or the GnRH receptor, kisspeptin or the kisspeptin receptor are associated with hypogonadotropic hypogonadism[4,5] resulting in the phenotype that includes low circulating levels of luteinizing hormone (LH) and follicle-stimulation hormone (FSH), low levels of estradiol and progesterone, absent ovulation and amenorrhea.

Leptin
Leptin is secreted by adipocytes and its concentration in the circulation correlates with total body adipocyte mass and thus with obesity. Leptin acts on the brain and causes a reduction in appetite. Leptin acts on neurons in the hypothalamus that secrete kisspeptin.[6,7] In very lean animals, leptin levels are low and this results in reduced secretion of kisspeptin, in turn, causing a decrease in GnRH secretion and anovulation. Women with hypothalamic amenorrhea (hypothalamic hypogonadism) often have low levels of leptin. Two clinical trials reported that the administration of exogenous leptin or a leptin analog (metreleptin) to these women, resulted in the resumption of ovulatory menses in some of the subjects.[8,9]

Steroidal Regulation (Long Loop)

Estradiol, progesterone, and testosterone act on both the hypothalamus and pituitary. Estradiol has both positive and negative effect on GnRH secretion. During follicular phase, Estrogen (E2) exerts a predominant inhibitory action on KISS1 expression at the ARC and contributes to negative-feedback control of GnRH/LH. In preovulatory period, rise of E2 levels in the presence of activated receptors for progesterone, stimulates *KISS1* gene expression in the AVPV and results positive feedback contributing to preovulatory surge of LH.

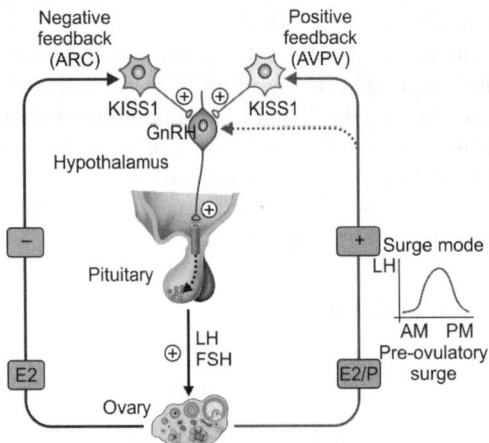

Fig. 1.1 Steroidal feedback on GnRH release

Thus, in early follicular phase when the levels of estradiol is low, negative feedback is diminished resulting in increased GnRH pulse frequency which further increases LH and FSH secretion. Progesterone in the luteal phase decreases GnRH pulse frequency (Fig. 1.2). In the early follicular phase, with low estrogen (E2) level, pulsatility is every 90 min, and with rise in E2 level, the frequency rises to every 60 minutes. In the luteal phase, the frequency slows down to 1 in 3 hour.

Pituitary Gland

Pituitary gland lies in the sella turcica. The anterior pituitary gland originates at the roof of the embryonic pharynx called Rathke's pouch and contains chromophil and chromophobe cells. The posterior lobe develops from the floor of the brain. Anterior lobe consists of three histologically distinguishable cells: (i) the chromophobe or parent cell, (ii) the chromophil cells described as eosinophil or alpha (α) cells and (iii) basophil or beta (β) cells. The β-cells secrete the gonadotropins that control the ovarian function and menstrual cycles.

Gonadotropins

Gonadotropins secreted from pituitary are FSH, LH, thyroid-stimulating hormone (TSH) and corticosteroid hormone.

Follicle-stimulating Hormone
It is a water-soluble glycoprotein of high molecular weight and is secreted by the β-cells. The FSH receptor is expressed in granulosa cells

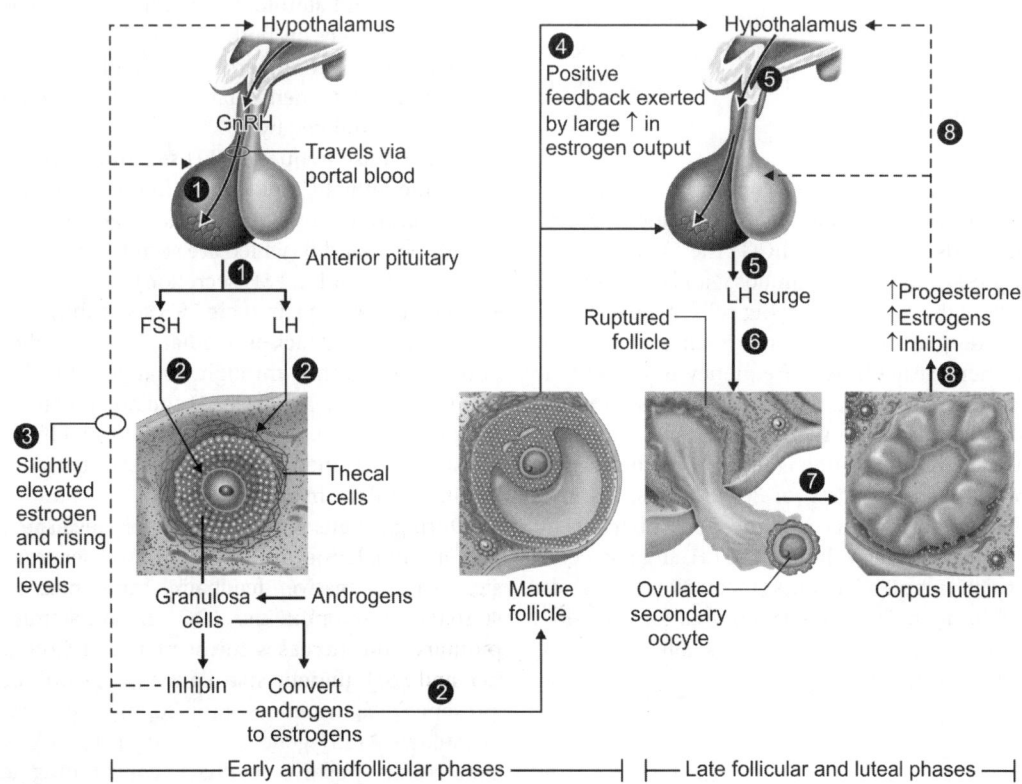

Fig. 1.2 Endocrine regulation of menstrual cycle

of the ovary and the Sertoli cells of the testis. Role of FSH are given further.
- Controls the ripening of the primordial follicles.
- In conjunction with the LH, it activates the secretion of estrogen.
- It helps in development of LH receptors in the granulosa cells, which secretes progesterone under the influence of LH.

Its activity builds up as the bleeding starts to cease, reaches a peak around the seventh day of the and then declines to disappear around the 18th day. Follicle growth is directly dependent on FSH stimulation. In women with amenorrhea due to hypothalamic hypogonadism (insufficient calorie intake, excessive exercise, excessive stress), the pituitary secretion of FSH is very low. In the absence of FSH stimulation, the small secondary follicles do not grow and no dominant follicle develops. In the absence of a dominant follicle, estrogen secretion is insufficient to trigger an LH surge, thereby resulting in anovulation and amenorrhea. Low FSH causes defective folliculogenesis and short or defective corpus luteal phase.

Luteinizing Hormone

It is a water-soluble glycoprotein of high molecular weight secreted by β-cell. The LH receptor binds both LH and hCG. The LH receptor is expressed in thecal, granulosa, and corpus luteal cells of the ovary and Leydig cells of the testis.

The gonadotropin surge is characterized by an increase in LH pulse frequency and amplitude resulting in a marked increase in serum LH. During this LH surge, there is small increase in FSH also. LH surge is initiated by high levels of estrogen and lasts for 36–48 hours. LH level doubles in 2 hours and the peak plateaus for 14 hours before declining. The LH surge precedes ovulation by 24–36 hours (mean 30 hours) and a minimum of 75 ng/mL is required for ovulation. Progesterone secretion begins after LH peak. Actions of LH are:

- In conjunction with FSH, it activates the secretion of estrogen, brings about the maturation of the ovum and causes ovulation.
- Stimulates the secretion of testosterone and androstenedione in the ovarian stroma (theca cells), which diffuse into the follicular fluid and are aromatized into estradiol.
- Increase in intrafollicular proteolytic enzymes (e.g. plasmin), which destroys the basement membrane of the follicle and results in follicular rupture.
- Stimulates the completion of the reduction division of the oocyte.
- Following ovulation, it produces luteinization of the granulosa and the theca cells and initiates progesterone secretion.
- Growth of blood vessels into the follicle, which prepares it to become a corpus luteum.

Regulation of Gonadotropins

Secretion of gonadotropins is regulated by both GnRH and steroidal hormones. GnRH has stimulatory effect on both LH and FSH release, but both gonadotropins are differentially released throughout the menstrual cycle. Differential release is modulated by
- GnRH pulse frequency (LH secretion favored by moderately rapid pulse frequencies and FSH secretion by slow pulse frequencies),
- Inhibin A and B (which are secreted from the ovary and inhibit FSH secretion),
- Activins (which stimulate FSH secretion).

Negative feedback is mediated by estradiol and progesterone through changes in the hypothalamic release of GnRH and not directly at the pituitary level. The positive feedback effects of estradiol are mediated at the level of both the pituitary and the hypothalamus.

During menses, estradiol, progesterone, and inhibin levels are low. In the absence of significant negative feedback from ovarian steroids and proteins, the hypothalamic-pituitary unit increases the secretion of GnRH, LH, and FSH, thereby stimulating the growth of a cohort of small follicles. Among the cohort of growing small follicles, one follicle achieves more rapid growth and secrete increasing quantities of estradiol and inhibin A and B. This will result in the suppression of FSH and the cessation of growth in all but the largest, dominant follicle. A rising level of estradiol will eventually trigger an LH surge initiating the ovulatory process. Within 12 hours of the initiation of the LH surge, progesterone levels start to rise due to luteinization of the follicle and estradiol levels begin to fall. During the luteal phase of the cycle, FSH levels are low, preventing the growth of a new cohort of the follicles. LH pulse frequency slows considerably and progesterone levels peak during the mid-luteal phase (Fig. 1.3). If pregnancy does not occur, the corpus luteum begins to undergo luteolysis with a decrease in inhibin, estradiol, and progesterone production and a subsequent rise in pituitary secretion of LH and FSH, initiating a new round of follicle growth.

Ovaries

Selection and Dominance

At the beginning of follicular phase, there are approximately five antral follicles (range 0–15 follicles) measuring 4 mm in diameter (range 2–9 mm in diameter) in each ovary.[10] One antral

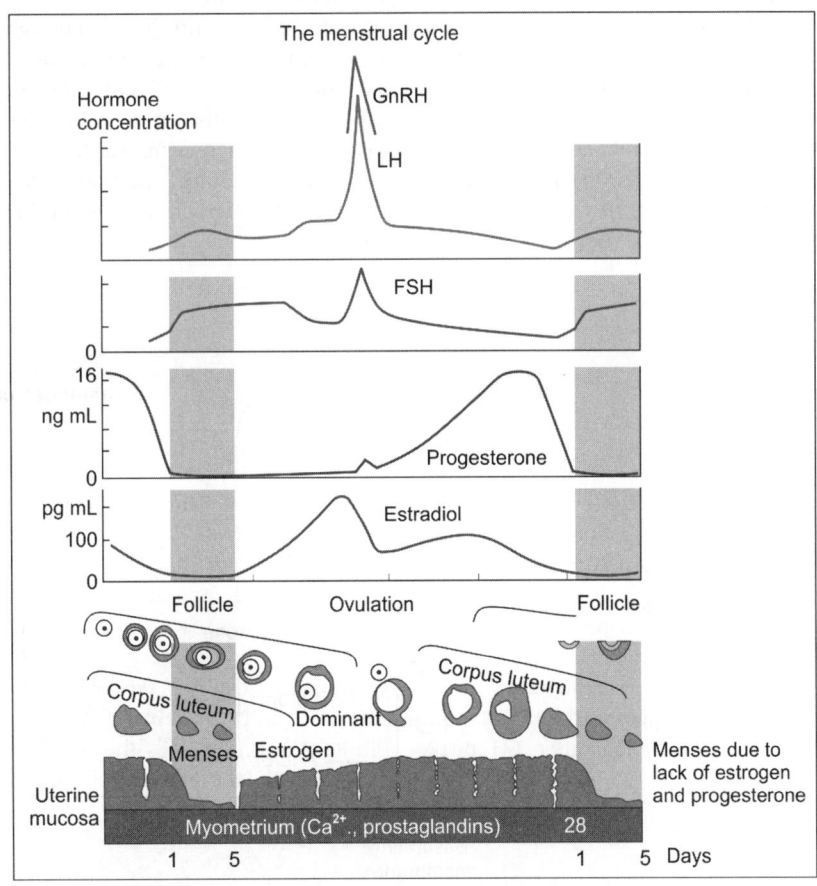

Fig. 1.3 Hormonal changes in menstrual cycle

follicle which is destined to ovulate becomes dominant and starts to grow rapidly, achieving a preovulatory diameter of approximately 20–25 mm. The process by which one small antral follicle is selected among its peers to develop into the large preovulatory follicle is called selection. The dominant follicle prevents the growth of other new large follicles by secreting inhibin-B inhibin-A and estradiol, which markedly suppress FSH secretion, thereby blocking the growth of other follicles.

Two Cell Theory

The follicle has three main components: theca cells, granulosa cells and the oocyte. Theca cells express LH receptors and secrete androgens, and a small amount of progesterone, in response to LH stimulation. Granulosa cells from small follicles express FSH receptors and respond to FSH stimulation by synthesizing aromatase, the aromatase enzyme, which converts thecal androstenedione to estradiol. Granulosa cells from large follicles also have LH receptors, in preparation for responding to the LH surge.[11] There is a delicate balance between LH and FSH stimulation of the thecal and granulosa cell compartments (Fig. 1.4). In polycystic ovary syndrome, excessive pituitary secretion of LH (evidenced by an elevated ratio of LH to FSH) results in excess stimulation of androstenedione production from the theca cells and insufficient conversion of the androstenedione to estradiol. Consequently, the follicular microenvironment is characterized by excessive androstenedione and low estradiol concentration in the follicular fluid. These androgen dominant follicles contain a suboptimal number of granulosa cells for their size and an oocyte that has difficulty resuming meiosis, which leads to anovulatory cycles characteristics of polycystic ovary syndrome (PCOS).

The timing of ovulation is determined by the dominant ovarian follicle. When the dominant ovarian follicle produces enough estradiol to sustain levels in the range of 200–300 pg/mL for 48 hours, it has positive feedback effect on hypothalamus. The hypothalamus responds by increasing kisspeptin and GnRH secretion resulting pituitary secretion of LH and FSH, which results in LH and FSH surge.

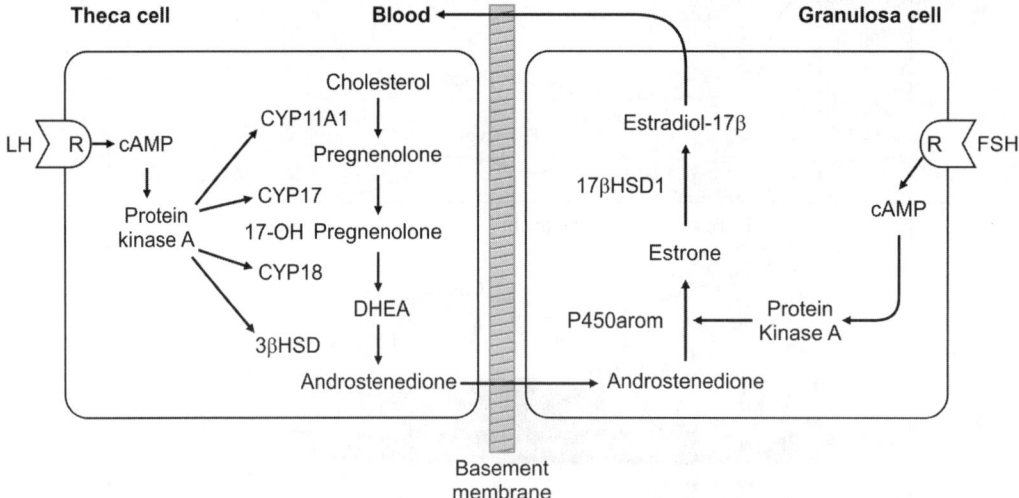

Fig. 1.4 Theca and granulosa cells interaction to synthesize androstenedione and estradiol

Corpus Luteum

The main purpose of the corpus luteum is to secrete progesterone to prepare the endometrium for embryo implantation. Progesterone secreted from corpus luteum maintains a developing pregnancy until the placenta becomes the main source of progesterone. During the luteal phase, pituitary LH stimulates the corpus luteum to make progesterone. Similarly, during early pregnancy, hCG secreted from the conceptus stimulates the corpus luteum, to make progesterone and support the growth of the conceptus within the endometrium. The corpus luteum is derived from both theca and granulosa cells. In the corpus luteum the small cells are thought to be derived from the theca and the large cells from the granulosa cells. Both cell types produce progesterone. Theca-derived luteal cells produce androgen precursors that are aromatized to estradiol by the granulosa-derived luteal cells.[12]

Ovarian Regulatory Proteins (Fig. 1.5)

- *Estrogens* are secreted from theca and granulosa cells of the Graafian follicles and corpus luteum. Estrogen is secreted in the form of estradiol. The plasma estradiol level rises approximately 6–7 days before ovulation and reaches its peak about 2 days before ovulation and approximately 24 hours before the LH peak. Thereafter, its concentration falls daily.

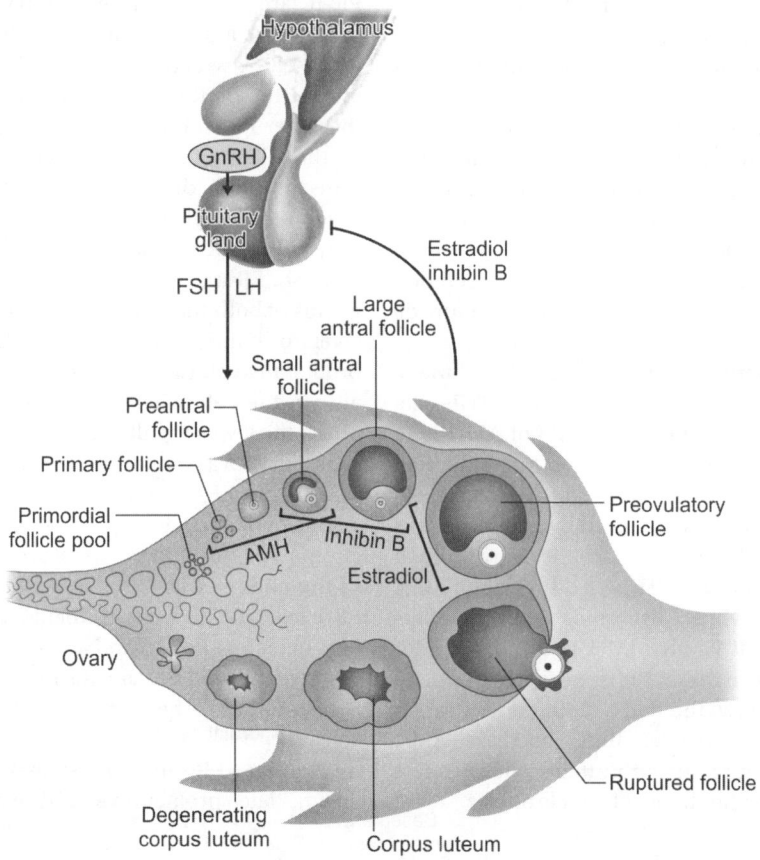

Fig. 1.5 Ovarian regulatory proteins

- *Inhibin A:* Secreted by the granulosa cells of the large dominant follicles in the preovulatory phase and the luteinized granulosa cells in the corpus luteum in the luteal phases of the menstrual cycle.
- *Inhibin B:* Secreted by small developing follicles in the follicular phase.
  The feedback of the inhibins on pituitary FSH secretion is critical to the development of a single dominant follicle. Once a dominant follicle is selected, it secretes sufficient quantities of Inhibin A and Inhibin B to suppress FSH and prevent the growth of other follicles, during that cycle. Thus, they play important role in development of single dominant follicle.
- *Follistatin*, a protein present in the pituitary and follicular fluid binds the activins, inactivating them, and therefore acts to suppress FSH secretion.
- *Leptin (adipocyte protein hormone):* Leptin is also found in the follicular fluid in the ovaries and triggers pulsatile secretion of GnRH around puberty. It is linked to nutrition and has a important role in the control of hypothalamic–pituitary–ovarian axis. A diet restriction has a negative impact on hypothalamus and decreases LH secretion causing amenorrhea as seen in anorexia nervosa.
- Anti-mullerian hormone (AMH) is a dimeric glycoprotein member of the TGF-beta superfamily. The classical role of AMH is to induce the degeneration of the mullerian ducts during male sexual differentiation. In addition, AMH is produced by granulosa cells of small follicles and acts in the ovary through two receptors, type II which is specific for AMH and type I which also binds other members of the BMP family. AMH is responsible for FSH responsiveness of growing follicles. As follicles grow, the antral fluid concentration of AMH decreases. Thus, decrease AMH results in a reduction in this responsiveness and an increased rate of follicle atresia.

Hormonal Sensors: Receptors

To exert their transcriptional actions both estrogen and progesterone recruit classical estradiol and progesterone nuclear receptors (ER and PR, respectively) whereas the non-genomic actions are brought about by alternative membrane receptors. Though these membrane receptors for estrogens and for progestins receptor family have been isolated and identified but their contribution in menstrual regulation is not yet clear. ER, PR along-with androgen receptors (ARs) and glucocorticoid receptors (GRs), belongs to the subfamily 3 of nuclear receptors. The major isoforms of ER and PR are: ER-a and ER-b; PR-A and PR-B. The two ER isoforms are derived from distinct genes on different chromosomes, whereas, PR-A and PR-B are derived from alternate promoters present on a single gene.[13] Another isoform of PR is PR-C, which lacks DNA binding domain, is specific for the uterus and can inhibit both the other PR isoforms PR-A and PR-B. Because of the differences in the ligand binding and transactivating domains, ER-a and ER-b exert different biological effects: ER-a is a potent transcriptional activator and can be inhibited by ER-b. ER-a is detected in the stroma and the glands of both the functional as well as the basal layers of human endometrium. During the late proliferative phase ER-α detection is maximal in all types of cell, whereas during early secretory phase the levels rapidly decreases in the stromal cells, but with a gradual fall in the glandular levels. Rise in the ER-a immune-staining is also seen during mid- and late secretory phases in decidual stromal cells around the spiral arterioles and also in the endometrial vascular wall. Expression of ER-b levels peaks in the epithelial cells during the peri-ovulatory period and in the stromal and the vascular cells in the late secretory phase. ER-b is also found to be present in endometrial NK cells.[14]

Nuclear PR immune-staining is highest during late proliferative and early secretory phases but consistently higher levels are also found throughout the proliferative phase in the glands of both the basal and functional layers. The glandular PR level reduces considerably during the mid and late secretory phases, with the staining remaining only in very few glands in the basal layer. In contrast to the glandular levels, the stromal levels of the PR immune-labeling fluctuates very minimally throughout the cycle in both the layers. There is also differential expression of both the major PR isoforms throughout the cycle. During the proliferative phase, both PR-A and PR-B are co-expressed in the glandular cells whereas, stromal cells are predominated by PR-A isoform. The immune staining during early secretory phase is highly heterogeneous, in the glandular cells and stains with either PR-A, PR-B or even both. During the mid secretory phase, expression of PR-B is predominant and is the only isoform expressing during the late secretory phase and at the time of menstruation in some glands. Whereas, PR-A expression predominates the stromal cells during the secretory phase, Though it reduces during late secretory phase, but still expression is found at the time of menstruation. These variations in the expression of both the PR-A and PR-B isoforms is mainly governed by estradiol and progesterone synthesis. High estradiol levels found during the proliferative phase induce the PR expression, whereas high progesterone levels, negatively regulates its receptors and reduces PR expression during the secretory phase.

Androgens, glucocorticoids and their receptors are also involved in the cyclic endometrial modifications. Because estradiol is synthesized from androgen, ovaries produce testosterone, although about 20 times less than testes.[15] Despite aromatase-mediated conversion of testosterone into estradiol, testosterone levels remain elevated throughout the cycle. Serum androgen levels peak around ovulation but tissue levels are increased in the secretory endometrium. Expression of AR is detected in the stroma throughout the cycle but decreases during the secretory phase. GR is also expressed in fibroblasts, lymphocytes (including NK cells) and endothelial cells of the human endometrial stroma throughout the cycle but is absent from the glandular compartment.

Uterus

Endocrinology of Endometrium

The proliferative phase of the endometrium represents the estrogenic part of the menstrual cycle. It is initiated and controlled by estrogen. The secretory phase of the endometrium is controlled by progesterone, although the effect of progesterone is obtained only after the endometrium has been sensitized with estrogen. This is because estrogen produces progesterone receptors on which progesterone acts.

Proliferative Phase

After bleeding is over endometrium regrows under stimulation of estrogen. This is called priming of endometrium. Proliferative period is divided into three phases, early proliferative, mid proliferative and late proliferative (Table 1.1).

Secretory Phase

Secretory phase starts with ovulation. In the secretory phase, the endometrium that is primed by estradiol differentiates under the effect of progesterone. Secretory phase is further divided into early and late phase (Table 1.2).

If pregnancy does not occurs, corpus luteum atrophies resulting in decrease of estradiol and progesterone which results in the collapse of the endometrial glands, constriction of the blood vessels, and the sloughing of the endometrium with resumption of menstrual bleeding. A fall in the level of these hormones also starts off a fresh positive feedback mechanism and triggers the hypothalamus to release gonadotropin. This is how a menstrual cycle is regulated. *The luteal phase, i.e. time between ovulation and menstruation, is fairly constant at 14 days in a menstrual cycle.*

Table 1.1 Division of proliferative phase		
Early proliferative	Mid proliferative	Late proliferative
• Extends from cycle day 4–7 • Endometrial thickness is less than 3 mm • Glands are short, narrow, tubular, and straight • A few mitoses are present in the glands • The stroma is compact and has few mitoses	• Extends from cycle 8–11 • Endometrial thickness is 4–8 mm • Glands are longer and have a slightly curved effect • There are numerous mitoses in the glands with early pseu-dostratification of the nuclei that appear superimposed in layers • The stroma increases with increased mitoses	• Extends from cycle day 11–14 • Endometrial thickness is 6–10 mm • Glands are tortuous as a result of active growth • There are numerous mitoses and pseudostrati-fication of the nuclei • The stroma is dense and has numerous mitoses

Table 1.2 Division of secretory phase	
Early secretory phase	Late secretory phase
• First 7 days • Appearance of basal vacuoles • Increase in glandular tortuosity with prominent subnuclear vacuoles • Initial accumulation of glycogen-rich vacuoles at the base of the luminal cells • Onset of prominent acidophilic • Secretions in the gland lumen	• Last 7 days • Maximal stromal edema • Development of highly coiled spiral arteries • Condensation of the stroma around the spiral arterioles • Lymphocytic infiltration of the stroma • Focal necrosis of the stroma around the spiral arterioloes

REGULATION OF MENSTRUATION

The important feature of the menstrual changes is the contraction and constriction of the coiled arteries. Vasoconstriction of the coiled arteries causes ischemia and the necrosis of the superficial layers of the endometrium. Menstrual bleeding occurs when the open arteries damaged by necrosis relax and discharge blood in the uterine cavity. Some degree of venous hemorrhage also occurs. Superficial layer of the endometrium is shed-off by the end of the first day. The regeneration of the vascular system is brought about by the development of anastomosing arteries. The re-epithelialization is brought about by glandular cells that remain in the unshed basal layer of the endometrium.

Induction of Menstruation: Progesterone Withdrawal

The process of menstruation or menstrual bleeding is basically an inflammatory process characterized by tissue destruction and recruitment of inflammatory cells. Just prior to menstrual bleed, inflammatory cell content (leukocytes: mainly neutrophils, NK cells and macrophages) rises in the endometrium and makes up about 40-45% of the of the stromal cells. This leukocytic infiltration is triggered by the progesterone withdrawal. It has been seen that induction of menstruation is blocked if progesterone is supplemented back, in a model of artificially cycling macaques even up to 36 hours after its withdrawal, though it is long known that tissue destruction is inevitable 36 hours after progesterone withdrawal. This leukocyte influx is probably induced by endometrial resident cells (like perivascular cells around the spiral arterioles) in response to the changes in the progesterone levels and hence produces inflammatory chemokines and prostaglandins. Spiral arterioles thus, brings about menstruation by vasoconstricting and promoting leukocyte influx that express PR and recruit further more inflammatory mediators. Many chemokines which are able to recruit inflammatory cells, including IL-8, MCP 1 are found to be up-regulated in response to progesterone withdrawal.[16] Once activated, these inflammatory cells locally secrete proteases which are capable of degrading ECM components. This inflammatory cells triggered ECM proteolysis is the mandate for the menstrual shedding. Most classes of proteinases are expressed in the human endometrium and hence participate in menstruation *in vivo* to name a few: plasmin, lysosomal enzymes and caspases. Though they play important role in ECM proteolysis and hence menstrual shedding, but the major role is played by matrix metalloproteinase (MMP) family of enzymes.[17]

Thus, we have seen that normal menstruation results from estrogen-progesterone withdrawal, so any decrease in serum level of estrogen and progesterone may initiate bleeding, and this is known as *withdrawal bleeding*.

Estrogen Withdrawal Bleeding

Midcycle bleeding may be seen in some women due to abrupt fall in estrogen levels just before the ovulation.[18]

Progesterone Withdrawal Bleeding

Progesterone withdrawal bleeding is seen in cases of luteal phase defect, which is characterized by spotting before the menstruation be as a result of insufficient progesterone secretion.[18]

Estrogen Breakthrough Bleeding

In normal menstruation cycle, estrogen and progesterone stimulus is balanced leading to stable endometrial epithelium, stroma, and microvasculature. Random breakdown is avoided, and endometrial shedding occurs uniformly in whole of the endometrial cavity.

Prolonged hyperestrogenism unopposed by progesterone in cases of anovulatory cycles, leads to proliferative endometrium and hyperplasia without proper stromal support.[19] This leads to focal stromal breakdown and bleeding is initiated and is called 'estrogen breakthrough bleeding'.[18] Endometrial shedding in this case is irregular and not throughout the endometrial cavity. Also, the sensitivity of abnormal vasculature in hyperestrogenic endometrium is suspected to be greater to vasodilation by prostaglandins than to their vasoconstrictor counterparts. In addition, a potent vasoconstrictor, angiotensin-2 is decreased in endometrial hyperplasia. As tissue loss involves the superficial endometrium only focally, vasoconstriction of basal and radial arteries does not occur and this causes abnormalities in hemostasis. This is the mechanism of bleeding in chronic anovulation. The amount and duration of bleeding can vary according to the amount and duration of unopposed estrogen exposure.[20] Low level chronic estrogen stimulation typically results in intermittent spotting, whereas sustained high level estrogen exposure commonly results in acute episodes of profuse bleeding.

Progesterone Breakthrough Bleeding

Hyperprogestogenism may be seen in cases of continuous progestin or low-dose oral contraceptive users. Due to hyperprogesteronism, there is defective proliferative phase leading to glandular atrophy and thining of endometrium. There is a decrease in the number and turtuosity of spiral arterioles and many of the subepithelial microvessels are dilated and lined by a very thin endothelial cell layer. Since the basement membrane is poorly formed or absent, and there are gaps between endothelial cells, pools of extravasated red blood cells are often seen. These structural alterations and vascular fragility lead to breakdown and bleeding and is known as progesterone breakthrough bleeding.[18]

Serum levels of steroid hormones during different phases of menstrual cycle in reproductive age

Menstrual phase	Serum estradiol	Serum progesterone	Serum FSH	Serum LH
Follicular phase	27–123 pg/mL	• Early follicular: 0.6 ng/mL • Late follicular: 14.5 ng/mL	3.1–7.9 mIU/mL	1–18 mIU/dL
Ovulation peak	96–436 pg/mL	16.1 ng/mL	2.3–18.5 mIU/mL	20–105 mIU/mL
Luteal phase	49–294 pg/mL	31.4 ng/mL	1.4–5.5 mIU/mL	0.4–20.0 mIU/mL
Post-menopausal	<20 pg/mL	0.2 ng/mL	30.6–106.3 mIU/mL	15.0–62.0 mIU/mL

Menstrual parameters and its variation

Menstrual parameters	Normal menstruation	Abnormal menstruation (The FIGO Recommendations on Terminologies of Abnormal Uterine Bleeding)
Frequency of menses (days)	21–35 days	<21 days-polymenorrhea >35 days-oligomenorrhea
Duration of flow	3–7 days	< 3days-shortened menstrual bleeding >7 days-prolonged menstrual bleeding
Volume of monthly blood loss	20–80 mL	<20 mL-light menstrual bleeding >80 mL-heavy menstrual bleeding

Factors Affecting Menstruation

- *Stress:* Stress may be associated with short or long menstrual cycles or there may be no association.[21,22] Stress, via corticotropin-releasing hormone, inhibits LH and may lead to poor follicular development, resulting in abnormal corpus luteum function.[23]
- *Obesity:* Although a minimal amount of body fat is necessary to initiate and maintain ovulatory menstrual cycles. Excess number of fat cells in obese women results in extraglandular aromatization of androgen to estrogen. Circulating levels of sex hormone binding globulin is also less in these women, which leads accumulation of larger proportion of free androgen, which gets converted into estrogen. These altered levels of esrogen and androgen is the basis for menstrual irregularity in obese women.[24]
- *Exercise:* Exercise is reduces stress, and improves the quality of life. The incidence of menstrual is highly variable and depends on the intensity, volume, and type of exercise. High intensity exercise causes decrease in GnRH pulstality due low levels of leptin or high levels of ghrelin/corticotropin releasing hormone.[24]
- *Smoking:* Smoking is associated with short cycle length, especially in those who smoke at least 1 pack per day.[25,26] The greater the smoking, the more likely is the risk of anovulation and shorter luteal phase.
- *Sleep hygiene:* Night-time ambient light exposure have pronounced effects on menstrual cycle through the influence of melatonin secretion.[27] Melatonin is found in the follicular fluid surrounding the egg and is associated with gonadotropin levels and influences ovulation. Thus, female shift workers have more menstrual irregularity and longer cycle lengths.[28,29]
- *Emotional disturbances:* Hypothalamus is influenced by the higher cortical centers, especially the temporal lobe. Emotional disturbances are known to stimulate or depress the H-P-O axis and disturb the menstrual cycles.
- *Hormones:* Growth hormone, insulin-like growth factor, epidermal growth factor, adrenal cortex and TSH also participate in the endocrinological functions in a woman,

through their action on the hypothalamus and anterior pituitary gland.
- *Hyperprolactenemia:* In hyperprolactinemia, various menstrual disorders such as irregular bleeding, insufficient luteal phase, anovulatory cycles, oligomenorrhea to amenorrhea may be found. Hyperprolactinemia acts at the hypothalamic level affecting the GnRH secretion, which leads to altered LH and steroidal secretion.[31]
- *Hypothyroidism:* A high level of TSH is associated with menstrual irregularities. Hypothyroidism is commonly associated with ovulatory dysfunction due to various interactions of thyroid hormones on the female reproductive system. In hypothyroidism, there is increase in thyroid-releasing hormone (TRH) due to negative feedback, this increased TRH results in hyperprolactinemia. Ovulatory dysfunction in hypothyroidism is caused both due to TRH-mediated hyperprolactenemia and altered GnRH pulsatile secretion, leading to a delay in LH response and inadequate corpus luteum.[30] Thyroid hormones also synergize with the FSH-mediated LH/hCG receptor to exert direct stimulatory effects on progesterone secretion.[31]

> Thus, if both hypothyroidism and hperprolactenemia are present, hypothyroidism is to be treated first, because prolactin level often normalizes with treatment of hypothyroidism because TRH is elevated in hypothyroidism which stimulates prolactin secretion.

REFERENCES

1. Allen K. The Reluctant Hypothesis: A History of Discourse Surrounding the Lunar Phase Method of Regulating Conception. Lacuna Press; 2007.p.239.
2. Buckley T. Menstruation and the power of Yurok women: Methods in cultural reconstruction. American Ethnologist. 1982;9 (1):47-60
3. Chan YM, Butler JP, Pinnell NE, et al. Kisspeptin resets the hypothalamic GnRH clock in men. J Clin Endocrinol Metab. 2011;96:E908-E15.
4. Mimri R, Lebenthal Y, Lazar L, et al. A novel loss of function mutation in GPR54/ KISS1R leads to hypogonadotropic hypogonadism in a highly consanguineous family. J Clin Endocrinol Metab. 2011;96:E536-E45.
5. Pitteloud N, Durrani S, Raivio T, et al. Complex genetics in idiopathic hypogonadotropic hypogonadism. Front Horm Res. 2010;39:142-53.
6. Bjorbaek C, Kahn BB. Leptin signaling in the central nervous system and the periphery. Recent Prog Horm Res. 2004;59:305-31.
7. Castellano JM, Bentsen AH, Mikkelsen JD, et al. Kisspeptins: bridging energy homeostasis and reproduction. Brain Res. 2010;1364:129-38.
8. Welt CK, Chan JL, Bullen J, et al. Recombinant human leptin in women with hypothalamic amenorrhea. N Engl J Med. 2004;351:987-97.
9. Chou SH, Chamberland JP, Liu X, et al. Leptin is an effective treatment for hypothalamic amenorrhea. Proc Natl Acad Sci USA. 2011;108(16):6585-90.
10. Haadsma ML, Groen H, Fidler V, et al. The predictive value of ovarian reserve tests for spontaneous pregnancy in subfertile ovulatory women. Hum Reprod. 2008;23:1800-7.
11. Young JM, McNeilly AS. Theca: the forgotten cell of the ovarian follicle. Reproduction. 2010;140:489-504.
12. Kohen P, Castro O, Palomina A, et al. The steroidogenic response and corpus luteum expression of the steroidogenic acute regulatory protein after human chorionic administration at different times in the human luteal phase. J Clin Endocrinol Metab. 2003;88:3421-30.
13. Giangrande PH, Pollio G, McDonnell DP. Mapping and characterization of the functional domains responsible for the differential activity of the A and B isoforms of the human progesterone receptor. J Biol Chem. 1997;272 (52):32889-900.
14. Snijders MP, de Goeij AF, Debets-Te Baerts MJ, Rousch MJ, Koudstaal J, Bosman FT. Immunocytochemical analysis of oestrogen receptors and progesterone receptors in the human uterus throughout the menstrual cycle and after the menopause. J Reprod Fertil. 1992;94 (2):363-71.
15. Federman DD. The biology of human sex differences. N Engl J Med. 2006;354 (14):1507-14.
16. Kelly RW, King AE, Critchley HO. Cytokine control in human endometrium. Reproduction. 2001;121 (1):3-19.
17. Patrick H, Héloïse P, Gaide C, Etienne M. The endocrine and paracrine control of menstruation. Molecular and Cellular Endocrinology. 2012;358:197-207.

18. Speroff L, Fritz MA. Abnormal uterine bleeding. In: Clinical Gynecologic Endocrinology and Infertility, 8th edn. Philadelphia. Lippincott Williams and Wilkins; 2010.pp.547-73.
19. Ferenczy A. Pathophysiology of endometrial bleeding. Maturitas. 2003;45:1-14.
20. Speroff L, Fritz MA. Dysfunctional uterine bleeding. In: Clinical Gynecologic Endocrinology and Infertility, 6th edn. Philadelphia. Lippincott Williams and Wilkins; 2005.pp.547-73.
21. Barsom S, Mansfield P, Koch P, Gierach G, West S. Association between psychological stress and menstrual cycle characteristics in perimenopausal women. Women Health Issues. 2004;14(6):235-41.
22. Fenster L, Waller K, Swan S, et al. Psychological stress in the workplace and menstrual function. Am J Epidemiol. 1999;149(2):127-34.
23. Olive D. Exercise and fertility: an update. Curr Opin Obstet Gynecol. 2010;22(4):259-63.
24. Baker VL, Schillings WJ. Amenorrhea. Berek and Novak's Gynecology, 15th edn. Wolters Kluwer: Lippincott Williams and Wilkins; 2012.pp.1035-60.
25. Rowland A, Baird D, Sandler D, et al. Influence of medical conditions and lifestyle factors on the menstrual cycle. Epidemiology. 2002;13(6):668-74.
26. Windham G, Elkin E, Swan S, Waller K, Fenster L. Cigarette smoking and effects on menstrual function. Obstetr Gynecol. 1999;93(1):59-65.
27. Barron M. Light exposure, melatonin secretion, and menstrual cycle parameters: an integrative review. Biol Res Nurs. 2007;9(1):49-69.
28. Baker F, Driver H. Circadian rhythms, sleep, and the menstrual cycle. Sleep Med. 2007;8(6):613-22.
29. Lawson C, Whelan E, Lividoti HE, et al. Rotating shift work and menstrual cycle characteristics. Epidemiology. 2011;22(3):305-12.
30. Thomas R, Reid RL. Thyroid disease and reproductive dysfunction: a review. Obstetrics and Gynecology. 1987;70:789-98.
31. Cecconi S, Rucci N, Scaldaferri ML, Masciulli MP, Rossi G, Moretti C, et al. Thyroid hormone effects on mouse oocyte maturation and granulosa cell aromatase activity. Endocrinology. 1999;140:1783-8.

2

Ultrasonography in Gynecology

Niharika Dhiman

INTRODUCTION

Ultrasonography (USG) has significant role in gynecology. It has both diagnostic and therapeutic values. The abdominal and transvaginal evaluation of pelvic organs with USG is valuable to confirm the clinical diagnosis and manage the case in follow-up. Ultrasound transducers usually range from 2 MHz to 10 MHz, with higher-frequency transducers providing better resolution and image quality but at the expense of attenuation and reduced penetration. Transvaginal ultrasound (TVS) uses higher frequency probes than transabdominal ultrasound (TAS), as the organs of interest are nearer the transducer, and provides more information and improved definition as a result. Transvaginal pelvic assessment should always be performed in conjunction with transabdominal ultrasound, as the limited penetration and field of view may mean that a large mass, such as an ovarian mass or serosal fibroid, can be missed.

The common indication for USG in gynecoloy are listed in Table 2.1.

CONSENT

The written request for an ultrasound examination should provide sufficient information to allow for the appropriate performance and interpretation of the examination. All the documentation should be completed as per Preconception, Prenatal Diagnostic Techniques (PCPNDT) act before doing a scan in a pregnant female (Form F).

Table 2.1 Indications of ultrasonography

- Pelvic pain
- Dysmenorrhea (painful menses)
- Amenorrhea
- Menorrhagia (excessive menstrual bleeding)
- Metrorrhagia (irregular uterine bleeding)
- Menometrorrhagia (excessive irregular bleeding)
- Follow-up of a previously detected abnormality
- Evaluation, monitoring, and/or treatment of infertility patients
- Delayed menses, precocious puberty, or vaginal bleeding in a prepubertal child
- Postmenopausal bleeding
- Abnormal or technically limited pelvic examination
- Signs or symptoms of pelvic infection
- Further characterization of a pelvic abnormality noted on another imaging study
- Evaluation of congenital anomalies
- Excessive bleeding, pain, or signs of infection after pelvic surgery, delivery, or abortion
- Localization of a intrauterine contraceptive device
- Screening for malignancy in patients at increased risk
- Urinary incontinence or pelvic organ prolapse and
- Guidance for interventional or surgical procedures

The standard examination of female pelvis requires a combined approach of performing a TAS followed by a TVS. The TAS uses a sectoral transducer ranging from 3 MHz to 5 MHz and the TVS uses a probe frequency ranging from 5 MHz to 12 MHz. The higher frequency probes are useful in achieving higher resolution scans in the near field whereas low frequency probes are used in areas requiring higher penetrations.

The TAS requires a full bladder and gives a wider view of the pelvic organs. A full bladder act as an acoustic window (posterior enhancement due to fluid) through which a better view of the pelvic organs can be made moreover it displaces the airfilled bowel upwards and straightens the uterus thus giving a clearer view. It provides a better visualization of structures superficial and remote from the vagina. A TVS provides an enhanced and better visualization of the adnexal structures and the uterus which can be obscured during a TAS scan. The only contraindications for a TVS are:
- Premenarchal/Virginal patients
- Patient not consenting for a TVS.

TECHNIQUE

Before undertaking a pelvic scan one should be well versed with the pelvic anatomy in order to identify and correlate the structures and to differential normal findings from abnormal ones. During a transabdominal and TVS the probe should be held in proper position to prevent misinterpretation of the side. Images should be taken in the following planes for studying the normal and abnormal structures: sagittal, coronal and oblique. These images can be obtained moving the probe in the following directions:
- Side to side movement [Sagittal plane]
- Rotation of probe from 0° to 90° [Coronal plane]
- Angulation [Oblique plane].

UTERUS

The vagina and uterus provide anatomic landmarks that can be used as reference points for the other pelvic structures, whether normal or abnormal. In examining the uterus, the following should be evaluated:
- The uterine size, shape, and orientation
- The endometrium
- The myometrium
- The cervix.

Table 2.2 Normal dimensions during reproductive age

Uterus (length × breadth × width)	7.5–8 × 4.5–5 × 2.5–3 cm
Cervix (length)	4–5 cm
Ovary (length × breadth × width); volume	3.5 cm × 2.5 cm × 1.5 cm (10–12 cm^3)

The overall uterine length (Table 2.2) is evaluated in a sagittal view from the fundus to the cervix (to the external os). The depth of the uterus (anteroposterior dimension) is measured in the same sagittal view from its anterior to posterior walls, perpendicular to the length. The maximum width is measured in the transverse or coronal view. If volume measurements of the uterine corpus are performed, the cervical component should be excluded from the uterine length measurement.

ENDOMETRIUM

The endometrium is usually best seen on transvaginal scans. Endometrial thickness is measured from one echogenic border to the other echogenic border across the endometrial cavity in a sagittal plane.
- *During menstruation:* The endometrium appears thin, echogenic line 1–4 mm. Intrauterine blood or sheets of sloughed endometria may be identified.
- In the *proliferative phase* of the menstrual cycle (days 6–14), the endometrium becomes thicker (5–7 mm) and more echogenic relative to the myometrium, because of the development of glands, blood vessels, and stroma (*Bilaminar appearance*).
- In the *late proliferative (periovulatory) phase*, the endometrium develops a multilayered appearance with an echogenic basal layer and hypoechoic inner functional layer, separated

by a thin echogenic median layer arising from the central interface and measures measure up to 11 mm in thickness. The layered appearance usually disappears 48 hours after ovulation (*Trilaminar appearance*).

During the secretory phase: The endometrium becomes even thicker (7-16 mm) and more echogenic. This increased echogenicity is related to the stromal edema and glands distended with mucus and glycogen. Stromal edema also accounts for the increased posterior acoustic enhancement.

THE POSTMENOPAUSAL ENDOMETRIUM

The normal postmenopausal endometrium has the following characteristics i.e. *thin, homogeneous*, and *echogenic*. In general, a double-layer, smooth, homogeneous thickness of less than 5 mm without focal thickening excludes significant disease and correlates with an atrophic endometrium. The endometrium in a patient undergoing hormonal replacement therapy may vary up to 3 mm if cyclic estrogen and progestin therapy is being used. The endometrium will appear thickest prior to progestin exposure and thinnest after the progestin phase. Imaging should be performed at the beginning or end of a cycle of treatment, when the endometrium will be at its thinnest and any pathologic thickening will be most prominent. A patient undergoing unopposed estrogen therapy with endometrial thickening exceeding 8 mm should be considered for biopsy, whereas patients receiving progesterone in addition to estrogen can be rescanned at the beginning or end of the following cycle to determine if there has been a change in endometrial thickness.[1] Any thickness greater than 5 mm with postmenopausal bleeding or any endometrial heterogeneity or focal thickening seen at TVS should be investigated further with sonohysterography, biopsy, or hysteroscopy.[2]

Endometrial Polyps

Endometrial polyps may be visualized at transvaginal ultrasonography as focal non-specific endometrial thickening. Polyps appear as echogenic, smooth, intracavitary masses outlined by fluid. A polyp may be broad-based or sessile or pedunculated and the point of attachment does not disrupt the endometrial lining. Fibroids or foci of endometrial hyperplasia or carcinoma can mimic a sessile polyp. Foci of atypical hyperplasia are sometimes found within polyps.

Submucosal Fibroids

They are commonly identified at USG as hypoechoic solid masses, but they may be heterogeneous or hyperechoic, depending on the degree of degeneration and calcification. Fibroids usually do not interrupt the endometrium unless they become submucosal in location (Table 2.3). Submucosal fibroids distort the uterine cavity with a varying degree of intracavitary extension. Hysteroscopy can depict only the intracavitary portion of the fibroid.[3]

Endometrial Hyperplasia

Endometrial hyperplasia is an abnormal proliferation of endometrial stroma and glands and represents a spectrum of endometrial changes

Table 2.3 ESGE: Classification of submucous myomas

Type 0
- Entirely within endometrial cavity
- No myometrial extension (pedunculated)

Type I
- <50% myometrial extension (sessile)
- <90° angle of myoma surface to uterine wall

Type II
- ≥50% myometrial extension (sessile)
- ≥90° angle of myoma surface to uterine wall

Abbreviation: ESGE, European Society of Gynaecological Endoscopy

ranging from glandular atypia to frank neoplasia. All types of endometrial hyperplasia (cystic, adenomatous, atypical) can cause diffusely smooth or, less commonly, focal hyperechoic endometrial thickening. The USG appearance can simulate that of normal thickening during the secretory phase, sessile polyps, submucosal fibroids, cancer, and adherent blood clots, yielding potentially false-positive results. Endometrial hyperplasia is considered whenever the endometrium appears to exceed 10 mm in thickness, especially in menopausal patients, although it can be reliably excluded in these patients only when the endometrium measures less than 6 mm. Endometrial hyperplasia may also cause asymmetric thickening with surface irregularity, an appearance that is suspicious for carcinoma. Because endometrial hyperplasia has a nonspecific appearance, any focal abnormality should lead to biopsy if there is clinical suspicion for malignancy.

Endometrial Adenocarcinoma

Ultrasonographic signs of endometrial carcinoma include heterogeneity and irregularly thickened endometrium with irregularity of the endometrium myometrium border, which indicates an invasive disease. However, these signs can also be seen in endometrial hyperplasia and polyps. Polypoid tumors tend to cause more diffuse and irregular thickening than a polyp and more heterogeneity than endometrial hyperplasia an intrauterine fluid collection in a postmenopausal patient, can be associated with cervical stenosis and should raise a suspicion for endometrial or cervical carcinoma. Increased focal vascularity may be seen at color Doppler ultrasonography in both benign and malignant diseases of the endometrium. Significant overlap in Doppler indices (i.e. peak systolic velocity, resistive index, pulsatility index) in benign and malignant endometrial processes reduces the value of Doppler ultrasonography in characterizing endometrial masses.

Fibroids

Leiomyomas (fibroids) are the most common benign tumors of the female genital tract, affecting half of all women aged 30 or more. Fibroids are composed of smooth muscle fibers and fibrous tissue arranged in concentric whorls, which accounts for the typical appearance on ultrasound. Typically, fibroids appear as well-defined, solid masses with a whorled appearance. These are usually of similar echogenicity to the myometrium, but sometimes may be hypoechoic. Degenerate fibroids may have a complex appearance, with areas of cystic change. The heterogenicity increases with increased growth, fibrosis, degenation and calcification of a fibroid. Doppler USG typically shows circumferential vascularity; however, fibroids which are necrotic or have undergone torsion will show absence of flow. Transvaginal ultrasound is highly accurate in detecting intramural and subserosal fibroids, with a sensitivity of 99% and a specificity of 91%,[4] and can be used to categorise the number, size and position of each. When fibroids are multiple, large, or predominantly anterior, the image quality is often poor. Fibroids are associated with adenomyosis (50% of women with adenomyosis having coexistent fibroids), can also reduce image quality. This lack of clarity can complicate assessment of the posterior uterine wall and endometrial cavity, and inadvertently lead to a missed diagnosis. An area of adenomyosis or a solitary adenomyoma may be misdiagnosed as a fibroid, but Doppler ultrasound can be applied to differentiate these pathologies as fibroids have a peripheral vasculature, vessels run straight through areas of adenomyosis and present as diffuse hypervascularity. Pedunculated subserosal fibroids may also be misinterpreted as ovarian lesions, however identification of ovary on the same side can help in differentiating it from any ovarian lesion.

Ultrasound is less useful in the delineation of submucous fibroids, however, for which the sensitivity falls to 58.3% for a specificity of

94.8%.[4] Saline infusion sonohysterography (SIS) increases the diagnostic accuracy as the injected saline distends the uterine cavity and provides an echo-free, negative-contrast medium and improves the sensitivity and specificity to 81.3%[4] and 98.0%, respectively.

Adenomyosis

Adenomyosis is defined by the presence of ectopic endometrial glands and stroma within the myometrium. The presence of ectopic endometrial glands and stroma induces a hypertrophic and hyperplastic reaction in the surrounding myometrial tissue and presents most commonly as a diffuse disease involving the entire myometrium. It can also present in a focal area of the uterus, known as adenomyoma. Almost 70% of the hysterectomised specimens will have adenomyosis. A recent meta-analysis on the accuracy of sonography in the diagnosis of adenomyosis showed that it had sensitivity of 82.5% and specificity of 84.6%. A probe tenderness is generally present while performing a TVS in adenomyosis.[5]

The sonographic findings of adenomyosis, is best obtained by transvaginal sonography and include the following:
- Uterine enlargement—Globular uterine enlargement that is generally up to 12 weeks size without any mass or contour deformity.
- Abnormal heterogeneous myometrium.
- Cystic anechoic spaces or lakes in the myometrium representing dilated glands with collection.
- Uterine wall thickening—The uterine wall thickening can show anteroposterior asymmetry, especially when the disease is focal.
- Subendometrial echogenic linear striations/ "Venetian Blinds"—Invasion of the endometrial glands into the subendometrial tissue induces a hyperplastic reaction, which appears as echogenic linear striations fanning out from the endometrial layer.
- Obscure endometrial/myometrial border

- Thickening of the transition zone—there is pseudo-widening of the endometrial echo because of the extension of the endometrial tissue into the stratum basale. Normally this zone is a layer that appears as a hypoechoic halo surrounding the endometrial layer. A thickness of 12 mm or greater has been shown to be associated with adenomyosis.

A globular uterus, cystic spaces, and linear striations are the most specific findings in the diagnosis of adenomyosis.

Ultrasonographic Features of Ovarian Mass[6,7]

A number of prediction models have been created to maximize the predictive capability of ultrasonography in differentiating between the various types of ovarian lesions. However, more recently logistic regression models and simple rules created by the International Ovarian Tumor Analysis (IOTA) group have been shown to perform better than the risk of malignacy index (RMI) [which is a product of ultrasound score (U); menopausal status and serum CA125 (IU/mL) U × M× CA125]. The most recent systematic review and meta-analysis has concluded that based on currently available evidence, these IOTA rules and models should now be used in clinical practice.

The International Ovarian Tumor Analysis (IOTA) framework is a pattern recognition approach that has been frequently used to present large-scale multicenter-based consensus results. It includes a standardized methodology for the USG evaluation of ovarian masses and definitions of the ultrasonographic parameters of ovarian masses.

Five ultrasonic features to predict a malignant tumor (M features):
1. Irregular solid tumor (M1).
2. Ascites (M2).
3. At least four papillary structures (M3).
4. Irregular multilocular solid tumor with a largest diameter of at least 100 mm (M4).

5. Very high color content on color Doppler examination (M5).

Five ultrasonic features to predict a benign tumor (B features):
1. Unilocular cyst (B1).
2. Presence of solid components for which the largest solid component is <7 mm in largest diameter (B2).
3. Acoustic shadows (B3).
4. Smooth multilocular tumor (B4).
5. No detectable blood flow on Doppler examination (B5).

If one or more M features were present in the absence of a B feature, we classified the mass as malignant (rule 1).

If one or more B features were present in the absence of an M feature, we classified the mass as benign (rule 2).

If both M features and B features were present, or if none of the features was present, the simple rules were inconclusive (rule 3).

Predictors of Malignant Ovarian Lesions on Ultrasonography

- *Solid component:* USG demonstration of a solid component within a cystic mass is the most important predictor of malignancy, it also includes papillary projection, excrescence, vegetation, and nodule. Small solid areas that protrude 3 mm or more from the cyst wall are considered as papillary projections. Solid component can also be present in a dermoid or hemorrhagic cyst. The solid nodule in a dermoid cyst is hyperechoic whereas the echogenicity is similar to the cyst wall in a malignancy. Clot, however, often has concave borders, while a true mural nodule has outwardly convex borders. Color or power Doppler USG can be helpful in this distinction; with absent flow characteristic for clot and definite visible flow typical for neoplasm.
- *Septa:* Septa in a cystic ovarian mass are more likely to indicate malignancy if they are greater than 2–3 mm in thickness or have detectable flow on Doppler USG scans.
- *Ascites:* Ascites, an indirect indicator of malignancy, occurs with advanced malignancy. A small amount of fluid in the cul-de-sac is normal in premenopausal women, an increased risk of malignancy has been reported if it measures more than 15 mm in anteroposterior dimension.
- *Doppler:* The vessels in a malignant ovarian tumor have a lower pulsatility index, lower resistive (PI < 0.8 and RI < 0.6). The IOTA group has suggested a scoring system for the Doppler color:
  - Score 1—No detectable flow,
  - Score 2—Minimal vascularization,
  - Score 3—Moderate vascularization, and
  - Score 4—Abundant vascularization.

Metastatic Tumors to the Ovary

Ovarian metastasis from breast, gastric, and uterine cancers as well as lymphomas appear as solid tumors in contrast, ovarian metastasis from the colon, rectum and biliary tract, tend to be multilocular-solid or multilocular with anechoic or low-level. The latter group demonstrate a larger diameter and more frequently the presence of an irregular external surface. The detection of papillary projections is rare in metastatic tumors. The presence of rich vascularity (color score 3–4) is characteristic of all metastatic tumors, but metastatic tumors from the colon, rectum and biliary tract tend to be less vascular compared to those from the stomach, breast, uterus or lymphomas.

ULTRASONOGRAPHIC FEATURES OF BENIGN OVARIAN CYST

Polycystic Ovary[7]

Current recommended sonographic criteria for polycystic ovarian morphology:
- 25 or more follicles per (superseding the earlier Rotterdam criteria of 12 or more follicles)
- *Increased ovarian size (>10 cc):* Less sensitive than the follicle number criteria, but has a role when image resolution does not allow

accurate follicle count, e.g. transabdominal scanning, older equipment.

Other morphologic features include:
- Hyperechoic central stroma
- *Peripheral location of follicles:* Which can give a string of pearl appearance
- Follicles of similar size measuring 2–9 mm
Endometrium may appear thickened resembling that of a proliferative endometrium.

Benign Ovarian Cyst

- *A simple cyst* (defined as having anechoic fluid, a thin wall, no solid area or septa, and distal acoustic enhancement) is usually easily recognizable. Most simple ovarian cysts are follicular cysts, occur in premenopausal patients, and will resolve within 1–2 months. Large cysts may mimic a serous cystadenoma.
- *Hemorrhagic corpus luteum cyst:* A reticular pattern of internal echoes due to fibrin strands is a strong predictor of a hemorrhagic cyst. This pattern has also been referred to as having a fishnet, lacy, cobweb, or spider web appearance. While a clot may occasionally simulate a solid nodule, it is usually recognizable by its concave outer margin and/or absence of detectable flow at color or power Doppler. These require a follow-up scan after 6–12 weeks.
- *Endometriomas* typically appear as complex cysts, either unilocular or multilocular, that have a ground glass appearance due to diffuse, homogeneous, low to medium level internal echoes. Additionally endometriomas may include echogenic foci in the wall and small solid areas along the wall, making it difficult to distinguish endometriomas from neoplasms. A small percentage (probably, 15%) of endometriomas have less typical USG features such as anechoic fluid, a fluid-fluid level, heterogeneity, or calcification and can be confused with dermoid cyst, abscesses, ovarian fibromas, mucinous and serous cystadenomas and hemorrhagic cysts. Rarely, endometrioid or clear cell carcinoma may develop within an endometrioma; this is more likely in women older than 45 years of age and in endometriomas larger than 9 cm.
- *Dermoid cyst (mature teratoma):* The most characteristic features of a dermoid cyst on ultrasound are the presence of:
  - A *white ball* (corresponding to hair and sebum) sometimes occupying the entire cyst.
  - Long echogenic white lines and prominent echogenic dots in cyst fluid (corresponding to hair floating in the non-sebaceous material).
  - Distal acoustic shadowing.

  The Rokitansky pouch area or dermoid plug can be seen as a hyperechoic with acoustic shadow due to hair, fat or calcifications. Rarely a dermoid may not have all of these characteristic USG features.
- *Serous cystadenomas:* These appear as smooth, thin walled, anechoic, fluid-filled structures. They are bilateral in 15% of cases and their mean size is 5–8 cm. Some contain fine septations whilst others have areas of hemorrhage appearing as small echogenic areas.
- *Mucinous cystadenomas:* Mucinous cysts are classically thin walled, large and unilateral. They consist of internal thin-walled locules containing mucin which appears as fluid with low level echogenicity. In general neither serous nor mucinous cystadenomas are associated with significant vascularity on Doppler.
- *Ovarian fibrothecoma:* Ovarian fibroma is the most common sex-cord stromal neoplasm and is mostly benign. A thecoma is another sex-cord stromal neoplasm, and occasionally there will be histologic features of both fibroma and thecoma giving rise to the term *fibrothecoma*. Fibromas typically occur in middle-aged women and appear as heterogeneous or homogeneous solid masses, similar to pedunculated fibroids. On occasion, they may have a small cystic component. Marked acoustic shadowing is a predictive feature that occurs in 18–52% of fibromas. With fibromas, the acoustic shadowing

does not originate from an area of increased echogenicity due to calcification or from the hyperechoic nodule of a dermoid, instead, the shadowing occurs because of marked attenuation of sound by the hypoechoic mass of the fibroma. A minority of ovarian fibromas grow exophytically from the ovary, which may mimic a pedunculated uterine leiomyoma.

Benign Extraovarian Masses

- *Paraovarian cyst:* It appears as a clear hypoechoic mass not more than 9 cm in diameter, near to the broad ligament, separate from the ovary. In case the extraovarian location is not obvious, gentle pressure with the transvaginal transducer and/or with the examiner's hand on the lower abdomen may show separation of the cyst from the ovary. Paraovarian cystadenomas are uncommon cystic lesions and typically have a small solid nodule or septum within and are usually larger than 5 cm.
- *Hydrosalpinx:* The Fallopian tube is 10 cm long and is usually not visible on an ultrasonographic examination. Hydrosalpinx which refers to a fluid filled diseased tube has the following characteristic appearance on gray scale: (A) fluid filled sausage shaped structure. (B) Presence of incomplete septa (referred to as the *"waist sign"* which is a strong predictor of Hydrosalpinx). (C) On a transverse view the mucosal folds give a *'Cogwheel appearance'* when the tube is thick and *'beads on a string'* when the tube is thin. When a hyperechoic material fills the tube it corresponds to pyosalpinx.
- *Tubo-ovarian abscess:* It may have the appearance of a unilocular cystic structure or a complex multicystic structure with thick walls and thick septae, filled with echogenic material (*'ground glass' appearance*). Probe tenderness while performing a TVS can be helpful in differentiating it from a malignancy and endometriomas.
- *Torsion of adnexal mass:* It is the fifth most common gynecological emergency with a prevalence of 2.7%. In adnexal torsion various degree of arterial, venous and lymphatic occlusion occurs leading to massive congestion and edema of the involved structures. The involved ovary becomes round and globular; torsion of normal ovary in an adolescent girl gives a typical picture of enlarged ovary with peripherally arranged cysts. The wall of a diseased tube becomes thicker. On Doppler the flows are compromised depending upon the degree of torsion.

Ultrasonographic Features of Ectopic Pregnancy

In suspected cases of ectopic pregnancy a transabdominal scan should always be done before a tranvsvaginal scan is taken up.

Uterus

- Empty uterine cavity with no evidence of intrauterine pregnancy.
- Presence of psuedogestational sac or decidual cast (20%).
- Thick echogenic endometrium.

Tube and Ovary

- Extrauterine sac containing yolk sac or fetal pole, with or without heart motion.
- Complex adnexal mass—95% chance of a tubal ectopic (if no intrauterine pregnancy).
- Moderate amount of anechoic free fluid (or any echogenic free fluid).
- Tubal ring sign—5% chance of a tubal ectopic if seen described in 49% of ectopics and in 68% of unruptured ectopics.
- *Ring of fire:* It can be seen on color Doppler in a tubal ectopic, but can also be seen in a corpus luteum.

Peritoneal Cavity

The presence of free intraperitoneal fluid with positive beta-human chorionic gonadotropin (hCG) and empty uterus is ~70% specific for an ectopic pregnancy and ~63% sensitive for ectopic pregnancy.[9]

Heterotopic pregnancy: In patients with in vitro fertilization (IVF), there is a possibility of a coexisting ectopic pregnancy in ~1:500. In patients not receiving IVF, the risk of heterotopic pregnancy is rare (1:30,000).

Molar Pregnancy

Complete Hydatidiform Mole

- Classic sonographic appearance is that of a solid collection of echoes with numerous small (3-10 mm[6]) anechoic spaces (Snowstorm appearance) with a normal interface between abnormal trophoblastic tissue and myometrium.
- No identifiable fetal tissue or gestational sac is seen.
- Color Doppler may show high velocity, low impedance flow.

Partial Mole

- Placenta is enlarged and contains areas of multiple, diffuse anechoic lesions.
- Fetus with severe structural abnormalities or growth restriction, oligohydramnios or a deformed gestational sac may be noted.
- Color Doppler interrogation may show high velocity, low impedance flow.
- *Theca lutein cysts:* It may be seen bilaterally in 25-60% of cases

In patients where transvaginal scan cannot be performed or is contraindicated a transrectal or transperineal ultrasonography can be performed.

SAFETY PROFILE OF ULTRASONOGRAPHY

According to the AIUM Bioeffects Committee the following parameters where identified to study the biological effects on mammalian tissues: Free Field Spatial Peak Temporal Average (SPTA of 100 mW/cm^2); thermal index (TI) <2 and mechanical index (MI) <0.3. These biological parameters allow the operators to apply the as low as reasonably achievable (ALARA) principle for ultrasonographic exposure.[10]

REFERENCES

1. Fong K, Kung R, Lytwyn A, et al. Endometrial evaluation with transvaginal US and hysterosonography in asymptomatic postmenopausal women with breast cancer receiving tamoxifen. Radiology. 2001; 220:765-73.
2. Ascher SM, Imaoka I, Lage JM. Tamoxifen-induced uterine abnormalities: the role of imaging. Radiology. 2000;214:29-38.
3. AAGL practice report: practice guidelines for the diagnosis and management of submucous leiomyomas. J Minim Invasive Gynecol. 2012;19(2):152-71. doi: 10.1016/j.jmig.2011.09.005
4. Walker K, Jayaprakasan K, Fenning NJR. Ultrasound in Benign Gynaecology. OGRM. 2007;17(2):33-4.
5. Sakhel K1, Abuhamad A. Sonography of adenomyosis. J Ultrasound Med. 2012;31(5):805-8.
6. Schwarzler P, Collins WP, Claerhout F, Coenen M, Amant F, et al. Subjective assessment of adnexal masses with the use of ultrasonography: an analysis of interobserver variability and experience. Ultrasound Obstet Gynecol. 1999;13:11-6.
7. Timmerman D, et al. Simple ultrasound rules to distinguish between benign and malignant adnexal masses before surgery: prospective validation by IOTA group BMJ. 2010; 341 doi: http://dx.doi.org/10.1136/bmj.c6839 (Published 14 December 2010) Cite this as: BMJ. 2010;341:c6839.
8. Balen AH, et al. Ultrasound assessment of the polycystic ovary: international consensus definitions. Hum Reprod Update. 2003;9(6):505-14.
9. Kaakaji Y, et al. Songraphy of Obstetric and Gynecologic emergencies; Part I, Obstetric Emergencies, AJR. 2000;174(3):641-9.
10. American Institute of Ultrasound in Medicine. 2008. As Low as Reasonably Achievable (ALARA) Principle. Available from http://www.aium.org/publications/guidelinesStatementsX.aspx#statements [September 2008].

3
Endoscopies in Gynecology: Principles and Equipment

Leena Wadhwa, Shubhi Yadav, Pooja Rani

INTRODUCTION

Endoscopy is a procedure in which, with the use of telescope, the interior of a viscus or preformed space is visualized. The use of endoscopy has been more popularized in past three-four decades. In gynecology, laparoscopy and hysteroscopy are used to diagnose and treat various conditions. Laparoscopy involves the direct visualization of the peritoneal cavity and hysteroscopy involves the visualization of the inside of the uterus and endocervix. Endoscopic procedure appears to reduce the cost and morbidity associated with surgery in some conditions as compared to the traditional operations.

HISTORY

First description of endoscopy is attributed to Phillip Bozzini in 1805, when he viewed the mucosa of urethra with a candlelight and simple tube. First gynecologic endoscopic procedure was hysteroscopy, when Panteloni visualized uterine polyp with a cystoscope. First laparoscopy was done by Jacobaeus in 1910. In early 1930s, laparoscopy was used for various diagnostic and surgical procedures by Kalk of Germany. By the end of 1930s, it was used for diagnosis of ectopic pregnancy and for tubal sterilization. Harry Reich in 1989 performed first laparoscopic hysterectomy.

INDICATIONS OF LAPAROSCOPY

Tubal Surgery

Adhesiolysis, dilatation of phimotic fimbrial end, tuboplasty, tubal sterilization.

In ectopic pregnancy-linear salpingotomy, salpingostomy, segmental resection, salpingectomy, intrasac instillation of potassium chloride (KCL), methotrexate, polyglutamates (PGs), etc.

Ovarian Surgery

Ovarian biopsy, cyst aspiration, ovarian drilling, cystectomy, ovariolysis, excision of paraovarian cyst, salpingo-oophorectomy, oophorectomy, ovariotomy.

Uterine Surgery

Treatment of uterine perforation, myomectomy, hysterectomy (total laparoscopic hysterectomy (TLH), laparoscopic-assisted vaginal hysterectomy (LAVH), radical hysterectomy) adenomyomectomy.

Endometriosis

Fulguration and excision of endometriotic implants, cystectomy, adhesiolysis.

Infertility

Tubal patency, pelvic adhesiolysis.

Miscellaneous

Laparoscopic vaginoplasty, sling surgery for prolapse, cervicopexy, laparoscopic uterosacral nerve ablation (LUNA), presacral neurectomy, aortic and pelvic lymphadenopathy, mullerian anomalies, gonadal biopsy.

SURGICAL TECHNIQUE OF LAPAROSCOPY

Position

Laparoscopy is performed in low lithotomy position, thighs at the level of the trunk with hips in extension and abduction, knees slightly flexed, stirrups low, arms flushed with body and buttocks protruding beyond the edge of the table. The patient should be in an unaltered supine position during placement of the Veress needle/primary cannula to avoid the injury to intra-abdominal structures and vessels. The position of patient is to be changed to Trendelenburg position for secondary port insertion allowing the abdominal contents to move away from the sites.

Procedure

Primary Port

The common site of insertion of Veress needle is the base of the umbilicus. The abdominal wall is lifted manually to avoid injury to abdominal organs and vessels, and needle is advanced at a 45° angle from the horizontal directly into the peritoneal cavity in the sagittal plane. During insertion of needle, the surgeon must listen to the "double clicks" as the needle obturator retracts when it passes through the rectus fascia and the peritoneum. Excessive lateral movements of the needle should be avoided as they may convert small point of bowel injury into a complex one or cause tear in omentum.

Test for Confirmation of Proper Positioning of Needle

A drop of saline placed over the open, proximal end of the needle, if the needle is appropriately positioned, due to negative intra-abdominal pressure, the saline drop gets aspirated inside.

The other reassuring sign is the loss of liver "dullness" over the lateral aspect of the right costal margin. The other valuable test of correct placement of the needle is to observe that the initial insufflation pressure is relatively low (less than 8 mm Hg).

In patients known or suspected to have periumbilical adhesions, or after failure to establish pneumoperitoneum after three attempts, alternative sites for Veress needle insertion may be considered.

LEFT UPPER QUADRANT (PALMER'S POINT)

In patients with previous laparotomy, Palmer advocated insertion of the Veress needle 3 cm below the left subcostal border in the mid-clavicular line. This technique is especially useful in obese as well as the very thin patient, patients with large pelvic mass dense adhesions and second trimester of pregnancy. Before insufflation stomach should be emptied with nasogastric suction and Veress needle is inserted perpendicular to the skin-relative contraindications include patients with ascites, previous splenic or gastric surgery, significant hepatosplenomegaly, portal hypertension.

PNEUMOPERITONEUM

After Veress needle insertion pneumoperitoneum to about 18–20 mm Hg is established followed by insertion of trocar with cannula without elevation of the anterior abdominal wall. The high-pressure setting used during initial insertion of the trocar is lowered as soon as abdominal entry is documented. The higher pressure entry technique has the advantage of reducing intra-abdominal trocar-related injuries by producing greater splinting of the anterior abdominal wall and a deeper intra-abdominal CO_2 bubble. The amount of gas transmitted into the peritoneal cavity should depend on the measured intraperitoneal pressure, not the volume of gas.

Gases used for pneumoperitoneum include carbon dioxide (CO_2), air, oxygen, nitrous oxide (N_2O), argon, helium and mixtures of these gases CO_2 is the most popular gas used because of its high solubility, low cost and suppression of combustion. N_2O is readily available, provides better analgesia (appears to decrease postoperative pain in patients with low anesthetic risk) and is physiologically more inert. Nitrous oxide (N_2O) has unpredictable pattern of absorption and supports combustion. Helium pneumoperitoneum decreases the cardiopulmonary changes associated with laparoscopic surgery but it is relatively insoluble in blood compared to CO_2. Oxygen and air are not readily absorbed through the peritoneum and can result in air embolism. Argon has a more significant depressant effect on hemodynamics than CO_2.

Transuterine Veress CO_2 Insufflation

Using a long Veress needle, pneumoperitoneum has been established through the fundus of the uterus transvaginally. This is especially helpful in obese patients.

Trans-Cul-de-sac CO_2 Insufflation

Through posterior vaginal fornix pneumoperitoneum can be established.

After pneumoperitoneum is created, trocar and cannula is placed. The trocar is removed and laparoscope with camera and light source attached is introduced in the peritoneal cavity.

The intraperitoneal structures including under surface of diaphragm (to rule out Fitz-Hugh-Curtis syndrome) and abdominal cavity is examined. Patient is given Trendelenburg tilt. Pelvic side wall is inspected; position of ureter is determined. Once anatomical landmarks are established uterus, fallopian tubes, ovaries, uterosacral ligaments, and Pouch of Douglas are thoroughly examined. Any pathology, if present are noted and corrected accordingly.

Placement of Secondary Trocars

After identifying the epigastric vessels by transillumination and intraperitoneal observation, 1-3 secondary trocars are placed, depending on the procedure and the number of trocars required for the operation. The trocars are placed either in the midline, 3 cm above the pubic symphysis, or laterally, approximately 8 cm from the midline and 8 cm above the pubic symphysis to avoid the inferior epigastric vessels (Fig. 3.1).

DIRECT TROCAR INSERTION

It refers to inserting the primary trocar without inserting the Veress needle. The primary trocar is inserted similar to the Veress needle and abdomen is insufflated with CO_2. The advantage is it avoids extraperitoneal insufflation. Direct insertion of the trocar without prior pneumoperitoneum may be considered as a safe alternative to Veress needle technique. Direct insertion of the trocar is associated with less insufflation-related complications such as gas embolism, and it is a faster technique than the Veress needle technique.

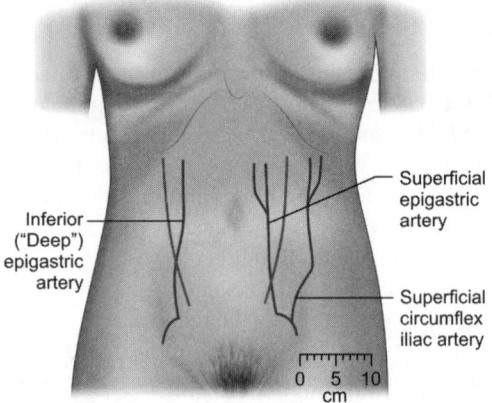

Fig. 3.1 Deep and superficial vessels of the anterior wall

OPEN LAPAROSCOPY (HASSON TECHNIQUE)

Hasson first described this technique in 1971. This technique uses a trocar fitted with cone-shaped sleeve, a blunt obturator and a second sleeve. A longitudinal or vertical incision is taken at the umbilicus, dissecting down to the anterior rectus fascia, incising it and bluntly entering the peritoneal cavity under direct vision. Trocar with sleeve is then inserted into the peritoneal cavity with obturator in place. For the Hasson technique, sutures are taken on the fascia through either side of trocar to hold the sleeve in place and seal the abdominal wall incision. This method almost completely avoids the risk of retroperitoneal vessel injury and there is decreased the risk of bowel injury. This method is used for patients with risk of abdominal adhesions. There is no evidence that the open entry technique is superior to or inferior to the other entry techniques currently available.

LAPAROSCOPIC INSTRUMENTS

Imaging System

Laparoscope

It has rod lens, optical fibers, objective lens and an eye piece. Images perceived at the tip of the scope are transmitted to the other end where camera is attached.

Diameter of the scope range from 1.8 mm to 12 mm. The viewing angle of 0° –provides straight forward view and 30° forward oblique view.

Light Cables

Transmit light from light source to the laparoscope. It has a diameter of >5.5 mm and length of >160 cm. These are of two types: fiber optic and fluid filled cables. Cables should be handled carefully and there excessive bending should be avoided as this may damage the fiber optic fibers and cause deterioration in the amount of transmission of light.

Light Source

- Halogen—yellow light (causes color distortion), more economical.
- Xenon—light source of 175 or 300 watt may be used, resembles daylight. It is cold source of light.

Camera and Monitor

Full high definition digital camera with high resolution monitor provides better image clarity. A three-chip CCD (charged couple device) has separate chip for each primary color. A high resolution monitor 700 lines provide optimal visualization.

Insufflator

The insufflator delivers CO_2 from a gas cylinder to the patient through tubing connected to one of the ports on the laparoscope. Most insufflators can be set to maintain a constant intra-abdominal pressure of 12–14 mm Hg. All insufflators display intra-abdominal pressure, rate of flow of CO_2 and the volume of gas used.

Veress Needles

Veress needles are hollow needles with spring like action used to create pneumoperitoneum by closed technique. Veress needles vary from 12 cm to 15 cm in length, with an external diameter of 2 mm. A beveled tip enables the needle to pierce the tissues of the abdominal wall. It has aspiring loaded blunt stylet with subterminal opening for gases and proximal end is a stopcock with luer lock hub. Pressure of insufflators must be kept low while using this as the narrow passage of needle may damage insufflators if high pressure gas flow is used.

Veress Needle Modifications

- Pressure-sensor-equipped Veress needle
- Optical Veress needle.

Laparoscopic Trocar and Cannulas

Laparoscopic cannulas are available in different sizes. Cannulas are hollow tubes with a valve. The cannula has side ports for the attachment of tubing connected with the CO_2 insufflator. The cannula usually comes with the trocar, tip of trocar may be pyramidal, conical, blunt tipped bladed and optical access. The trocar is a longer instrument of slightly smaller diameter that is passed through the cannula, exposing its tip. It is positioned in the abdominal wall by twisting or screwing movements. Sleeves of trocar range from 2 mm to 15 mm in diameter. They are available as reusable made of stainless steel or disposable trocars.

DISPOSABLE SHIELDED TROCARS

These trocars are designed with a shield that partially retracts and exposes the sharp tip as it encounters resistance through the abdominal wall. As the shield enters the abdominal cavity, it springs forward and covers the sharp tip of the trocar.

Endopath Optiview Optical Trocar

It has a provision to visualize the layers of abdominal muscle while passing through these layers.

Visiport Optical Trocars

The Visiport optical trocar is a disposable visual entry instrument that comprises a hollow trocar and a cannula with a sharp cutting knife, which when advanced transects tissue in contact with the crystal tip and swiftly retract back.

Radially Expanding-access Cannulas

This technique involves the placement of a Veress needle surrounded by a expanding polymeric sleeve for insufflation. After insufflation, the Veress needle is removed and the sleeve is dilated to 10-12 mm in diameter by a blunt obturator with twisting motion. Advantages include avoidance of sharp trocars, decreased risk of injury to vessels and no need for suturing fascial defects.

Other laparoscopic operative instruments include:
- Grasper and dissector
- Scissors
- Suction/irrigation
- Suturing—needle holder, knot pusher
- Uterine manipulators and vaginal tube
- Endoscopic specimen bag is used for extraction of specimens like dermoid cyst, endometrioma, suspected malignant mass without contaminating the peritoneal cavity.

Energy Sources

Different types of energy sources are used in laparoscopic surgeries. These are:
- Electrical energy sources
- Ultrasonic energy sources
- Laser energy source.

Electrosurgical Resources

They are of two types monopolar and bipolar:
1. In *monopolar electrosurgery*, the current flows start from the active electrode, through the patient and the return electrode to complete the circuit.
2. In *bipolar electrosurgery*, both active and return electrodes are located at the same field and heating occurs in tissue held between two electrodes. In monopolar, patient's body is a part of circuit; whereas in bipolar the space between two electrodes is part of circuit.

Dispersive electrode (grounding pad): It reduces the risk of injury during monopolar surgery. It should be placed over a large muscle with adequate blood supply on the same side of surgery and as close to the surgery site as possible. The difference between the active and return electrode is in their size and conductivity. Concentrated electrons at the active electrode produce high current and the same current is dispersed over larger area in return electrode and produces lesser heat. Suitable placement sites include: (1) the left and right anterior thigh; (2) the left and right buttock; or (3) the left and right bicep.

The following steps using the grounding pad should be taken:
- Inspect the skin area on the patient where the pad is being placed.
- Place the pad over a large area of skin, close to the operative site after the patient is positioned on the surgical table.
- Avoid placing the pad over bony prominences, on top of burned, scarred or hairy tissue or distal to the tourniquet.

In electrosurgical procedures, a high frequency current is passed through the body which does not cause neuromuscular stimulation and so the patient is protected from electrocution.

Electrothermal injury may result from insulation failure, direct coupling, capacitive coupling direct application, etc.
- *Direct application:* Electrosurgical injury may happen via direct application
- *Insulation failure:* It occurs when there is damage to the covering of the active electrode, allowing the current to pass through non-target tissue, which is outside the view of the surgeon. Major causes of insulation failure include manufacturing defect, the use of high voltage currents, mechanical trauma and re-sterilization of instruments which weakens and break the insulation. Breaks in the insulation create alternate pathways for current to flow. With a high enough concentration of current, injury to adjacent organs occur preoperative careful inspection of the equipment before and after use is the best means of identifying defective insulation.
- *Coupling:* Direct coupling occurs when activated electrode touches other instruments and transfers current to tissue outside the laparoscopic field of the electrosurgical unit current from the active electrode flows through the secondary instrument, and damages adjacent structures or organs in direct contact with the secondary instrument. Direct coupling can be prevented with visualization of the electrode in contact with the target tissue and avoiding contact with any other conductive instruments prior to activating the electrode.

Capacitive coupling is a mechanism where current in the electrode induces a current in nearby conductors despite an intact insulation. An electrostatic field is created when high frequency alternating current induces a magnetic field, which itself induces electrical current in nearby objects. The electric current is transferred from one conductor, through intact insulation, into adjacent conductive materials without direct contact. This results in capacitive coupling. Capacitor coupling may be minimized by activating the active electrode only when it is in contact with target tissues, and by using metal cannulas that allow stray current to be dispersed through the patient's abdominal wall, not internal tissue.

Vessel Sealing Devices

Harmonic Scalpel

Uses high frequency waves (more than 55,000 Hz) to induce mechanical vibration which generates heat by friction and shear to cause thermal destruction. They work on piezoelectric effect. Heat and vibration together denature proteins by disrupting hydrogen bonds, forms sticky coagulum in a localized area round instrument, so blood vessels are coagulated with minimum heat transmission, less tissue trauma and superior visualization. Ultrasonic cutting, harmonic blade oscillates back and forth in a linear fashion at very high speed; resulting in cutting as well as coagulating the tissue.

Enseal Tissue Sealing and Hemostasis System

Uses bipolar energy. Enseal has temperature sensitive matrix (nanopolar thermostats) in the jaws of the device that controls the energy transmitted to the electrode tissue interface. Jaws can cut and seal vessels up to 7 mm with high compression to have uniform effect.

LigasureV (Valley Lab)

This bipolar electrosurgical device delivers high current and low voltage to the tissues. Collagen and elastin fibers in the compressed vessels are denatured but during cool down phase cross linking re-occurs. It generates computer algorithm to adjust current and voltage according to the tissue impedance and determines optimal time and energy to achieve constant seal. This can seal vessels to a depth of 7 mm.

Gyrus Plasma Kinetic (PK) Tissue Management System (PKS Cutting Forceps and Plasma Trissector)

This bipolar electrosurgical device uses plasma kinetic energy. They deliver a high current and very low voltage to the tissue. Electrosurgical energy is delivered through a series of rapid pulses with a brief cool down phase during coagulation thus, limiting lateral thermal spread. Lumen of the vessel is occluded with a coagulum formed from denaturation of proteins.

Laser Energy

When focused on tissue it causes tissue vaporization, cutting and, to varying degree of coagulation. The commonly used lasers are CO_2 laser, the potassium-titanyl-phosphate (KTP) and neodymium:yttrium, aluminum, garnet (Nd:YAG) lasers.

SINGLE INCISION LAPAROSCOPIC SURGERY

Single-incision surgery has been known with acronyms and names, including single-incision laparoscopic surgery (SILS), single-port access (SPA) surgery, laparoscopic endoscopic single-site surgery (LESSS), single laparoscopic incision transabdominal (SLIT) surgery, one-port umbilical surgery (OPUS), natural orifice transumbilical surgery (NOTUS), and embryonic natural orifice transumbilical endoscopic surgery (E-NOTES). A single small incision is used as the entry point. All surgical instruments are placed through this small incision and also the incision site is located in the left abdomen or umbilicus. This can be done in a number of ways: multiple fascial defects are made through a single umbilical skin incision and raising skin flaps, or utilization of newly developed systems, like the Uni-X™ Single Port System, TriPort™, or GelPort® requiring a larger but single fascial incision for passage of multiple instruments. Benefits include fewer incisions, less wound infection-related complications, less scarring, better cosmetic result and faster recovery Difficulties in surgery are a loss of triangulation, clashing of instrument, and a lack of maneuverability reduced visibility, increased complexity technical difficulty and raised cost when custom ports are used.

Natural Orifice Transluminal Endoscopic Surgery

Natural orifice transluminal endoscopic surgery (NOTES) involves placing flexible endoscope through among the body's natural orifices, like the mouth, anus, vagina, or urethra, to access abdominal cavity. This ultimate form of non-invasive surgery has potential benefits decreased postoperative pain and recovery period, minimal anesthesia and analgesia, and no external scar.

Robotic Surgery

Da Vinci robotic system is used today for gynecological procedures as simple and radical hysterectomy, pelvic lymphadenectomy, adnexal surgery, myomectomy, endometriosis, sacrocolpopexy/hysteropexy, vesicovaginal fistula repair. Recent indications for robotics include ovarian cancers and anterior pelvic exenteration.

Da Vinci robotic system has three major components:
1. A console where the surgeon sits unscrubbed, views the operative field through a stereoscopic viewer three dimensionally, and controls the robotic instruments and camera via finger graspers and foot pedals.

2. A patient side cart which has three or four telerobotic arms that hold instruments.
3. A insite vision system which allows visualization of surgical field. It includes Endowrist instruments with computer interfaces that translate the movements of the surgeon's hands into computer algorithms. These surgical instruments have seven degree of freedom of movement surgery with 90° of articulation.

Robotic-assisted surgery offers the benefit of reduced postoperative pain, decreased length of stay, quick recovery. Specific benefits include short learning curve, improved ergonomics and less technical. Well-designed randomized controlled trials or comparably rigorous nonrandomized prospective trials are required for comparing techniques, outcomes and establishing efficacy of robotic-assisted surgery.

Morcellation

The FDA called for its strongest warning on this device, known as a "black-box." Laparoscopic power morcellation in cases of hysterectomy or myomectomy in women with uterine fibroids, poses a risk of spreading unsuspected cancerous tissue, notably uterine sarcomas, beyond the uterus. The FDA is warning against using laparoscopic power morcellators.

COMPLICATIONS

Due to laparoscopy itself:

Extraperitoneal insufflation of gas (surgical emphysema), gas embolism, hypotension cardiac arrhythmias, cardiac arrest.

Injury to blood vessels (0.3–0.5%), injury to intestine (0.5%) or abdominal and pelvic organs. Thermal injuries during electrosurgical procedures and anesthetic complications as hypoventilation, gastroesophageal reflux, bronchospasm.

Prevention of Complications

- Patient should be flat position during primary trocar insertion and angle of insertion should change from 45° to 90° in very thin to obese patients. Alternate site for trocar insertion can be used in patients with previous surgery and secondary trocars should be placed under direct vision.
- Approximately half of bowel injuries occur during entry (bowel preparation helps). Entry-related bowel injuries are mostly lacerations, and intraoperative injuries are mostly thermal (monopolar/bipolar forceps should be in the center of the screen during activation), plate should be in proper position.
- Injury to blood vessels. These injuries usually occur in relation to the positioning of accessory ports. Practical technique for hemostasis is direct compression. If bleeding is not controlled in this way, tamponade and suturing may be used.

In case of major vascular injury—do not remove the Veress needle/instruments. Through a midline incision, access the bleeding site, and repair the injury.
- Ureteral injury during laparoscopic hysterectomy is more common (0.2–6.0%) than in abdominal hysterectomy. Ureteral injury accounts for 4.3–7% of the total laparoscopy complications.
- Electrocautery (unipolar or bipolar) has been identified as the leading cause of laparoscopic ureteral injury. To minimize ureteral injury, use of sutures should be preferred instead of staplers or electrocautery in close proximity to ureters. Visualization of ureters during the operation, use of ureteral catheters, and creating hydroprotection by injection of saline to parietal peritoneum are the other protective measures to prevent bladder injuries:
  - Perform a very careful dissection of the vesicovaginal pouch and use uterine cannulation.
  - Fill the bladder with a methylene blue dye solution to visualize its limits in case of difficult dissection, such as previous surgery (cesarean delivery, endometriosis surgery, conization, and others).
  - Perform very careful and restricted use of bipolar coagulation in the vesicovaginal space for hemostasis.

  In bladder injury, which is small size, catheterization for 7–10 days help

otherwise bladder repair in two layers with Foleys catheterization.
- *Gas embolism:* It results from introduction of CO_2 into the large veins through the Veress needle. Its earliest sign is a drop in end-tidal carbon dioxide concentration, due to diminished blood flow to the lungs. Cardiopulmonary resuscitation is required.

CONTRAINDICATIONS

Absolute

- Advanced intrauterine pregnancy
- Large abdominal mass
- Paralytic ileus
- Hemodynamically unstable patient
- Severe cardiopulmonary disease
- Obstructive intestinal disease
- Generalized peritonitis.

Relative

- Gross obesity
- Abdominal wall sepsis
- Ischemic heart disease
- Multiple abdominal procedures
- Patient on anticoagulation therapy.

HYSTEROSCOPY

Hysteroscopy involves inspection of uterine cavity and the cornual ends of the fallopian tube with an endoscope inserted through the cervix. Subtle changes in the form of small polyps, adhesions and subendometrial fibroid seedling, which influences fertility are better picked-up on magnification with hysteroscopy. Hysteroscopy is done for diagnostic or therapeutic purposes. Diagnostic hysteroscopy can be performed in an office or clinic with minimal discomfort and lower cost.

Indications for Diagnostic Hysteroscopy

- Unexplained abnormal uterine bleeding (premenopausal and postmenopausal)
- Abnormal hysterography or transvaginal ultrasonography
- Unexplained infertility
- Recurrent spontaneous abortion.

Indications for Operative Hysteroscopy

- Removal of foreign body from uterine cavity
- Uterine septum resection
- Endometrial polyp
- Uterine fibroid resection
- Endometrial ablation
- Asherman syndrome
- Hysteroscopic sterilization.

Technique of Hysteroscopy

Hysteroscopy is usually performed along with laparoscopy in operation theater under anesthesia. It is performed in lithotomy position. Size and position of the uterus is confirmed by bimanual examination. Preoperative administration of prostaglandin E1 (*misoprostol*) to ripen the cervix 12 hours before the procedure (400 µg orally or 200 µg vaginally) may facilitate cervical dilation. The hysteroscope is connected to the source of distending medium and introduced into endocervical canal and uterine cavity after ensuring that there are no air bubbles in the distending fluid. The endocervical and uterine lining is studied and both uterine ostia are identified. Any abnormality of uterine cavity, endometrium and uterine ostia are noted and corrective measures are taken accordingly. The procedure can be performed without anesthesia, or under local anesthesia and general anesthesia or spinal anesthesia. Spinal anesthesia is preferred as mental status of patient (altered consciousness or irritating behavior) can be assessed in case of electrolyte imbalance (e.g. hyponatremia) occurring due to use of distension media.

Distending Media

They can be gaseous or liquid.

Gaseous Medium

Only CO_2 is used as gaseous distending medium. It is used only for diagnostic hysteroscopic procedures because of risk of gas embolism at large volumes. CO_2 is unsuitable distension medium specially if there is bleeding because it is highly soluble in blood and there is no effective way to remove blood and other debris from the endometrial cavity. Hence, whenever used it should be used with low pressure hysteroscopic insufflator, which regulates the pressure.

Liquid/Fluid Medium

- *High viscosity distending media:* Most commonly used high viscosity medium is; *a hyperosmolar solution of 32% dextran 70 in 10% glucose (Hyskon)*. It does not mix with the blood, so can be used in patients with bleeding. Its use has declined due to risk of vascular overload leading to heart failure and pulmonary edema; risk of anaphylactic reaction and risk of instruments damage because of it getting caramelized on instruments.
- *Low viscosity distending media:* These can be electrolytes rich (normal saline) and electrolytes free (3% sorbitol, 1.5% glycine, 5% mannitol). The commonly used media are:
  - *Normal saline* is an isotonic electrolyte rich solution. It is a useful and safer media. It does not cause electrolyte imbalances and is a good choice for minor procedures and for diagnostic procedures. Because saline is a good conductor of electricity hence this media is not suitable for operative procedures requiring monopolar electrical energy. It can be safely used with instruments using bipolar energy and mechanical energy.
  - *Glycine* 1.5% is nonconductive media. Its advantage is that it can be used with monopolar electrical energy sources. Glycine gets metabolized in liver to water and ammonia. Ammonia causes further reduction of osmolarity and causes increased absorption. This can result in hyperammonemia, excessive fluid absorption and sometimes coma. *Techniques and equipment for uterine distension.*
  - *Media delivering system:* Gravity is the simplest method of instilling fluid under constant hydrostatic pressure. Positioning a pressure cuff around the bag filled with distension media is an extension of gravity method. This has a disadvantage of poor control of pressure which increases the risks related to injury to myometrium and excessive extravasation of fluid; especially if pressure exceeds the mean arterial pressure.
  - *Infusion pump (Hysteromat):* It maintains a constant preset intrauterine pressure and simultaneous continuous fluid. It helps in optimal view at all the times because the uterine cavity remains sufficiently dilated and rinsed all the times.

Hysteroscopic Instruments

Hysteroscopes are available in two basic types—flexible and rigid. Flexible hysteroscopes are most useful for cannulation of the fallopian tube. For other uses, rigid hysteroscopes are more durable. Endoscopes for hysteroscopy and are available in 0°, 12-15°, and 25-30° models.

- *Diagnostic hysteroscopes:* The most commonly used diagnostic hysteroscopes are 3-4 mm diameter with detachable external sheath to deliver the distending media. 0° is used for diagnostic procedures.
- *Operative hysteroscope:* Operative hysteroscope has a larger diameter with larger outer sheath than diagnostic hysteroscope. Operative sheaths allow the space for instillation of medium, telescope and instruments. About 25°-30° angled hysteroscopes are mostly used for operative procedures like tubal cannulation of the fallopian tubes or placement of sterilization devices. The instruments available for use through operative hysteroscopes include grasping, cutting and punch-biopsy devices.

- *Uterine resectoscope:* The uterine resectoscope works with radiofrequency electrical energy in the endometrial cavity resulting in cutting and coagulation of endometrial tissue. It has an inner sheath and outer sheath. Inner sheath provides a common channel for instruments like telescope, electrode and medium; whereas outer sheath is for medium return. A variety of electrode tips can be used like pointed electrode, loop, roller bar and Colin's knife for septum resection.

  Use of resectoscope requires a continuous-flow system with distension media, most commonly used media is glycine. During operation the lowest intrauterine pressure necessary for adequate distension should be used; usually in range 70–80 mm Hg. This pressure can be achieved with a specially designed pump. At a fluid deficits of more than 1 L measurement of electrolyte levels should be done. If the deficit is more than a 1.5–2 L then procedure should be terminated.

- *Bipolar resectoscope electrosurgical system:* It is used for operative procedures. Its advantage is that it works under normal saline; so it is safely tolerated by the patients. The risk of fluid overload is minimal with this. It has accessible and visible outflow and inflow valve levers. The disadvantage of this system is that it is not intended for tubal sterilization procedures.

- *Hysteroscopic morcellator:* It is used for removing the tissues during operative hysteroscopic procedures. It uses a blade and suction tube to cut and remove the tissue (like polyps and selected submucosal myomas) simultaneously. It shortens the time of surgery. As it does not use any energy hence risks like thermal injury and perforation are minimized. The disadvantage is morcellators cannot cauterized the blood vessels hence there is slight increased risk of bleeding. This is not of much help in removing the intramural fibroids of type 1 and type 2. In such cases resectoscope is preferred.

Available Hysteroscopic Morcellation Systems

Currently, two morcellation systems are available: the TRUCLEAR™ Hysteroscopic Morcellator and the MyoSure® Tissue Removal System. The TRUCLEAR™ 5.0 with an outer diameter 5 mm and a 2.9 mm morcellator and MyoSure® system uses a 2 mm morcellator and has an outer dimension of 6.25 mm.

Recent Advances

Hysteroscopic Sterilization

There are two methods of hysteroscopic tubal occlusion Essure and Adiana which can be done as an office procedure. Hysteroscopic sterilization has been reported by several authors to lead to rapid recovery without unacceptable postprocedure pain, as well as high long-term patient tolerability, satisfaction and effective permanent contraception.

Essure Sterilization Procedure

Essure is a coiled spring device that is inserted through the uterine cavity into the interstitial portion of each fallopian tube. The Essure microinsert consists of a stainless steel inner coil, a super-elastic outer coil, and polyethylene fibers wound in and around the inner coil. When released, the outer coil expands to anchor the microinsert in the fallopian tube. As the device expands to fill the tubal opening, it gradually becomes scarred in place and forms a barrier causing complete tubal occlusion. A hysterosalpingogram (HSG) is performed 12 weeks later to ensure the fallopian tubes are completely blocked. According to the phase II multicenter trial of effectiveness, no pregnancies were reported in 6015 women-months of exposure to intercourse following documented bilateral tubal occlusion with bilateral micro-inserts. For women with significant medical problems (such as severe cardiac disease), who require permanent contraception, but might otherwise carry considerable surgical risks, Essure has been shown to be a safe alternative to tubal ligation.

Adiana Sterilization Procedure

Adiana is another new hysteroscopic sterilization procedure. It was approved for use in the US by the FDA in July, 2009. Adiana uses radiofrequency (RF) energy and a polymer micros insert that together result in tubal blockage in the interstitial segment of the fallopian tube that is within the uterine muscle.

Under hysteroscopic guidance, a delivery catheter is introduced into the tubal os, the distal tip of the catheter delivers RF energy, causing a lesion within the fallopian tube following which the silicone matrix is deployed in the region of the tube where the lesion was formed and the catheter and hysteroscope are removed. Over the next few weeks, occlusion is achieved by fibroblast ingrowth into the matrix, which serves as permanent scaffolding and allows for "space-filling." Occlusion of tubes is assessed by HSG 3 months after device placement. Essure and Adiana reversal if required need to be performed by the technique of tubouterine implantation.

HYSTEROSCOPY AND ITS ROLE IN CANCERS

Hysteroscopy helps in evaluation of endometrium to assess its proper growth maturity or dysmaturity. Use of the panoramic and contact microcolpohysteroscope, facilitated by use of biological dyes such as methylene blue, may help in the evaluation of tissues at cellular level and may be of assistance in predicting normal proliferation and maturity of endometrium. Hysteroscopically directed sampling for receptor assay may provide information necessary to tailor therapy to these disorders.

Hysteroscopy has recently been confirmed as an accurate diagnostic method for endometrial carcinoma. Several retrospective studies have found increased positive peritoneal cytology in women who underwent hysteroscopy, but recent studies have indicated that there is currently no evidence to suggest that diagnostic hysteroscopy increases the risk of malignant cells spreading into the peritoneal cavity, or worsens the prognosis in women with endometrial carcinoma.

As prognosis is based on early diagnosis and screenings, devices analogous to cervical pap smears have yet to be achieved for endometrial neoplasia, new methodology is urgently required. The future will see appearance of 1–2 mm disposable viewing devices with sampling brushes for direct viewing and sampling of endometrial cavity.

Contraindications

- Active uterine infection
- Severe systemic illness
- Pregnancy
- Heavy uterine bleeding
- Cervical cancer.

Risk

- Uterine perforation
- Pelvic infection
- Failure to visualize cavity.

Complications

- Incidence serious complications in diagnostic hysteroscopy 0.012%.
- Failed procedure (<2%) due to
  - Cervical stenosis
  - Blood, gas bubbles
- Problems due to distension media
  - Fluid overload
- Problems due to procedure itself
  - Infection
  - Bleeding
  - Cervical/uterine damage/perforation
- Anesthetic problems.

BIBLIOGRAPHY

1. Principles of gynaecologic surgical techniques & management of endoscopy; Te Linde's operative gynecology, 10th edn.

2. Robotic assisted surgery in gynaecology and urogynaecology: Current progress in obstetrics & gynaecology (volume-1); John Studd; 2013.
3. Robotic surgery in gynecology. Committee Opinion No. 628. American College of Obstetricians and Gynecologists. Obstet Gynecol. 2015;125:760-7.
4. Royal College of Obstetricians and Gynaecologists (RCOG), British Society for Gynecological Endoscopy. Best practice in outpatient hysteroscopy. London (UK): Royal College of Obstetricians and Gynaecologists (RCOG); 2011 Mar. 22 p. Green-top guideline; no. 59).
5. Royal College of Obstetricians and Gynaecologists (RCOG) Green-top Guideline No. 49); 2008.
6. SOGC clinical practice guideline; 2013.

4

Minor Procedures in Gynecology

Bidhisha Singha

Minor procedures are the surgical procedures which are of short duration, has minimal risk, done under local anesthesia, sedation or oral analgesic. These procedures are usually done in outpatient department (OPD) minor operation theater (OT) as day care procedure. These procedures help in diagnosis and further management of the case.

Following is the list common procedures done in gynecology:
- Pap's test
- Visual inspection with acetic acid (VIA)
- Visual inspection with Lugol's iodine (VILI)
- Colposcopy
- Cervical biopsy
- Endometrial biopsy
- Dilatation of cervix
- Dilatation and curettage
- Office hysteroscopy
- Hysterosalpingogram
- Intrauterine insemination (IUI).

General principals: Prior to any procedure:
- Proper and detail history to be elucidated—chief complaints, menstrual history, any significant past and family history.
- General and systemic examination—to rule out any associated medical or surgical disorders.
- Gynecologic examination—Per speculum examinations are done first. Condition of cervix and vagina are noted. Any abnormal discharge, growth, amount of bleeding if present are to be noted.
- Bimanual pelvic examination done to assess the size, position, mobility of uterus, to rule out any adnexal mass.
- Patient explained about the procedure she has to undergo. The indication, risk, benefits, duration required, need of any anesthesia and interpretation of the test are explained.
- Consent for the surgical procedure is a must. The consent form should include the indication, risk associated and consent for any type of anesthesia.
- The position of the patient during the procedure is important.
- Bladder has to be emptied.
- Aseptic and *Universal* precautions are to be taken during the procedure. Proper cleaning and sterile drapping to be done wherever needed. Perineal area to be cleaned with savlon and betadine solution.

Type of analgesia depends on procedure, set-up and patient choice.

CONVENTIONAL PAP TEST

Ideal Screening test for cervical malignancy as it is inexpensive, easy to administer, well tolerated, poses no significant risk to patients. Detects both precancerous and cancerous cells.

For detection of cervical cancer and its precursors, conventional cytology has a high test specificity (range 79–100%, mean ~95%) and an acceptable test sensitivity (range 30–80%, mean 47%).[1]

Recommendations

- Pap's smear to be done for women from 21 years to 65 years every 3 yearly or for women 30 to 65 years every 5 yearly if Pap's and HPV testing done together.[2]
- Mandatory for the high risk group
  - Early intercourse
  - Early marriage
  - Smoking habits
  - Multiple sexual partners.

Patient Prerequisites[1]

- After the menstrual period
- Absteinance for 48 hours prior to test
- Avoid use of tampons, vaginal creams, contraceptive foams or jellies or vaginal medications for 48 hours prior to test
- Should be done prior to any vaginal examination.

Procedure

- Patient to be placed in dorsal position. No antiseptic solution or any lubricant should be used.
- Labia separated.
- Cusco's speculum gently introduced without any lubricant or jelly.
- Cervix is exposed and any discharge or growth or any bleeding should be checked.
- Whole of squamo—columnar junction is scraped using Ayre's spatula (wood/plastic). Ayre's spatula is rotated 360° firmly against the cervix keeping the longer tongue inside the endocervix.
- The spatula sample is quickly applied on the slide through a rotating motion of the cervical sampling face of the spatula across the glass slide. The slide should be initially marked for patient identification.
- Slide should be immediately fixed with a spray fixative or by placing in a jar containing 95% ethanol. It is important that the cellular debris are not air dried.
- Endocervical brush device—used to sample the endocervix. Combined sampling technique (conventional paps and endocervical sample with endocervical brush) has demonstrated the lowest false negative rates.
- Endocervical brush inserted into the endocervix until the junction of the bristles of the brush with the end of the handle is at the external os. The brush should be rotated only 180° (one-half turn) in the endocervical canal. Additional rotations not required. The sample is rolled at right angles to the slide near the frosted end. The sample is immediately fixed as in Pap's smear.[1]

The adequate sample should have both endocervical and ectocervical cells of cervix.

Visual Inspection with Acetic Acid[3-7]

Physiological basis of VIA: Acetic acid causes reversible coagulation of intracellular proteins (nuclear proteins and cytokeratins). Areas of CIN or invasive cancer undergoes maximal coagulation due to higher content of nucleoproteins (large number of undifferentiated cells present in the epithelium) and prevent light from passing through the epithelium, as a result of which the subepithelial vessel pattern is obliterated and epithelium appears densely white.[3]

Other conditions where aceto-white areas seen are:
- Immature squamous epithelium
- Inflammation
- Leukoplakia
- Condyloma.

Differentiating points:
- *CIN/invasive carcinoma*: Acetowhite areas are dense, thick, opaque, well-demarcated margins, appear rapidly reverse slowly and last longer for 3–5 minutes.
- *Inflammation*: Aceto—white areas distributed widely in cervix and disappear quickly (within 1 minute).

- *Leukoplakia/condyloma*: Stain intensely greyish white.
- **VIA negative**—means no acetowhite areas.
- **VIA positive**—means presence of acetowhite areas which are distinct, well defined, dense with regular/irregular margins.

VILI (Visual inspection with Lugol's iodine)[3-7]

Physiological basis of VILI: Iodine is glycophilic so there is uptake of iodine in glycogen containing epithelium on iodine application. Squamous metaplastic epithelium is glycogenated whereas CIN/invasive cancer cells contain little/no glycogen.[3]

- Naked eye visualization of cervix after application of acetic acid is simple test used for early detection of precancerous lesions and early invasive cancer.
- Used in low resources area as an alternative to cytology.
- Done after 5–12 days of menstruation.
  Normal glycogen containing squamous cells—stain mahogany brown/black.
  CIN/invasive cancer—appear as thick mustard yellow/saffron colored areas.
- **VILI negative**—normal uptake of iodine
- **VILI positive**—suggest presence of dense, thick, bright mustard yellow or saffron yellow iodine nonuptake areas seen in transformation zone or in the whole of cervix.

Procedure of VIA/VILI

- Procedure explained to patient.
- Consent taken.
- Patient placed in modified lithotomy position
- Inspection of perineal area and external genitalia for vesicles, papules, ores, ulceration or warts. Perineal area cleaned with antiseptic solution.
- Sterile Cusco's vaginal speculum inserted and cervix visualized. Any abnormality in cervix is to be noted. Identify the external os, columnar epithelium, squamous epithelium, squamo-columnar junction (SCJ) and transformation zone (TZ).
- Application of acetic acid 3–5% (VIA)/Lugol's iodine (VILI) gently over the cervix with cotton swabs. In VIA after application of acetic acid, wait for 1 minute in case of any doubt in VIA, acetic acid can be reapplied and test can be repeated.
- Squamocolumnar junction and the transformation zone to be assessed for any acetowhite areas (VIA)/Lugol's negative uptake areas (VILI).
- Any findings are to be recorded.
  Biopsy to be taken from VIA positive/VILI positive areas.

COLPOSCOPY[8-11]

Colposcopy is a magnified illumination of lower genital tract including vulva, vagina and cervix. Colposcopic examination involves the systemic evaluation of lower genital tract with special emphasis on the superficial epithelium and blood vessels of the underlying stroma.

Role

- To locate abnormal appearing epithelium
- To direct biopsies of areas in which CIN or invasive cancer is suspected.

Indications

- Suspicious looking cervix
- Invasive carcinoma on cytology
- CIN-2 and CIN-3 on cytology
- Persisting low grade abnormalities (CIN-1) on cytology for more than 12–18 months
- Infection with oncogenic HPV
- Acetopositivity on visual inspection with acetic acid (VIA)
- Positive on visual inspection with Lugol's iodine (VILI).

Colposcopic Examination

- Procedure to be explained to the patient.
- History to be reviewed, consent to be taken.

- Patient placed in dorsal lithotomy position. Perineal area cleaned with antiseptic solution.
- Cusco's self-retaining vaginal speculum inserted. If vaginal side wall retraction required, condom or latex glove finger can be applied over the speculum (tip of glove and condom must be cut).
- Cervix must be adequately visualized. Cervix to be inspected for any obvious findings and to be noted. Excess mucus to be removed with saline swabs. Transformation zone to be identified. Squamocolumnar junction should be visualized, if not endocervical speculum to be used. Colposcopy is considered unsatisfactory if SCJ is not visualized.
- Green filter to be used to evaluate the vessel pattern. Green filter absorbs certain wavelengths of light making the red color of vessel black.
- *Application of acetic acid (3–5%)*: Liberally applied over the cervix with swabs. Excessive rubbing or patting to be avoided. Second application should follow the first to ensure an appropriate acetowhite reaction. Acetic acid coagulates the mucus and remove it, facilitating penetration of acetic acid into cells. Cervix is assesed for acetowhite reaction after 1 minute of application.
- *Application of Lugol's iodine*: Lugol's solution stains normal mature nonkeratinized squamous epithelium, dark mahogany color which indicates presence of glycogen in cells. Absence of staining indicates a non-glycogenated state or a keratinized surface. Squamous metaplasia shows variegated staining and cloumnar epithelium stains mustard yellow color. Cervix is assessed for any Lugol's negative areas.
- Colposcopic-guided cervical biopsy and endocervical curettage to be taken if required. Biopsy is taken with punch biopsy forceps and it should be taken from posterior to anterior to prevent blood from obscuring the biopsy sites. Small lesions can be completely excised. In case of an ulcer biopsy should include an edge of the intact epithelium as well as portion of the ulcer. Monsel's solution (ferric subsulphate) can be used to achieve hemostasis.
- Speculum is removed gradually and the vagina is grossly inspected.

Findings are documented and tissues sent for biopsy if taken.

CERVICAL BIOPSY (PUNCH BIOPSY)

Indications

- Growth in the cervix
- Suspicious area in the cervix
- Ulcer in the cervix.

Procedure

- Patient placed in lithotomy position.
- Perineal area cleaned and sterile draping done.
- Vaginal speculum inserted and cervix visualized.
- Biopsy taken from growth if visible or aided with VIA/VILI/Colposcopy with a punch biopsy forceps. Biopsy should be taken in such a manner that it includes both the normal and abnormal area. Biopsies to be taken from posterior to anterior to prevent obscuring of the site with blood.
- Speculum removed.

Complications

- Bleeding—if bleeding is excessive, vaginal packing to be done
- Infection.

Random biopsies from the transformation zone increases the detection rate of high grade cervical disease by 20% in women who have negative colposcopy.[10]

Studies have shown that multiple directed biopsies during colposcopy increases detection of HSIL.[11]

DILATATION OF CERVIX[12]

Indications

As a preliminary step to other procedures:
- Uterine curettage
- Early termination of pregnancy
- Intracavitary radiotherapeutic procedure
- Manchester repair
- Cervical conization
- Hysteroscopic procedures.

As a single procedure
- Post-traumatic stenosis of cervix
- Atrophic stenosis of cervix
- Postsurgical hematometra
- Pyometra.

Procedure

- Patient to be placed in lithotomy position.
- Perineal area cleaned and sterile draping done.
- Bladder to be emptied aseptically.
- Per speculum and bimanual pelvic examination done. This step of the procedure is important as the direction of uterine sound and cervical dilators are inserted according to the position of the uterus. Misdirection leads to complications like perforation.
- Posterior vaginal speculum inserted, cervix visualized. Anterior vaginal wall to be used if required.
- Paracervical block can be given if required.
- Anterior lip of cervix held with vulsellum and held with the left hand and gentle downward traction applied.
- Uterine sound is gently passed and utero cervical length measured. Contraindicated in pyometra as it increases risk of perforation.
- Dilatation of cervix—done gradually in order. Dilators are held on the right hand with the thumb posteriorly and first three fingers along the length of the dilator. Degree of the dilatation depends on the procedure. For curettage procedures dilated up to 7 mm. Dilators should not be passed more than the uterocervical length and excessive force to be avoided.

Complications[12]

- *Tear and laceration of cervix*: Occur due to excessive force used. If tear is suspected or seen, procedure to be abandoned immediately. If bleeding noted, suture is mandatory. If there is no bleeding, suturing helps to restore the anatomy. Late complications in lacerations—infection, bleeding, cervical incompetence.
- *Perforation of the uterus*: Sudden release of pressure suggestive of perforation. Position of the dilator or sound to be noted. Procedure to be abandoned immediately. Perforation can occur into—peritoneal cavity, broad ligament, bladder or an adherent viscus (rarely).
  - Monitoring of vitals are very crucial (half hourly pulse, blood pressure).
  - If vitals are normal, observation to be done
  - If infection is suspected, antibiotic coverage for 7 days.
  - If malignancy is demonstrated, early treatment recommended.
  - Perforation into broad ligament—occurs secondary to lacerations of cervix at or close to internal os. Uterine arteries or their major branches may be damaged. The most ommon symptom is pain. On examination doughy mass felt in broad ligament. If vessels not involved and no presence of infection or carcinoma.
- Conservative management is advised. In presence of significant hemorrhage—immediate laparotomy is required.
- *Peritonitis*: It may occur following perforation, rupture of pyosalpinx or tubo-ovarian abscess.
- *Pelvic cellulitis and parametritis*: Complaints of pain in lower abdomen, dyspareunia. On examination, there is tenderness during pelvic examination and movement of cervix, thickening of parametrium noted. Conservative management with antibiotics. In case if any mass is palpable, fine needle aspiration to be done to confirm presence of pus, which requires drainage.
- *Bleeding*: Early bleeding may be due to a tear, ruptured branch of cervical arteries. Offending vessel to be sutured if visible or

pressure packing to be done if not. Strict vitals monitoring is necessary. If bleeding is profuse and site not detected, cervix can be split to demonstrate the bleeding point and if bleeding point still not visualized uterine artery ligation to be done.
  - Late bleeding are usually consequences of an unnoticed laceration or hematoma which are infected. Conservative management with broad spectrum antibiotics, packing and blood transfusion. If bleeding still persist—laparotomy with internal iliac ligation or hysterectomy.
- Vasovagal attack and even cardiac arrest.

DILATATION AND CURETTAGE[13]

Minor surgical procedure where the cervix is dilated and endometrial tissues are curretated and sent for biopsy.

Indications

- Abnormal uterine bleeding at any premenopausal age
- Postmenopausal bleeding
- Prehysterectomy in postmenopausal at risk for endometrial or endocervical carcinoma
- Hemorrhage not responsive to hormone therapy (therapeutic).

Contraindications

- Pregnancy
- Acute pelvic inflammatory disease
- Pyometra
- Acute cervical or vaginal infections
- Clotting disorders.

Procedure

- Bladder to be emptied
- Patient placed in lithotomy position
- Perineal area cleaned and sterile draping done
- Per speculum and bimanual pelvic examination done
- Vaginal speculum inserted, cervix visualized
- Anterior lip of cervix held with vulsellum
- Curettage of endocervix done
- Sounding of uterus
- Dilatation of cervix
- Curettage of anterior, posterior and lateral walls of uterus done
- Tissues send for histopathological examination.

Complications

- Uterine perforation—most common. If perforation by a blunt instrument–vitals monitoring and to watch for signs of peritonitis. If perforation suspected by a sharp instrument—intra-abdominal injury has to be ruled out by laparoscopy. If active bleeding is present—immediate laparotomy
- Bleeding
- Infection—is rare unless cervicitis is present during the procedure.

ENDOMETRIAL BIOPSY[14-17]

Indications

- Abnormal uterine bleeding
- Postmenopausal bleeding
- Endometrial dating
- Cancer screening
- Evaluation for infertility (rule out endometrial tuberculosis)
- Follow-up of patients on hormonal treatment
- Follow-up of previously diagnosed endometrial hyperplasia
- Abnormal Pap smear with atypical cells favouring endometrial origin

Contraindications

- Pregnancy
- Acute pelvic inflammatory disease
- Clotting disorders
- Cervical and vaginal infections.

Premedication

- NSAIDs given 30 minutes prior to the procedure
- No anesthesia required.

Procedure

- Bladder to be emptied
- Patient placed in lithotomy position
- Perineal area cleaned and sterile draping done
- Per speculum and bimanual pelvic examination done
- Vaginal speculum inserted and cervix visualized
- Anterior lip of the cervix held by vulsellum, downward traction applied
- Uterine sounding done
- Endometrial biopsy catheter (either metallic or plastic) is gently inserted until the fundus or resistance is felt. Karman's cannula no. 4 can be used for endometrial aspiration
- The end of the catheter tip is fixed to a syringe whose piston is pulled out to create a suction pressure. The catheter with the suction maintained in moved with a in and out movement and rotated 360°. Atleast 4-5 excursions are made to obtain adequate tissues
- Once the catheter is filled with tissue, it is withdrawn and sample is collected
- Vulsellum is removed, check for bleeding, speculum removed.

Complications

- Infection
- Cervical injury
- Asherman syndrome
- Uterine perforation.

Drawback

- Inadequate sampling—site of pathology can be missed
- Endometrial polyp/pedunculated submucous fibroid may escape detection.

OFFICE HYSTEROSCOPY[18,19]

Direct visual inspection of the cervical canal and uterine cavity through a rigid or a flexible hysteroscope.

Indications

- Evaluation of unexplained abnormal uterine bleeding
- Prior to IVF
- Postoperative evaluation
- Recurrent spontaneous abortion
- Suspected intrauterine adhesions
- Preoperative surgical planning
- Suspected intrauterine growth
- Suspected mullerian anomalies.

Contraindications

- Pregnancy
- Pelvic inflammatory disease
- Uterine or cervical malignancy.

Risk

- Bleeding
- Perforation.

Analgesia

- NSAIDs to be given 1 hours prior to the procedure
- Routine use of opiate analgesia should be avoided
- Routine intracervical/paracervical block not indicated. Should be given if cervical dilatation is anticipated or larger size hysteroscope (outer diameter > 5 mm) is used.

Hysteroscope

- Miniature hysteroscope—2.7 mm with 3-3.5 mm sheath to be for diagnostic outpatient hysteroscopy
- Choice of hysteroscope—size and type (flexible/rigid) hysteroscope should be left to the discretion of the operator.

Distension Media

- Carbon dioxide or normal saline can be used
- Normal saline has lesser incidence of vasovagal episodes and gives an improved image quality.

Procedure

- Patient placed in modified dorsal lithotomy position
- Vaginal speculum inserted gently and cervix visualized
- Anterior lip of cervix held with tenaculum
- Hysteroscope is gently inserted
- Pressure of 45 mm Hg is to be maintained for adequate distension of uterine cavity by the distension media
- Visualization of the cervical canal with the uterine cavity done.

HYSTEROSALPINGOGRAM[20-23]

- Diagnostic radiographic study of the uterine cavity and fallopian tube
- Requires 20–30 mins for the procedure
- Three basic flims taken
  - Scout
  - One flim to document the uterine cavity and tubal patency
  - Postevaluation film to detect any areas of contrast loculation
- Additional oblique films taken if uterus obscure the tube or if uterine cavity appears abnormal
- Timing—day 7 —day 12 of menstrual cycle.

Premedication

- NSAIDs 30 minutes to 60 minutes prior to procedure
- Routine prophylactic antibiotic can be given if hydrosalpinx suspected 2 days prior to hysterosalpingogram (HSG) for 5 days (Tab doxycycline 100 mg BD for 5 days).

Indications

- Tubal patency in cases of infertility
- Previous recurrent spontaneous abortion
- Postoperative evaluation of patients who had tubal ligation/tubal recanalization.

Contraindications

- Pregnancy
- Current or suspected PID
- Allergy to contrast material
- Lower genital tract infection.

Procedure

- Bladder to be emptied
- Patient placed in dorsal lithotomy position
- Perineum cleaned with antiseptic solution and sterile draping done
- Sterile vaginal speculum inserted and cervix visualized
- Anterior lip of cervix held by vulsellum
- Metallic cannula (Leisch Wilkinson's/Rubin's cannula) or a balloon catheter is inserted through the cervix and internal os crossed
- Speculum is removed
- Contrast dye injected under fluoroscopic guidance
- Visualization of uterine cavity, fallopian tube and tubal patency noted.

Complications

- Allergic response to contrast dye
- Vascular intravasation—procedure to be stopped immediately
- Cervical laceration
- Uterine perforation
- Hemorrhage
- Vasovagal reaction.

INTRAUTERINE INSEMINATION

Intrauterine Insemination (IUI), or artificial insemination, is a fertility treatment wherein sperm are placed directly into a woman's uterus to facilitate fertilization. The goal of IUI is to increase the number of sperm that reach the fallopian tubes and subsequently increase the chance of fertilization.

Indications

- Low sperm count or decreased sperm mobility
- Sexual dysfunction
- Unexplained infertility
- A hostile cervical condition, including cervical mucus problems
- Cervical scar tissue from past procedures which may hinder the sperms' ability to enter the uterus
- Ejaculation dysfunction
- Need of donor sperm insemination.

The success of IUI increases when used in conjunction with controlled ovarian stimulation using fertility drugs. Follicular monitoring is necessary to determine when the eggs are mature. The IUI procedure is performed around the time of ovulation, for which injection hCG for trigger is given and IUI is performed about 24–36 hours later which coincides with the time of ovulation.

Procedure

Essentially, an IUI involves the 3 steps:
1. Collection of a sperm sample by masturbation or into a seminal collection device (a special sperm collection condom)
2. Sperm processing (a sperm wash procedure) and
3. Then placing the "washed" sperm sample through the cervical canal into the uterus with a small catheter.

Universal precautions and aseptic techniques should be followed by the clinician as body fluids are being handled and sample itself may introduce infection in endometrial cavity. Patient is asked to empty the bladder to make the insertion of the speculum easier. The washed sperm specimen is kept ready. It is drawn into a sterilized catheter that has a syringe attached to it. As the physician presses the plunger on the syringe, the sperm specimen that it is holding inside it, readily flows through the catheter straight inside the uterus. After this, the physician withdraws the catheter and removes the speculum. The patient is now allowed to remove her legs from the stirrups.

She is asked to relax for about five minutes. This marks the completion of the intrauterine insemination. There are no restrictions for the woman after this procedure and couple is advised to have intercourse as it enhances the chances of pregnancy.

The IUI process takes only minutes and is pain free and does not require sedation or anesthesia, although there may be some temporary cramping during the IUI process and there is a one percent risk of infection following the procedure.

Overall, the IUI procedure is a less invasive and less expensive fertility alternative than its counterparts, including in vitro fertilization (IVF), and is popular because it utilizes the body's natural fertilization process.

REFERENCES

1. Drew Peter A, Wilkinson Edward. Conventional cytology. Colposcopy Principles and Practice. Saunder's. 2008.pp.59-63.
2. Pap's smear. AAFP clinical recommendations. U.S Preventive Task Force Report; 2012.
3. R Sankaranarayanan, Ramani S Wesly. A practical manual on visual screening for cervical neoplasia. (WHO): IARCP. 2003;41.
4. Sarian LO, Derchian SF, Naud P, et al. Evaluation of visual inspection with acetic acid (VIA), Lugol's iodine (VILI), Cervical cytology and HIV testing as cervical screening tools in Latin America. J Med Screen. 2005;12(3):142-9.
5. WHO Guidelines for screening and treatment of precancerous lesions for cervical cancer prevention; 2013.
6. Meghan J Huchko, Jennifer Sneden, Hannah H Lestea. A comparison of two visual inspection methods of cervical cancer screening among HIV infected women in Kenya. Bulletin of World Health Organisation. 2014;92:195-203.
7. Katherine Camacho Carr, John W Sellors. Cervical cancer screening in low resource settings using visual inspection with acetic acid. J. Midwifery Women's Health. 2004;49(4): 329-37.
8. Barbara S. Apgar, Gregory L Brotzman, Mary M Rubin. Principles and technique of colposcopic exam. Colposcopy principles and practice. Saunder's. 2008.pp.101-19.

9. John W Sellors, R Sankaranarayanan. Colposcopy and treatment of cervical intraepithelial neoplasia: A Beginner's manual (WHO):IARC Press; 2003.
10. Huh Warner K, Sideri Mario. Relevance of random biopsy at the transformation zone when colposcopy is negative. Obstetrics and Gynaecology. 2014; 124(4):670-73.
11. Andrews M. Kaunitz. Colposcopic cervical biopsies: more is usually better, Medscape; 2015.
12. Monaghan JM, Lopes T, Naik R. Operations on the cervix. Boney's Gynaecological Surgery. Blackwell Publishing USA; 2004.pp.27-33.
13. Janice L, Bacon Christine Isaacs. Diagnostic dilatation and curettage: Medscape; updated; 2015.
14. Baugham DM. Office endometrial aspiration biopsy. Fam Pract Res. 1993;15:45-55.
15. Chambers JT, Chambers SK. Endometrial sampling: Who? Where? Why? With What? Clin Obstet Gynaecol. 1992;35(1):28-39.
16. Endometrial intraepithelial neoplasia. Committee on gynaecologic practice society of gynaecologic oncology (ACOG); No. 631;2015.
17. Dijkhuizen FP, Mol BW, Brolmann HA, Heintz AP. The accuracy of endometrial sampling in the diagnosis of patients with endometrial carcinoma, hyperplasia: A meta-analysis. Cancer. 2002-2015;89(8):1765-72.
18. Best practice in outpatient hysteroscopy. Green Top guidelines, No. 59, March; 2011.
19. Shah PK, V Lakshmi. Indications and contraindications of hysteroscopy; Textbook of hysteroscopy. Japyee. 2013.pp.28-31.
20. Marc A Fritz, Leon Speroff. Female infertility: Hysterosalpingography. Clinical gynaecologic endocrinology and infertility. Wolter's Kluwer. 2011.pp.1178-80.
21. Ryan G Steward, Richard Scott Lucidi. Hysterosalpingogram periprocedural care. Medscape update; 2014.
22. William L Simpson, Laura G Butia, Jolinda Mester. Hysterosalpingography: A reemerging study. RSNA Radiographics. 2006;26(2):419-31.
23. Victor Gomel. Reconstructive Tubal Surgery. TeLinde's operative gynaecology. Wolters Kluwer. 2015.pp.366-7.

5
Recent Advances in Contraceptions

Rachna Sharma, Siddhidatri Mishra

INTRODUCTION

Contraception has been in practice since ancient times. Field of contraception has made tremendous advances to fulfil the needs of individuals. Contraceptive methods may be temporary or permanent, assisting in controlling fertility. Permanent methods include male and female sterilization. Temporary methods include natural methods, barrier contraceptives, IUCD, hormonal methods. Newer methods include vaginal rings, transdermal methods (patch, spray on), implants, combined injectables, hormonal releasing IUCD. Newer delivery systems are more effective, fewer side effects, easier to deliver than current options.

VAGINAL RINGS

Vaginal contraceptive rings are of two types, combined estrogen progesterone rings and progesterone only rings.

Combined Vaginal Ring (NuvaRing)

It is a flexible, soft transparent ring made of ethylene vinyl acetate (EVA) with outer diameter of 54 mm and cross section of 4 mm (Fig. 5.1). Each ring contains ethinyl estradiol 2.7 mg and etonogestrel 11.7 mg (active metabolite of desogestrel) and releases 15 µg EE and 120 µg ENG per day.

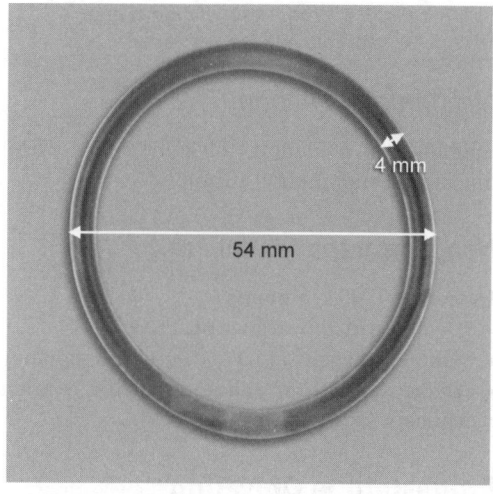

Fig. 5.1 NuvaRing *(For color version, see Plate 1)*

Timing and Position of Insertion

NuvaRing is inserted and removed by women herself. It can be inserted in any position which allows her to insert ring easily by squatting, lying or standing with one leg raised, within first 5 days of menstrual cycle. Each cycle comprises of 3 weeks of ring followed by a 1-week ring free period.

Failure Rate

0.65% per 100 women year.[1]

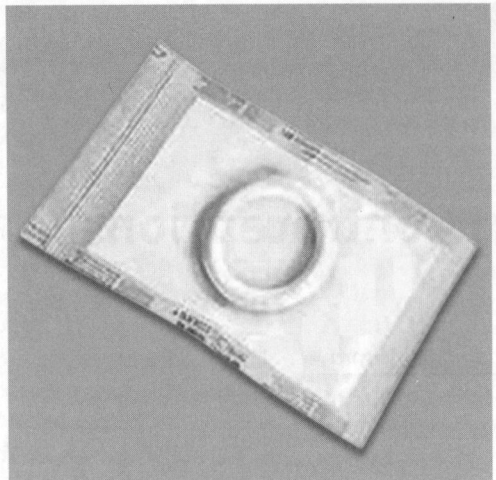

Fig. 5.2 Progesterone vaginal ring *(For color version, see Plate 1)*

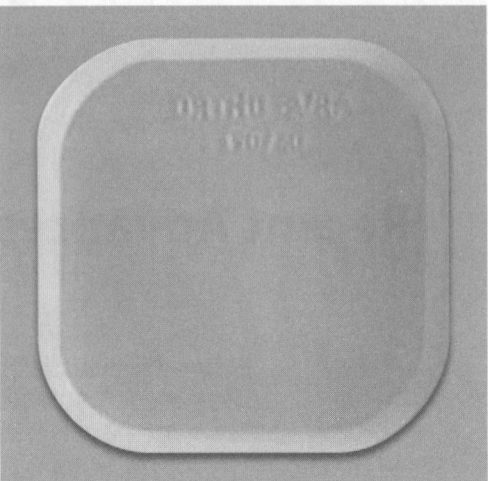

Fig. 5.3 Ortho Evra *(For color version, see Plate 1)*

Mechanism of Action

Inhibition of ovulation, thickening of cervical mucus and endometrial atrophy.

Noncontraceptive Benefits

Decreased PMS symptoms
- Decrease in appearance of acne
- Protection against PID and ectopic pregnancy
- Decreased risk of endometrial and ovarian cancers.

Progesterone Only Ring

This is more useful for breast feeding mothers (Fig. 5.2). It releases 20 μg of levonorgesterol daily. It is left in the vagina for 3 months then replaced.

Mechanism of Action

Thickening of cervical mucus, decidualization of endometrium.

TRANSDERMAL CONTRACEPTION

Works slowly by releasing a combination of progestin and estrogen through skin. Transdermal contraceptives could be patches, spray on or gel.

Transdermal Patch

In 2002, the FDA approved the use of a combination contraceptive patch (Fig. 5.3) that releases 20 mcg of ethinylestradiol and 150 mcg of norelgestromin per day.

Mechanism of Action

Similar to OCPs which include inhibition of ovulation, thickening of cervical mucus, decidualization of endometrium.

Timing of Application

The patch is applied weekly for three weeks, followed by a patch-free week during which withdrawal bleeding occurs. Recommended application sites include the upper arm, buttocks, lower abdomen, and upper torso (excluding the breasts).

Failure Rate

The overall failure rate for the contraceptive patch has been reported to be only 0.88 pregnancies per 100 women-years, with a method failure rate of 0.7 pregnancies per 100 women-years.[2] However, this form of contraception may be less effective in women weighing more than 90 kg.

Advantage

Weekly application encourages compliance
- Does not require vaginal insertion
- Nonoral route of administration
- Contraceptive effects are rapidly reversible
- Excellent cycle control after 3 months.

Spray on Contraceptives

Progestin nestorone (Fig. 5.4), appropriate for breastfeeding women, can be delivered through a spray or gel also. Nesterone Metered Dose Transdermal System under phase I trial.

Contraceptive Gel

Nestorone gel is used. It is applied to the skin daily for 3 months and suppresses ovulation in 83% cases.

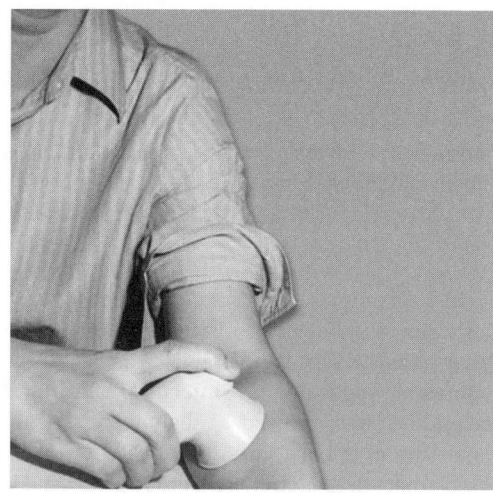

Fig. 5.4 Spray on contraceptive *(For color version, see Plate 1)*

IMPLANTS

Implants are progesterone containing devices inserted subcutaneously. Implants available are Norplant, Norplant II (Jadelle), Implanon.[3]

Norplant

Progestin only delivery system containing LNG which is effective for 5 years. Contains 6 flexible closed capsules of polydimethylsiloxane (Fig. 5.5), each containing 36 mg of LNG. It releases 85 µg LNG initially and later on 30 µg/day over 5 years.

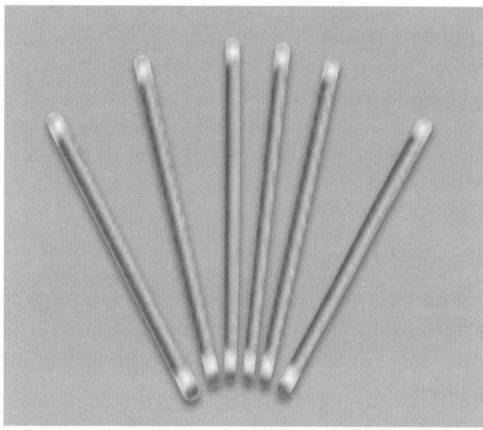

Fig. 5.5 Norplant *(For color version, see Plate 1)*

Mechanism of Action

Includes inhibition of ovulation in 90% of the cycles, endometrial atrophy, thickening of cervical mucus.

Insertion

Inserted subcutaneously on inner side of forearm in a fan shaped manner.

Failure Rate

Its failure rate is 0.05% within first year of use.

Advantage

Highly effective with reversible contraceptive effect.
- Easy to use with no after care
- No estrogenic effects
- Does not affect quality and quantity of breast milk.

Disadvantages

Include its cost, insertion and removal by trained health professional and irregular bleeding.

Norplant II (Jadelle)

Contains 2 silastic rods, each containing 70 mg LNG.

Insertion and removal: Same as Norplant. It is effective for 5 years.

Failure rate is 0.05% within first year of use.

Implanon

It is a single rod device containing 67 mg 3-keto desogestrel which is inserted from a sterile preloaded applicator by injection/withdrawal technique and placed subcutaneously on inner side of upper arm under local anesthesia (Fig. 5.6). It releases etonogestrel 30 μg/day and is effective for 3 years.

Mechanism of Action

Similar to Norplant.

Failure Rate

Highly effective with a failure rate of 0.01% in clinical trials.[4]

Advantages

Low androgenic effect: Can be used in women with hypertension, diabetes mellitus, endometriosis. Also safe in adolescents and breastfeeding mothers.

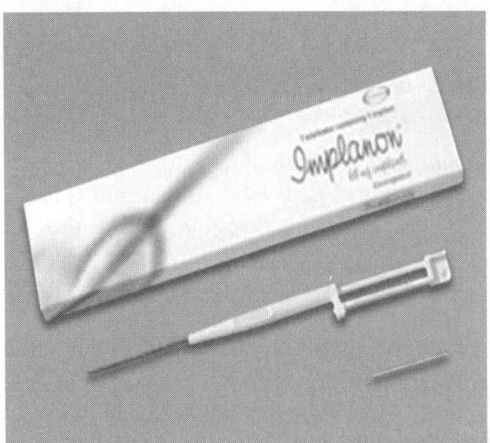

Fig. 5.6 Implanon *(For color version, see Plate 1)*

Disadvantage

Irregular vaginal bleeding and amenorrhea.[4]

HORMONAL INJECTABLE CONTRACEPTIVES

Combined Injectable Contraceptives

Monthly injectable contaceptives containing estrogen and progesterone. Cyclofem contains 25 mg medroxyprogesterone acetate DMPA and 5 mg of estradiol cypionate. Mesigna contains 50 mg NET EN and 5 mg estradiol valerate. Lunelle is a monthly combined injectable, is available as a aqueous suspension of medroxyprogesterone 25 mg and estradiol 5 mg.

Mechanism of Action

Similar to OCPs which include ovulation inhibition, cervical mucus thickening and endometrial atrophy.

Timing

The first injection should be given during the first 5 days of a normal period. Repeat injections be given 28–30 days after the previous injection, without exceeding 33 days.

Advantage

Over progesterone only injectables include less common irregular bleeding patterns which decrease with length of use.

Failure Rate

Its failure rate is around 0.2–0.4%.[5]

Subcutaneous DMPA (Figs 5.7A and B)

DMPA-SC provides slower, more sustained absorption of the progestin than conventional DMPA and is available in a prefilled syringe. Contains 104 mg of medroxyprogesterone acetate (30% lower dose as compared to DMPA).

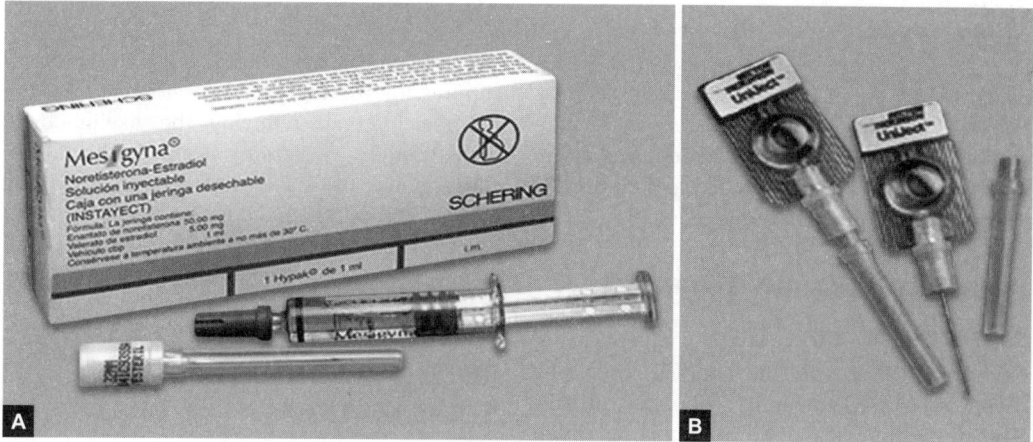

Figs 5.7A and B Subcutaneous DMPA *(For color version, see Plate 2)*

Mechanism of Action

Similar to injectable progesterone which include thickening of cervical mucus, endometrial atrophy.

Advantage

Rapid onset of action as compared to DMPA and is effective for 3 months.

INTRAUTERINE CONTRACEPTIVE DEVICES

Hormone Releasing IUCD (3rd Generation)

Mirena (Fig. 5.8)

It is a long acting levonorgesterol containing IUCD with T-shaped polyethylene frame and steroid reservoir around vertical stem which contains 52 mg LNG with a release rate 20 µg/day.

Mechanism of Action
It stimulates inflammatory response in the uterine cavity that is toxic to sperm. Progestin-releasing IUDs also thicken cervical mucus and suppress endometrial growth.

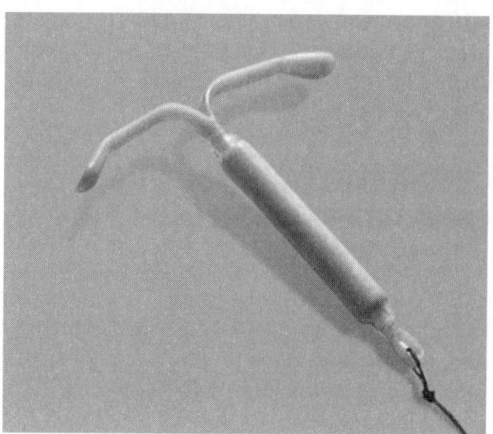

Fig. 5.8 Mirena *(For color version, see Plate 2)*

Failure Rate
Mirena is effective for 5 years with a pregnancy rate of <0.5%.[5,6]

Advantages[5]
- *Reduction of blood loss:* DUB and anaemia.
- *Reduction of pain and dysmenorrhea:* Endometriosis and adenomyosis.
- Beneficial effect on fibroids.
- Lower risk of PID.[7]
- Can be used in HRT for endometrial protection.

Does not influence lactation, introduced 6 weeks postpartum.

Skyla

It is another hormone releasing IUCD which contains 13.5 mg of LNG which is released at a rate of 14 µg/day. Skyla must be removed by the end of the third year and can be replaced at the time of removal with a new Skyla if continued contraceptive protection is desired.

Frameless IUCD (4th Generation) (Fig. 5.9)

Frameless IUCD can be copper containing (Gynaefix) or LNG containing (fibroplant) IUCD. Gynaefix is frameless IUCD, 3 cm long which contains 6 Copper sleeves (330 sq mm of Cu) strung on a surgical polypropylene nylon thread knotted at the upper end. The Knot is pushed 9–10 mm into myometrium of fundus by a special stylet. Fibroplant is frameless LNG releasing IUCD which releases 14 µg of LNG/day and it is effective for 3 years.

CHEWABLE LOW DOSE ORAL CONTRACEPTIVE PILLS

A new chewable combined oral contraceptive pill (OCP) containing ethinylestradiol (EE) 0.025 mg and norethindrone (NE) 0.8 mg in a 24/4 regimen was approved for marketing in December 2010. Each of the four inactive tablets contains 75 mg ferrous fumarate.

Mechanism of Action

Similar to other combined hormonal contraceptive.

Advantage

The advantage of a 24/4 regimen is better suppression of follicular development in the pill-free interval, reducing the likelihood of breakthrough ovulation even further.[8] The convenience of a low-dose pill that can be chewed without the need for water will be useful in allowing women who have forgotten a pill to take it whenever they remember, provided they carry it with them.

RECENT METHODS OF FEMALE STERILIZATION

Hysteroscopic methods of sterilization include Adiana and Essure.

Adiana

Controlled thermal damage to the lining of the fallopian tube followed by insertion of a non-absorbable biocompatible silicone elastomer matrix within the tubal lumen (Fig. 5.10).

Essure

Micro insert placed inside the fallopian tubes under hysteroscopic guidance (Fig. 5.11). Loaded

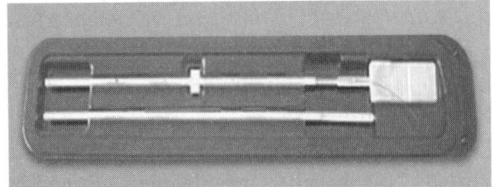

Fig. 5.9 Frameless IUCD
(For color version, see Plate 2)

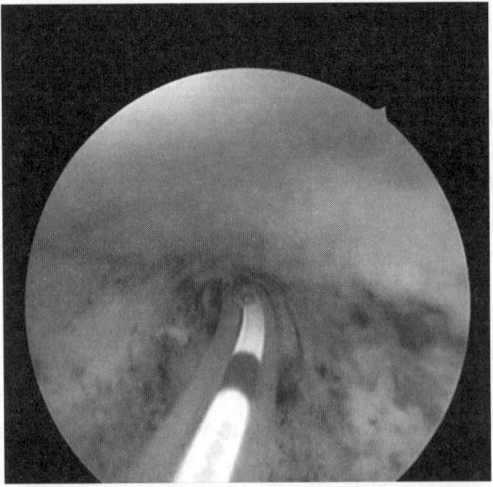

Fig. 5.10 Adian introduced in fallopian tube to cause thermal damage *(For color version, see Plate 2)*

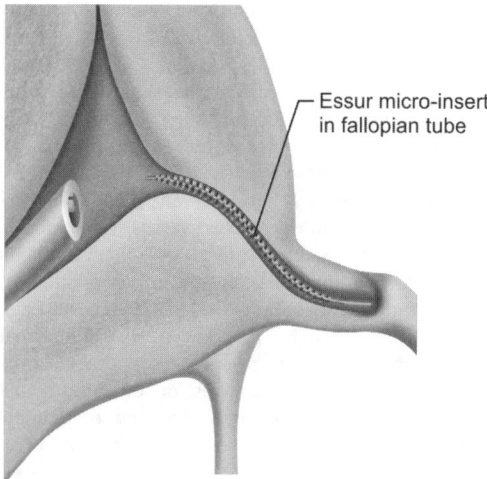

Fig. 5.11 Essure

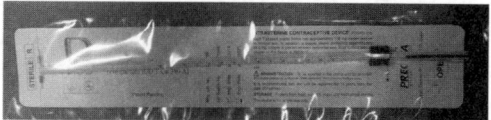

Fig. 5.12 PPIUCD inserter *(For color version, see Plate 2)*

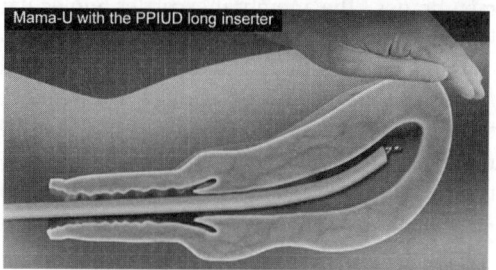

Fig. 5.13 Mama-U (PPIUCD) from Pregna international company *(For color version, see Plate 2)*

with a single-use inner coil of stainless steel and polyethylene terephthalate (PET) fibers and an outer coil of nickel-titanium (nitinol).

NEWER EMERGENCY CONTRACEPTIVES

Ulipristal

Ulipristal (Ella) is a progesterone agonist/antagonist marketed for emergency contraception.

Mechanism of Action

Its mechanism of action varies based on time of administration. When taken before ovulation, ulipristal delays or inhibits ovulation.[9,10] Administration in the early luteal phase may decrease endometrial thickness and affect implantation of a fertilized egg.[9,11] Ulipristal is labeled for use as an emergency contraceptive following unprotected sexual intercourse or contraceptive failure.[9]

Failure Rate

When given within 72 hours of unprotected sexual intercourse, ulipristal is at least as effective as levonorgestrel, with pregnancy rates of 0.9–1.8%.[12,13] whereas the effectiveness of levonorgestrel declines when given more than 48 hours after unprotected sexual intercourse, ulipristal maintains consistent effectiveness when administered up to 120 hours after unprotected intercourse.[9,10,12] In the 72- to 120-hour window, ulipristal is more effective than levonorgestrel.[13]

POSTPARTUM INTRAUTERINE CONTRACEPTIVE DEVICE

Postpartum intrauterine contraceptive device (PPIUCD) insertion is traditionally done with kelly's forceps. There are new advances in insertion techniques where CuT 380A (Fig. 5.12) is inserted with a long, wide inserter (Fig. 5.13) and has longer thread. Due to its thickness it is easy to use. Its efficacy compare to traditional method is yet to establish as its undergoing phase 3 trial.

NEWER MALE CONTRACEPTIVE

Reversible Inhibition of Sperm Under Guidance (RISUG)

The RISUG is an injectable compound that partially blocks the vas deferens providing effective contraception for up to 10 years per dose. It is composed of styrene maleic anhydride (SMA) complexed with the solvent dimethyl sulfoxide (DMSO). RISUG has two contraceptive effects: partial blockage of the vas deferens and disruption of the sperm that pass through it.[14] It is under Phase III trial.

Sperm that are present in the ejaculate after RISUG has been administered have broken cell membranes. The membrane carries molecular keys that are needed to attach to an egg. It also contains packets of enzymes that are needed to dissolve the outer coating of an egg. Without those keys or enzymes, the sperm are functionally infertile.[15] Researchers postulate that RISUG ruptures the membranes by stressing their ion exchange mechanisms.

Contraceptive Vaccines (CVs)

- Sperm antigens constitute the most promising targets for CVs
- hCG vaccine is the first vaccine to undergo clinical trials in humans
- Gene-based approaches promise dramatic change in contraception.

CONCLUSION

Developing countries like India have an overwhelming need to control fertility and there is no shortage of potential contraceptives available. Recent methods of contraception have increased the birth control choices for female and their partners. Most of the above mentioned contraceptives are available in India except transdermal patch, combined injectable contraceptives, implants and ulipristal.

REFERENCES

1. Roumen FJ, Apter D, Mulders TM, Dieben TO. Efficacy, tolerability, and acceptability of a novel contraceptive vaginal ring releasing etonogestrel and ethinyloestradiol. Hum Reprod. 2001;16: 469-75.
2. Zieman M, Guillebaud J, Weisberg E, Shangold G, Fisher AC, Creasy GW. Contraceptive efficacy and cycle control with the Ortho Evra/Evra transdermal system: the analysis of pooled data. Fertil Steril. 2002;772(suppl 2):S13-8.
3. Winner B, Peipert JF, Zhao Q, Buckel C, Madden T, Allsworth JE, et al. "Effectiveness of Long-Acting Reversible Contraception". New England Journal of Medicine. 2012;366(21):1998-2007.
4. Power J, French R, Cowan F. Subdermal implantable contraceptives versus other forms of reversible contraceptives or other implants as effective methods of preventing pregnancy. Cochrane Database. Syst Rev. 2007;18(3):CD001326.
5. Power J, French R, Cowan F. Subdermal implantable contraceptives versus other forms of reversible contraceptives or other implants as effective methods of preventing pregnancy. Cochrane Database Syst Rev. 2007;18(3):CD001326.
6. Power J, French R, Cowan F. Subdermal implantable contraceptives versus other forms of reversible contraceptives or other implants as effective methods of preventing pregnancy. Cochrane Database Syst Rev. 2007;18(3):CD001326.
7. Andersson K, Odlind V, Rybo G. Levonorgestrel-releasing and copper-releasing (Nova T) IUDs during five years of use: a randomized comparative trial. Contraception. 1994;49:56-72.
8. Read CM. New regimens with combined oral contraceptive pills-moving away from traditional 21/7 cycles. Eur J Contracept Reprod Health Care. 2010;15(Suppl 2):S32-41.
9. Ella (ulipristal acetate) tablet. Highlights of prescribing information. Morristown, NJ: Watson Pharma, Inc.; 2010.
10. Fine P, Mathé, Ginde S, Cullins V, Morfesis J, Gainer E. Ulipristal acetate taken 48–120 hours after intercourse for emergency contraception. Obstet Gynecol. 2010;115(2 pt 1):257-63.
11. Stratton P, Hartog B, Hajizadeh N, et al. A single mid-follicular dose of CDB-2914, a new antiprogestin, inhibits folliculogenesis and endometrial differentiation in normally cycling women. Hum Reprod. 2000;15(5):1092-9.
12. Creinin MD, Schlaff W, Archer DF, et al. Progesterone receptor modulator for emergency contraception: a randomized controlled trial. Obstet Gynecol. 2006;108(5):1089-97.
13. Glasier AF, Cameron ST, Fine PM, et al. Ulipristal acetate versus levonorgestrel for emergency contraception: a randomised non-inferiority trial and meta-analysis. Lancet. 2010;375(9714):555-62.
14. Chaudhury K, Bhattacharyya AK, Guha SK. "Studies on the membrane integrity of human sperm treated with a new injectable male contraceptive." Human Reproduction. 2004;19(8):1826-30.
15. Guha SK, Singh G, Anasari S, Kumar S, Srivastava A, Koul V. "Phase II clinical trial of a vas deferens injectable contraceptive for the male." Contraception. 1997;56(4):245-50.

6

Menopause

Poonam Kashyap

DEFINITION

Menopause is a natural and inevitable event that happens on average at age 51 years in white Caucasians with ethnic and regional variations. Menopause is a retrospective clinical diagnosis, as the final menstrual period can only be defined if followed by 12 months of amenorrhea. Menopause is not just cessation of menstruation it is "depletion of ovarian follicles" leading to decrease in ovarian hormones. It is characterized by the menstrual changes that reflect oocyte depletion and reduction in ovarian hormone production. Menopause before the age of 40 years is considered to be premature, whether occurring naturally or as a result of surgery or some other intervention (e.g. chemotherapy). Therefore, it is stressed to understand the pathophysiology of menopause as its implications may be different in various age group.[1]

Premature ovarian insufficiency (POI) is defined as primary hypogonadism before the age of 40 years in women with a normal karyotype who previously had normal menstrual cycles. It is characterized by typical menopausal symptoms and signs, oligomenorrhea or amenorrhea and FSH >40 IU/L. The diagnosis of POI should only be confirmed after a minimum of two elevated FSH test results (>40 IU/L) at least 4–6 weeks apart. The incidence of spontaneous POI is 1% of women under the age of 40 years and 0.1% of women under the age of 30 years. There is an increased burden of surgical menopause in India.[2] Nowadays, the number of hysterectomies with bilateral oophorectomies are on rise. The reason may be to avoid follow-up with other options of conservative management by these women.

The factors which influence age at menopause are smoking, history of ovarian drilling, ovarian cystectomies, unilateral oophorectomies, pelvic chemotherapy or radiotherapy.

In India, mean age of menopause is 49.4 years and 130 million Indian women are expected to live beyond menopause into old age by 2015.[2] In India, 19% of women aged 40–41 years have already reached menopause, and the incidence of menopause increases rapidly after the age of 41 years. By age of 48–49 years, two-thirds of women are in menopause. So, the number of women in menopause is increasing with increase in life expectancy and so is the increase in reported problems.[3] Therefore, quality of life of this population becomes a major issue and understanding of menopause is very important issue for all the clinicians as most of the time it is multidisciplinary approach to the problems of menopause.[3]

There are various staging systems described for menopause. Stages of Reproductive Aging Workshop + 10 (STRAW + 10) describes stages of reproductive aging as Reproductive, menopausal transition, and postmenopause. Each stage is broken down further into early, peak (reproductive stage only) and late stages (Table 4.1). STRAW + 10 made a substantial contribution to women's health by providing a standardized and consistent staging system for reproductive aging for studies of midlife. Altogether, there are a total of ten specific stages, labeled from –5 to +2. Stage –1 corresponds to the late stage of the menopausal transition, with the principal criterion of an interval of amenorrhea of >60 days and other supportive criteria such as FSH >25 IU/L.[1]

The criteria cannot be used in women with polycystic ovarian syndrome and premature ovarian insufficiency and those who have had endometrial ablation or removal of a single ovary and/or hysterectomy. In such women, the supportive criteria should be used to determine reproductive stage.

HORMONAL CHANGES

A subtle rise in the concentration of FSH is the earliest and most consistent clinically measurable hormonal change. A FSH level measured during the early follicular stage of the menstrual cycle that is greater than two standard deviations above the mean level in women of reproductive age is a marker of impending menopausal transition. A slow rise in FSH followed by LH (luteinizing hormone) and a decline in estradiol and estrone. In menopause ovarian theca cells are producing androstenedione and testosterone under the influence of increased levels of LH and they are the source of androgens in menopause. When oophorectomy is done, there is sudden fall of androgens because of loss of this source of androgens. But gradually as aging of adrenal gland occurs, levels of androgens fall up to 50% at 60 years of age as compared with women at 40 years of age and after age 70, levels of dehydroepiandrosterone sulfate (DHEAS) are 20% or less.

CLINICAL PRESENTATION

Most of the problems associated with menopause are mainly because of deficiency of estrogens but some problems may be because of deficiency of other hormones also such as testosterone (Table 4.2). Women with premature ovarian insufficiency have high risk of endothelial function impairment, ischemic heart disease, ischemic stroke, a higher incidence of osteoporotic fractures, impaired cognition and diminished sexual well-being. Menopause is a physiological phenomenon but can produce problems later in life. So, when women come to us in menopausal transition we have to assess her for the high-risk factors which would influence her quality of life later on and this includes the following:

- Asses her weight and height and calculate her BMI which should be between 19 and 23 for the Asians and 20–25 for others.
- Take family history of osteoporosis or fragility fractures or other risk factors for osteoporosis.
- History of diabetes, hypertension.
- History of previous fracture.
- History of any drug intake.
- Family or past history of chronic heart disease.
- Any history of breast cancer in the family.
- Do her pap smear if not already done and then every year till the age of 50 years.
- Do TVS if not already done or if dysfunctional bleeding.
- There is no need to do FSH or hormonal levels for diagnosis of menopause.
- Advise mammography and BSE (breast self-examination) once in month.
- Clinical breast examination (CBE) once in a year.
- Mammography 1–2 years after 40 years and every two year after the age of 50 years.

Table 6.1 The stages of reproductive aging workshop + 10 staging system for reproductive aging in women[1]

Stage	-5	-4	-3b	-3a	-2	-1	+1a	+1b	+1c	+2
Terminology	Reproductive				Menopausal transition		Postmenopause			
	Early	Peak	Late		Early	Late	Early			Late
					Perimenopause					
Duration	Variable				Variable	1–3 years	2 years (1+1)		3–6 years	Remaining lifespan
Principal criteria										
Menstrual cycle	Variable to regular	Regular	Regular	Subtle changes in flow length	Variable length persistent ≥7-day difference in length of consecutive cycles	Interval of amenorrhea of ≥60 days				
Supportive criteria										
Endocrine										
FSH			Low	Variable*	↑Variable*	↑ >25 IU/L**	↑Variable*	Stabilizes		
AMH			Low	Low	Low	Low	Low	Very low		
Inhibin B				Low	Low	Low	Low	Very low		
Antral follicle count			Low	Low	Low	Low	Very low	Very low		
Descriptive characteristics										
Symptoms						Vasomotor symptoms likely	Vasomotor symptoms most likely		Increasing symptoms of urogenital atrophy	

* Blood draw on cycle days 2–5
**Approximate expected level based on assays using current international pituitary standard

Abbreviations: FMP, final menstrual period; FSH, follicle stimulating hormone; AMH, anti-mullerian hormone

Table 6.2 Clinical presentation

Symptoms	Signs
• Hot flashes, night sweats and/or cold flashes • Irritability, mood swings • Dry vagina • Trouble sleeping through the night • Irregular periods • Anxiety, depression • Difficulty concentrating, disorientation • Disturbing memory lapses • Incontinence, stress and urge incontinence • Weight gain • Breast tenderness • Sudden tears • Loss of libido • Joint pains • Hair loss • Gastrointestinal disturbances-flatulence, gas, pain, nausea • Easy fatigue • Skin changes, cracking of nails	• Weight gain • Breast tenderness • Osteoporosis • Vaginal atrophy • Senile endometritis • Senile dementia

Investigations for Premature Ovarian Insufficiency

It should include detailed history taking including family history, vaginal examination. Information on hot flushes, vaginal dryness, lack of libido, arthralgia, loss of concentration, insomnia and fertility issues should be obtained in a sensitive and caring manner.[4] The following investigations are to be done:
- *Hormone analysis:* FSH, LH, estradiol, anti-mullerian hormone (AMH), inhibin B, prolactin, testosterone, free thyroxine, TSH, cortisol, adrenocorticotropic hormone (ACTH), dehydroepiandrosterone sulfate (DHEAS)
- Autoimmune screen for polyendocrinopathies
- Chromosome analysis for women younger than 30 years
- Pelvic and breast ultrasound
- Dual X-ray absorptiometry (optional).

(FSH, follicle stimulating hormone; LH, luteinizing hormone; AMH, anti-mullerian hormone; TSH, thyroid stimulating hormone; ACTH, adrenocorticotropic hormone; DHEAS, dehydroepiandrosterone sulfate).

MANAGEMENT

Menopausal Hormone Therapy

The recommendations for the use of hormone therapy has been given by International Menopausal Society in 2016 to help health care professionals to optimize management of menopause.[4] The aim of hormone therapy is for treating menopausal symptoms and also in the prevention of disease of aging.
- It is offered to only those women who have full blown symptoms of menopause. The menopausal symptoms mainly comprise of vasomotor symptoms and clinical manifestation of urogenital atrophy. The other important issue is that of osteoporosis which is not manifest clinically but makes the bones prone to fractures on minimal trauma. Menopausal hormone therapy (MHT) is very effective therapy for treating vasomotor symptoms and urogenital atrophy. Other complaints, such as joint and muscle pains, mood swings, sleep disturbances and sexual dysfunction (including reduced libido) may improve during MHT. There may be improvement in quality of life and sexual function by the administration of individualized MHT like androgenic preparations.
- Before considering MHT, overall strategy should be made and various parameters including diet, exercise, avoidance of smoking and alcohol use should be made.

- Menopausal hormone therapy (MHT) must be individualized and tailored according to symptoms and should be started in lowest dose. The use of hormone therapy for prevention of symptoms should also be considered. The need of therapy also depends on family and personal history and also on basis of results of investigations. The benefits and risks of hormone therapy are different for women during the menopause transition compared to those for older women. There are no mandatory limitations as regards the duration of MHT. It has been suggested from women's health initiative (WHI) Trial and other studies that MHT can be safely used for 5 years in healthy women starting treatment before age 60.[5]
- Women with primary ovarian insufficiency (POI) should receive hormonal treatment after exclusion of contraindications and they usually need higher doses of estrogens compared to women over 40 years old.
- The dosage of MHT should be titrated to the lowest effective dose.

Contraindications of Menopausal Hormone Therapy

Absolute

- Existing breast cancer or endometrial cancer (any estrogen dependent tumor).
- Undiagnosed abnormal genital bleeding.
- History of venous thromboembolism, stroke or coronary heart disease
- Acute liver or gallbladder disease.

Relative

- Presence of fibroid
- History of benign breast disease
- Chronic liver disease
- Migraine.

VASOMOTOR SYMPTOMS

- Counseling the woman is most important
- Medical therapy.

The gold standard of treatment for vasomotor symptoms relating to menopause is systemic hormone therapy. Hormone therapy either estrogens alone or in combination with progestogen, in minimum dosage and for the shortest period of time are prescribed, they can be either by oral route or transdermal route or transvaginal route or pellets of estrogen. No other therapy, other than estrogen has been approved by US Food and Drug Administration (FDA) for the treatment of hot flashes.[5] Although HT is well-tolerated by most women, standard doses may cause adverse effects, such as vaginal bleeding, breast tenderness, bloating, and headaches. Lower doses of hormones are not as effective as traditional doses of in treating vasomotor symptoms. It is recommended that healthcare providers should individualize care and women should be started with the lowest effective dose and for the shortest duration required to relieve vasomotor symptoms.[6]

There may be recurrence of symptoms in 50% of women after stopping hormone therapy. Therefore, the decision to discontinue should be based on individual women's risk versus benefit ratio and also on clinical parameters. The American College of Obstetricans and Gynaecologists recommends that there is no need to discontinue systemic estrogen at the age of 65 years.[5]

- Standard hormonal therapy
  - Conjugated equine estrogen (CEE) 0.625 mg/day orally
  - Micronized estradiol 1 mg/day orally.
  - Estradiol patch 0.0375–0.05 mg/week
- Low dose therapy
  - Conjugated equine estrogen 0.3–0.45 mg/day orally.
  - Micronized estradiol 0.5 mg/day orally.
  - Ethinylestradiol 5 µg/day orally
  - Estradiol patch 0.025–0.0375 mg/week
- Ultra low dose therapy
  - Micronized estradiol 0.25 mg
  - Estradiol transdermal 0.014 mg
- Estrogen combined with estrogen agonist/antagonist
  - CEE 0.45 mg/day and bazedoxifene 20 mg/day

- Progestin
  - Depot medroxyprogesterone acetate 10 mg, 5 mg, 2.5 mg
  - Norethindrone 5 mg, 1 mg

  Tibolone 2.5 mg/day

  It is a synthetic steroid with tissue specific estrogenic and progestogenic effects but it is not FDA approved. Tibolone is effective for vasomotor symptoms, and vaginal symptoms and also beneficial for bone density. It does not have estrogenic effects on the uterus or breasts. It is not a first line drug but can be used where hormone therapy is contraindicated.[5]

Nonhormonal Medications

- *Bazedoxifene:* It is a third generation selective estrogen receptor modulator. It is used in combination with conjugated estrogen and it is FDA approved.
- Serotonin and norepinephrine reuptake inhibitors— Venlafaxine (75 mg/day) has also been shown to decrease hot flushes similar to a low dose of oral estradiol (0.5 mg) in a randomized trial.[7] Venlafaxine (37.5 mg per day increasing to 75 mg controlled release) is equally effective but better tolerated than gabapentin (300 mg once per day increasing to 300 mg three times per day) in breast cancer patients. Both products reduced the frequency and severity of hot flushes by 65%.[8] Paroxetine 7.5 mg/day is the only nonhormonal therapy that is approved by the FDA for the treatment of vasomotor symptoms. Women with a history of breast cancer represent an important category of patients where non-hormonal treatments are useful for the treatment of VMS.
- *Gabapentin:* It may be specifically useful in patients experiencing night-time flushes with nocturnal sweats and repeated awakenings, due to its sedating effect. High doses of gabapentin (300 mg three times per day) have been shown to reduce hot flushes similar to 0.625 mg estrogen. However, at this dose gabapentin is associated with significant side effects.[9] Intake of a single dose of gabapentin at bedtime has been suggested in these patients and this treatment schedule may help decrease side-effects.
- Clonidine 0.1 mg/day but not FDA approved. Clonidine, an α-2 adrenergic agonist, is slightly more effective than placebo is reducing hot flushes in a meta-analysis of ten trial. Clonidine use is associated with significant side effects (dry mouth, dizziness, constipation, hypotension and sedation) that limit its clinical use.[10]
- Phytoestrogens are plant derived substances with estrogenic biologic activity. Examples are isoflavones geistein and daidzein which are found in high amounts in soybeans, soy products, and red clover. But there has been no evidence of benefit in studies done for this.
- Vitamins.
- Herbal remedies.
- Reflexology.
- Stellate ganglion block.

BONE LOSS (OSTEOPOROSIS) AND FRACTURE RISK

Osteoporosis is a systemic skeletal disease characterized by decreased bone strength with the risk of sustaining a fracture when falling from own body height (fragility fracture). Postmenopausal osteoporosis results from a failure to attain peak bone density, accelerated bone loss after menopause, age-related bone loss or a combination of factors. Accelerated postmenopausal bone loss is induced by estrogen deprivation.[11] It has been responsible for big financial burden to health care systems especially hip fractures and vertebral fractures.[8] Osteopenia and osteoporosis are problems of concern in Indian women. Almost all women over 65 years have been found to have either osteopenia or osteoporosis. Out of all 35–40% of women between 40 and 65 years have been found to be suffering from osteopenia whereas 8–30% suffer from osteoporosis. The higher incidence of this because of low calcium intake in, lack of exercise in all ages and also, to lack of exposure to sunlight in women living in urban areas.

The diagnosis of osteoporosis is based on assessment of bone mineral density (BMD) by dual X-ray absorptiometry (DXA). The value obtained is compared to peak bone density and expressed as the T-score. Osteoporosis is defined when T-score <−2.5 or the presence of a fragility fracture. It is not a cost-effective to screen whole population with BMD but selectively done on women, having risk factors such as a personal or family history of fractures, based on age, history of amenorrhea, primary ovarian insufficiency, low body mass, diet, smoking, alcohol abuse, the use of bone toxic medication and rheumatoid arthritis.[12]

The goal of osteoporosis treatment is the prevention of fracture. Choice of therapy should be based on considering various parameters benefit of drug, risks associated with use and also on cost of therapy. Treatment should depend on the 10-year fracture probability but it may vary in various countries. Alternatively, treatment can be given to all patients who are prone to fracture or a T-score of <−2.5 (osteoporosis), or a T-score of <−1> −2.5 (osteopenia) with additional risk factors. Monitoring of therapy can be done by serial DXA and its interpretation is very important.

Therapeutic Options

Menopausal Hormone Therapy

Menopausal hormone therapy is effective in decreasing the incidence of all fractures, including vertebral and hip fractures. Age at the initiation of MHT is important in preventing fractures. It can be considered as first line of therapy in the age group 50–60 years or within 10 years after menopause when the benefits of MHT are most likely to outweigh any risk. In the age group 60–70 years, individual calculation of risk versus benefit, availability of other drugs and the lowest effective dose should be considered. MHT should not be initiated after age 70 years. There is no mandatory time limit for duration of MHT considering the risk factors and also the necessity of treatment required. Although the protective effect of hormone therapy gradually declines after stopping hormone therapy but some effect may be there.[13] Therefore, while considering hormone therapy for the purpose of fracture prevention, long-term benefits and risks should be considered. It has been seen that the standard dosages of CEE and medroxyprogesterone acetate (MPA) are only effective in preventing fractures. In women with premature ovarian insufficiency, higher doses hormones are given. The recommended estrogen doses are: 17β-estradiol 2 mg/day or 1.25 mg conjugated equine estrogen (CEE) or transdermal estradiol 75–100 mg/day or 10 mg ethinylestradiol. The aim is to achieve the typical mean serum estradiol levels of approximately 100 pg/mL (400 pmol/L) in regularly menstruating women.

Bisphosphonates

Alendronate, risedronate, and ibandronate are commonly used for both prevention and treatment of osteoporosis. For maximum GI absorption and to reduce the incidence of esophageal irritation, alendronate must be taken in the morning on an empty stomach (½ hour before breakfast) with about 240 mL of plain water and the patient must remain upright for ½ hour after ingestion. Bisphosphonates in combination with estrogen are more effective than either agent alone. For prevention of osteoporosis, Alendronate is available as daily tablet of 5 mg and weekly tablet of 35 mg. For treatment of postmenopausal osteoporosis, alendronate is given in 10 mg daily dose and 70 mg weekly. Zoledronic acid is new drug approved by FDA. It has been seen that a single intravenous infusion of zoledronic acid 5 mg over 15-minute period once in a year decreases bone turnover and improves bone density in reducing fractures.

Tibolone is a synthetic preparation metabolized to molecules that have affinity for the estrogen, progesterone and androgen receptors and it has been evident from studies that it prevented vertebral and nonvertebral fractures.[14]

Calcium and Vitamin D

The daily requirement of calcium in postmenopausal women is 1000–1500 mg of elemental calcium daily. Calcium supplementation should be just adequate to meet the demand as its excessive intake may be associated with increased cardiovascular risk, renal calculi and constipation.[15] The daily intake of vitamin D should be 800–1000 IU in the postmenopausal period. As the major source of vitamin D is dependent on sunlight exposure, the need for supplementation may vary. In selected individuals, the measuring of the blood 25 hydroxyvitamin D level may be helpful in screening individuals for calcium deficiency.[16] Studies have shown that vitamin D supplementation has been shown independently to lower the risk of fracture and of falling in elderly patients.[17]

Selective Estrogen Receptor Modulators

The selective estrogen receptor modulators (SERMs), raloxifene and bazedoxifene, reduce vertebral fractures in postmenopausal women with or without vertebral fracture.[18] It has been seen that bazedoxifene prevents hip fracture in a select group of women at high risk of hip fracture. Raloxifene prevents ER positive breast cancer in osteoporotic women. The SERMs do not have effect on vasomotor symptoms associated with menopause. They have a favorable effect on lipid profile. History of venous thrombosis is an contraindication for their use. Raloxifene available as 60 mg tab/day for prevention as well as treatment.

Parathyroid Hormone

Parathyroid hormone (PTH) is an anabolic agent that significantly reduces risk of vertebral fractures by stimulation of bone formation. PTH is indicated for severe cases of osteoporosis or in patients who sustain fracture while on other forms of therapy. PTH is given as a daily subcutaneous injection for a maximum of 18 months. After this period, the use of an antiresorptive agent must be considered. The use of PTH is limited by its higher cost. Bisphosphonate therapy should not be given along with parathormone as it blunts the effect of latter. It is FDA approved.[19]

Strontium Ranelate

Treatment with strontium ranelate significantly reduces the risk of vertebral and nonvertebral fractures in osteoporotic patients, irrespective of the presence of a fracture or age. Studies have shown its adverse effect on cardiovascular profile, therefore, its use is limited to severe cases of osteoporosis in patients at low risk of cardiovascular disease.[16]

Denosumab

Denosumab is a human monoclonal antibody to the receptor activator of nuclear factor-kappa B ligand (RANKL). It is given at a dose of 60 mg subcutaneously 6-monthly, it significantly reduces the risk of vertebral, nonvertebral and hip fractures. Denosumab is generally safe and well-tolerated.[20]

Others

Exercises—weight bearing and resistance exercises should be done. Exercises for back muscles, at wrist, thigh and buttocks should be advised.

POSTMENOPAUSAL VULVOVAGINAL ATROPHY

Atrophic vaginitis is an inflammation which develops when there is a significant decrease in estrogen levels after menopause. The onset of symptoms may not be immediate and may take 3–4 years after menopause. A new definition for vulvovaginal atrophy (VVA) has been proposed named genitourinary syndrome of menopause (GSM) to describe more accurately the group of urogenital symptoms and signs associated with menopause and also to remove the negative stigma of atrophy.[21] Postmenopausal vaginal atrophy commonly causes distressing symptoms which severely affect quality of life but they can be easily treated.

Treatment should be started early, before irreversible atrophic changes occur, and the therapy has to be continued till the symptoms are there. The principles of treatment is to restore the urogenital physiology and removal of symptoms. Local estrogen treatment should be the first choice when VVA is the main symptom. The choice for local estrogen use should take into account various factors like preference of patient, such as ease of administration, dosage and cost of therapy. Estrogen creams are most economical and widely used. The estradiol tablets avoid the messiness of the cream and is preferred by some. The estradiol ring is long acting and does not need daily application but requires skill to insert and remove.

Local estrogen therapy minimizes the degree of systemic absorption and, although vaginal administration can increase plasma levels of estrogens during chronic administration, the observed levels are not above the normal range of <20 pg/mL for postmenopausal women. The adverse effects of vaginal estrogen are vaginal bleeding, breast pain, nausea and perineal pain. A cochrane review has shown no significant differences among the various delivery methods if we compare risk of hyperplasia, endometrial thickness and the other side effects.[22] Additional use of progestogen is not indicated when low-dose, local estrogen is used, although the data is not sufficient to prove this. If estrogen therapy is not effective or if patient not willing then vaginal lubricants and moisturizers can be used to relieve symptoms due to vaginal dryness. Sexual activity should be recommended on a regular basis.

Use of local estrogen treatment following breast and gynecological cancers: As the data on the use of vaginal estrogens in women with gynecological hormone-responsive cancers is less so they should be used carefully. A risk benefit analysis is needed in women with severe symptoms and they should be counseled for the same taking into account their individual risk factors. Those who want to avoid can use alternative therapy and if required, vaginal estrogens can be used at the lowest effective doses. Use of local estrogen in women on tamoxifen or aromatase inhibitors requires careful evaluation and discussion with the patient as efficacy of vaginal estrogen is decreased by tamoxifen.[5] Combination of bazedoxifene and conjugated estrogen is also effective in treating moderate to severe vaginal atrophy in patients developing side effects with the use of progestogens. Although this combination has been found to reduce breast density but data are not sufficient to confirm its effect on breast cancer incidence. Daily topical use of DHEA has been effective in the treatment of sexual symptoms especially in women where there is contraindication to hormone therapy.[23]

Ospemifene, an SERM recently approved drug at the dose of 60 mg orally. It is indicated for the systemic treatment of moderate to severe dyspareunia associated with VVA in women who are unable to tolerate to take local or systemic estrogens. It has also been found to be positive effective on other sexual symptoms. Another SERM, lasofoxifene, is under investigation.[24]

Systemic estrogen therapy is indicated when a women has other symptoms of menopause, like hot flushes which also need to be treated.

Local estrogen therapy—the various preparations available are equine estrogen, estriol and estradiol and available in the form of pessaries, creams or rings.

Intravaginal estradiol tablets: Containing 25 μg of estradiol to be used once a day for 2 weeks and thereafter inserted every 3 days high up in vagina for maintenance therapy.

Estriol vaginal suppository contains 3.5 g estriol.

Estrogen vaginal cream each gram of conjugated equine estrogen cream contains 0.625 mg to be given once daily to two or three times weekly.

Sustained-release intravaginal estradiol ring is a flexible silicon ring with an estradiol - loaded core containing 2 mg of micronized estradiol, and it releases 7.5 μg of estradiol every 24 hours over 3 months.

Nonhormonal Therapy

It is indicated where patients have mild symptoms and do not want to use hormonal therapy or when hormones are contraindicated. Lubricants are used to relieve the symptoms of vaginal dryness and may help to alleviate dyspareunia. However, the effects are temporary and often require repeated applications.

Vaginal moisturizers can be safely used long-term with no serious side effects, but they need to be used regularly for adequate effect.

Lifestyle modifications: Avoidance of smoking as smoking causes increased metabolization of estrogen and affects vaginal epithelium by increasing atrophic changes. Regular sexual activity and masturbation are known to decrease the incidence of vaginal atrophy, by increasing blood flow.

CARDIOVASCULAR DISEASE

Cardiovascular disease is the principal cause of morbidity and mortality in postmenopausal women. The incidence of cardiovascular disease (CVD) in Indian women has been noted to have significantly risen in recent time. The estimated deaths from cardiovascular diseases by 2020 would be 42% of the total deaths. The major primary prevention measures for cardiovascular disease are reducing obesity, blood pressure reduction, regular exercise, avoidance of smoking, diabetes control.[25] Hormone therapy has proved to be beneficial for improving the cardiovascular risk profile through its effects on vascular function, lipid levels and glucose metabolism. It has also been shown to reduce the incidence of new-onset diabetes mellitus.[26] There is strong and consistent evidence that estrogen therapy may be cardioprotective if started around the time of menopause (often referred to as the 'window of opportunity' or[6] 'timing' hypothesis), and may be harmful if started more than 10 years after menopause. In Women Health Initiative (WHI), the data has shown that in the age group 50–59 years, there was reduction of coronary artery disease and also risk of myocardial infarction was also much reduced.[27]

Coagulation, Venous Thromboembolism Disease and MHT

The risks of systemic estrogens are mainly venous thromboembolism events in recently postmenopausal women. This risk increases with age and also in the presence of other risk factors like obesity and thrombophilia. The studies have not found any increased risk of VTE with use of transdermal estrogen. In women at high VTE risk, it is better to use transdermal estrogen with progesterone. The risk of such events may also be affected by the type and duration of progestogen. Medroxyprogesterone acetate may be associated with greater risk when used in oral therapy. Continuous combined regimens are associated with higher risks than sequential regimens.

Venous Thrombosis (VTE) and Oral Estrogen with or without Progestogen

Various studies have shown that the incidence of VTE is higher during the first year of oral estrogen use, with or without progestogen.[28] Whether the type of estrogen molecule is associated with different levels of venous risk remains controversial. In recent study of oral hormone therapy users, conjugated equine estrogen (CEE) use was associated with a higher risk of incident VTE than estradiol use. These results need to be confirmed.

Cognitive Aging

It is well-known that estrogens play a important role in the neurobiology of cognitive functions. Although some studies have shown that certain forms of hormonal therapy are effective when started early during menopause transition, but they should not be used to enhance cognitive function. Estrogen therapy may be of short-term cognitive benefit to surgically menopausal women when initiated at the time of oophorectomy. In cases of Alzheimer's disease, hormone therapy does not benefit cognitive function or slow disease progression once the symptoms of dementia appear.[29] Other nonhormonal therapies like phytoestrogens supplements have no effect on cognition.

Other problem associated with menopause is of depression. For treatment of depression clozapine, imipramine, and amitriptyline should be avoided as they lead to weight gain.[8]

Weight gain at midlife can be managed by caloric restriction and maintenance of physical activity. With estrogen therapy, there is reduction in overall fat mass, improved insulin sensitivity and a lower rate of development of type 2 diabetes.

All women complaining of stress urinary incontinence will benefit from pelvic floor muscle training. The cases requiring drug therapy will benefit from duloxetine along with other conservative surgeries. Some women not responding to drugs may require surgery, and retropubic and transobturator tapes are currently the most popular procedures.

Cancers

The incidence of cancers in Indian women is rising. Most of the cancers occur in women between 36 and 65 years. The common cancers in women in India are breast, cervix, ovary, endometrium, oral cancer. For early diagnosis of breast cancer, all women should be told about the benefits of breast self-examination and to be supplemented with clinical breast examination by a health professional every year after the age of 40 years. In some instances, screening mammography may be advised before 40 years in women having high-risk factors of breast carcinoma.

Lifestyle Changes

There has been strong recommendation on lifestyle changes for menopausal age group. These are adequate exercise, taking diet rich in calcium, low fat and consumption of diet rich in phytoestrogens. These measures are to be started in childhood and continued lifelong. They have additional benefits on bone health, diabetes and cardiovascular diseases. Utilization of yoga and meditation has shown to be helpful in such cases.

For treatment of hot flashes avoidance of triggering factors like stress, caffeine, alcohol, spicy foods, beverages, staying in cold environment are helpful.

DIFFERENTIAL DIAGNOSIS

- There are multiple different etiologies for hot flushes apart from menopause, carcinoid syndrome is one that is essential to suspect and exclude given the underlying association with malignancy. This is associated with systemic symptoms and elevated levels of urinary 5-HIAA.
- Serum pooled prolactin levels are useful in differentiating hyperprolactinemia from menopause. After 1 to 3 years of menopause LH levels reach to over 30 IU/L.

MONITORING OR FOLLOW-UP

Women taking hormone therapy should have at least an annual consultation. This should include the following:
- Physical examination
- Medical and family history
- Relevant laboratory and imaging investigations
- Discussion on lifestyle
- Strategies to prevent or reduce chronic disease.

The most important sociomedical change of the present era has been the dramatic increase in life expectancy and the rise of older population. The menopause should be taken as a positive change and awareness should be spread regarding the benefits of lifestyle changes thus improving the quality of life.

KEY POINTS

The key principles are as follows:
- Informed consent should be done before starting hormone therapy. Women should be

told about the facts, need of therapy and new state of art therapies available to enable them to make proper choice.
- The risks and benefits of MHT vary widely in individual situations. Therefore, to have maximum benefits and to minimize risks, optimal regime to be selected at appropriate time.
- The safety of MHT largely depends on age and time since menopause.
- Menopause hormone therapy (MHT) should be given for the shortest period in the smallest doses possible for symptomatic relief only.
- Progestogens added to the MHT regimen largely eliminate any increased risk of endometrial cancer. In hysterectomized women only estrogen can be given.
- Studies have strongly suggested that it is the progestogen component of MHT that is more significant in any increase in breast cancer risk rather than the estrogen but this can be optimized with the use of modern progestogens, natural progesterone and SERMs.
- Recent randomized trials such as the Danish Osteoporosis Prevention Study (DOPS), Kronos Early Estrogen Prevention Study (KEEPS) and the Early versus Late Intervention Trial with Estradiol (ELITE) are now confirming the window of opportunity in early menopause when cardiovascular harm is avoided and benefits can be achieved.
- The various studies have shown that MHT has found to be very effective for primary prevention of fractures and coronary artery disease who initiate therapy around the time of menopause.

REFERENCES

1. Harlow SD, Gass M, Hall JE, et al. Executive Summary: Stages of Reproductive Aging Workshop+10: addressing the unfinished agenda of staging reproductive aging. Climacteric. 2012;15:105-14.
2. Kumar P, Malhotra N. Menopause. In: Jeffcoates (7th International ed). New Dellhi, India: Jaypee Brothers Medical Publishers; 2008.pp.862-63.
3. Sternfeld B, Wang H, Quesenberry CP Jr, et al. Physical activity and changes in weight and waist circumference in midlife women: findings from the Study of Women's Health Across the Nation. Am J Epidemiol. 2004;160:912-22.
4. Baber RJ, Panay N, Fenton A. The IMS Writing Group (2016) 2016 IMS Recommendations on women's midlife health and menopause hormone therapy, Climacteric. 2016;19:109-50.
5. The American College of Obstetricians and Gynecologists Practice Bulletin: Management of Menopausal Symptoms; No 141. 2014:123:202-16.
6. Honjo H, Taketani Y. Low-dose estradiol for climacteric symptoms in Japanese women: a randamised, controlled trial. Climacteric. 2009; 12:319-28.
7. Reddy SY, Warner H, Guttuso T Jr, et al. Gabapentin, estrogen, and placebo for treating hot flushes: a randomized controlled trial. Obstet Gynecol. 2006;108:41-8.
8. Joffe H, Guthrie KA, LaCroix AZ, et al. Low-dose estradiol and the serotonin-norepinephrine reuptake inhibitor venlafaxine for vasomotor symptoms: a randomized clinical trial. JAMA Intern Med. 2014;174:1058-66.
9. Loprinzi CL, Sloan J, Stearns V, et al. Newer antidepressants and gabapentin for hot flashes: an individual patient pooled analysis. J Clin Oncol. 2009;27:2831-7.
10. Rossouw JE, Anderson GL, Prentice RL, et al. Risks and benefits of estrogen plus progestin in healthy postmenopausal women: principal results from the Women's Health Initiative randomized controlled trial. JAMA. 2002;288:321-33.
11. deVilliers TJ, Gass MLS, Haines CJ, et al. Global Consensus Statement on Menopausal Hormone Therapy. Climacteric. 2013;16:203-4.
12. Bagger YZ, Tanko LB, Alexandersen P, et al. Two to three years of hormone replacement therapy in healthy women have long-term prevention effects on bone mass and osteoporotic fractures: the PERF study. Bone. 2004;34:728-31.
13. Shane E, Burr D, Abrahamsen B, et al. Atypical subtrochanteric and diaphyseal femoral fractures: Second Report of a Task Force of the American Society for Bone and Mineral Research. J Bone Miner Res. 2014;29:1-23.
14. Cummings SR, Ettinger B, Delmas PD, et al. For the LIFT Trial Investigators. The effects of tibolone in older postmenopausal women. N Engl J Med. 2008;359:697-708.

15. Bolland MJ, Avenell A, Baron JA, et al. Effect of calcium supplements on risk of myocardial infarction and cardiovascular events: meta-analysis. BMJ. 2010;341:c3691.
16. Recommendation to restrict the use of Protelos/Osseor (strontium ranelate). European Medicines Agency. EMA/258269/2013.
17. Bischoff-Ferrari HA, Dawson-Hughes B, Staehelin HB, et al. Fall prevention with supplemental and active forms of vitamin D: a meta-analysis of randomised controlled trials. Br Med J. 2009;339:b3692.
18. Ettinger B, Black DM, Mitlak BH, et al. Reduction of vertebral fracture risk in postmenopausal women with osteoporosis treated with raloxifene: results from a 3-year randomized clinical trial. Multiple Outcomes of Raloxifene Evaluation (MORE) Investigators. JAMA. 1999;282:637-45
19. Neer RM, Arnaud CD, Zanchetta JR, et al. Effect of parathyroid hormone (1-34) on fractures and bone mineral density in postmenopausal women with osteoporosis. N Engl J Med. 2001;344:1434-41.
20. Cummings SR, Martin JS, McClung MR, et al. Denosumab for prevention of fractures in postmenopausal women with osteoporosis. N Engl J Med. 2009;361:756-65.
21. Portman DJ, Gass ML. Vulvovaginal Atrophy Terminology Consensus Conference Panel. Genitourinary syndrome of menopause: new terminology for vulvovaginal atrophy from the International Society for the Study of Women's Sexual Health and the North American Menopause Society. Climacteric. 2014;17:557-63.
22. Sucklinng J, Kennedy R, Lethaby A, Roberts H. Local estrogen therapy for vaginal atrophy in postmenopausal women. Cochrane Database Syst Rev. 2006(4):CD 001500.
23. Archer DF, Labrie F, Bouchard C, et al. other participating members of the VVA Prasterone Group. Treatment of pain at sexual activity (dyspareunia) with intravaginal dehydroepiandrosterone (prasterone). Menopause. 2015;22:950-63.
24. Nappi RE, Panay N, Bruyniks N, Castelo-Branco C, de Villiers TJ, Simon JA. The clinical relevance of the effect of ospemifene on symptoms of vulvar and vaginal atrophy. Climacteric. 2015;18:233-40.
25. Maruthur NM, Wang NY, Appel LJ. Lifestyle interventions reduce coronary artery disease risk. Results from the PREMIER trial. Circulation. 2009;119:2026-31.
26. Lobo RA, Davis SR, de Villiers TJ, et al. Prevention of diseases after menopause. Climacteric. 2014;17:540-56.
27. Cushman M, Kuller LH, Prentice R, et al. Women's Health Initiative Investigators. Estrogen plus progestin and risk of venous thrombosis. JAMA. 2004;292:1573-80.
28. Smith NL, Blondon M, Wiggins KL, et al. Lower risk of cardiovascular events in postmenopausal women taking oral estradiol compared with oral conjugated equine estrogens. JAMA Intern Med. 2014;174:25-31.
29. Henderson VW. Alzheimer's disease: review of hormone therapy trials and implications for treatment and prevention after menopause. J Steroid Biochem Mol Biol. 2014;142:99-106.

SECTION 2

Benign Gynecological Diseases

Chapters

- Vaginal Discharge
- Pelvic Inflammatory Disease
- Genital Tuberculosis
- Viral Infections in Gynecology
- Abnormal Uterine Bleeding
- Fibroid Uterus
- Endometriosis and Adenomyosis
- Chronic Pelvic Pain
- Ectopic Pregnancy
- Amenorrhea
- Polycystic Ovary Syndrome
- Hirsutism
- Female Infertility
- Ovarian Stimulation Protocols in *In Vitro* Fertilization and Ovarian Hyperstimulation Syndrome
- Pelvic Organ Prolapse
- Urodynamics in Stress Urinary Incontinence
- Benign Adnexal Masses

7

Vaginal Discharge

Sangeeta Gupta, Bhavya Sareen

The most common gynecological complaint is vaginal discharge.[1] This discharge can vary from a physiological symptom to one which may indicate a severe ailment. The causes of vaginal discharge vary according to the age group of the patient (Table 7.1).

DIAGNOSTIC APPROACH TO VAGINAL DISCHARGE

Clinical Profile of the Patient

- *Age:* The causes of vaginal discharge vary according to age—prepubertal, reproductive or postmenopausal.[1,2]
- *Relevant history:* Information on sexual behaviors and practices, gender of sex partners, menses, vaginal hygiene practices (such as douching), and other medications should be elicited.
- *Pelvic examination:*[3]
  - *Nature of discharge:* Color, amount, consistency, blood stained or not
  - *Vulva:* Edema, erythema, ulcer or lesion
  - *Vagina:* Inflammation, growth
  - *Cervix:* Erosion, strawberry appearance, mucopurulent discharge, growth, consistency
  - *Uterus:* Size, consistency
  - *Adnexa:* Any mass, tenderness.

INVESTIGATIONS

Investigations should be advised depending on the basis of the history and examination findings
- *pH:*
  - Less than 4.5—physiological or candidiasis
  - Between 5 and 6—bacterial vaginosis or trichomonal vaginitis
  - More than 6—trichomonal vaginitis, atrophic vaginitis, genitourinary fistula, normal vagina in nonestrogenized state.
- *Amine test or whiff test*[4]*:* Fishy odor on addition of 10% potassium hydroxide (KOH) is diagnostic of bacterial vaginosis.
- *Wet smear*[4]*:* Add normal saline to the discharge and examine under microscope.
- *KOH smear*[4]*:* Add 10% KOH solution to the discharge and examine under microscope, presence of hyphae or pseudomycelia confirms *Candida vaginitis*.
- *Gram staining.*
- *Culture:* The patient should abstain from douching, intravaginal medication and intercourse prior to obtaining cultures.[4]
  - *Trichomonas vaginalis:* Culture is the gold standard for diagnosis. Special media like Feinberg-Whittington, Diamond's or Kupferberg's medium is required.
  - *Candida species:* The medium used is Sabouraud's agar. It is indicated when symptomatology persists but KOH smear

Table 7.1 Common causes of vaginal discharge

Etiology	Prepubertal	Reproductive years	Postmenopausal
Physiological (leukorrhea)	• Postnatal • Premenarchal	• Midcycle • Premenstrual	
Infections STDs	N. gonorrhoeae • C. trachomatis • Trichomonas vaginalis • HSV • Condyloma acuminata	• Trichomonas vaginalis • Bacterial vaginosis • N. gonorrhoeae • C. trachomatis • HSV • Condylomata acuminata • Genital ulcers	
Non-STDs	• Enterobius vermicularis • Shigellosis • Mixed enteric organisms • Streptococcal and staphylococcal • Candidiasis	• Candidiasis • PID • Tubo-ovarian abscess • Septic abortion • Puerperal sepsis	
Postoperative		• Cryotherapy • Uterine artery embolization	• Posthysterectomy vault sepsis
Malignancy of the genital tract	• Vaginal adenosis	• Cervical cancer	• Cervical cancer • Endometrial cancer • Vaginal cancer • Vulvar cancer • Fallopian tube cancer
Atrophic vaginitis		• Following castration/premature ovarian failure • Drugs: Danazol, GnRH analogs • Postpartum atrophic vaginitis	• Postmenopausal
Miscellaneous	• Ectopic ureter • Fistula • Meningocele	• Fibroid polyp • Vulvar dystrophy • Postradiation	• Vulvar dystrophy • Postradiation
Pyometra		• Endometritis • Cervical stenosis • Endometrial tuberculosis	• Senile endometritis • Endometrial or cervical cancer
Foreign body	+	+	+
Allergy, chemical irritants	+	+	+
Skin disorders	+	+	+

is negative before excluding fungal vulvovaginitis. It identifies the non-albicans species of *Candida*.[5]
- *N. gonorrhoeae:* It is a fastidious organism and requires Thayer-Martin culture medium for isolation. If special media is not available stuart medium should be used for transportation.
- Pus from pyometra can be sent for analysis of pyogenic organisms and Mycobacterium.
- *Endocervical smear:* To detect microscopic cervicitis by Gram staining and culture.
- *Stool examination:* Especially in prepubertal girls for pinworms or *Enterobius vermicularis*. Diagnosis is confirmed by demonstration of eggs collected on cellophane paper from the perineal area.
- *Urine sediments: T. vaginalis* microscopy and culture can be done. This specimen is preffered sample in males.
- *Immunological tests:* These are indicated in work-up of genital ulcers especially syphilis. For trichomonal and *Candida* infections ELISA and latex agglutination tests are still under research. Detection of viral antigens of HSV by ELISA and immunofluorescent technique is gaining popularity.
- *Molecular testing:* For gonorrhea, LCR (ligase chain reaction) and PCR (polymerase chain reaction) have promising results. PCR is a highly sensitive technique for detecting HSV and *Candida*.[6]
- *Pap smear:* The conventional role of pap smear is for screening of dysplasia and cervical cancer.
- *Colposcopy:* Indicated particularly in peri-menopausal patients with vaginal discharge to screen for malignancy of cervix.
- *Biopsy:* Taken from any apparent growth or suspicious area on the cervix, vagina or vulva. Endometrial aspiration or curettage is required when there is suspicion of endometrial or endocervical malignancy.
- *Imaging techniques:* Ultrasonography is of help in diagnosing pyometra or tubo-ovarian masses and to assess endometrial thickness and uterine size. Intravenom pyelogram (IVP) helps to diagnose ectopic ureter.

The CDC 2015[7] guidelines recommend the following clinical criteria for diagnosis of bacterial vaginosis. The presence of three of the following four criteria is necessary for diagnosis:
1. Homogeneous milky or creamy discharge.
2. Presence of clue cells on microscopic examination.
3. pH of secretions above 4.5
4. Fishy or amine odor with or without 10% KOH.

TREATMENT

The mainstay of management lies in identification of the cause and its treatment.

Nonspecific Vulvovaginitis

Caused by enteric organisms due to faulty wiping technique and fecal contamination of vulva and vagina, especially seen in prepubertal girls.
- *Treatment:*
  - Good hygiene
  - Cotton and loose fitting undergarments
  - Proper wiping technique of perineum (from front to back)
  - Avoid harsh soaps and bubble bath.

Trichomonal Vaginitis

CDC 2015[7] recommendations:
Metronidazole 2 g orally in a single dose
Or
Metronidazole 500 mg orally twice daily for 7 days
(Cure rates: 90–95%)
Or
Tinidazole 2 g orally single dose
(Cure rates: 86–100%)
No role of metronidazole gel in treatment of trichomonal vaginitis.
Treat the sex partners and observe the abstinence till both the patient and the sex partner are cured.

Treatment failure: Metronidazole 500 mg orally twice daily for 7 days.

Pregnancy: Metronidazole 2 g orally in a single dose.

HIV positive patients: Same treatment as for HIV negative cases (multidose regime better).

Vulvovaginal Candidiasis[8]

Features	Uncomplicated	Complicated
Severity	Mild or moderate	Severe
Frequency	Sporadic	Recurrent
Organism	*Candida albicans*	Nonalbicans
Host	Normal	Abnormal

CDC 2015[7] recommendations for uncomplicated vulvovaginal candidiasis (VVC):

Over-the-counter intravaginal[9] agents:
 Butoconazole 2% cream 5 g intravaginally for 3 days.
 OR
 Clotrimazole 1% cream 5 g intravaginally for 7–14 days.
 OR
 Clotrimazole 2% cream 5 g intravaginally for 3 days.
 OR
 Miconazole 2% cream 5 g intravaginally for 7 days.[10]
 OR
 Miconazole 4% cream 5 g intravaginally for 3 days.
 OR
 Miconazole 100 mg vaginal suppository, one suppository for 7 days.
 OR
 Miconazole 200 mg vaginal suppository, one suppository for 3 days.
 OR
 Miconazole 1,200 mg vaginal suppository, one suppository for 1 day.
 OR
 Tioconazole 6.5% ointment 5 g intravaginally in a single application.

Prescription Intravaginal Agents

 Butoconazole 2% cream (single dose bioadhesive product), 5 g intravaginally for 1 day.
 OR
 Nystatin 100,000-unit vaginal tablet, one tablet for 14 days.
 OR
 Terconazole 0.4% cream 5 g intravaginally for 7 days.
 OR
 Terconazole 0.8% cream 5 g intravaginally for 3 days.
 OR
 Terconazole 80 mg vaginal suppository, one suppository for 3 days.

Oral agent: Fluconazole 150 mg oral tablet, one tablet in single dose

CDC Recommendations for Complicated VVC

Recurrent VVC: Four or more episodes of VVC every year.[5,11] *C. glabrata* and other nonalbicans species are found in 10–20% of patients with recurrent VVC. Vaginal cultures are done. Recurrent VVC caused by *Candida albicans*.[12]

Initial therapy: Topical azole therapy for 7–14 days or oral dose of fluconazole repeated after 3 days.

Maintenance therapy: Given for 6 months.
 Clotrimazole 500 mg vaginal suppository once weekly or ketoconazole 100 mg once daily or fluconazole 100–150 mg once weekly or itraconazole 400 mg once monthly or 100 mg once daily.

Severe VVC: Topical azole for 7–14 days or fluconazole 150 mg in two sequential doses 72 hour apart.

Nonalbicans VVC: Optimal treatment remains unknown. Non-fluconazole azole drug for 7–14 days is recommended. If infection recurs 600 mg boric acid in gelatin capsule is administered vaginally daily for 2 weeks or topical 4% flucytosine once a day for 14 days or 100,000 units nystatin vaginal suppository daily.[13]

Compromised host[14]: Women with underlying debilitating disease like uncontrolled diabetes or corticosteroid therapy. Conventional antimycotics treatment for 7–14 days and correction of the underlying disorder is the usual treatment.

Recently it has been shown that vulvovaginal candidiasis in diabetic women is more often due to *C. glabrata* than *C. albicans* and only one-third of these patients respond to single dose 150 mg fluconazole. Boric acid 600 mg capsule placed intravaginally for 14 days is more effective in these cases.

Pregnancy: Topical azole for 7 days.[14,15]

HIV infection: Same regime as for seronegative women. Fluconazole 200 mg weekly in cases of recurrent VVC in HIV infected patients is recommended.

Besides the CDC recommendations, 1% aqueous gentian violet applied locally on vagina and perineum is an effective remedy *C. glabrata*, with the only disadvantage of staining undergarments.

Bacterial Vaginosis[16]

CDC 2015 recommendations in nonpregnant women
Metronidazole 500 mg orally 2 times a day for 7 days.
OR
Clindamycin cream 2% 5 g intravaginally twice a day for 7 days.
OR
Metronidazole gel 75% 5 g intravaginally twice a day for 5 days.

Alternative regime
Tinidazole 2 g orally once daily for 2 days
OR
Tinidazole 1 g orally once daily for 5 days.
OR
Clindamycin 300 mg orally twice daily for 7 days.
OR
Clindamycin ovules 100 mg intravaginally once at bedtime for 3 days.

Treatment of sex partners is not recommended.

CDC 2015 recommendations in pregnant women
All symptomatic pregnant women should be treated.

Women for high-risk at preterm labor are screened in second trimester and those with established diagnosis of bacterial vaginosis are treated.[17]

Recommended regime
Metronidazole 500 mg orally twice a day for 7 days.
OR
Metronidazole 250 mg orally three times a day for 7 days.
OR
Clindamycin 300 mg orally twice a day for 7 days.

Pyometra

It is drained by daily dilatation or dilatation followed by insertion of Foley's catheter or Malecot's catheter. Suitable antibiotic is administered to control the infection. The underlying pathology like malignancy, atrophic endometritis or tuberculosis, if present, has to be managed accordingly.

Atrophic Vaginitis

Estrogen is administered either locally or systemically. Estrogen cream is applied locally daily for one week and then twice weekly.

Pinworms

Oral mebendazole 100 mg single dose and repeat after 2 weeks.

Foreign Body

In the prepubertal girls small foreign body maybe lavaged from the vagina using a 5 mm irrigating endoscope or gentle irrigation with saline or water instilled through no. 12 urethral catheter or infant feeding tube. Larger foreign bodies warrant exploration and removal under general anesthesia.

Syndromic Management of Vaginal Discharge

In a low resource setting, like India where diagnostic facilities are not usually easily available, NACO has prescribed guidelines for syndromic management of vaginal discharge.[18] It includes:
- Diagnosis and treatment on symptoms
- Education on risk reduction
- Condom provision
- Counseling
- Partner notification
- Follow-up.

Recommended treatment
Azithromycin 2 g orally single dose under supervision
    Plus
    Metronidazole 2 g orally single dose
    Plus
    Fluconazole 150 mg orally single dose.

Vaginal discharge in prepubertal girls
The increased susceptibility of prepubertal girls to vulvovaginitis is attributed to the following:
- Unestrogenized thin vaginal mucosa
- Absence of acidic environment
- Lack of labial fat pad and pubic hair
- Proximity from anus to vagina.

Sexually transmitted disease in prepubertal girls[19] is associated with sexual abuse and the child should be investigated for other STDs.
- *N. gonorrhoeae:* In this age group, vagina is the site of infection (unlike cervix in adults).
- *Trichomonas vaginalis:* Rare in this age group as organism prefers estrogenic environment.

Non-STDs
- *Shigellosis:* Spreads through GIT infection. Diagnosis is confirmed by positive stool culture.
- *Respiratory pathogens:* Streptococcal and staphylococcal infections spread by manual transmission from the primary ear, nose and throat. Diagnosis is confirmed when vaginal cultures are positive for the same organisms identified in the primary infection site.
- *Candidiasis:* Uncommon in prepubescent females unless she has diabetes mellitus, recent antibiotic use or is immune-compromised.

Treatment: Topical antifungal cream for 10–14 days and remove the underlying cause.

LEUKORRHEA

It is an excessive normal discharge and has the following features:
- Vulvar moistness and staining of undergarments
- Non-irritant, non-foul smelling
- No pruritus.

Cause
Related to physiologically high estrogen levels.

Treatment
Reassurance, local hygiene, improvement of general health.

REFERENCES

1. Dai Q, Hu L, Jiang Y, Shi H, Liu J, Zhou W, Shen C, Yang H. An epidemiological survey of bacterial vaginosis, vulvovaginal candidiasis and trichomoniasis in the Tibetan area of Sichuan Province, China. Eur J Obstet Gynecol Reprod Biol. 2010;150(2):207-9.
2. Onyekonwu CL, Olumide YM, Oresanya FA, Onyekonwu GC. Vaginal discharge: aetiological agents and evaluation of syndromic management in Lagos. Niger J Med. 2011;20(1):155-62.
3. Quan M. Vaginitis: diagnosis and management. Postgrad Med. 2010;122(6):117-27.
4. Nenadić D, Pavlović MD. Value of bacterial culture of vaginal swabs in diagnosis of vaginal infections. Vojnosanit Pregl. 2015;72(6):523-8.
5. Sobel JD. Recurrent vulvovaginal candidiasis. Am J Obstet Gynecol. 2016;214(1):15-21. doi: 10.1016/j.ajog.2015.06.067. Epub 2015 Jul 9. Review.
6. Sobel JD, Akins RA. The role of PCR in the diagnosis of Candida vulvovaginitis-a new gold standard? Curr Infect Dis Rep. 2015;17(6):488.

7. Centers for Disease Control and Prevention. Sexually Transmitted Diseases Treatment Guidelines, 2015.
8. Mendling W, Brasch J, Cornely OA, Effendy I, Friese K, Ginter-Hanselmayer G, Hof H, Mayser P, Mylonas I, Ruhnke M, Schaller M, Weissenbacher ER. Guideline: Vulvovaginal candidosis (AWMF 015/072), S2k (excluding chronic mucocutaneous candidosis). Mycoses. 2015;58(Suppl 1):1-15. Erratum in: Mycoses. 2015;58(5):324.
9. Palmeira-de-Oliveira R, Palmeira-de-Oliveira A, Martinez-de-Oliveira J. New strategies for local treatment of vaginal infections. Adv Drug Deliv Rev. 2015;92:105-22.
10. Fan S, Liu X, Liang Y. Miconazole nitrate vaginal suppository 1,200 mg versus oral fluconazole 150 mg in treating severe vulvovaginal candidiasis. Gynecol Obstet Invest. 2015;80(2):113-8.
11. Dovnik A, Golle A, Novak D, Arko D, Takač I. Treatment of vulvovaginal candidiasis: a review of the literature. ActaDermatovenerol Alp Pannonica Adriat. 2015;24(1):5-7.
12. Boatto HF, Girão MJ, de Moraes MS, Francisco EC, Gompertz OF. The role of the symptomatic and asymptomatic sexual partners in the recurrent vulvovaginitis. Rev Bras Ginecol Obstet. 2015;37(7):314-8.
13. Powell AM, Gracely E, Nyirjesy P. Non-albicans Candida Vulvovaginitis: Treatment experience at a tertiary care vaginitis center. J Low Genit Tract Dis. 2016;20(1):85-9.
14. Mølgaard-Nielsen D, Svanström H, Melbye M, Hviid A, Pasternak B. Association between use of oral fluconazole during pregnancy and risk of spontaneous abortion and stillbirth. JAMA. 2016;315(1):58-67.
15. Mucci MJ, Cuestas ML, Cervetto MM, Landaburu MF, Mujica MT. A prospective observational study of vulvovagintis in pregnant women in Argentina, with special reference to candidiasis. Mycoses. 2016;59(7):429-35.
16. Romero Herrero D, Andreu Domingo A. Bacterial vaginosis. EnfermInfecc Microbiol Clin. 2016;34(Suppl 3):14-8.
17. Afolabi BB, Moses OE, Oduyebo OO. Bacterial vaginosis and pregnancy outcome in Lagos, Nigeria. Open Forum Infect Dis. 2016;3(1):11-22.
18. Sexually transmitted infections-treatment guidelines. NACO. http//www.nacoonline.org/publication/stiguideline.pdf.
19. Rahman G, Ocampo D, Rubinstein A, Risso P. Prevalence of vulvovaginitis and relation to physical findings in girls assessed for suspected child sexual abuse. Arch Argent Pediatr. 2015;113(5):390-6.

8
Pelvic Inflammatory Disease

Ashok Kumar, Gunjan Bhatnagar

INTRODUCTION

Pelvic inflammatory disease or pelvic inflammatory disorder (PID) is an *infection* of the upper part of the *female reproductive system* namely the *uterus, fallopian tubes, ovaries*, and the *pelvis*. It may include any combination of endometritis, salpingitis, tubo-ovarian abscess, and pelvic peritonitis.[1]

Pelvic inflammatory disease (PID) is has clinical significance in gynecology due to following reasons:
- Increasing prevalence in younger women
- Varying clinical manifestations
- Long-term sequelae.

More alarming is that untreated PID can result in long-term complications including infertility, ectopic pregnancy, chronic pelvic pain, and cancer.[2]

Pelvic inflammatory disease (PID) may produce tubo-ovarian abscess (TOA) and may progress to peritonitis and Fitz-Hugh-Curtis syndrome (perihepatitis).

Pelvic inflammatory disease (PID) is initiated by infection that ascends from the vagina and cervix into the upper genital tract. *Chlamydia trachomatis* and *Neisseria gonorrhoeae* are the predominant sexually transmitted organisms associated with PID. Contrary to the popular teaching, recent studies suggest that the proportion of PID cases attributable to *N. gonorrhoeae* or *C. trachomatis* is declining, of women who received a diagnosis of acute PID, <50% test positive for either of these organism.[3] Other organisms implicated in the pathogenesis of PID include *Gardnerella vaginalis, Haemophilus influenzae*, and Anaerobes such as *Peptococcus* and *Bacteroides* species. Laparoscopic studies have shown that in 30–40% of cases, PID is polymicrobial. In addition, cytomegalovirus (CMV), *Mycoplasma hominis, U. urealyticum*, and *M. genitalium* might be associated with some PID cases.

Newer data suggest that *M. genitalium* might play a role in the pathogenesis of PID and might be associated with milder symptoms, although one study failed to demonstrate a significant increase in PID following detection of *M. genitalium* in the lower genital tract.[4]

All women who receive a diagnosis of acute PID should be tested for human immunodeficiency virus (HIV), as well as gonorrhea and *Chlamydia*, using nucleic-acid amplification testing (NAAT).

The CDC has estimated that more than 1 million women experience an episode of PID every year.[5] No specific international data are available for PID incidence worldwide. In 2005, however, the World Health Organization (WHO) estimated that approximately 448 million new cases of curable sexually transmitted infections (STIs) occur annually in individuals aged 15–49 years.[6]

In India and other developing countries, the incidence of PID is much higher. Multiple reasons like poor sexual education and high prevalence of sexually transmitted diseases (STDs), illegal abortions, puerperal sepsis and low awareness about contraceptive usage increase the risk of PID. Studies have reported prevalence ranging from 5.2% to 17.2% PID in various parts of country.[7]

CLINICAL PRESENTATION

The diagnosis of acute PID is primarily based on historical and clinical findings. Clinical manifestations of PID vary widely, however: many patients exhibit few or no symptoms, whereas others have acute, serious illness.

A low threshold should be used for the diagnosis of PID.

Symptoms include
- Abnormal vaginal discharge
- Pain in the lower abdomen (often a mild ache)
- Pain in the upper right abdomen
- Abnormal menstrual bleeding
- Fever and chills
- Painful urination
- Nausea and vomiting
- Painful sexual intercourse.

Signs

Centers for Disease Control and Prevention (CDC) guidelines for PID 2015 state that presumptive treatment for PID should be initiated in sexually active young women and other women at risk for STDs if they are experiencing pelvic or lower abdominal pain, no other cause for the illness can be identified other than PID and if one or more of the following minimum clinical criteria are present on pelvic examination:
- Cervical motion tenderness
- Uterine tenderness
- Adnexal tenderness.

One or more of the further given additional criteria can be used to enhance the specificity of the minimum clinical criteria and support a diagnosis of PID:

- Oral temperature >101°F (>38.3°C);
- Abnormal cervical mucopurulent discharge or cervical friability;
- Presence of abundant numbers of white blood cell (WBC) on saline microscopy of vaginal fluid;
- Elevated erythrocyte sedimentation rate;
- Elevated C-reactive protein; and
- Laboratory documentation of cervical infection with *N. gonorrhoeae* or *C. trachomatis*.

The most specific criteria for diagnosing PID include:
- Endometrial biopsy with histopathologic evidence of endometritis;
- Transvaginal sonography or magnetic resonance imaging techniques showing thickened, fluid-filled tubes with or without free pelvic fluid or tubo-ovarian complex, or Doppler studies suggesting pelvic infection (e.g. tubal hyperemia); or
- Laparoscopic findings consistent with PID.

Laparoscopy is the current criterion standard for the diagnosis of PID. Clinical diagnosis of symptomatic PID has a positive predictive value (PPV) for salpingitis of 65–90% compared with laparoscopy.[8] However, this diagnostic tool frequently is not readily available, and its use is not easily justifiable when symptoms are mild or vague.

DIFFERENCE BETWEEN ACUTE AND CHRONIC PELVIC INFLAMMATORY DISORDERS

Chronic PID often causes vague symptoms that may be present for months or years. The symptoms are mild and may disappear in a few days. In a few weeks the symptoms recur, and they may continue recurring off and on for years. Chronic PID is accompanied by the following signs and symptoms:
- Mild, recurrent pain in the lower abdomen
- Backache
- Irregular menstrual periods
- Pain during intercourse
- Infertility
- Heavy, unpleasant smelling vaginal discharge
- Abnormal uterine bleeding.

Acute PID means an active infection is present and causing severe symptoms. Acute PID is accompanied by the following signs and symptoms:
- Pain and tenderness in lower abdomen
- Vaginal discharge
- Fixed retroversion of uterus
- Adnexal tenderness and thickening
- Parametrial fibrosis
- Adnexal mass.

DIFFERENTIAL DIAGNOSIS

The differential diagnosis includes appendicitis, cervicitis, urinary tract infection, endometriosis, and adnexal tumors. Ectopic pregnancy can be mistaken for PID. Hence, a pregnancy test is mandatory in the work-up of women of child-bearing age who have lower abdominal pain.

Grading of Acute PID

Grade 1: Uncomplicated—limited to tubes ± peritonitis.

Grade 2: Complicated—with inflammatory mass ± peritonitis.

Grade 3: Spread to structures beyond pelvis, to mass or abscess.

TREATMENT

In women with PID of mild or moderate clinical severity, outpatient therapy yields short- and long-term clinical outcomes similar to inpatient therapy. The decision for hospitalization is based on the clinical scenario and whether the patient meets any of the following suggested criteria:
CDC 2015 criteria for hospitalization:
- Surgical emergencies (e.g. appendicitis) cannot be excluded;
- The patient is pregnant;
- The patient does not respond clinically to oral antimicrobial therapy;
- The patient is unable to follow or tolerate an outpatient oral regimen;
- The patient has severe illness, nausea and vomiting, or high fever; or
- The patient has a tubo-ovarian abscess.

Intramuscular/Oral Treatment

Intramuscular/oral therapy can be considered for women with mild-to-moderately severe acute PID, because the clinical outcomes among women treated with these regimens are similar to those treated with intravenous therapy. Failure to respond to IM/oral therapy within 72 hours warrants re-evaluation to confirm the diagnosis and intravenous therapy.

Recommended Intramuscular/ Oral Regimens

Ceftriaxone 250 mg IM in a single dose
- Plus doxycycline 100 mg orally twice a day for 14 days
- With or without metronidazole 500 mg orally twice a day for 14 days; or Cefoxitin 2 g IM in a single dose and Probenecid, 1 g orally administered concurrently in a single dose.
- Plus Doxycycline 100 mg orally twice a day for 14 days
- With or without metronidazole 500 mg orally twice a day for 14 days; or Other parenteral third-generation cephalosporin (e.g. ceftizoxime or cefotaxime)
- Plus Doxycycline 100 mg orally twice a day for 14 days.
- With or without metronidazole 500 mg orally twice a day for 14 days.

Alternative Oral Regimens

Azithromycin is effective when used as monotherapy (500 mg IV daily for 1–2 doses, followed by 250 mg orally daily for 12–14 days) or in combination with metronidazole.[9]

Or

1 g orally once a week for 2 weeks in combination with ceftriaxone 250 mg IM single dose.[10]

As a result of the emergence of quinolone-resistant *N. gonorrhoeae*, regimens that include a quinolone agent are no longer routinely recommended for the treatment of PID. Use of fluoroquinolones for 14 days:
- Levofloxacin 500 mg orally once daily; or
- Ofloxacin 400 mg twice daily; or moxifloxacin 400 mg orally once daily.

With metronidazole for 14 days (500 mg orally twice daily) can be considered if patient is allergic to first line of drugs and community prevalence of *Gonococcus* is low.[11]

Recommended Parenteral Regimens

Parenteral treatment is usually required in severe cases for 24–48 hours following which transition to oral therapy, can usually be initiated if there is clinical improvement. In women with tubo-ovarian abscesses, at least 24 hours of inpatient observation is recommended.

Regimens

Cefotetan 2 g IV every 12 hours
- Plus doxycycline 100 mg orally or IV every 12 hours; or

Cefoxitin 2 g IV every 6 hours
- Plus doxycycline 100 mg orally or IV every 12 hours; or
- Clindamycin 900 mg IV every 8 hours

Plus gentamicin loading dose IV or IM (2 mg/kg), followed by a maintenance dose (1.5 mg/kg) every 8 hours. Single daily dosing (3–5 mg/kg) can be substituted.

Doxycycline should be administered orally when possible as IV injections are painful. Oral and IV administration of doxycycline provide similar bioavailability.

When using the parenteral cefotetan or cefoxitin regimens, oral therapy with doxycycline 100 mg twice daily can be used 24–48 hours after clinical improvement to complete the 14 days of therapy.

For the clindamycin/gentamicin regimen, oral therapy with clindamycin (450 mg orally four times daily) or doxycycline (100 mg twice daily) can be used to complete the 14 days of therapy.

However, when tubo-ovarian abscess is present, clindamycin (450 mg orally four times daily) or metronidazole (500 mg twice daily) should be used to complete at least 14 days of therapy with doxycycline to provide more effective anaerobic coverage than doxycycline alone.

Alternative Parenteral Regimen

Ampicillin/sulbactam 3 g IV every 6 hours
Plus Doxycycline 100 mg orally or IV every 12 hours.

Ampicillin/sulbactam plus doxycycline is effective against *C. trachomatis*, *N. gonorrhoeae*, and anaerobes in women with tubo-ovarian abscess.

Surgical Intervention in Acute PID

Indications of surgery
- Ruptured pelvic abscess
- Adhesions—intestinal obstruction/general peritonitis.
- Failed response to medical treatment in cases of tubo-ovarian masses.
- Uncertain diagnosis as when suspecting a malignancy.

Types of Surgery

Colpotomy for drainage of pelvic abscess.

The requirements for colpotomy drainage are following:
- Midline pelvic abscess (Approachable from pouch of Douglas)
- Abscess should be adhered to cut de sac peritoneum and should dissect the rectovaginal septum.
- Cystic or fluctuant abscess.

The colpotomy can be done under local anesthesia or intravenous sedation. Use of corrugated drain or Malecot's tube is advised to prevent collapse and incomplete drainage.

Percutaneous Drainage/Aspiration

Transabdominal ultrasonographic guided aspiration of abscess can be done if it is single. Commonly, aspiration is done to confirm that it is abscess. Multiloculated or pyoperitoneum require laparotomy.

Exploratory laparotomy and direct drainage.

Extent of Surgeries

- Conservative—if fertility desired
- U/L or B/L Salpingo-oophorectomy with/without hysterectomy
- Drainage of abscess at laparotomy.

Complications during Surgery

During operation
- Septic shock
- Injury to small bowel or rectum
- Injury to bladder.

Postoperative
- Repeated pus collection
- Chest empyema
- Septicemia
- Septic shock
- Recto-vaginal fistula
- Wound abscess or infection
- Pneumonia
- Renal failure
- Liver failure.

Role of Laparoscopy

It has a role in chronic PID but limited role in acute PID. Incidental finding of PID is noticed during diagnostic laparoscopy performed for infertility.

Laparoscopic grading of salpingitis
- *Mild:* Hyperemic, mobile tubes, no purulent exudate from fimbrial end.
- *Moderate:* Edematous tubes with purulent exudates from fimbria or adherent fimbria.
- *Severe:* Pyosalpinx, inflammatory tubo-ovarian mass or abscess.

FOLLOW-UP

Women should demonstrate clinical improvement (e.g. defervescence; reduction in direct or rebound abdominal tenderness; and reduction in uterine, adnexal, and cervical motion tenderness) within 3 days after initiation of therapy. If no clinical improvement has occurred within 72 hours after outpatient IM/oral therapy, hospitalization, assessment of the antimicrobial regimen and additional diagnostics (including consideration of diagnostic laparoscopy for alternative diagnoses) are recommended.

All women who have received a diagnosis of chlamydial or gonococcal PID should be retested 3 months after treatment, regardless of whether their sex partners were treated. If retesting at 3 months is not possible, they should be retested whenever they next present for medical care in the 12 months following treatment.

PELVIC INFLAMMATORY DISEASE PREVENTION

- Use of barrier contraceptives, even if other methods of birth control are used.
- Avoiding multiple sexual partners.
- Abstaining from sexual intercourse until therapy is completed, symptoms have resolved and sex partners have been adequately treated.

KEY POINTS

- Pelvic infection is one of the most common causes of morbidity in young women.
- Results in short-term physical pain and psychological stress and in the long-term, causes chronic pelvic pain, ectopic pregnancy and infertility.
- *Chlamydia trachomatis* and *Neisseria gonorrhoeae* are the two mainly implicated organisms.
- Recurrent and resistant cases must point towards atypical causes like HIV and genital tuberculosis.

REFERENCES

1. Wiesenfeld HC, Sweet RL, Ness RB, et al. Comparison of acute and subclinical pelvic inflammatory disease. Sex Transm Dis 2005;32: 400-5.
2. Mitchell C, Prabhu M. Pelvic inflammatory disease: current concepts in pathogenesis, diagnosis and treatment. Infect Dis Clin North Am. 2013;27(4): 793-809.
3. Cohen CR, Mugo NR, Astete SG, et al. Detection of Mycoplasma genitalium in women with laparoscopically diagnosed acute salpingitis. Sex Transm Infect. 2005;81:463-6.
4. Bjartling C, Osser S, Persson K. Mycoplasma genitalium in cervicitis and pelvic inflammatory disease among women at a gynecologic outpatient service. Am J Obstet Gynecol. 2012;206:e471-8.
5. Ness RB, Smith KJ, Chang CC, Schisterman EF, Bass DC. Prediction of pelvic inflammatory disease among young, single, sexually active women. Sex Transm Dis. 2006;33(3):137-42.
6. World Health Organization. Sexually transmitted infections. Available at *http://www.who.int/mediacentre/factsheets/fs110/en/*. Accessed: February 2, 2010.
7. Bhatia. Self reported symptom of gynecological morbidity and their treatment in India. Studies in Family Planning. 1994;26(4).
8. Gaitan H, Angel E, Diaz R, et al. Accuracy of five different diagnostic techniques in mild-to-moderate pelvic inflammatory disease. Infect Dis Obstet Gynecol. 2002;10:171-80.
9. Bevan CD, Ridgway GL, Rothermel CD. Efficacy and safety of azithromycin as monotherapy or combined with metronidazole compared with two standard multidrug regimens for the treatment of acute pelvic inflammatory disease. J Int Med Res. 2003;31:45-54.
10. Savaris RF, Teixeira LM, Torres TG, et al. Comparing ceftriaxone plus azithromycin or doxycycline for pelvic inflammatory disease: a randomized controlled trial. Obstet Gynecol. 2007;110:53-60.
11. Heystek M, Ross JD. A randomized double-blind comparison of moxifloxacin and doxycycline/metronidazole/ciprofloxacin in the treatment of acute, uncomplicated pelvic inflammatory disease. International Journal of STD and AIDS. 2009;20:690-5.

9

Genital Tuberculosis

Pushpa Mishra, Nupur Ahuja, Deepali Dhingra

INTRODUCTION

Tuberculosis continues to be a major health problem throughout the world affecting about 9.4 million people annually with about two million deaths.[1]

India is a country with one of the highest burden of tuberculosis (TB) accounting for one fifth of the global incidence annually. Although pulmonary TB is the primary and the most common presentation of tuberculosis, there are a significant number of cases of extra-pulmonary TB reported annually. Among these, tubercular meningitis is the gravest manifestation while female genital tract TB poses a diagnostic challenge.

The actual incidence of genital TB cannot be determined accurately in any population because it is estimated that at least 11% of patients are asymptomatic and the disease is discovered incidentally. Genital TB affects about 12% of patients with pulmonary tuberculosis and represents 15–20% of extrapulmonary tuberculosis.[2] The incidence is very high in women seeking assisted reproduction being 24.5% overall but as high as 48.5% with tubal factor infertility.[3]

PATHOGENESIS

Mycobacterium tuberculosis accounts for 90–95% of cases of genital TB. However, *Mycobacterium bovis* may be the causal agent (5–10%), especially when the organisms are acquired from the gastrointestinal tract.[4] Predisposing factors for TB include factors reducing personal immunity like poverty, overcrowding with improper ventilation, inadequate access to health care, malnutrition, diabetes mellitus, smoking, alcohol and drug abuse, end-stage renal disease, cancer treatment, hemodialysis patients and patient with HIV infection.

MODE OF SPREAD

Tuberculosis of the female genital tract is nearly always secondary to a focus elsewhere in the body. The TB bacilli reach the genital tract by three principal routes.
1. Hematogenous spread represents about 90% of cases, with the primary focus being the lungs, lymph nodes or skeletal system.
2. Descending direct spread occurs, with infection reaching the genital organs via the lymphatic system or directly from the gastrointestinal tract, mesenteric nodes or the peritoneum.
3. Primary infection of the vulva, vagina and cervix may result from direct inoculation at sexual intercourse with persons having genitourinary TB. Ascending spread of infection from the vagina, cervix and the vulva may occur.

If the primary infection occurs close to the time of menarche, there is an increased likelihood of genital tract involvement.

Tuberculosis of Fallopian Tubes

Hematogenous spread of TB bacilli to the tubes results in involvement of the submucosa (endosalpingitis) at the outer ends with gradual spread medially to the endometrium. Direct spread of infection to the fallopian tubes results in exosalpingitis with tubercles on the surface. During active infection they appear red and edematous and in chronic infection they appear fibrosed. In more than 90% of patients with genital TB, the tubes are involved bilaterally. Although only one tube appears infected, there probably are microscopic lesions in the other. The gross appearance varies and is nondiagnostic. In the early stages, the tubes show little change, but as progression occurs, the diameter of the tube becomes larger. The ampullary region shows the earliest and most extensive changes and the fimbrial processes become greatly swollen. In 25-50% of cases of genital TB, the tubes remain patent with recognizable everted fimbriae, even if the remaining tube is enlarged and distended, the so-called tobacco-pouch appearance. The peritoneal surfaces of the tubes can be studded with tubercles. Tubal obstruction may result in pyosalpinx or hydrosalpinx.

Tuberculosis of Endometrium

Grossly, the endometrium appears unremarkable in most cases, probably because of the cyclic menstrual shedding. The myometrium is not usually involved. Most extensive areas are present areas at the fundus and decrease towards the cervix. When extensive involvement of the endometrium occurs, ulcerative, granular or fungating lesions are present in endometrial cavity or it may be obliterated with intrauterine adhesions. Total destruction of the endometrium with resulting amenorrhea secondary to end-organ failure and predisposition to pyometra is there if the internal os becomes occluded.[5]

Tuberculosis of Ovaries

The tough tunica albuginea protects the ovaries from infection, hence, there is less frequent involvement of the ovary compared with the tube. Extension of the lesion spreads from the periphery towards the center of the ovary.

CLINICAL PRESENTATION

The clinical diagnosis of genital TB requires a high index of suspicion. About 20% of patients with genital TB give a history of TB in their immediate family. Approximately 50% of patients might have had tuberculous pleurisy, peritonitis or renal, osseous, or pulmonary TB. Although genital TB can occur in any age group, the majority of patients are in the reproductive age group, 75% being in the 20-45 years of age. Postmenopausal women account for 7-11% of cases of genital TB.[6]

Genital TB may be asymptomatic and the majority of women are diagnosed during investigations for infertility. Genital TB may present with a variety of gynecological symptoms of infertility, menstrual disturbance and chronic pelvic pain (Fig. 9.1).[6,7] In the postmenopausal woman, genital TB presents with postmenopausal bleeding, persistent leukorrhea and pyometra. Tuberculous lesions of the cervix present with postcoital bleeding, abnormal discharge and on examination, have appearances similar to cancer of the cervix. Lesions on the vulva appear as shallow ulcers, which may be painful, especially with secondary bacterial infection. Vaginal lesions are often painless and are usually sited at the introitus. Both can result in blood stained purulent discharge and may be identified as sexually transmitted infection. The Bartholin's gland may be affected, presenting with pain and

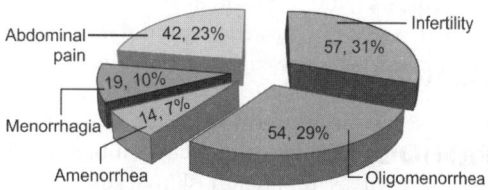

Fig. 9.1 Clinical presentation

fistula formation despite adequate antibiotic cover. Involvement of the ovaries may result in an adnexal ovarian mass. Fistula formation to the bowel, skin or vagina may be seen. Peritoneal involvement may give rise to ascites. This, in addition to an adnexal mass and a raised serum CA125 level, can be mistaken for ovarian cancer and can result in unnecessary surgical intervention.

Tuberculosis in Infertility Patients

Genital tuberculosis is a major risk factor leading to infertility and the infection can be silent without causing any signs or symptoms at all. Therefore, investigations for tuberculosis should be carried out in the initial stages of management of infertility.

DIAGNOSIS

As the clinical presentation of genital tuberculosis is nonspecific, the care provider should have a high suspicion for diagnosing tuberculosis due to its endemic existence in the country. Failure to respond to routine medical management for various gynecological symptoms should raise the suspicion of tuberculosis.

INDIRECT TESTS

These tests provide an indirect evidence of acute or chronic infection necessitating the need for further investigations.

Routine Tests

- Complete blood count
- Erythrocyte sedimentation rate
- Chest X-ray PA view for evidence healed or active TB.

Mantoux Test

This test has been used worldwide as an aid to diagnose both latent and active tuberculosis. Also termed as tuberculin skin testing (TST), i.e. intradermal injection of purified protein derivative (PPD) of tuberculin. An induration of >15 mm is considered as positive with no risk factors.[8] A positive result increases the risk of current and future risk of tuberculosis. However, a positive test is to be interpreted with prior history of BCG vaccination as tuberculin share common antigens with BCG.[9] False negative results are observed in the setting of immunosuppression, liver disease and malignancy. Sensitivity of Mantoux test is 55% and specificity is 80% in laparoscopically diagnosed tuberculosis.

Interferon Gamma Release Assays (IGRAs)

Interferon gamma (IFN-γ) is recognized now to play important role in mounting cell mediated immunity (CMI) against *Mycobacterium tuberculosis*. So assays detecting interferon gamma were developed. Initially QuantiFERON test was developed in 2002 and later QuantiFERON-TB Gold test (QFT-G) was developed in 2005. Later to improve specificity QuantiFERON-TB Gold In-Tube test (QFT-GIT) and the T-SPOT. TB test (T-Spot) were developed to improve specificity in 2008. All these tests are approved by FDA as indirect tests for detection of *M. tuberculosis* infection and should be used in conjunction with risk factors for disease, chest X-ray, and other tests for detection of tuberculosis.[10,11] The antigens used in IGRTs is absent in BCG strain and most nontubercular mycobacteria.

DIRECT TESTS

Microscopy

Endometrial biopsy specimens taken in premenstrual period is collected and sent for histopathology in formalin and AFB smear examination. In unmarried females presenting with symptoms of tuberculosis, menstrual blood is taken on the first day, can be sent for histopathology and PCR. Presence of caseating granulomas, lymphocytes, giant cells, plasma cells and epithelioid cells are diagnostic of tuberculosis. Staining with Ziehl-Neelsen stain for examination of acid-fast bacilli (AFB) may provide rapid diagnosis but requires the large amount of bacilli in a given sample. Detection rate by AFB smear range from 0.4% to 2.5%.[12,13]

Culture

Gold standard for diagnosing tuberculosis is culture on Lowenstein-Jensen (LJ) media. It requires culture for nearly 4–5 weeks. If the bacillary count is near 1000 bacilli colonies can be seen. With improvements in media conditions colonies can be grown when the count is near 100 bacilli. Use of radiometric growth detection in liquid based cultures such as BACTEC 460 or nonradiometric CO_2 growth detection with BACTEC ALERT 3D has reduced culture time to 2 weeks. As genital tuberculosis is paucibacillary these methods have limitations and sensitivity of around 30–35%.[14]

PCR-Based Rapid Detection of *Mycobacterium tuberculosis*

Polymerase chain reaction (PCR) is rapid technique for diagnosis of both pulmonary and extrapulmonary tuberculosis. PCR is highly specific and sensitive to diagnose mycobacteria. It can detect as low as 10 bacilli per mL in specimen and results are obtained within a day. DNA is extracted from specimen and specific gene is identified and amplified to be detected. False negative result is obtained because of contamination of sample with blood and heparin, both of which act as PCR inhibitor. It has high sensitivity (83–100%), positive predictive value (94–100%), and negative predictive value (96–100%).[15-17] Recently menstrual blood is gaining popularity as noninvasive, quick painless method to replace tissue samples.[18] But false negatives are high as blood is thought to be PCR inhibitor. Further large scale studies are needed to replace tissue samples from endometrial biopsy with menstrual blood. The sensitivity approaches 95% PCR for AFB smear-positive patients and 48% for smear negative patients.[18]

Hysterosalpinography

As a part of infertility work-up hysterosalpinography (HSG) is done to evaluate patency of tubes. It should be performed after ruling out tuberculosis on endometrial sample to avoid flare of the disease.

Some findings on HSG raise the suspicion of genital tuberculosis. Tuberculous salpingitis leads to edematous thickening of the tubal walls and later tubal dilatation. It manifests as hydrosalpinx, i.e. dilated or tortuous tubes. It may or may not be associated with tubal patency. Tubes are crowded, dilated and folded upon themselves giving corkscrew appearance. As the disease progresses, it leads to fibrosis and scarring which appears as alternate areas of constriction and terminal dilatation seen as beaded appearance on HSG. Peritubal adhesions are seen following multiple episodes of acute salpingitis. They are seen as loculated spill of contrast and "halo sign" which is seen in between hydrosalpinx and loculated spill, which is actually thickened wall of tube. Tubercular endometritis is seen as deformed countour of uterine cavity. Fibrosis and scarring leads to uterine adhesions, which are seen as irregular filling defects on HSG.

Ultrasonography

On ultrasonography, hydrosalpinx is seen as anechoic oblong cystic mass near the ovary or if internal echoes are present suggests pyosalpinx. The thickened mucosal folds produce the appearance of incomplete septa. In cross-section, it appears as the "cogwheel sign." Tubo-ovarian mass presents as heterogeneous complex mass on ultrasonography.

Role of Endoscopy in Genital Tuberculosis

In patients presenting with infertility, diagnostic and operative hysterolaparoscopy is performed to access uterine, tubal and peritoneal status as well as to identify evidence suggestive of tuberculosis, endometriosis, adenomyosis or any other pathology leading to infertility.

When the diagnosis of pelvic tuberculosis cannot be made by other ways, laparoscopy can be used. It should be done with particular care because numerous adhesions may be present making the introduction of trochar hazardous. Biopsy specimen from tubal fimbriae or other suspicious areas should be obtained.

Hysteroscopy

Endoscopic visualization of the uterine cavity in may show a normal cavity (if no endometrial TB or early stage TB) with bilateral open ostia. More often, however, following findings can be observed:
- Pale looking endometrium
- Partially or completely obliterated cavity by adhesions
- Fibrosis of ostia
- Small shrunken cavity
- Increased difficulty to distend the cavity
- Increased chances of complications like excessive bleeding, perforation and flare-up of genital TB.

Laparoscopy

- Tubercles on the peritoneal surface
- Inflamed or blue-colored uterus
- Salpingitis, oophoritis or a tubo-ovarian mass
- Tubal occlusion with hydrosalpinx
- Dye dripping (instead of free flowing) from the fimbreal opening on
- Chromopertubation
- Free peritoneal fluid looking like blood
- Caseation in the Pouch of Douglas
- Frozen pelvis
- Omental adhesions.

MANAGEMENT

Antitubercular Treatment

Female genital tuberculosis comes under WHO category 1 being seriously ill extrapulmonary. It is given as four drugs, i.e. isoniazid (H), rifampicin (R), pyrazinamide (Z) and ethambutol (E), daily or thrice a week for two months (intensive phase) and isoniazid (H), rifampicin (R) for four months daily or thrice a week. In directly observed treatment, (DOTS) short course therapy, fixed dose combipacks are given thrice a week.

Role of Surgery in Genital Tuberculosis

Surgery is reserved for patients who have an adequate trial of medical therapy, which includes the following:[19]
- Persistence or enlargement of an adnexal mass after 4–6 months of antitubercular therapy, though the rare possibility of an ovarian tumor must also always be considered.
- Persistence of pelvic pain or recurrence of pelvic pain while on medical therapy.
- Primary unresponsiveness of the tuberculous infection to antibiotic therapy, as shown by persistent spiking temperature, leukocytosis, elevated ESR and evidence on biopsy of continued endometrial infection.
- Difficulty in obtaining patient cooperation for continued long-term therapy. In these cases, a brief course of streptomycin, 0.5 g every 12 hours intramuscularly for 1 week before surgery is given, followed by 0.5 g every 24 hours for 2 weeks in the postoperative period.

The preferred surgical treatment includes total abdominal hysterectomy with bilateral salpingo-oophorectomy. The nature of this inflammatory disease may make this operative procedure difficult, with an increased risk of bladder and bowel injury. Consequently in the event of frozen pelvis, it is necessary to perform a subtotal hysterectomy and adnexectomy.

Conservation of an ovary at the time of operation for pelvic surgery is occasionally done if the ovary is involved only on its surface.

FERTILITY PROGNOSIS

Genital tuberculosis leads to permanent scarring and damage to fallopian tubes. IVF-ET remains the only option for these patients. If tubercular endometritis is present prognosis is poor as the cavity becomes narrow and shrunken and gestational surrogacy or adoption is only treatment option.

KEY NOTES

- India is a country with one of the highest burden of tuberculosis accounting for one fifth of the global incidence annually.
- The clinical diagnosis of genital TB requires a high index of suspicion.
- Genital TB may be asymptomatic and the majority of women are diagnosed during investigations for infertility.
- Failure to respond to routine medical management for various gynecological symptoms should raise the suspicion of tuberculosis.
- Gold standard for diagnosing tuberculosis is culture on Lowenstein-Jensen (LJ) media.
- Female genital tuberculosis comes under WHO category 1 extra-pulmonary.
- Failure of an adequate trial of medical therapy is an indication for surgery which involves total abdominal hysterectomy with bilateral salpingo-oophorectomy.

REFERENCES

1. World Health Organization. Global tuberculosis control: a short update to the 2009 report. WHO/HTM/TB 2009, 426. Geneva: WHO; 2009.
2. Aka N, Vural TZE. Evaluation of patients with active pulmonary tuberculosis for genital involvement. J Obstet Gynaecol Res. 1997;23:337-40.
3. Singh N, Sumana G, Mittal S. Genital tuberculosis: a leading cause for infertility in women seeking assisted conception in North India. Arch Gynecol Obstet. 2008;278:325-7.
4. Haas DW. Mycobacterial diseases. In: Mandell GL, Bennet JE, Dolin R (Eds). Principles of Practice of Infectious Diseases. Philadelphia, PA: Churchill Livingstone; 2000. pp. 2576-607.
5. Gaur BM, Meheshwari B, Lal N. Tuberculous endometritis: a clinico-pathological study of 1000 cases. Br J Obstet Gynaecol. 1983;90:84-6.
6. Qureshi RN, Sammad S, Hamd R, Lakha SF. Female genital tuberculosis revisited. J Pak Med Assoc. 2001;51:16-8.
7. Samal S, Gupta U, Agarwal P. Menstrual disorders in genital tuberculosis. J Indian Med Assoc. 2000;98:126-7.
8. Edwards PQ, Edwards LB. Story of the tuberculin skin test from an epidemiologic viewpoint. Am Rev Respir Dis. 1960;81:1-47.
9. Centers for Disease Control and Prevention. Targeted tuberculin testing and treatment of latent tuberculosis infection. MMWR. 2009;49(RR06):1-54.
10. Food and Drug Administration. QuantiFERON-TB Gold In-Tube - P010033/S011. Available athttp://www.fda.gov/MedicalDevices/Products andMedicalProcedures/DeviceApprovalsand Clearances/PMAApprovals/ucm106548.htm. Accessed June 16, 2010.
11. Food and Drug Administration. T-SPOT-TB - P070006. Available at *http://www.fda.gov/ MedicalDevices/ProductsandMedicalProcedures/ DeviceApprovalsandClearances/PMAApprovals/ ucm102794.htm*. Accessed June 16, 2010
12. Bhanu NV, Urvashi B, Chakraborty SM, Naga S, Arora J, Rana T, et al. Improved diagnostic value of PCR in the diagnosis of female genital tuberculosis leading to infertility. Journal of Medical Microbiology. 2005;54:927-31.
13. Agarwal J, Gupta JK. Female genital tuberculosis: A retrospective clinicopathological study of 501 cases. Indian J Pathol Microbiol. 1993;36:389-97.
14. Shrivastava, Bahatambare GS, Deshmukh AB, Rajpai P, Rajpai T, Singh T, et al. Genital tuberculosis: evaluating microscopy, culture, histopathology and PCR for diagnosis all play their role. Int J Curr Microbiol Appl Sci. 2014;3(4):439-45.
15. Gamboa F, et al. Comparative evaluation of initial and new versions of the Gen-Probe Amplified *Mycobacterium tuberculosis* direct test for direct detection of *M. tuberculosis* in respiratory and nonrespiratory specimens. J Clin Microbiol. 1998;33:2699.
16. Vlaspolder F, Singer P, Roggeveen C. Diagnostic value of an amplification method (Gen-Probe) compared with that of culture for diagnosis of tuberculosis. J Clin Microbiol. 1995;33:2699-703.
17. Chedore Pn, Jamieson FB. Routine use of the Gen-probe MTD2 Amplification Test for detection of *M. tuberculosis* in clinical specimens in a large public mycobacteriology laboratory. Diagn Microbiol Infect Dis. 1999;35:185-91.
18. Catanzaro A, Davidson BL, Fujiwara PI, Goldberger MJ, Gordin F, Salfinger M, et al. Rapid diagnostic tests tuberculosis: what is the appropriate use? Am J Resp Crit Care Med. 1997;155:1804-14.
19. Martens MG. Pelvic Inflammatory Disease—chapter 30. In: Rock JA, Jones III HW, (Eds). Te Linde's Operative Gynecology, 10th edition. Lippincott William & Wilkins Wolters Kluwer Press; 2008.

10

Viral Infections in Gynecology

Shakun Tyagi

INTRODUCTION

Viral infections in gynecology are important cause of morbidity in patients. Virus has to invade host cells to manifest its genome and replication. Amongst the viruses that are sexually transmitted some viruses have only local manifestations while others have limited or no local affection but severe long standing systemic ramifications. Viral sexually transmitted diseases (STD) with predominantly local manifestations are genital herpes, genital warts and molluscum contagiosum while HIV/AIDS, Hepatitis B, C and D are systemic disorders.

National AIDS Control Organization advocates the syndromic management of all STDs.[1] This encompasses following common approach while evaluating and managing the patients of STD's:
- *History taking and clinical examination:* General examination, genital/oral and ano-rectal.
- Appropriate syndromic diagnosis.
- Minimal and appropriate laboratory tests, wherever available.
- Early and effective treatment, preferably single dose and directly observed.
- Promotion and provision of condoms and counseling for behavior change and risk reduction.
- Referral for syphilis screening and HIV counseling and testing.
- Partner's notification and management.
- Follow-up as per schedule.
- Documentation of case details and laboratory results.

Although genital herpes is the only STD amongst viral STDs that is included in the syndromic approach the above mentioned approach holds good for all STD's.

HERPES SIMPLEX VIRUS

Genital herpes is a chronic disease and once a person is infected, the viral infection remains lifelong. Both HSV-1 and HSV-2 viral types can cause genital herpes but is mostly caused by HSV-2. The importance of this infection lies in the fact that the infection is mostly subclinical and asymptomatic but the person may continue to intermittently shed the virus and be a source of infection for his or her sexual partners.

The virus may lie latent in the proximal nerve ganglion with reactivation due to stimuli such as fever, trauma, emotional stress, sunlight, menstruation.

Clinical Presentation

The ulcerative lesions may persist for 4–15 days and usually heal without scarring.

Differential Diagnosis

Primary syphilis ulcer (Chancre), chancroid, Crohn's disease.

Investigations

Clinical picture usually raises high degree of suspicion and treatment needs to be initiated without waiting for Laboratory reports. The clinical suspicion can be confirmed by virological (cell culture and polymerase chain reaction [PCR]) and serological tests if facilities are available. Virological tests have low sensitivity. Serologic test also helps in differentiating an HSV-1 infection from HSV-2 infection which is useful in prognostication and counseling.[2] HSV-2 virus is more frequently associated with recurrences and subclinical shedding as compared to HSV-1. Tzanck smear and direct immune-fluorescence assay were earlier performed as a confirmatory test but are no longer preferred due to low sensitivity.[2] Type-specific HSV serologic assays based on the herpes simplex virus-specific glycoprotein G2 (HSV-2) and glycoprotein G1 (HSV-1) are the most sensitive and specific. Table 10.1 lists the clinical presentation of HSV in gynecology.

Table 10.1 Clinical presentation of herpes simplex virus in gynecology

Symptoms	Signs
• Primary infection may be asymptomatic • May have severe systemic manifestations similar to any viral infection with fever myalgia. • Dysuria • Multiple painful vesicular or ulcerative lesion over genital area • Recurrent episodes are less severe with regards to number of lesions and pain with no systemic features	• Multiple tender vesicular or superficial ulcerative lesion over labia majora, minora, vestibule, vagina and cervix • Tender Lymphadenopathy

According to CDC, guidelines 2015, the indications for type specific testing are:[2]
- Atypical or recurrent genital symptoms with negative culture or HSV PCR
- When diagnosis is made based on clinical picture only without a confirmatory laboratory report
- Patient whose partner also has genital herpes.

Additional serological testing for HIV and syphilis should also be done.

Treatment

Antiviral therapy must be started in case of primary herpes at the earliest as it reduces the severity as well as duration of symptoms.

Drugs: Tablet acyclovir 200 mg five times a day orally for 7–10 days; or tablet acyclovir 400 mg TDS orally for 7–10 days; or tablet valacyclovir 1 g BD orally for 7–10 days; tablet famciclovir 250 mg TDS orally for 7–10 days. In case of incomplete relief the treatment will need to be extended in accordance with symptomatic relief till 2–3 weeks.

- Local hygiene should be maintained with warm saline fomentation along with pain relief with oral analgesics.
- In case of severe systemic disease during primary herpes infection (pneumonitis, hepatitis, disseminated infection or CNS manifestations) hospitalization and intravenous therapy is required. Injection acyclovir in the dose of 5–10 mg/kg IV every 8 hours is advised for 2–7 days or till clinical improvement is present. This is followed by oral antiviral therapy so that at least 10 days of total therapy is completed.[1] Twenty one days intravenous therapy with acyclovir is advocated in case of HSV encephalitis. Dose of acyclovir is adjusted according to renal functions in case of renal function impairment.
- In case of recurrence treatment of that episode will be required. The treatment must be started during prodrome itself or within one day of lesion. The recommended dosage regimen is: tablet acyclovir 400 mg TDS orally for 5 days or tablet acyclovir 800 mg orally twice a day

for 5 days or tablet acyclovir 800 mg BD orally for 2 days or tablet valacyclovir 500 mg BD orally for 3 days or tablet valacyclovir 1 g once a day orally for 5 days or tablet famciclovir 125 mg orally BD for 5 days or tablet famciclovir 1 g BD orally for one day.
- For recurrent genital herpes lesions long-term suppressive treatment is better than intermittent treatment if there are more than six episodes in one year. The recommended therapy is tablet acyclovir 400 mg BD orally; or tablet valacyclovir 500 mg once a day or tablet valacyclovir 1 g orally once a day or tablet famciclovir 250 mg twice a day orally. It reduces chances of recurrent disease and also reduces the spread to the partner. Suppressive therapy is also indicated near term in pregnant women, starting at 36 weeks of gestation, to prevent intrapartum transmission of HSV to the newborn leading to encephalitis.
- Counseling is of utmost importance in these patients and while prognosticating and advising further follow-up. Following points must be dealt with during counseling:
  - Suppressive therapy needs to be advised to avoid recurrent disease and asymptomatic viral shedding in case of repeated recurrent episodes.
  - The partner must be informed and either abstinence must be practiced or adequate precautions—latex condom must be used during the period of active lesion to reduce transmission to the partner.
  - Suppressive antiviral therapy does not reduce the increased risk for HIV acquisition in the patients associated with HSV-2 infection.

GENITAL WARTS

Genital warts are caused by infection with non oncogenic human papilloma virus (HPV) infection. HPV serotypes 6 and 11 are the most important cause of anogenital warts.

Clinical Presentation

Table 10.2 depicts the clinical presentation of genital warts.

Table 10.2 Clinical presentation of genital warts

Symptoms	Signs
• Asymptomatic and incidentally detected on examination • Patient may present with singular or multiple warty growths	Single or multiple flat, papular, or pedunculated lesions may be present on labia majora, labia minora, vagina and/or cervix

Differential Diagnosis

Condylomata lata, vulval intraepithelial neoplasia, squamous cell carcinoma, molluscum contagiosum.

Investigation

Usually no diagnostic investigations are required in characteristic lesions. However, in atypical presentations diagnostic biopsy is required such as when the lesion is pigmented, affixed to underlying tissue, indurated, bleeding, or ulcerated to rule out malignant or premalignant lesion. Also in the event of the lesion not responding to standard therapy or worsening of lesion on therapy biopsy needs to be performed. HPV testing is not indicated according to CDC.[2]

Pap smear along with testing for HIV and syphilis must be performed as there are high chances of co-infection with oncogenic HPV.

Treatment

Spontaneous resolution of warts may take place but may take up to one year duration to resolve. Considering the psychological impact of the lesion on patient and the high chances of transmission to the partner, it is preferable to treat the genital warts.

Main treatment comprises of removal of the lesion. Both medical and surgical modalities may need to be initiated according to the size, site, type of lesion and associated conditions like pregnancy. Cesarean section is only indicated in case of vaginal or vulval warts if they are obstructing the delivery of fetus and prelabor

LSCS does not prevent laryngeal papillomatosis in the baby.

Medical Management

- *Imiquimod:* It is a topically active immune enhancer and stimulates production of cytokines and interferons. It is category C in pregnancy and should be used only when benefits outweigh side effects. After 6–10 hours the area of drug application should be thoroughly washed with water and soap. Local excoriation and irritation is the main side effect of this therapy.
    - Imiquimod 5% cream local application HS on alternate days for up to 16 weeks.
    - Imiquimod 3.75% local application HS daily upto 16 weeks.
- Podophyllotoxin (Podophyllin 0.5%) gel or solution. It is an antimitotic drug and causes wart necrosis. The solution or gel is applied over the warts twice a day for three days. This is followed by a break of 4 days. Up to four cycles can be repeated. Not more than 10 cm^2 of area should be treated with this modality. Maximum dose of Podophyllin is 0.5 mL/day. It is contraindicated in pregnancy.
- Sinecatechins 15% ointment. It is a green-tea extract. The active product is catechins. It is applied as 0.5 cm strand of ointment in a thrice a day regimen till the response is complete and need not be washed off. It causes erythema, ulceration, induration, and vesicular rash. Its safety and efficacy with HIV and pregnancy is not known.

Surgical Management

- Ablation with cryotherapy or electrocautery can be done. Carbon dioxide laser, fine scissors or knife can also be used for excision of the lesions. Smaller lesions can be ablated using weekly application of trichloroacetic acid (TCA) 80% solution. In case of an exophytic cervical lesion HSIL/malignancy should be ruled out by colposcopic directed biopsy.

- Most warts respond within three months of therapy. Sometimes they may resolve without any therapy over period of time.

> *Counseling* is important in these patients regarding following points:
> - The excision does not remove the virus from the epithelium and therefore the warts might recur. Recurrence is maximum within 3–6 months of treatment.
> - The latex condoms reduce the transmission but does not fully prevent transmission to the partner.
> - Risk management and testing of other STD's should also be performed.

HPV Testing

As 99% of all cervical cancers are associated with high risk oncogenic HPV (16, 18, 31, 33, 35, 39, 51, 52, 45, 56, 58, 73, 59, 68, 82) its testing is being inculcated in protocols for screening and management of cervical premalignant lesions. Table 10.3 lists the various HPV kits that have been approved by FDA for clinical use.

The HPV testing for oncogenic types may be used in for following indications:

Triage of Abnormal Cytology Report

Triage of cytology results of ASC-US is the most common indication of HPV testing. If oncogenic HPV is ruled out in these cases colposcopic examination can be avoided and the patient can go for further follow-up as part of routine cervical screening. A report positive for high risk oncogenic type requires colposcopy and a directed biopsy of high risk lesion. This approach is more sensitive in detecting high grade CIN in women with LSIL, ASCUS and AGUS reports than repeat pap smear.[3]

For Follow-up, Following CIN Treatment-test of Cure

A negative combined test of cytology and high risk HPV at 6 months after treatment of CIN2 or higher grade allows return to routine 3-yearly

Table 10.3 FDA approved human papillomavirus tests for cervical cancer screening clinical tests for oncogenic types of human papillomavirus

- The Hybrid Capture 2 High-Risk HPV DNA test (manufactured by Qiagen, Gaithersburg, Maryland)
- The Digene HC2 HPV DNA test (manufactured by Qiagen, Gaithersburg, Maryland) detects 13 oncogenic or five nononcogenic HPV types.
- APTIMA HR HPV (manufactured by Gen Probe, San Diego CA) test detects 14 oncogenic HPV types of HPV mRNA.
- Cervista HPV High-Risk DNA test (manufactured by Hologics, Bedford, Massachusetts) detect presence of 13–14 oncogenic HPV types.
- Cervista HPV 16/18 DNA test only detects oncogenic HPV types 16 and 18.
- The Cobas 4500 (manufactured by Roche, Pleasanton, California) test detects 14 oncogenic HPV DNA types and can detect individual types HPV 16 and 18.
- Aptima HPV 16/18/45 test is also FDA-cleared to triage its pooled Aptima HR HPV test further, although there are no algorithms for HPV 16/18/45 testing in any clinical guidelines.

Abbreviation: FDA, food and drug administration

follow-up as compared to up to 10 years of annual cytology when only cytology is used to manage these patients. Following a positive report of high risk HPV patient continues yearly cytology, colposcopy and further management and as indicated by cytology, colposcopy and biopsy.

Primary Screening for Cervical Cancer along with Cervical Cytology

As there is high negative predictive value of HPV and Pap test, women who test negative for both should not be screened again for 5 years. Reflex HPV testing is the process when the HPV testing is performed on a part of the same sample in which cytological abnormality such as LSIL, ASCUS or AGUS is detected.

HPV as a Primary Screening Test[4]

Currently stand alone HPV testing for cervical cancer screening is not advocated but various researchers are evaluating its utility as a standalone method. It is less labor intensive, more automated as well as more sensitive than pap smear and therefore longer screening interval of 5 years is possible. However, its low specificity compared to cytology especially in younger women (less than 30 years of age) is a big disadvantage towards using it as only test.

Women who test positive for high risk HPV will require reflex cytology as triage and those with positive results on cytology (abnormal cells) will be referred directly to colposcopy. Reflex cytology is comparable to reflex HPV testing and is the performance of cytological review of the patient's liquid-based cellular sample acquired at HPV testing, which is routinely stored until after HPV results are available. Women who are high risk HPV positive but have negative cytology will have early recall at 12 months for repeat HPV testing. This will be in anticipation that at least half will then be high risk HPV negative and can return to routine recall of 5 yearly testing.

Complementary Biomarker such as p16InK4A (p16) or p16 Combined with the Minichromosome Maintenance Protein Family (MCM)

As HPV testing has low specificity newer oncogenic markers with high specificity are being studied. When these markers are combined with HPV testing it will reduce the number of patients that need to follow up with cytology/colposcopy.
- *Dual p16 staining in cytology (CINtec®, Roche, Basel, Switzerland):* It improves specificity of triage of minor cytological abnormalities compared with HPV testing alone (63.2% versus 37.8% for borderline cytological

abnormalities and 37.3% versus 18.5% for low-grade dysplasia).[5]
- Dual testing of proliferation marker Ki-67 with p16 in CINtec® PLUS: It Identifies CIN2+ at risk of progression. The specificity is equivalent to cytology (95.2% versus 95.4%; P = 0.15) in women of all ages, but more sensitive (86.7% versus 68.5%; P < 0.001) for detecting CIN2+.[6] HPV testing in women 30 years or older was less specific than CINtec® PLUS (93.0% versus 96.2%; P < 0.001) but more sensitive (93.3% versus 84.7%; P = 0.03) in detecting high grade lesion.[7]

The HPV testing (including oncogenic HPV and HPV 16/18 tests) is not helpful in following clinical situations and should not be performed:
- Deciding whether to vaccinate against HPV
- Conducting STD screening in women or men at risk for STDs
- Providing care to persons with genital warts or their partners
- Testing women aged <30 years as part of routine cervical cancer screening.

MOLLUSCUM CONTAGIOSUM (TABLE 10.4)

It is a benign cutaneous lesion caused by Pox virus. Sexually transmitted molluscum contagiosum lesions may be present on the abdomen, inner thighs, and genital area of sexually active adults.

Clinical Presentation

It is a self-limited infection. The usually disappear spontaneously within 6–12 months.

Table 10.4 Clinical presentation of molluscum contagiosum

Symptoms	Signs
Main complaint is small superficial cutaneous eruptions that are usually painless	Characteristic lesion is a 2–5 mm pearly papule with a central depression. The core may be expressed to produce a white cheesy material. The lesions may undergo secondary infection and become inflamed

Patient needs to be investigated for other coexisting STDs. No specific investigations are required for molluscum contagiosum.

Treatment

As it is self-limited and resolves over time. Treatment is only required to prevent transmission and remove the visible lesion. Ablation of the lesion can be carried out using cryotherapy, curettage and trichloroacetic acid (80%) application weekly.

HUMAN IMMUNODEFICIENCY VIRUS

Human immunodeficiency virus/acquired immune deficiency syndrome (HIV/AIDS) impacts the gynecological health of a woman by causing menstrual alterations and increased chances of vaginal infections. HIV infection also alters the course of HPV infection resulting into increased chances premalignant and malignant lesions of cervix. Prevention of mother to child transmission of HIV is an important component of antenatal care (ANC) care. It involves universal screening for HIV, antiretroviral therapy (ART) [Tenofovir 300 mg OD, lamivudine 300 mg OD and efavirenz 600 mg OD (TLE)] preferably continued lifelong, Nevirapine/Zidovudine prophylaxis for the baby: for six weeks for non breastfeeding babies and till one week after the cessation of breastfeeding in breastfeed babies.

Menstrual Abnormalities

Menstrual abnormalities can be related to conditions associated with HIV, including weight loss, comorbid psychiatric illnesses and psychotropic medications, illicit substance use, thrombocytopenia and renal dysfunction. Secondary amenorrhea is more commonly seen than menorrhagia.

Co-infection with HPV

Co-infection with oncogenic human papillomavirus (HPV) and HIV exponentially increases a woman's risk for development of cervical neoplasia.[8] US Department of health and human services (HHS) recommends cytology screening every six months until two consecutive negative tests, and then annually thereafter in HIV positive women.

Vaginitis

There is higher prevalence of pelvic inflammatory disease (PID) and vaginitis in HIV positive women. Any episode of vaginitis is known to increases the HIV viral load in the patient's vaginal secretions and hence there are higher chances of HIV transmission to the partner. In pregnant women vaginitis and cervicitis is associated with increased intrapartum mother to child transmission of HIV. HIV increases the chances of colonization of vagina by *Candida*. Among women with lower CD4+ counts, the rates of colonization and symptomatic infection with candidiasis are tripled.[9] Bacterial vaginosis is also significantly associated with HIV seropositivity.[10]

Postexposure Prophylaxis for Human Immunodeficiency Virus

Postexposure prophylaxis (PEP) against HIV needs to be considered in cases of exposure to the operating surgeon or following episode of sexual assault.
- *Assessment of the exposure is made:*
  - All cases of exposure require PEP except exposure code one. Exposure code one includes the situation when exposure to mucous membrane or intact skin is present with low titer of exposure, i.e. of only few drops of contaminated fluid from source person who is asymptomatic with High CD4 count.
  - All other scenario requires ART prophylaxis
  - Any exposure more than exposure code one from unknown source, PEP is prescribed if prevalence of HIV is high in that population and the source person belongs to high risk category like commercial sex worker or intravenous drug abuser.
  - First-aid is provided after adequate counseling regarding possible side effects, adherence and follow-up protocol.
- First dose of postexposure prophylaxis is provided at the earliest, preferable within two hours of exposure with antiretroviral therapy (ART) [Tenofovir 300 mg OD, lamivudine 300 mg OD and efavirenz 600 mg OD (TLE)] for six weeks.
- If the source is already on ART, TLE should be started immediately and expert opinion should be urgently sought by phone/e-mail from center of excellence (CoE)/ART Plus center.
- The event should be reported to the appropriate authority.

Operating Theater Preparation in HIV/HBsAg/HCV Positive Cases

The risk of acquiring HIV/HBsAg/HCV is 0.3% in surgical operation. Although special precautions are advisable when operating women who are HIV or HBsAg positive it is advocated that all patients must be treated as potentially infectious and all precautions must be followed universally. The following guidelines are advised during the operation and cleaning after the surgery:
- It is preferable that the HIV and HBV status of the patient is known before the operation with prior consent of the patient. It is advisable that the patient is scheduled at the end of the operating list. The theater or labor ward staff should be informed prior to the scheduled operation so that appropriate precautions are taken.
- Protective gear should worn by the staff who are exposed to the surgical field. This includes—plastic aprons double gloves, and eye protection. Appropriate footwear/shoe cover should be worn to avoid contact with blood or body fluids.
- Only essential equipment and staff should be exposed to the operating field. Disposable

equipment should be used as far as possible. Inexperienced staff should also be excluded.
- Sharps should not be passed in a kidney tray and not hand-to-hand. Needles should never be guided with fingers. All waste must be disposed off according to its category. All disposable items used during the operation, e.g. IV cannulae need to be disposed of in the sharps container.
- All disposable, incinerable waste is put in clearly labeled yellow bags.
- In case of blood soaking paper, linen or gauze is put over the spill; freshly prepared 2% sodium hypochlorite/7.5% bleach solution is put over the spill; leave for contact time ideally 20 minutes but if the spill area is very busy then at least 5 minute contact time should be there. After contact another paper or gauze covering the soaked paper is put and then removed and put in red bag. The area is then cleaned with soap/detergent and water.
- In between surgery if there is spill of blood or body fluid on the OT table it is managed like a spill. Without a spill the OT table is wiped with surface disinfectant (0.5% Bacillocid)
- Walls should be washed up to a 3-4 feet height with water and detergent.

Bacillocid/equivalent product: Each 100 g contains:
- 1,6 dihydroxy 2,5-dioxahexane (chemically bound form of formaldehyde) @11.2 g
- Glutaraldehyde 5.0 g
- Benzalkonium chloride 5.0 g
- Alkylurea derivative 3.0 g

Preparing solution for use
0.5%: 50 mL of bacillocid made up to 10 L with water
2%: 200 mL bacillocid made up to 10 L with water

KEY POINTS

- Genital herpes is a recalcitrant lifelong disease with recurrent episodes.
- Symptoms of primary disease (HSV) as well as recurrent episodes are reduced by antiviral therapy. Suppressive therapy reduces both recurrent and disease and asymptomatic shedding
- Genital warts are due to low risk HPV infection and there might be coexisting other STDs and High risk HPV
- Medical therapy or surgical excision may be used depending upon the size and location of the genital warts. In atypical or nonresponding lesion diagnostic biopsy is important.
- HPV testing is gradually being incorporated into the protocols for cervical screening.
- Molluscum contagiosum is self-limited superficial cutaneous lesion that is treated by ablation with cryotherapy or TCA to prevent further transmission.
- Universal precautions and the protocols that are followed during OT cleaning of all surgeries need to be practiced for OT cleaning following surgery in patients with HIV/HBsAg seropositivity.
- Further extracaution may be taken while collecting and disposal of waste in these patients. According to various guidelines no extracleaning or increase in the contact period of disinfectants is required when cleaning OT's following surgery in patients with positive HIV/HBsAg positive status as compared to routine disinfection.[11]

REFERENCES

1. National STI/RTI Control and Prevention Programme NACP, Phase-III, India http://www.naco.gov.in/sites/default/files/STI-Report_7.pdf. Accessed on 16 July, 2016.
2. Sexually Transmitted Diseases Treatment Guidelines, 2015 Recommendations and Reports/Vol. 64/No. 3 June 5, 2015 http://www.cdc.gov/mmwr/pdf/rr/rr6403.pdf. Accessed on 15 July, 2016.
3. Arbyn M, Roelens J, Simoens C, Buntinx F, Paraskevaidis E, Martin-Hirsch PP, et al. Human papillomavirus testing versus repeat cytology for triage of minor cytological cervical lesions. Cochrane Database Syst Rev. 2013;(3):CD008054.
4. Progress in Cervical Screening in the UK, Scientific Impact Paper No. 7 March 2016 https://www.rcog.org.uk/globalassets/documents/guidelines/scientific-impact-papers/sip_7-progress-in-cervical-screening.pdf. Accessed on 15 July, 2016.

5. Denton KJ, Bergeron C, Klement P, Trunk MJ, Keller T, Ridder R; European CINtec Cytology Study Group. The sensitivity and specificity of p16INK4a cytology vs HPV testing for detecting high-grade cervical disease in the triage of ASC-US and LSIL pap cytology results. Am J Clin Pathol. 2010; 134:12-1.
6. Ikenberg H, Bergeron C, Schmidt D, Griesser H, Alameda F, Angeloni C, et al. PALMS Study Group. Screening for cervical cancer precursors with p16/Ki-67 dual-stained cytology: results of the PALMS study. J Natl Cancer Inst. 2013;105:1550-7.
7. Malinowski D. Molecular diagnostic assays for cervical neoplasia: emerging markers for the detection of high-grade cervical disease. Biotechniques. 2005;38 (Suppl 4):S17-23.
8. Palefsky JM. Cervical human papillomavirus infection and cervical intraepithelial neoplasia in women positive for human immunodeficiency virus in the era of highly active antiretroviral therapy. Curr Opin Oncol. 2003;15:382-8.
9. Duerr A, Sierra MF, Feldman J, et al. Immune compromise and prevalence of *Candida* vulvovaginitis in human immunodeficiency virus-infected women. Obstet Gynecol. 1997;90:252-6.
10. Cohen CR, Sinei S, Reilly M, et al. Effect of human immunodeficiency virus type 1 infection upon acute salpingitis: A laparoscopic study. J Infect Dis. 1998;178:1352-8.
11. Guideline for Disinfection and Sterilization in Healthcare Facilities, 2008 *https://www.cdc.gov/hicpac/pdf/guidelines/Disinfection_Nov_2008.pdf.* Accessed on 15 July, 2016.

11
Abnormal Uterine Bleeding

Krishna Agarwal

Abnormal uterine bleeding (AUB) is a menstrual disorder which comprises of abnormal menstrual bleeding in term of quantity, duration and the timing of bleeding.

When uterine bleeding is outside the following normal menstrual pattern it is labeled as AUB:
- Duration of bleeding >7 days
- Menstrual blood flow more than 6 full pads per day
- Period comes earlier than 21 days or later than 38 days
- Intermenstrual bleeding or postcoital bleeding

The AUB is a common gynecologic complaint and almost one-third of the outpatient visits are due to AUB. It can be caused by variety of disorders ranging from local pathology to systemic illnesses or it may be a side effect of a medication. Most common causes of AUB are uterine pathology (fibroid, polyp, adenomyosis); anovulation, coagulation disorders and gynecologic malignancies.

Since the common causes of AUB are different in different age group, it is important to divide AUB according to the age in following categories:
- AUB in adolescents
- AUB in reproductive age and premenopausal women
- AUB in postmenopausal women.

In year 2011, International Federation of Gynecology and Obstetrics (FIGO) introduced a classification and revised terminology for AUB in nongravid reproductive age group women.

This classification system is referred by the acronym PALM-COEIN (polyp, adenomyosis, leiomyoma, malignancy and hyperplasia, coagulopathy, ovulatory dysfunction, endometrial, iatrogenic and not yet classified). This classification includes initial four categories (PALM) which include structural anomalies. The next four categories (COEI) do not have any structural anomaly and the last category (N) includes all other conditions which are not included in any of the categories.

In revised terminology, term menorrhagia is replaced by heavy menstrual bleeding (HMB). This term refers to cyclic heavy and or prolonged bleeding and it does not include heavy and prolonged noncyclic bleeding in women with ovulatory dysfunction.

CAUSES AND CLASSIFICATIONS OF ABNORMAL UTERINE BLEEDING IN A REPRODUCTIVE AGE WOMAN

The first step is to rule out pregnancy irrespective of the history by performing urine pregnancy test and if there is doubt then serum beta-hCG should be performed.

History

Then a detailed menstrual history will give important formation about the source of bleeding and cause of bleeding. History is asked regarding the duration of bleeding, amount of bleeding and the color of bleeding.

Pattern of bleeding provided important information and helps in reaching to some diagnosis. There is typical pattern of menstrual bleeding in different causes of AUB. Following patterns are usually seen.
- Heavy menstrual bleeding (HMB)
- Intermenstrual bleeding
- Bleeding of ovulatory dysfunction
- Other types of bleeding which also includes amenorrhea

Heavy Menstrual Bleeding

Heavy menstrual bleeding (HMB) is cyclical bleeding which is heavy and prolonged. It refers only to the ovulatory cycles. Previously term menorrhagia was used for any heavy cycle and it did not differentiate between the ovulatory (cyclical bleeding) and anovulatory (noncyclical) uterine bleeding. Under the revised terminology of AUB by FIGO term menorrhagia been replaced with new term HMB which includes only the cyclical bleeding

The common causes of HMB are endometrial polyp; adenomyosis; leiomyoma uteri; endometrial hyperplasia or malignancy. Sometimes Cu T may be responsible for HMB.

Intermenstrual Bleeding

This type of bleeding may be caused by are endometrial polyp; endometrial hyperplasia or malignancy; endometritis and PID.

Irregular Uterine Bleeding

This bleeding pattern is due to ovulatory dysfunction and under the PALM-COEIN classification it is labeled as AUB-O. This is characterized by periods of no bleeding for 2 or more months followed by spotting or heavy bleeding.

It usually happens at the extremes of age—at the time of puberty for few years and before menopause for few years. It also occurs in cases of anovulation in polycystic ovarian syndrome and other endocrinological dysfunctions such as thyroid disorders and hyperprolactinemia.

Usually after excluding the structural causes of intermenstrual bleeding and based on the bleeding pattern diagnosis of ovulatory AUB is made. Further investigations are done to find out the cause of anovulation.

Other Patterns of Bleeding

It may be amenorrhea or decreased amount of bleeding. This pattern is seen in women on oral contraceptive pills (OCPs), Asherman syndrome or cervical stenosis. There may be another pattern where there is increase in the frequency of cycle.

After menstrual history, obstetric, contraceptive and drug history is asked in detail.

Physical Examination

Thorough general physical and gynecological examination is performed. General physical examination should focus on pallor, thyroid enlargement, galactorrhea, ecchymosis and, abnormal body hair growth. Per abdominal examination should be performed to look for any abdominal lump or organomegaly.

Per speculum and per vaginal examination is done with a focus to find out the amount and source of bleeding, any growth in vagina or cervix, size of the uterus, tenderness mobility, and adnexal masses.

Investigations

Following investigations are done in a woman who presents with AUB:
- Pregnancy test is always done irrespective of history, if still in doubt; serum beta human chorionic gonadotropin (hCG) test should be done.
- Hemogram-hemoglobin is done in patients with heavy and frequent bleeding. Platelet count is done if bleeding disorder is suspected. White blood cell count is performed if pelvic inflammatory disease (PID) or acute endometritis is suspected.

- *Hormones*
  - Serum thyroid stimulating hormone (TSH) is tested in cases of HMB where other causes have been ruled out.
  - Serum prolactin is performed in a woman who has anovulatory bleeding, amenorrhea, and galactorrhea or on drugs that cause hyperprolactinemia.
  - Serum testosterone is done in patients with AUB and signs of hyperandrogenism which occur in polycystic ovarian syndrome (PCOS) or congenital adrenal hyperplasia or rarely androgen secreting tumors of ovary or adrenal gland.
  - Serum follicle-stimulating hormone (FSH) and luteinizing hormone (LH) - FSH is advised if premature ovarian failure is suspected. In women with suspected hypothalamic dysfunction due to poor nutrition or intense exercise LH and FSH and estrogen progestogen withdrawal is advised.
  - *Estrogen levels:* It is advised in women whom all other causes of HMB have been ruled out and have an adnexal mass. This may occur rarely in estrogen secreting tumor.
- *Coagulation test:* Prothrombin time (PT) and activated partial thromboplastin time (APTT) are advised in women who have a history of heavy bleeding since the time of menarche, family history of bleeding disorder or history of easy bruisability or bleeding from other mucosal sites.
- *Pap smear:* It should be done in all patients of AUB.
- Endometrial sampling in women with AUB
  It needs to be done under following conditions:
  - In women between 45 years of age to menopausal age
  - In reproductive age women < 45 years of age who have persistent AUB-O of more than 6 months, women who are obese, who have failed on medical management and the ones who are at risk of endometrial carcinoma.
  - In adolescents aged 13–18 years of age- risk of cancer in these girls is rare but endometrial cancer may develop in obese girls with PCOS particularly in women not responding to the medical treatment.
  - *Postpartum and postabortal period:* In these women if endometritis is suspected the endometrial sampling may be done to help in confirming the diagnosis.
- *Imaging*
  - *Pelvic ultrasound:* It is indicated in following conditions:
    * PV examination show uterine enlargement or an adnexal mass
    * Symptoms persist in spite of the treatment and there is no clinical finding.
  It can be omitted if the cause of AUB is identified on clinical examination such as endometrial polyp, infection or anovulation. Usually TVS is performed, TAS may be required in few cases with a large pelvic mass.
  - *CT scan and MRI:* Usually these are not done and only indicated when initial USG does not provide adequate information.
  - *Saline infusion sonography (SIS) and hysteroscopy:* When a lesion is suspected in the uterine cavity SIS or hysteroscopy is required. Advantage of SIS over hysteroscopy is that it is less painful and at the same time it is possible to delineate the myometrial and the serosal components of lesions such as fibroids which is not seen in hysteroscopy.

Treatment

Treatment of AUB should not be started until the etiology of AUB is identified and premalignant and malignant lesions of genital tract have been excluded. Broadly treatment can be categorized under following categories:
- Treatment of the primary cause
- Medical treatment
- Surgical treatment.

Treatment of Primary Cause

Structural lesions of the uterus such as endometrial polyp or submucosa fibroid can be removed hysteroscopically.

Woman with AUB-O and PCOS, who does not desire pregnancy, should be started on OCPs.

In case of suspected endometritis, antibiotic course is given. Woman with hypothyroidism is started on thyroxine and one with hyperprolactinemia is given cabergoline or bromocriptine.

Patient with a bleeding disorder should be started on tranexamic acid.

Medical Therapy

In HMB due to fibroid or adenomyosis, initial treatment with medical therapy is given and the first line medicine is combine oral contraceptive pill or LNG-IUD. Both are effective, have minimal side effects and also provide contraception. Choice between the two medical therapies would depend on the profile and choices of the woman (Table 11.1).

In women where the estrogen dose present in OCPs is contraindicated, ultra-low dose postmenopausal hormonal formulations can be used.

High dose of oral progestins, norethisterone acetate or medroxyprogesterone acetate is also effective. Out of these two, norethisterone acetate is more potent because it has more androgenic action but for prolonged use medroxyprogesterone acetate is safer as compared to norethisterone acetate.

Although the cause of bleeding in HMB and AUB-O is completely different, same drugs are effective in both the conditions. Therefore the first line of treatment in AUB-O is also the oral or nonoral combined contraceptives, oral or injectable progestins or LNg-20. In PCOS patients this therapy though does not correct the primary pathology; it helps in regularizing the menses and also reduces the risk of endometrial carcinoma.

Second line drugs: It include nonhormonal noncontraceptive drugs, the nonsteroidal anti-inflammatory drugs and antifibrinolytic agent.

Medical therapy options
Estrogen-progestin contraceptives: Different formulations of combined oral contraceptives (COCs) can be given in different schedules depending on the patient's preference. COC has the advantage of making cycles lighter and regular and also decreases the incidence of dysmenorrhea. It reduces menstrual bleeding up to 35–69%. Another advantage is contraception.

Most commonly used formulation is COC in usual 21 day cycle with 7 days pill-free period works quite effectively. COC Mala N which freely available in all government hospitals is effective.

Other preparations with different routes of administration are also effective but there is no comparative study. Depending on the patient's preference, other preparations such as transdermal estrogen progestin contraceptive patch (Ortho-Evra) or vaginal ring (Nuva ring) can be used.

Women with relative contraindications for COCs (diabetes, hypertension, smoking, >35 years of age, obesity), may be given preparations containing ultra-low dose of estrogen and progestin which are used for treatment of postmenopausal symptoms. Jinteli 1/5 is a preparation which is approved for treatment of vasomotor symptom in postmenopausal women contains 5 mcg ethinyl estradiol and 1 mg norethisterone. It does not provide contraception

Table 11.1 Use of COC versus LNg-20 in women with heavy menstrual bleeding

	COC	LNg-20
Hypertension, risk of thromboembolism	Contraindicated	Safe
Mode of administration	If willing to take daily pill	Does not want daily intake
Menstrual control	Wants regular menses	Accepts initial irregular bleeding followed by reduced bleeding

Abbreviations: COC, combined oral contraceptive; LNg-20, levonorgestrel-20

and a barrier contraceptive is needed in these women.

High dose oral progestins: The usual oral preparations used in women with AUB are:
- Norethisterone acetate (NET)—given in dose of 5 mg once to 3 times daily
- Medroxyprogesterone acetate (MPA)—given in dose of 10 mg once to thrice daily

Both can be used from 5th to 25th day of cycle in HMB. In AUB-O it is effective even from 15th to 25th day of cycle.

Injectable progestins: These are used in women in where estrogens are contraindicated due to risk of venous thromboembolism (VTE) and when the woman also desires contraception.

Depot medroxyprogesterone acetate 150 mg is used IM every 3 monthly.

LNg20: It is effective in treatment of both HMB and AUB-O and improves quality of life more than when oral medications are used. Mostly effectiveness of LNg20 in HMB has been studied. It reduces menstrual blood loss up to 71–95%. It works by causing endometrial atrophy by increasing local progestin concentration.

However there are some concerns when LNG 20 is used for treatment of HMB:
- Effectiveness of LNg20 reduces after 3 years of use in contrast with its effectiveness for 5 years as a contraceptive. Thus it needs replacement after three years for it to remain effective for controlling HMB.
- Expulsion rate is higher in patients of HMB with fibroid uterus, so it requires proper counseling before its use.

Progestin preparations (oral, injectable, intrauterine system) can be safely used in women with HMB on anticoagulants. They do not increase the risk of venous thrombosis in women on anticoagulants however progestins should be stopped before discontinuation of anticoagulant therapy because effect of progestins may last up to six months after the stopping them.

Tranexamic acid: It is an effective nonhormonal treatment of HMB. It prevents conversion of plasminogen to plasmin and reduces fibrinolysis.

Dose—500 mg 3–5 times daily for 3–5 days during periods. It can be given orally, intramuscularly or intravenously.

There is risk of thromboembolism in women who have history of VTE or are at high risk of thrombosis.

Nonsteroidal Anti-inflammatory Drugs

The common NSAIDs used in treatment of HMB are mefanamic acid, ibuprofen and naproxen. They are not used in AUB-O. These drugs reduce synthesis of prostaglandin E2 and F2 alpha in the endometrium which leads to vasoconstriction and reduction in bleeding. These drugs are cheaper, have minimal side effects, no risk of thromboembolism, also effective in dysmenorrhea and required to be taken only during periods.

Dose: Mefanamic acid—500 mg 3 times a day for 3–5 days during periods

Ibuprofen—600 mg daily for 3–5 days during periods

Naproxen—500 mg twice daily for 3–5 days during periods

Surgical Methods

If the patient does not respond to medical treatment or she desires a definite treatment, surgical treatment is required. In women with HMB, adenomyosis and fibroid uterus is the main indication for surgery. Surgical options depend on the age of the woman, desire for fertility and willingness to come for follow up. If the woman desires fertility in a case of AUB-L, myomectomy is the option.

If woman does not desire fertility, then minimally invasive surgery like endometrial ablation or uterine artery embolization are the options.

If the woman desires definitive treatment, then hysterectomy is the option.

TREATMENT OF ABNORMAL UTERINE BLEEDING IN ADOLESCENTS

The main causes of AUB in this age group are same as in reproductive age group only difference is that the most common cause differs. AUB in adolescents can be categorized based on the pattern of bleeding as anovulatory bleeding, heavy menstrual bleeding, intermenstrual bleeding, amenorrhea same as in AUB in reproductive age woman.

- In adolescents, irregular bleeding is the common cause of AUB. In the initial 2 years after menarche, reason for anovulation is the immaturation of the hypothalamic-pituitary-ovarian axis. Therefore, the negative feedback effect of estrogen on the pituitary and it is mainly the estrogen withdrawal bleeding in the initial years. In between the girl may have ovulation and the endometrium thus gets stabilized by the progestogen. Usually in initial few years it gets settled and the periods get regularized.
- However if chronic anovulation persists then it evolves into PCOS which requires treatment as described above under the treatment of AUB in reproductive age group. PCOS is a common cause of chronic anovulation and AUB in adolescents.
- Other important cause is eating disorder such as bulimia nervosa or stress. Both may suppres ovulation and the girl will have amenorrhea and hyperestrogenism.
- HMB in disorders such as Von Willebrand disease, immune thrombocytopenia, platelet dysfunction or certain drugs.
- Other causes—hypo or hyperthyroidism, systemic illness like diabetes mellitus, SLE, renal failure, malignancy, cervical polyp or ectropion may cause irregular bleeding.

Treatment of AUB in adolescents is on the same lines as mentioned in the treatment of AUB in a reproductive age woman.

KEY POINTS

- A detailed menstrual history provide important information about the source of bleeding.
- Common causes of heavy menstrual bleeding are endometrial polyp, adenomyosis, leiomyoma uteri, endometrial hyperplasia and malignancy.
- Treatment of AUB should not be started until the etiology of AUB is identified and premalignant and malignant tissues of genital tract have been excluded.
- In women with heavy menstrual bleeding due to fibroid or adenomyosis, initial treatment with medical therapy is given and the first line medicine as combined oral contraceptive pill or LNG IUD.
- Tranexamic acid is an effective nonhormonal treatment in HMB. The common NSAIDs used are mefenamic acid, ibuprofen and naproxen.
- If patient does not respond to medical treatment or she desires a definite treatment, surgical treatment is required.

BIBLIOGRAPHY

1. Brahma PK, Martel KM, Christman GM. Future directions in myoma research. Obstet Gynecol Clin North Am. 2006;33:199-224.
2. Doherty L, Mutlu L, Sinclair D. Uterine fibroids: clinical manifestations and contemporary management. Reprod Sci. 2014;21:1067-92.
3. Fraser IS, Critchley HO, Broder M. The FIGO recommendations on terminologies and definitions for normal and abnormal uterine bleeding. Semin Reprod Med. 2011;29:383-90.
4. Kadir RA, Economides DL, Sabin CA. Frequency of inherited bleeding disorders in women with menorrhagia. Lancet. 1998;351:485-9.
5. Kouides PA, Conard J, Peyvandi F. Hemostasis and menstruation: appropriate investigation for underlying disorders of hemostasis in women with excessive menstrual bleeding. Fertil Steril. 2005;84:1345-51.
6. Lumsden MA, Hamoodi I, Gupta J. Fibroids: diagnosis and management. BMJ. 2015;351:h4887

7. Moulder JK, Yunker A. Endometrial ablation: considerations and complications. Curr Opin Obstet Gynecol. 2016;28(4):261-6.
8. Munro MG Classification of menstrual bleeding disorders. Rev Endocr Metab Disord. 2012;13:225-34.
9. Munro MG, Critchley HO, Fraser IS, for the FIGO Working Group on Menstrual Disorders. The FIGO classification of causes of abnormal uterine bleeding. Int J Gynaecol Obstet. 2011;113:1-2.
10. Naftalin J, Hoo W, Pateman K. Is adenomyosis associated with menorrhagia? Hum Reprod. 2014;29:473-9.
11. National heavy menstrual bleeding audit report. RCOG. 2014.
12. NICE. Clinical Guideline 44; Heavy menstrual bleeding 2007. National Institute for Health and Clinical Excellence (NICE); Available at:*http://www.nice.org.uk/nicemedia/pdf/CG44FullGuideline*.
13. Ogutcuoglu B, Karadag C, Inan C, Dolgun ZN, Yoldemir AT, Aslanova L. Diagnostic utility of saline infusion Doppler sonohysterography in endometrial mass lesions. Pak J Med Sci. 2016;32(2):284-8.
14. Preutthipan S, Herabutya Y. Hysteroscopic polypectomy in 240 premenopausal and postmenopausal women. Fertil Steril. 2005;83:705-9.
15. Roberts TE, Tsourapas A, Middleton LJ. Hysterectomy, endometrial ablation, and levonorgestrel releasing intrauterine system (Mirena) for treatment of heavy menstrual bleeding: cost effectiveness analysis. BMJ. 2011;342:d2202.
16. Sabbioni L, Zanetti I, Orlandini C, Petraglia F, Luisi S. Abnormal uterine bleeding unrelated to uterine structural abnormalities: management in the perimenopausal period. Minerva Ginecol. 2016.
17. Sangkomkamhang US, Lumbiganon P, Laopaiboon M. Progestogens or progestogen-releasing intrauterine systems for uterine fibroids. Cochrane Database Syst Rev. 2013;2:CD008994.
18. Shankar M, Lee CA, Sabin CA. von Willebrand disease in women with menorrhagia: a systematic review. BJOG. 2004;111:734-40.
19. Shapley M, Jordan K, Croft PR. An epidemiological survey of symptoms of menstrual loss in the community. Br J Gen Pract. 2004;54:359-63.
20. Stewart EA. Uterine fibroids. Lancet. 2001;357:293-8.
21. Van den Bosch T, Ameye L, Van Schoubroeck D. Intra-cavitary uterine pathology in women with abnormal uterine bleeding: a prospective study of 1220 women. Facts Views Vis Obgyn. 2015;7:17-24.
22. Wamsteker K, Emanuel MH, de Kruif JH. Transcervical hysteroscopic resection of submucous fibroids for abnormal uterine bleeding: results regarding the degree of intramural extension. Obstet Gynecol. 1993;82:736-40.
23. Zia A, Rajpurkar M. Challenges of diagnosing and managing the adolescent with heavy menstrual bleeding. Thromb Res. 2016;143:91-100.

12

Fibroid Uterus

Chetna Arvind Sethi, Divya Arora

INTRODUCTION

Uterine fibroids also known as leiomyomas are the most common benign uterine tumors, with an estimated incidence of 20–40% in women during their reproductive years. They are monoclonal tumors of the uterine smooth muscle cells and consist of extracellular matrix that contains collagen, fibronectin, and proteoglycan. Uterine fibroid tumors arise during the reproductive years and tend to enlarge during pregnancy and regress after menopause. The use of estrogen agonists is associated with an increased incidence of fibroid tumors. Conversely, progesterone appears to inhibit their growth.

In cases with abnormal uterine bleeding (AUB) following hysterectomy (any cause), 77% of uterine specimens show leiomyomas.[1] Leiomyomas are the most common indication for hysterectomy worldwide.[2] Mostly occur as asymptomatic tumors diagnosed during cervical examination or radiological investigation. On the other hand these may cause significant morbidity among women of reproductive age group, hence the importance in clinical practice.

Newer advances have been made in the diagnosis of this common condition with advent of SIS, 2D-3D USG, virtual hysteroscopy and MRI. However, challenges still exist in distinguishing leiomyomas from leiomyosarcomas.

Rapid advances have also been made in the management of fibroids, shifting focus from hysterectomy to conservative medical management, myomectomy with minimally invasive techniques and recently to radiological interventional therapy.

CLINICAL PRESENTATION

They are often asymptomatic but they can cause a multitude of symptom as:
- Asymptomatic ≥50% and may be diagnosed incidentally on sonography
- Abnormal uterine bleeding in the form of heavy menstrual bleeding due to intramural or submucosal fibroids (due to increased surface area, increased vascularity, distortion of shape leading to reduced contractility and compression of venous plexus and alteration in adjacent endometrium and myometrium. Intermenstrual or irregular HMB may be caused by ulceration and infection of a submucosal myoma or fibroid polyp. May at times be a cause of delayed menopause and rarely postmenopausal bleeding
- Pain in the form of dysmenorrhea—congestive due to increased vascularity in intramural myoma and spasmodic in a submucosal fibroid or polyp; dyspareunia—due to size, associated pelvic infections or endometriosis
- Acute pelvic pain may be due to torsion or hemorrhage from ruptured surface vessel in subserosal fibroid; inversion due to large fundal submucosal myoma; red degeneration

in pregnancy and rarely due to sarcomatous change
- Pelvic pressure symptoms due to large fibroids—urinary complaints like retention, constipation, tenesmus
- Vaginal discharge often blood stained in cases of submucosal polyp or cervical fibroids
- Pelvic or abdominal mass in case of large intramural or subserosal fibroid. May even cause respiratory discomfort and distress especially during pregnancy
- Infertility (*see* infertility and fibroid)
- Obstetric complication (see pregnancy and fibroid)—spontaneous abortion, fibroid growth, red degeneration.

Signs

The signs include anemia caused by AMB/HMB; vaginal discharge associated with polyp or cervical fibroid; abdominopelvic lump or only an enlarged uterus on bimanual examination; adnexal mass as in a broad ligament fibroid is rarely a large subserosal fibroid is associated with ascites—Pseudo-Meigs syndrome (Table 12.1).

Rarely fibroid may be associated with polycythemia, hypercalcemia or hyperprolactinemia due to ectopic secretions of erythropoietin, parathyroid hormone or prolactin.

Secondary Changes

- Atrophy or reduction in volume in menopause or postpregnancy

Table 12.1 Signs and symptoms of fibroid uterus	
Symptoms	Signs
• Asymptomatic	• Anemia
• Abnormal uterine bleeding	• Vaginal discharge
• Pelvic pain	• Abdominopelvic mass
• Pressure symptoms	
• Vaginal discharge	• Enlarged uterine size
• Pelvic or abdominal mass	
• Infertility	• Ascites in Pseudo-Meigs syndrome
• Obstetric complications	

- Hyaline, cystic and fatty degenerations which are not of much clinical significance occur with an increase in size in the central areas of fibroids
- Calcareous degeneration occurs peripherally in old long standing myomas
- Red degeneration during pregnancy
- Rarely malignant change (< 0.5%).

RISK FACTORS

- Nulliparity
- Early menarche
- Increased frequency of menses
- History of dysmenorrhea
- Family history of fibroids
- African descent
- Obesity
- Age (40-50 years)
- Hypertension
- Diabetes mellitus
- Increased intake of caffeine.

DIFFERENTIAL DIAGNOSIS

Feature of differentiation:
- Pregnancy—associated with amenorrhea and softer uterus
- Full bladder—more cystic feel and disappears on evacuation
- Adenomyosis—uterus uniformly enlarged and size generally <12 weeks
- DUB—no associated mass or uterine enlargement
- Endometrial polyp/hyperplasia/carcinoma
- Endometriosis—uterus normal in size with adherent adnexal masses and reduced mobility
- Chronic PID—tenderness and fixity of uterus
- Tubo-ovarian mass/ovarian tumors—may not be associated with menorrhagia, cystic or mixed consistency and fixity, (difficult to differentiate from pedunculated subserosal or broad ligament fibroid)
- Uterine sarcoma—rapid increase in size and pain
- Other pelvic masses—pelvic kidney/tumor of bowel/appendix/abscess/diverticular abscess.

TYPES OF FIBROIDS

Fibroids may be single or multiple varying in size, location, and perfusion.

Fibroid may arise in the uterine body, cervix (<4%), intraligamentary (round, broad ligament, utero-ovarian, uterosacral), vagina or vulva.

They are classified into 3 types according to their location: subserosal (protruding outside the uterine surface), intramural (lying inside the myometrium), and or submucosal (protruding inside the uterine cavity). A pedunculated subserosal fibroid may detach itself from the uterus and become a parasitic or wandering fibroid.

A newer, classification system has been devised and advocated by FIGO is given below.[3] It is especially useful in formulating the management and surgical selection of cases (Table 12.2).

Table 12.2 The FIGO leiomyoma sub-classification system:

S—Submucosal	0	Pedunculated intracavitary
	1	<50% intramural
	2	≥50% intramural
O—Other	3	Contacts endometrium; 100% intramural
	4	Intramural
	5	Subserosal ≥50% intramural
	6	Subserosal <50% intramural
	7	Subserosal pedunculated
	8	Other (specify, e.g. cervical, parasitic)
Hybrid leiomyomas (impact both endometrium and serosa)		Two numbers are listed separated by a hyphen. By convention, the first refers to the relationship with the endometrium while the second refers to the relationship to the serosa. One example is below
	2–5	Submucosal and subserosal, each with less than half the diameter in the endometrial and peritoneal cavities, respectively.

DIAGNOSIS

History

Important points to be noted in history taking are:
- Age (mainly reproductive age group)
- Presenting complaints (AUB/pain/pressure symptoms/vaginal discharge/mass or lump in the lower abdomen/urinary or bowel complaints)
- Menstrual history (age at menarche/AUB/HMB/dysmenorrhea)
- Obstetric history infertility/recurrent pregnancy loss/malpresentations/fetal growth restriction/preterm labor/post-partum hemorrhage
- Associated history for identifying risk factors (Hypertension/Diabetes mellitus/increase caffeine intake)
- Family history of fibroids.

EXAMINATION

- Signs of anemia
- Palpable abdominal mass arising from pelvis
- Per speculum examination—vaginal discharge/mass protruding through or distending os may be seen in cervical fibroids or pedunculated submucosal fibroids
- Bimanual pelvic examination reveals— Enlarged, often irregular, firm, nontender uterus, movements of cervix are transmitted to it unless it is a pedunculated or broad ligament fibroid.

INVESTIGATIONS

- Pregnancy test, if indicated
- Complete blood count, iron studies for anemia
- Endometrial sampling (EA+ECC) for histopathological examination in case of AUB and HMB
- PAP smear in case of AUB

- Imaging studies—most useful and preferred imaging technique is ultrasonography, TAS+TVUS. Computed tomography (CT) does not have much role in diagnosis and evaluation of leiomyomas. Magnetic resonance imaging (MRI) provides additional details and is accurate in assessing adnexa.

For submucous myomas hysteroscopy, infusion sonohysterography and MRI are all highly sensitive and specific. TVUS being less sensitive and specific for the same. MRI is superior to other imaging and endoscopic techniques for characterization of relationship of submucous fibroid to myometrium and uterine serosa (Level A).[4]

Ultrasonography

Ultrasonography using the transabdominal and transvaginal routes is best to assess fibroid growth and adnexa. Fibroids appear typically, as well-defined, hypoechoic lesions unless they have undergone degeneration leading to complex appearance. On Doppler studies circumferential vascularity is typically seen in myomas. It is at times difficult to differentiate focal adenomyosis from fibroids and pedunculated subserosal or broad ligament fibroids from adnexal masses where MRI offers an advantage.

Contrast Infusion (Saline/Gel) Sonography

This investigation acts as an adjunct to ultrasonography in evaluating submucosal and intracavitary fibroids, preventing overestimation of endometrial thickness, differentiating fibroids from mucosal polyps/blood clots/endometrial hyperplasia. Also 2D and 3D sonohysterography accurately diagnoses submucosal lesions with specificity and sensitivity of 98–100%.

Virtual Hysteroscopy

In this technique, carbon dioxide is used to distend and separate the walls of the uterus, a CT (computerized tomography) scan is then performed. 3D uterine image is then reconstructed, allowing accurate assessment of the size and impact of fibroids on the cavity of the uterus.

Virtual hysteroscopy is a safe technique which seems to offer a highly useful alternative to saline sonography and diagnostic hysteroscopy.

Magnetic Resonance Imaging

The MRI is accurate in diagnosing a leiomyoma with a sensitivity of nearly 100% and a specificity of 91%, it helps in fibroid mapping (localization, measurement, and characterization) which is helpful in preoperative assessment of the case. It is especially useful in conditions where ultrasound findings are doubtful regarding diagnosis as in differentiating leiomyoma from adenomyosis and adnexal masses. A 'bridging vascular sign': vessels/signal void ring seen from uterus to the pelvic mass is indicative of fibroid extending into the adnexa. A gadolinium enhanced MRI is useful in assessing vascularity of fibroid hence predicting a good UAE response. Main deterrents in its use are high cost and limited accessibility.

TREATMENT

Most fibroids being asymptomatic do not require any therapy. In the rest 20–50% symptomatic fibroids treatment modality depends on the following:
- Symptoms and severity
- Age of the woman
- Size and location of leiomyomas
- Patients desire for fertility or uterine preservation
- Availability of treatment modality
- Experience and expertise of the care provider.

Treatment Options for Symptomatic Fibroids

- Expectant management
- *Medical therapies:*
  - NSAIDs
  - GnRH agonists

- GnRH antagonists
- SPRM
- OCP
- Danazol
- LNG-IUS
- Tranexamic acid
- Vitamin D
- *Surgical therapies:*
  - *Hysterectomy:*
    - Abdominal
    - Laparoscopic
    - Vaginal
  - *Myomectomy:*
    - Abdominal
    - Laparoscopic
    - Hysteroscopic
    - Robotic assisted laparoscopic
- *Conservative treatments:*
  - UAE
  - Focus energy delivery system
  - Radiofrequency myolysis
  - Mr guided SFUS.

EXPECTANT MANAGEMENT

In premenopausal women imaging studies have shown regression in 3–7% of untreated fibroids over a period of 6 months to 3 years.[5] At menopause there is regression of fibroids and symptomatic relief, hence women nearing menopause may be left on expectant management.

MEDICAL MANAGEMENT

Medical therapies have a limited role mainly aiming at iron therapy for anemia, controlling AUB, improving hemoglobin before surgery and/or temporary reduction in volume of fibroids preoperatively. Recent therapies acting at receptor levels offer a scope for long-term management and are under evaluation.

GnRH agonist is the most well studied, has a role in short-term usage temporarily for perimenopausal women in anticipation of menopause. It is recommended for use as preoperative adjunct in correction of anemia, reducing fibroid size hence influencing the surgical modality and approach for therapy (a less invasive approach and cosmetically better incisions are possible). Its use preoperatively has shown reduction in peroperative blood loss, duration of surgery, duration of hospital stay and postoperative complications in hysterectomy. Usage prior to myomectomy leads to reduction of blood loss and number of vertical incisions. However, there is increased likelihood of fibroid recurrence after 6 months of myomectomy and the increased difficulty in dissection of myomas is still controversial.

SPRM have shown promising results in fibroid size reduction with least side effects. Also cause reduction in menstrual blood loss thus helping in ameliorating anemia.

SERMS and aromatase inhibitors have shown effectivity mainly in postmenopausal women.

LNG-IUS use has shown significant reduction in menstrual blood loss but seem to have a higher expulsion rate (Table 12.3).

SURGICAL THERAPIES

Surgical therapies are planned after complete evaluation of the patient; the number, location, size of fibroid and the indication for which the surgery is being performed. The surgeon before planning should personally view the images, ensure correction of anemia and appropriately counsel and inform patient about various options available.

Hysterectomy

It is indicated in:
- In symptomatic women who have completed their family and desirous of definitive therapy. It guarantees complete removal of fibroid with symptomatic relief.
- In asymptomatic women hysterectomy is done only for fibroids increasing in size after menopause due to concerns of uterine leiomyosarcomas.
- It may be required as the repeat therapy in patients who have failed or have recurrence of fibroids after previous conservative surgical therapy.

Table 12.3 Drugs for medical therapy of fibroid uterus

Category	Drug (Quality of evidence)[2]	Mechanism	Effects	Dose and duration	Side effect
NSAID	Mefenamic acid	Inhibit prostaglandin synthesis	• Reduce dysmenorrhea	500 mg three times daily	Gastric irritation
Antifibrinolytic agent	Tranexamic acid	Reversible block of the locus that connects with lysine on plasminogen molecules	• Reduces menstrual blood loss	500 mg three times daily up to maximum 5 days during menses	Nausea vomiting
Combined oral contraceptive pills	Oral contraceptive (II-2)	• Inhibits ovulation • Inhibit sex steroid secretion	• Reduces menstrual blood loss[6] • Decrease fibroid growth • Increase hematocrit	Cyclical low dose COC for 21 day	• Mastalgia • Headache
Progesterones	• Norethisterone • Medroxyprogesterone acetate (II-2)	• Inhibits insulin like growth factor-I • Down regulates ER and PR • Cause endometrial atrophy	• Reducing menstrual bleeding in 70% • Amenorrhea in 30% • Decrease uterine volume in 50%[7]	15 mg norethisterone or (20–30 mg/day) medroxyprogesterone acetate given from day 5 to 25 of menstrual cycle	• Weight gain • Breast tenderness
	LNG-IUS (I)	Local progesterone action inhibits endometrial growth	• Reduces menstrual blood loss in 99% • Reduces uterine volume up to 40%[6]	Release levonorgestrel @ 20 µg/day	• Amenorrhea • Spotting
GnRH agonist	• Leuprolide • Goserelin • Triptorelin (I)	Pituitary down-regulation of Gonadotropin production	• Shrink by up to 50% of their initial volume within 3 months of therapy[7]	• Leuprolide Subcutaneous injection 500–1000 mg/day • Intranasal 400 mg 4 days Intramuscular depot 3.75–7.5 mg/month 10.25 mg/3 months	• Bone demineralization requiring add back therapy after 3–6 months of use • Regrowth occurring within an year of stoppage
GnRH antagonist	• Cetrorelix • Ganirelix	Pituitary down-regulation of Gonadotropin production	• Shrink fibroid size • Lack initial "flare" as with GnRHa	Ganirelix 2 mg subcutaneous daily	Bone demineralization

Contd...

Contd...

Category	Drug (Quality of evidence)[2]	Mechanism	Effects	Dose and duration	Side effect
Androgen agonist	Danazol (II-2)	Inhibitory action over sex-steroids synthesis and directly inhibits the progesterone receptor	• Reduces fibroid volume up to 30%	100–400 mg/day for 4–6 months	Weight gain, acne, hirsutism
SERM	Raloxifene	Selectively inhibits estrogen receptor in uterus	Useful adjunct in inducing fibroid shrinkage	60 mg daily for 3–6 months	Hot flashes, sweating, headache
Estrogen receptor antagonist	Fulvestrant	Degradation and down-regulation of estrogen receptors	Reduce fibroid volume	500 mg intramuscular injection fortnightly	Injection site reactions (pain, swelling, redness),
SPRM	Ulipristal acetate Asoprisnil (I)	Exhibits antiproliferative effects on leiomyoma cells and the endometrium. Inhibits ovulation	• Reduces menstrual blood loss • Reduces fibroid volume	5 mg ulipristal acetate per day up to 6 months	• Vasomotor symptoms • Benign endometrial changes
Progesterone receptor antagonist	Mifepristone (RU486)	Inhibits progesterone receptor and prevents fibroid growth	• Reduces fibroid volume[8]	2.5 mg daily for 3–6 months	• Amenorrhea • Vasomotor symptoms
Aromatase inhibitor	• Letrozole • Anastrozole	Inhibits the conversion of androgen into estrogen	Reduces fibroid volume 45%	2.5 mg/day of letrozole and 1 mg/day of anastrozole up to 6 months	Bone loss
Testosterone derivatives	Gestrinone synthetic derivative of the 19-nortestosterone group	Antioestrogen and antiprogesterone activity at the cellular receptor	Reduce uterine size and fibroid volume	2.5–5 mg (orally or by vaginal pessary), two or three times weekly. Used for 6 months to 1 year	
Somatostatin analog	Lanreotide	Reduce growth hormone secretion	Reduce fibroid volume	60 mg subcutaneous depot injection	Cardiac side effects
Vitamin	Vitamin D	An antifibrotic factor and inhibits growth and induces apoptosis in cultured human leiomyoma cells	Reduce fibroid volume[9]		

- Hysterectomy may also be required for uncontrolled hemorrhage during myomectomy where facility for emergency UAE is not available.

Route

The hysterectomy should be performed by the least invasive approach, feasible in each case.
- Vaginal route is the most preferred. Increasing expertise and surgical skill in nondescent vaginal hysterectomies has made this route more popular for benign conditions including fibroids. It is used in uterine size of up to 12 weeks. For bigger sizes morcellation, uterine bisection, coring may be used by experts as it may carry a higher risk of adjacent organ damage and peroperative blood loss.
- Laparoscopic hysterectomies (TLH/LAVH) are preferred over vaginal in larger uteri or associated adnexal pathology or suspected adhesions due to previous pelvic or abdominal surgeries.
- Abdominal hysterectomy is only indicated in very large uterine sizes (>20–24 weeks uterus) or when laparoscopic route is deemed risky due to anatomic distortion, excessive adhesions, large broad ligament (ureter lies medial to a true broad ligament and lateral to a pseudo broad ligament fibroid) and in cervical fibroids not approachable by vaginal route.

Preservation versus bilateral oophorectomy is controversial in women with healthy ovaries and over the age of 45 years. For women less than 45 years of age, the ovaries should definitely be spared.

Supracervical/subtotal hysterectomy has limited acceptance, but if done one should ensure preoperative pap smear to confirm a normal cervix.

Myomectomy

It is the procedure performed for symptomatic women who are desirous of retaining uterus irrespective of fertility considerations. It involves higher blood loss, increased operative time in comparison to hysterectomy along with a chance of requiring hysterectomy in 10% women due to recurrence of myoma. Hence, myomectomy is the alternative for women who desirous of preserving uterus or enhancing their fertility, but there are chances of further intervention (II-2)[2]

In cases of unexplained infertility, submucosal myomas are required to be removed for improving conception and pregnancy rates (II-2A).[10]

Hysteroscopic Myomectomy

It involves reduced surgical morbidity and avoidance of abdominal incisions, thus is the mainstay of conservative operative therapy for women with symptomatic fibroids which are intracavitary. Women having type 0, I, and II submucous fibroids (FIGO classification, Table II), up to 5 cm in size can undergo hysteroscopic myomectomy. Type II submucous myomas may require a 2–staged procedure. It is imperative to be cautious in myomas with less than 5 mm myometrial thickness from serosa.

Indications

Intracavitary symptomatic myomas presenting mainly with:
- AUB/HMB
- Recurrent pregnancy loss.
- Infertility.

Contraindications

- Active pelvic infections
- Suspected malignancy
- Medical co-morbidities like cardiovascular disease.

Preoperative Preparation

GnRH agonist administered preoperatively for reducing time of surgery, absorption of distention media and incidence of incomplete resection is not yet proven (level B).[4]

Cervical preparation before hysteroscopic myomectomy is an option to avoid excessive

force during cervical dilatation causing cervical tears and uterine perforation (level A).[4]
- Misoprostol 200–400 mcg oral or vaginal, 12 hours before surgery helps easier cervical dilatation and reduces risk of trauma in premenopausal women[11]
- Luminaria tents placed through internal os a day prior to surgery is under trial
- Intracervical vasopressin 10 mL of dilute solution prepared by 4 units in 80 mL solution, injected at 3'o clock and 9'o clock position at time of surgery facilitates cervical dilatation[12] but is under trial.

Procedure involves distention of uterus with distending media, the input and output of which should be accurately measured and quantified to reduce risk of systemic absorption (level B).[4] A 1000 mL of absorption of distending media is considered as maximum permissible. Hypotonic solution (like 5% glycine, 3% sorbitol, 5% mannitol) is used while preparing for procedure with monopolar loop resectoscopy.

Isotonic fluid like normal saline/ringer lactate is used while performing procedure with bipolar resectoscopes.

The basic modalities for hysteroscopic resection are:
- Electrosurgical loop (monopolar/bipolar)
- Morcellation
- Vapourization.

All precautions should be taken to minimize thermal injury to endometrium adjacent to incision in case of fertility preservation. Ensure avoidance of loop touching adjacent areas of endometrium.

The incision should be started at most cephalad area of the fibroid. The direction of movement of resectoscope loop should always be towards surgeon and never away. The loop is to be kept under visualization at all times. Myoma is to be resected till the level of the adjacent endometrium.

The *complication* rate varies from 0.8% to 2.6% and the uterine perforation, excessive distention fluid absorption, burns, bleeding, adhesion formation and uncommonly infection.

Rate of recurrent fibroid and bleeding following hysteroscopic myomectomy is around 20% in 3–4 years.

Laparoscopic Myomectomy

Laparoscopy is superior to open myomectomy as there is reduced blood loss and postoperative pain, quicker postoperative recovery and cosmetically advantageous.

Indications for laparoscopic approach:
- Symptomatic fibroids—intramural/subserosal
- Fibroids appropriate for laparoscopic approach
  - Size (<10 cm)
  - Number (depends on surgical expertise)
  - Location (not in the lower segment or cervical)
- Submucous leiomyomas where hysteroscopic myomectomy is not appropriate (e.g. Type 2-5, or 2-6 lesions) or associated large intramural or subserosal lesions
- There is associated intra-abdominal pathology with fibroids.

Procedure involves: insertion of ports, measures for reducing blood loss, uterine incision—transverse are preferred, removal of myoma through port or morcellation, closing the defect with multilayer delayed absorbable suture.

Laparoscopic myomectomy has a longer duration of surgery and requires special training.

Laparoscopic and open myomectomy have comparable major complication rates of hemorrhage, visceral injuries and conversion to hysterectomy as also pregnancy outcomes, and recurrence.[13]

Abdominal Myomectomy

Limited indications and not a preferred route.

Indicated in:
- Symptomatic intramural/subserosal fibroids
- Hysteroscopic or laparoscopic myomectomy is not appropriate
  - Large >10 cm fibroid
  - Fibroid in lower segment or cervical

- Associated intra-abdominal pathology requiring laparotomy.

Basic Principles

- Consent for hysterectomy along with myomectomy to be taken for unforeseen peroperative problems
- Adequate blood to be arranged prior to surgery
- Intraoperative adjuncts for reducing blood loss are to be used
- Anterior uterine incision is preferred with an attempt to remove maximum fibroids through minimal tunneling incision
- Enucleation to be performed by incising capsule and identifying appropriate plane
- Hemostasis to be secured and thorough obliteration of myoma cavity by multilayering with delayed absorbable sutures
- Raw areas on surface should be peritonised well to prevent postoperative adhesions
- Anteversion to be assured if required by round ligament plication
- Complications are similar and comparable to laparoscopic myomectomy (Hemorrhage, trauma to adjacent viscera, infection, adhesions and recurrence).

Minilaparotomy for Myomectomy

It is a technique used as an alternative of laparoscopic myomectomy. It may offer an advantage of easier myometrial suturing simultaneously utilizing a less invasive technique than usual abdominal myomectomy. Minilaparotomy may also be used as adjunct to laparoscopic myomectomy.

Robotic-assisted Laparoscopy

Robotic surgery is gaining popularity since last 10 years. But studies have shown a longer duration of surgery, greater blood loss and is costlier than laparoscopic myomectomy.

Adjuncts for reduction of blood loss during myomectomy should be utilized (I-A).[2] These include:
- *Misoprostol:* PGE1 analogue in single dose of 400 µg per vaginum an hour before surgery reduces operative time, loss of blood, fall in hemoglobin and requirement for blood transfusion.
- *Vasopressin:* Intramyometrial into planned incision site before incision for each fibroid has shown to reduce 290 mL of blood loss[14] (20 units in 20 mL)
- *Bupivacaine and epinephrine:* Intramyometrial injection before myomectomy performed laparoscopically showed a reduction in blood loss and time of surgery, led to easier surgical enucleation of myoma as well as there is reduction in requirement of analgesia[15]
- *Tranexamic acid:* Up to 1 g when given intravenously 15 minutes, prior to skin incision during abdominal myomectomy shows a reduction in blood loss but clinically significant reduction is not yet demonstrated.
- Gelatin-thrombin matrix is a bovine extracted hemostatic agent which on application adheres to the bleeding wet tissues and seals it thus reducing blood loss both intra- and postoperatively.
- Occlusion of uterine arteries intraoperatively with or without ovarian artery occlusion has shown to reduce blood loss significantly and also the requirement of blood transfusion.[16]

MINIMALLY INVASIVE TECHNIQUES

Uterine Artery Embolization (UAE)[17]

- It is a percutaneous fluoroscopic procedure performed usually by interventional radiologist with special training and experience in vascular embolization.
- Cochrane review (2012)[18]—states regarding evidenced based use of UAE that "UAE appears to have an overall patient satisfaction rate similar to hysterectomy and myomectomy while offering an advantage with regards to routine activities. However, UAE is associated with a higher rate of minor complications and increased likelihood of requiring surgical intervention within two to five years of the initial procedure. There is very low level evidence suggesting that myomectomy may

be associated with better fertility outcomes than UAE, but more research is needed.
- Procedure is performed under local anesthesia and involves unilateral/bilateral femoral access with 4/5Fr catheter and injection of embolization agent with a diameter 300–750 micrometer (PVA/metal coil/gel foam) into one or both uterine arteries approached via the anterior division of internal iliac arteries. It causes irreversible ischemia, necrosis and shrinkage.
- It is a safe procedure with 80–90% women having improvement in symptoms becoming asymptomatic by 1 year. There is 40–70% reduction in fibroid size.[17]
- Indication: in fibroid uterus for embolization
  - Symptomatic fibroids with HMB, dysmenorrhea or causing pressure symptoms
  - May be used for adenomyosis when associated with fibroids after patient being well counseled.
  - Women with medical contraindication to surgery
  - In emergency situations like acute hemorrhage associated with fibroid during cesarean section or postpartum hemorrhage.
- *Contraindications:*
  - *Absolute:*
    - Active/current infection of genital tract
    - Asymptomatic myomas
    - Pregnancy
    - Patient not willing for hysterectomy even in emergency situation
  - *Relative:*
    - Women desirous of preserving fertility as RCTs show lowered rates of pregnancy and a higher rate of miscarriage as compared to myomectomy[17]
    - Thin stalked submucosal pedunculated fibroids or large submucosal fibroids which are intracavity as these might detach into the uterine cavity post procedure or slough causing sepsis
    - Large uterus (>20 weeks) with pressure symptoms as results might not be satisfactory.
- *Complications:*
  - *Immediate:* Hematoma, thrombosis, dissection or aneurysm, reaction to contrast medium, nontargeted embolization leading to ovarian failure and amenorrhea.
  - *Early (<30 days):* Pain, nausea, fever and malaise, rarely infection.
  - *Late (>30 days):* Vaginal discharge, expulsion of fibroid and its impaction, infection, amenorrhea and occasional changes in sexual function.

Magnetic Resonance-guided Focused Ultrasound Surgery (MRgFUS)

MRgFUS is a relatively new method of thermal ablation for treating fibroids, which uses high-intensity focused ultrasound that passes through the anterior abdominal wall and converges into a precise target point within the fibroid to cause a temperature rise (55–90°C) sufficient to induce coagulative necrosis within a few seconds. Concurrent MRI allows accurate tissue targeting and real-time temperature feedback, thereby achieving controlled localized thermal ablation. The advantages of MRgFUS are its completely noninvasive character and continuous imaging of fibroids and adjacent structures, which optimizes fibroid ablation and prevents injury to adjacent tissues. The disadvantage is that relatively few patients are eligible—only those with fibroids located immediately beneath the anterior abdominal wall without bowel interposition or scars in the region of interest. The average treatment time is however, long and the patient has to lie still for the duration of the treatment time.

Myolysis

Laparoscopic myolysis involves delivering of RF energy or laser energy or cryo probe or bipolar electrodes to myomas under ultrasonic guidance. it cause coagulative necrosis of the myoma and reduces the size of myoma. The mapping of myomas is performed prior to the procedure by ultrasound visualization. Myolysis has shown some efficacy in reducing fibroid size in some patients, but is associated with a risk of bowel adhesions and coagulation of the myometrium.

Laparoscopic Uterine Artery Occlusion

Laparoscopic uterine artery occlusion uses a laparoscopic lateral retroperitoneal approach to achieve uterine artery occlusion. Unlike with UAE, patients undergoing LUAO are placed under general anesthesia, and artery occlusion is performed using ultrasonically activated sheets, clips, or electrosurgery. This method is still under evaluation.

Doppler-guided Uterine Artery Occlusion

Dickner and colleagues[19] demonstrated that a Doppler-guided nonincisional transvaginal approach could be used to successfully identify uterine arteries in 108 of 109 healthy premenopausal women despite wide variability in the position and depth of these arteries. These findings were the basis for the development of a uterine device (D-UAO) composed of a cervical tenaculum incorporating a guiding monorail and a paracervical vascular clamp with integrated Doppler ultrasound crystals, connected to a battery-powered ultrasound transceiver to generate an audible Doppler signal. This method is still under evaluation.

GENERAL TREATMENT PLAN

Asymptomatic—No therapy

Mildly symptomatic perimenopausal women (tolerating symptoms well)—Expectant Management.
Symptomatic women:
- Desirous of fertility/preservation—medical therapy/myomectomy
- Desirous of retaining uterus—medical therapy/myomectomy/myolysis/UAE
- Infertile/pregnancy complications in previous pregnancy desirous of pregnancy—myomectomy
- Severe symptoms wanting definitive treatment—Hysterectomy.

Special Considerations

Infertility and Fibroids

The role of fibroids as a cause of infertility and myomectomy for the treatment of the same still remains controversial. Fibroids are found to be present in 5-10% of fertile women, when other causes are ruled out the percentage further falls to 1-2%.[20] It is nearly proven that subserosal fibroids do not have any role in causing infertility. Submucosal fibroids though shown a negative impact on implantation rates and are associated with higher rates of miscarriages. Role of intramural fibroids remains unclear.

Meta-analysis of the limited studies available shows that myomectomy for submucosal fibroids apparently benefits pregnancy rates.[21]

The various proposed mechanisms by which fibroids adversely impact fertility are:
- Increased association with PID, endometriosis and anovulation
- Direct mechanical corneal and tubal block
- Impairment of blood supply to endometrium and adjacent myometrium
- Atrophy and ulceration especially associated with intracavity fibroids
- Impaired gamete transport and migration of embryo due to distortion of cavity and altered contractility of uterus
- Implantation rates are decreased in intra-mural and submural fibroids due to endometrial change in vascularity and through secretion of growth/angiogenic factors, impairment of their normal secretion
- Mechanical pressure leading to changes in myometrial contractility in surrounding areas.

Pregnancy and Fibroids

The prevalence of fibroid has been variably reported in pregnancy, between 8% and 18%.[22] Most (60-70%) fibroids do not undergo any change in size during pregnancy. A few grow mainly in the 1st trimester and minimally in 2nd and 3rd trimesters. Maximum growth is around 25% increase in volume. 70% show a decrease in volume during puerperium.[23]

Most fibroids remain asymptomatic. Most common symptom if occurs is pain which may be acute and severe when it undergoes red degeneration, torsion or impaction (these generally occur in fibroids >5 cm in size).

Red degeneration causes a sudden severe pain in abdomen associated with febrile illness, moderate leukocytosis and a raised ESR. It is said to occur when:
- The fibroid outgrows its blood supply leading to anoxia, necrosis and infarction.
- Changes in uterine size causing kinking of blood vessels supplying the fibroid causing ischemia and thrombosis.

Prostaglandin release from necrotic tissue is responsible for the extreme pain associated with this condition.

It is generally relieved by rest, analgesia and adequate hydration.

Fibroids cause complication in 10–30% of pregnant women.

In early pregnancy, miscarriage rate is significantly increased and is more dependent on location and number of fibroids rather than the size of fibroid. It is more in multiple fibroids, those in uterine body and intramural or submucosal.[23] Bleeding has also been shown to be significantly increased more so if placental implantation is close to fibroid.

In late pregnancy fibroids are associated with higher rates of preterm labor, abruptio placentae and placenta previa.

Fetal growth restriction and fetal anomalies like dolichocephaly, torticollis, limb reduction defects have been reported.[24]

During labor and delivery, risk of malpresentation, dystocia (2 fold), cesarean delivery (3.7 fold) and retained placenta. Large cervical fibroids may lead to obstructed labor.

Incidence of postpartum hemorrhage is high due to distortion of cavity, reduced contractility leading to increased chances of cesarean hysterectomy. Bilateral UAE is effective in controlling PPH also if performed immediately after cesarean section is effective in reducing blood loss, risk of myomectomy and hysterectomy.

Myomectomy other than for symptomatic pedunculated fibroids should not be performed in pregnant women. Recently a number of case series have reported myomectomy during cesarean section as safe but should only be considered if clinically required.[25]

Scar rupture associated with previous myomectomy is an extremely rare occurrence. None occurs if uterine cavity is not entered. Incidence of 0.5–1% is reported with laparoscopic myomectomy. If cavity has been entered, an elective cesarean section is preferred before patient goes into labor.

Fibroids and Concerns for Malignancy

Leiomyosarcomas are rare tumors. The chances of finding a uterine sarcoma in women with intrauterine mass ~0.1–0.28%. The importance lies in differentiation of uterine sarcoma from fibroid uterus as both present as focal uterine myometrial masses.

Clinical presentations are not helpful in differentiating leiomyomas from sarcomas as both present with AUB and pain with pelvic mass. Uterine size being large is also not shown to be a marker for higher risk of sarcoma. Rapid growth in menopausal women is a risk factor for uterine sarcoma. MRI is somewhat helpful but not definitive. Absence of calcification, ill-defined margins and intralesional hemorrhage point towards uterine sarcomas.

Gadolinium enhancement on contrast MRI has reported high specificities for sarcoma detection. Raised LDH levels seem to be marker of uterine sarcoma.

Endometrial biopsy may detect a uterine sarcoma.

Another variant which poses a diagnostic and treatment dilemma are variants of these two extremes with some features of malignancy but not classified as benign or malignant. These are now labeled by WHO as 'Smooth muscle tumors of uncertain malignant potential/STUMP'.[26]

It is extremely rare for a myoma to undergo malignant change (0.5%).

Concerns Regarding Morcellation

Laparoscopically performed hysterectomy and myomectomy quite frequently require specimen to be morcellated for removal. The complications related to it are trauma to adjacent visceral organs and vascular injuries. The use of this technique may cause dissemination of small pieces of fibroid causing leiomyomatosis. It may further have a risk of upstaging an existing undiagnosed leiomyosarcoma.

The risk of having an incidental leiomyosarcoma in women undergoing surgery for leiomyoma is 1 per 400. Even though care may be taken to prevent spillage by use of endobags and enclosed morcellation its risk of spread remains.

Warning issued by USFDA in 2014 for laparoscopic power morcellation has discouraged its use during hysterectomy or myomectomy for fibroid uterus.[27]

KEY POINTS

- Uterine fibroids are the most common benign uterine tumors and ≥50% are asymptomatic
- They have varied clinical presentation like AUB, dysmenorrhea, infertility, pelvic or abdominal mass or pressure symptoms
- Ultrasound is the most useful and preferred imaging technique for diagnosis MRI provide a more accurate and specific diagnosis
- Medical management has limited role at present for correction of anemia, preoperative adjunct for size reduction and in perimenopausal women in anticipation of menopause
- Surgical management has to be selected according to symptoms and severity; fertility preservation; desire of uterine preservation and expertise of surgeon
- Minimally invasive and radiological interventions are gaining importance and have a promising future.

REFERENCES

1. Cramer SF, Patel A. The frequency of uterine leiomyomas. Am J Clin Pathol. 1990;94:435-8.
2. George AV, Catherine A, Philippe YL, et al. Society of Obstetrics and Gynaecology Canada Clinical Practice—Gynaecology Committee. The management of Uterine Leiomyomas. SOGC Clinical Practice Guidelines, No. 318, Feb. 2015. J Obstet Gynaecol Can. 2015;37(2): 157-78.
3. Munro MG, Critchley HO, Broder MS, et al. The FIGO Classification System ("PALM-COEIN") for causes of abnormal uterine bleeding in non-gravid women in the reproductive years, including guidelines for clinical investigation. Int J Gynaecol Obstet. 2011;113:3-13.
4. American Association of Gynecologic Laparoscopists (AAGL): Advancing Minimally Invasive Gynecology Worldwide. AAGL practice report: practice guidelines for the diagnosis and management of submucous leiomyomas. J Minim Invasive Gynecol. 2012;19:152-71.
5. Peddada SD, Laughlin SK, Miner K, et al. Growth of uterine leiomyomata among premenopausal black and white women. Proc Natl Acad Sci USA. 2008;105:19887-92.
6. Sayed GH, Zakherah MS, El-Nashar SA, et al. A randomized clinical trial of a levonorgestrel-releasing intrauterine system and a low-dose combined oral contraceptive for fibroid-related menorrhagia. Int J Gynaecol Obstet. 2011;112:126-30.
7. Carr BR, Marshburn PB, Weatherall PT, et al. An evaluation of the effect of gonadotropin-releasing hormone analogs and medroxyprogesterone acetate on uterine leiomyomata volume by magnetic resonance imaging: a prospective, randomized, double blind, placebo-controlled, crossover trial. J Clin Endocrinol Metab. 1993;76:1217-23.
8. Eisinger SH, Bonfiglio T, Fiscella K, et al. Twelve-month safety and efficacy of low-dose

mifepristone for uterine myomas. J Minim Invasive Gynecol. 2005;12:227-33.

9. Halder SK, Sharan C, Al-Hendy A. Vitamin D treatment induces dramatic shrinkage of uterine leiomyomas growth in the Eker rat model. Fertility and Sterility. 2010;94(4):S75-S76.

10. Belina CM, Jon H, Robert H, et al. Society of Obsterics and Gynaecology Canada Clinical Practaice—Reproductive endocrine and infertility committee. The management of uterine fibroids in women with otherwise unexplained infertility. SOGC clinical practice guidelines, No. 321, March, 2015. J Obstet Gynaecol Com. 2015;37(3):277-285.

11. Batukan C, Ozgun MT, Ozcelik B, et al. Cervical ripening before operative hysteroscopy in premenopausal women: a randomized, double-blind, placebo-controlled comparison of vaginal and oral misoprostol. Fertil Steril. 2008;89:966-73 (I).

12. Phillips DR, Nathanson HG, Milim SJ, et al. The effect of dilute vasopressin solution on the force needed for cervical dilatation: a randomized controlled trial. Obstet Gynecol. 1997;89:507-11 (I).

13. Jin C, Hu Y, Chen XC, Zheng FY, et al. Laparoscopic versus open myomectomy—a meta-analysis of randomized controlled trials. Eur J Obstet Gynecol Reprod Biol. 2009;145:14-21.

14. Fletcher H, Frederick J, Hardie M, et al. A randomized comparison of vasopressin and tourniquet as hemostatic agents during myomectomy. Obstet Gynecol. 1996;87:1014-8.

15. Zullo F, Palomba S, Corea D, et al. Bupivacaine plus epinephrine for laparoscopic myomectomy: a randomized placebo-controlled trial. Obstet Gynecol. 2004;104:243-9.

16. Taylor A, Sharma M, Tsirkas P, et al. Reducing blood loss at open myomectomy using triple tourniquets: a randomised controlled trial. BJOG. 2005;112:340-5.

17. Clinical recommendations on the use of uterine artery embolizaton (UAE) in the management of fibroids, 3rd edn. London: RCOG and RCR, 2013

18. Gupta JK, Sinha A, Lunsden MA, Hickey M. Cochrane database of systematic reviews: Uterine artery embolization of symptomatic uterine fibroids. http://onlinelibrary.wiley.com/doi/10.1002/14651858.CD005073pub3/full

19. Dickner SK, Cooper JM, Diaz D. A nonincisional, Dopplerguided transvaginal approach to uterine artery identification and control of uterine perfusion. J Am Assoc Gynecol Laparosc. 2004; 11: 55-8.

20. Cook H, Ezzati M, Segars JH, McCarthy K. The impact of uterine leiomyomas on reproductive outcomes. Minerva Ginecol. 2010;62:225-36.

21. Pritts EA, Parker WH, Olive DL. Fibroids and infertility: an updated systematic review of the evidence. Fertil Steril. 2009;91:1215-23.

22. Laughlin SK, Baird DD, Savitz DA, et al. Prevalence of uterine leiomyomas in the first trimester of pregnancy: an ultrasound-screening study. Obstet Gynecol. 2009;113:630-5.

23. Laughlin SK, Herrings AH, Savitz DA, et al. Pregnancy-related fibroid reduction. Fertil Steril. 2010;94:2421-3.

24. Klatsky PC, Tran ND, Caughey AB, et al. Fibroids and reproductive outcomes: a systematic literature review from conception to delivery. Am J Obstet Gynecol. 2008;198:357-66.

25. Park BJ, Kim YW. Safety of cesarean myomectomy. J Obstet Gynaecol Res. 2009;35:906-11.

26. Ip PP, Tse KY, Tam KF. Uterine smooth muscle tumors other than the ordinary leiomyomas and leiomyosarcomas: a review of selected variants with emphasis on recent advances and unusual morphology that may cause concern for malignancy. Adv Anat Pathol. 2010;17:91-112.

27. Food and Drug Administration. Quantitative assessment of the prevalence of unsuspected uterine sarcoma in women undergoing treatment of uterine fibroids: summary and key findings. Silver Spring, MD: FDA; 2014. Available at *http://www.fda.gov/downloads/MedicalDevices/Safety/AlertsandNotices/UCM393589.pdf*.

13

Endometriosis and Adenomyosis

Nilanchali Singh, Deepali Dhingra, Nupur Ahuja

ENDOMETRIOSIS

Endometriosis, one of the most common diseases encountered by gynecologists, is defined as the presence of endometrial glands and stromal tissue outside the uterus. This ectopic endometrial tissue induces chronic, estrogen dependent inflammatory response.[1] The most common sites affected are the ovaries, uterine ligaments, recto and vesicovaginal septae, pelvic peritoneum, cervix, labia, and vagina.

Prevalence

Endometriosis is one of the most common conditions encountered in gynecological practice and its incidence is on rise. Major studies have reported that 25–50% of infertile women have endometriosis and 30–50% of women with endometriosis are infertile.[2] The true prevalence of endometriosis is difficult to quantify as very wide ranges have been reported in literature. Endometriosis is found in 45–82% of women with chronic pelvic pain and in 2.1–78% of infertile women. It affects 6–10% of women of reproductive age, and it is present in approximately 38% of women with infertility and in up to 87% of women with chronic pelvic pain.[2] An Indian study found the frequency of endometriosis in women with infertility to be 48.38%.[3]

Symptoms[4]

- Pelvic symptoms—cyclical pelvic pain, dysmenorrhea and dyspareunia
- Heavy menstrual bleeding
- Infertility
- Intestinal complaints—periodic bloating, diarrhea or constipation
- Atypical presentations—cyclic leg pain or sciatica, cyclic rectal bleeding, hematuria and cyclic dyspnea secondary to catamenial pneumothorax suggesting more severe disease.

However, the predictive value of these symptoms for the presence of endometriosis is low.

The ESHRE Guidelines (European Society of Human Reproduction and Embryology), 2013 recommends that clinicians should consider the diagnosis of endometriosis in the presence of gynecological symptoms such as dysmenorrhea, noncyclical pelvic pain, deep dyspareunia, infertility, fatigue in the presence of any of the above (good practice point).[5] It also recommends that clinicians should consider the diagnosis of endometriosis in women of reproductive age with nongynecological cyclical symptoms (dyschezia, dysuria, hematuria, rectal bleeding, shoulder pain) (good practice point).

Signs

- Fixed, retroverted uterus
- Tender nodules on palpation of uterosacral ligaments
- Adnexal masses suggesting endometriomas.

The ESHRE Guidelines, 2013 recommends that clinicians should perform clinical examination in all women suspected of endometriosis, although vaginal examination may be inappropriate for adolescents and/or women without previous sexual intercourse. In such cases, rectal examination can be helpful for the diagnosis of endometriosis (good practice point). It also recommends clinicians may consider the diagnosis of deep endometriosis in women with painful induration and/or nodules of the rectovaginal wall found during clinical examination, or visible vaginal nodules in the posterior vaginal fornix. Clinicians may consider the diagnosis of ovarian endometrioma in women with adnexal masses detected during clinical examination. Clinicians may also consider the diagnosis of endometriosis in women suspected of the disease even if the clinical examination is normal (Grade C recommendation).[5]

Etiopathogenesis

The most widely accepted theory on endometriosis is Sampson's transplantation theory, which states that endometriosis is the result of retrograde menstruation of viable endometrial cells through patent fallopian tubes. This theory is supported by the anatomic distribution of implants of endometriotic tissue. But it does not explain why endometriosis is present in only 10% of patients when reflux menstruation is present in most of menstruating women. Other theories are metaplasia of peritoneal cells into endometriotic cells and spread of ectopic endometrial cells via lymphatic or vascular system.

Local increased production of estrogen and progesterone, resistance to progesterone and failure to clear ectopic endometrial tissue due to defective immune mechanism are some of proposed molecular basis of endometriosis.[4] There is overproduction of cytokines, prostaglandins and growth factors in ectopic endometrial tissue which is responsible for pain and subfertility.

Risk Factors

- Likelihood of endometriosis is increased in presence of following:
- Nulliparity
- Subfertility
- Presence of disease in first degree relative
- Reproductive tract anomalies
- Early menarche and late menopause
- Low body mass index (BMI)
- Alcohol consumption.

Diagnosis

Diagnosis of suspected endometriosis requires history, examination and imaging studies. The gold standard for diagnosis is direct visualization at laparoscopy and histologic study. Role of some biomarkers are also elucidated.

Ultrasonography

When suspected transvaginal ultrasound (TVS) is modality of choice to diagnose or exclude ovarian endometrioma.[6] The ESHRE Guidelines, 2013 recommends transvaginal ultrasonography with bowel preparation and transrectal ultrasonography can detect deep infiltrating lesions affecting the bowel, bladder, and rectovaginal pouch.[7] (Grade A recommendation) Clinicians should base the diagnosis of ovarian endometrioma in premenopausal women on the following ultrasound characteristics: ground glass echogenicity and one to four compartments and no papillary structures with detectable blood flow (good practice point). Clinicians should be aware that the usefulness of 3D sonography to diagnose rectovaginal endometriosis is not well established (Grade A recommendation).[5] Bladder endometriosis can be suspected from patient history and diagnosed by transvaginal sonography, ideally while the patient has a full bladder.

Magnetic Resonance Imaging

If there is suspicion of deep infiltrative disease the involvement of abdominal organs like bladder, ureter, or bowel should be evaluated by additional imaging studies like MRI. Magnetic resonance imaging (MRI) or sonography, with or without barium enema studies can be performed to map the extent of the disease, which may be multifocal. Endometriosis involving the ureter can be visualized by MRI or CT urogram. The usefulness of magnetic resonance imaging to diagnose peritoneal endometriosis is not well established.

Role of Biomarkers

Serum CA-125 has been proposed as a noninvasive diagnostic biomarker. The role of serum CA-125 in diagnosis of early stages endometriosis is limited, whereas its utility in the diagnosis of high grade endometriosis is better. Despite its limited diagnostic performance, routine use of serum CA-125 measurement in patients with infertility might be of some relevance, as early laparoscopy might be helpful in these women. There are currently no known immunological biomarkers in endometrial tissue, menstrual or uterine fluids, which are able to diagnose endometriosis in a noninvasive way (The ESHRE Guidelines, 2013, Grade A recommendation).[5] Future studies may show a potential of biomarkers in endometriosis, including prognosis, disease staging, identifying subgroups of patients and differentiation from other ovarian abnormalities.

Laparoscopic Findings

Laparoscopy and directed biopsy forms the gold standard for diagnosis of endometriosis. In the absence of signs and symptoms of ovarian endometrioma, invasive disease or infertility, laparoscopy is not mandatory before commencing medical therapy. Again, laparoscopy should be considered when symptoms are severe and/or persistent despite medical treatment.

Typical lesions: Powder burn or gunshot black, dark-brown, or bluish puckered lesions, nodules or small cysts containing old hemorrhage surrounded by a variable extent of fibrosis (Fig. 13.1).

Atypical lesions: Red implants (petechial, vesicular, polypoid, hemorrhagic, red flame-like) and serous or clear vesicles (Fig. 13.2).

Endometrioma: These arise from the ovary, contain thick chocolate colored fluid. There is often surrounding fibrosis with involvement of fallopian tubes or bowel (Fig. 13.3).

Deep infiltrative disease: The endometriotic nodules extend >5 mm beneath the peritoneum and may involve the uterosacral ligaments,

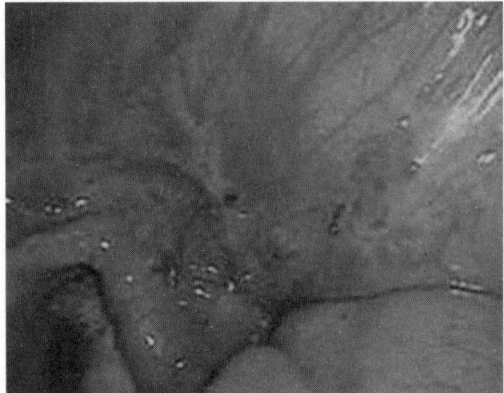

Fig. 13.1 Bluish puckered lesions and small vesicles surrounded by some fibrosis (typical lesion) *(For color version, see Plate 3)*

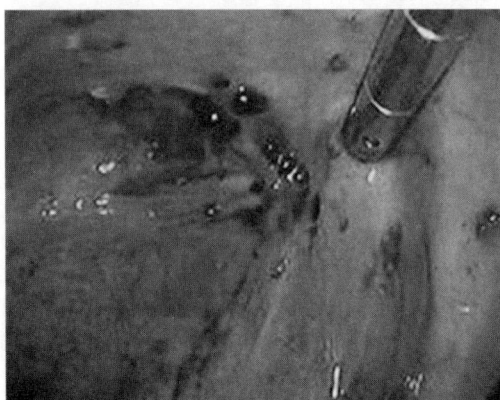

Fig. 13.2 Red implants with petechiae and vesicles (atypical lesion) *(For color version, see Plate 3)*

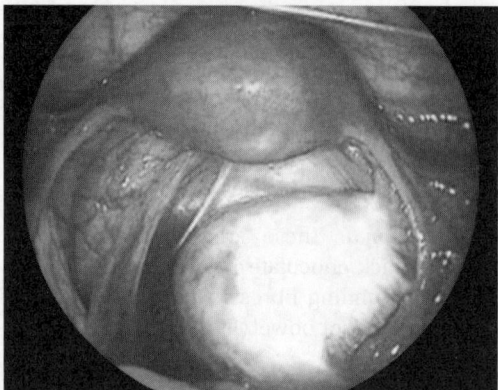

Fig. 13.3 Large endometrioma arising from right ovary *(For color version, see Plate 3)*

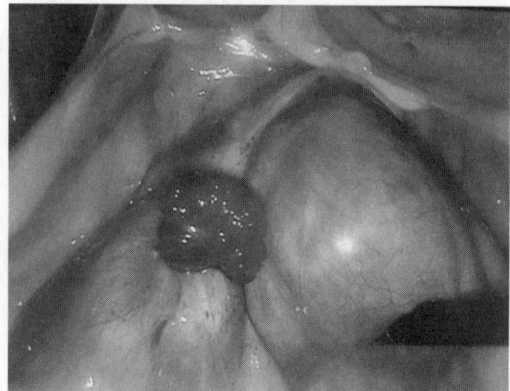

Fig. 13.5 Dense adhesions due to endometriosis leading to tubo-ovarian mass formation, suggestive of moderate-to-severe disease *(For color version, see Plate 3)*

Histology

It is recommended to obtain tissue for histology in women undergoing surgery for ovarian endometrioma and/or deep infiltrating disease, to exclude rare instances of malignancy (The ESHRE Guidelines, 2013, good practice point). The gold standard for diagnosis is direct visualization at laparoscopy and histologic study.[5]

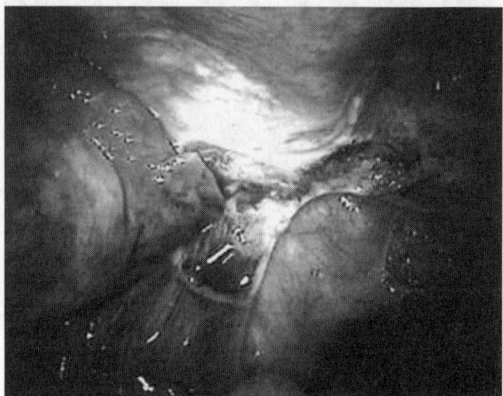

Fig. 13.4 Infiltrative lesion of the uterosacral ligament obliterating the pouch of Douglas *(For color version, see Plate 3)*

Staging of Endometriosis

vagina, bowel, bladder, or ureters. Depth of invasion is proportional to severity of symptoms[5] (Fig. 13.4).

The ESHRE Guidelines, 2013 recommends that clinicians perform a laparoscopy to diagnose endometriosis, although evidence is lacking that a positive laparoscopy without histology proves the presence of disease. It is also recommended that a positive laparoscopy should be confirmed by histology, since positive histology confirms the diagnosis of endometriosis, even though negative histology does not exclude it (good practice point).[5]

American Society for Reproductive Medicine (ASRM) has classified endometriosis into different stages depending on location, extent, and depth of endometriosis implants; presence and severity of adhesions; and presence and size of ovarian endometriomas. Minimal and mild endometriosis is characterized by few superficial implants and mild adhesions. Moderate and severe endometriosis is characterized by deep implants, presence of endometriomas and dense adhesions (Figs 13.5 and 13.6).

Adamson developed the endometriosis fertility index (EFI) in 2010, a scoring system consist of historical factors at the time of surgery, adnexal function after the intevention of surgery and assessment of endometriosis.

Stage I (Minimal)

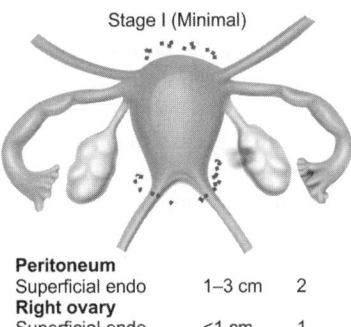

Peritoneum
Superficial endo 1–3 cm 2
Right ovary
Superficial endo <1 cm 1
Flimsy adhesions 1/3 1
Total points 4

Stage II (Mild)

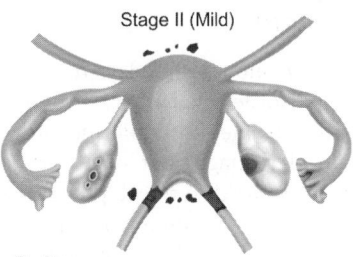

Peritoneum
Deep endo >3 cm 6
Right ovary
Superficial endo <1 cm 1
Flimsy adhesions <1/3 1
Left ovary
Superficial endo <1 cm 1
Total points 9

Stage III (Moderate)

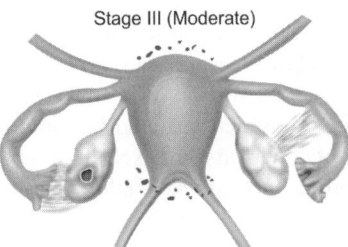

Peritoneum
Deep endo >3 cm 6
Cul-de-sac
Partial obliteration 4
Left ovary
Deep endo 1–3 cm 16
Total points 26

Stage III (Moderate)

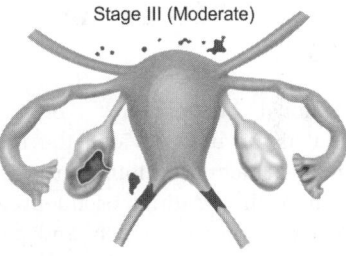

Peritoneum
Superficial endo >3 cm 4
Right tube
Flimsy adhesions <1/3 1
Right ovary
Flimsy adhesions <1/3 1
Left tube
Dense adhesions <1/3 16*
Left ovary
Deep endo 1–3 cm 4
Dense adhesions <1/3 4
Total points 30

Stage IV (Severe)

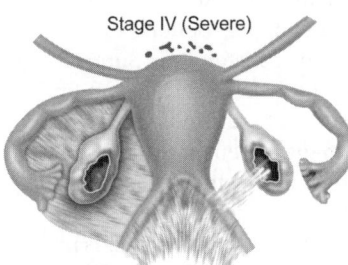

Peritoneum
Deep endo >3 cm 6
Cul-de-sac
Complete obliteration 40
Right ovary
Deep endo 1–3 cm 16
Dense adhesions <1/3 4
Left tube
Dense adhesions >2/3 16
Left ovary
Deep endo 1–3 cm 16
Dense adhesions >2/3 16
Total points 114

*Point assignment changed to 16

Stage IV (Severe)

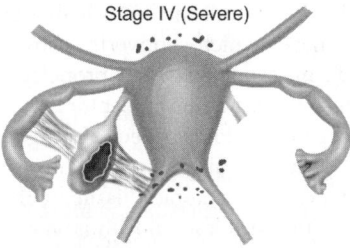

Peritoneum
Superficial endo >3 cm 4
Left ovary
Deep endo <1 cm 32**
Dense adhesions <1/3 8**
Left tube
Dense adhesions <1/3 8**
Total points 52

**Point assignment doubled

Fig. 13.6 Revised American Society of Reproductive Medicine Classification (r-ASRM) for Endometriosis, 1996

Management

Endometriosis should be viewed as chronic, progressive disorder characterized by presence of pain and associated with infertility. It requires individualized management plan with goal of minimizing repeated surgical procedures and taking in account of women preferences, age, presenting symptomatology and presence of infertility. The current modalities are medical management, surgical management or combination of both.

Medical Management of Endometriosis Related Pain (Table 13.1)

The hormonal dependence of ectopic endometrial tissue has provided the basis for medical management of endometriosis. Ovarian suppression with creating pseudopregnancy state can reduce disease activity and pain. An overview of 19 cochrane reviews has shown efficacy of oral contraceptives, progestogens including medroxyprogesterone acetate, norethisterone, cyproterone acetate, or dienogest for pain associated with endometriosis.[8] Oral contraceptives are not universally effective in every case. Estrogen receptors are normal in ectopic endometrial tissue but that the progesterone receptor isoforms PRA and PRB are markedly diminished. 17β-hydroxysteroid dehydrogenase which converts estradiol to inactive form is not activated properly due to diminished Progesterone receptors.[9,10] So the local estrogen antagonist effect of progesterone is absent.[11] There is also increased local activity of aromatase in ectopic tissue converting androgens to estradiol and thus more local estradiol concentrations.

Second line treatment for endometriosis is GnRH agonists and levonorgestrel releasing intrauterine device (IUD).[11-15] Nonsteroidal anti-inflammatory drugs (NSAIDs) are initial empirical treatment of endometriosis but the efficacy has not been more compared to placebo.[8] Danazol although extremely efficacious in decreasing disease activity and pain, it is not used in clinical practise due to its androgenic side effects. Clinicians are recommended to prescribe hormonal treatment hormonal contraceptives (level B), progestagens (level A), antiprogestagens (level A), or GnRH agonists (level A)] as one of the options, as it reduces endometriosis-associated pain. Patients' preferences, side effects, efficacy, costs and availability should be taken into consideration when choosing hormonal treatment for endometriosis-associated pain. (The ESHRE Guidelines, 2013).

Surgical Management

Surgery for endometriosis associated pain is indicated when medical management fails, patient declines, severe side effects of medical therapy, or suspicion of invasive disease Peritoneal endometriosis can be eliminated by division of adhesions and excision or ablation of endometrial implants with either electosurgery or laser.

Laparoscopic Surgery

Laparoscopy is preferred surgical route for surgical management in view of magnified view, short hospital stay, and quick return to routine activities. Excision of implants could be seen as better option as it will retrieve samples for histology. Surgical treatment of endometriosis associated pain has been compared with diagnostic laparoscopy and medical management in a Cochrane trial and it is shown to be more effective in relieving pain at 6 and 12 months.[16] In presence of advance disease involving other abdominal organs patient should be managed with multidisciplinary approach. When endometriosis is identified at laparoscopy, surgically treatment of endometriosis is recommended, as this is effective for reducing endometriosis-associated pain, i.e. 'see and treat'.

Ablation versus Excision of Endometriosis

ESHRE guidelines 2013, recommends that either ablation or excision of peritoneal endometriosis

Table 13.1 Drugs used in medical management of endometriosis

Drug	Mechanism of action in endometriosis	Dosage	Side effects	Notes
Oral contraceptives	Ovarian suppression, Decidualization of ectopic endometrium. Decrease retrograde menstruation with continuous use	Continuous/cyclical use. Oral formulation, ring, patch[10]	Nausea, Headaches fluid retention and irregular spotting or bleeding	Most commonly used initial management. Not universally effective in every case. Decrease non-menstrual pain, dysmenorrhea, less impact on dyspareunia[9,10]
Oral progestins	• Suppression of ovarian steroidogenesis, antiproliferative effect by causing initial decidualization of endometrial tissue followed by atrophy, reduce the elevated activity of metallo-proteinases and growth factors • Dienogest inhibits angiogenesis and proliferation of stromal cells in ectopic endometrium[11]	Continuous use	Weight gain, bloating, acne, breakthrough bleeding	Lower cost, better side effect profile. First choice for treatment of endometriosis. No evidence which progestin is better than another
• Norethindrone acetate		5–20 mg daily		
• Medroxyprogesterone acetate	Most extensively studied	30 mg/day, 150 mg monthly		The time to resumption of ovulation is longer and variable with depot preparations
• Dienogest		2 mg/day		Comparable to GnRH agonists in relieving dysmenorrhea, dyspareunia, and pelvic pain with no side effects of the former.[12]
Levonorgestrel intrauterine device (LNG)	Levonorgestral has potent anti-estrogenic effects on the endometrium	Intrauterine device releases 20 µg/day		Causes atrophic endometrium and amenorrhea.[13] Decrease pelvic pain similar to GnRH analogous,[14] better side effect profile. Effective for rectovaginal endometriosis.

Contd...

Contd...

Drug	Mechanism of action in endometriosis	Dosage	Side effects	Notes
Antiprogestins–Gestrinone	19-nortestosterone derivative with androgenic, anti-progestagenic, anti-estrogenic, and anti-gonadotropic properties, degeneration of endometriotic implants	1.25–2.5 twice a week	Nausea, muscle cramps, weight gain, acne, seborrhoea, oily hair/skin, and irreversible voice changes	As effective as GnRH agonists for the treatment of pelvic pain,[15] severe androgenic side effects
GnRH analogs	Initial stimulation causes increased FSH, LH later prolonged stimulation results in receptor desensitization and decreased FSH, LH thus creating reversible pseudo-menopause	All analogs are inactive orally Buserelin—nasal spray, daily injection Goserelin—monthly or 3-monthly injection Leuprolide acetate—monthly or 3-monthly Naferelin—nasal spray Triptorelin—monthly or 3-monthly	Hypo-oestrogenic side effect- hot flushes, vaginal dryness, reduced libido, and reduction in bone density	Bone density loss is reversible. Side effects can be reduced by add-back with progestogens only or with added estrogens. Aim is to reduce side effects without decreasing efficacy

can be done to reduce endometriosis-associated pain.[5] Ablation and excision of peritoneal disease are equally effective for treatment of endometriosis-associated pain. Excision of lesions could be preferred with regard to the possibility of retrieving samples for histology. Furthermore, ablative techniques are unlikely to be suitable for advanced forms of endometriosis with deep endometriosis component.

Surgical Management of Endometriomas

Endometriomas are formed by invagination of the cortex containing blood from bleeding of endometrial implants, which are located superficially on the ovarian surface. The presence of endometrioma implies severe disease and it is important to consider the patient's reproductive desire and her fertility potential. Surgical options include excision of the cyst wall or drainage and coagulation of the cyst bed.[17] Cystectomy is superior in terms of recurrence of pain and recurrence of endometrioma when compared to drainage and coagulation.[18]

The procedure begins with freeing the cyst by adhesiolysis and mobilizing ovary. Then the cortex of the endometrioma is held by grasper and incision is made along antimesenteric border away from hilum of ovary. Then by creating plane between capsule of ovary and cyst, cystectomy is done. Should the spillage of contents of cyst occurs, irrigation and drainage of peritoneal cavity is done to prevent chemical peritonitis. The cyst is then decompressed by suction drainage and cyst wall from inside is inspected. By using traction and counter traction technique cyst wall is removed and bed of remaining ovary is inspected for bleeders. Recurrence rate of 23.6% has been reported.[19] Cystectomy instead of drainage and coagulation should be performed, as cystectomy reduces endometriosis-associated pain.

Surgical Interruption of Pelvic Nerve Pathways

Laparoscopic uterosacral nerve ablation (LUNA), as an additional procedure to conservative surgery, is not recommended to reduce endometriosis-associated pain. Presacral neurectomy (PSN) is effective as an additional procedure to conservative surgery to reduce endometriosis-associated midline pain, but it requires a high degree of skill and is a potentially hazardous procedure. (The ESHRE Guidelines, 2013, Level A recommendation).[5]

Surgery for Deep Endometriosis

Surgery improves pain and quality of life in women with deep endometriosis and improves quality of life. However, surgery in women with deep endometriosis is associated with substantial intraoperative and postoperative complication rates. One should refer women with suspected or diagnosed deep endometriosis to a center of expertise that offers all available treatments in a multidisciplinary context.

Hysterectomy for Endometriosis-associated Pain

There are no RCTs on hysterectomy (with or without oophorectomy) for the treatment of endometriosis-associated pain. Many clinicians believe that hysterectomy with oophorectomy would lead to regression of endometriotic lesions. The ESHRE guidelines, 2013 recommends that one should consider hysterectomy with removal of the ovaries and all visible endometriosis lesions, in women who have completed their family and failed to respond to more conservative treatments. Women should be informed that hysterectomy will not necessarily cure the symptoms or the disease.[5]

Adhesion Prevention in Endometriosis Surgery

Oxidized regenerated cellulose can be used during operative laparoscopy for endometriosis, for prevention of adhesion formation. Other anti-adhesion agents (polytetrafluoroethylene surgical membrane, hyaluronic acid products) have not been studied and proven effective for adhesion prevention in the context of pelvic surgery.[5]

Preoperative and Postoperative Hormonal Therapies

Preoperative hormonal treatment to improve the outcome of surgery for pain in women with endometriosis is not useful. Postoperative hormonal therapies for treatment of endometriosis associated pain can be divided into two: adjunctive short-term (< 6 months) hormonal treatment after surgery and long-term (> 6 months) hormonal treatment. The latter is is useful in secondary prevention. Adjunctive hormonal treatment for endometriosis-associated pain after surgery does not improve the outcome.

Endometriosis and Infertility

Endometriosis is found in up to 38% of patients of infertility. Ovulatory abnormalities distorted pelvic anatomy, altered peritoneal function, and altered hormonal and cell-mediated functions in the endometrium are some of the proposed mechanisms of infertility in endometriosis. These patients tends to have endocrine and ovulatory disorders, including luteinized unruptured follicle syndrome, impaired folliculogenesis, luteal phase defect, and premature or multiple luteinizing hormone (LH) surges.[20]

Table 13.2 ESHRE guidelines for management of endometriosis-related infertility, 2013[5]

- In infertile women with endometriosis, hormonal treatment for suppression of ovarian function to improve fertility should not be prescribed (Level A)
- In infertile women with AFS/ASRM stage I/II endometriosis, operative laparoscopy (excision or ablation of the endometriosis lesions) including adhesiolysis, rather than performing diagnostic laparoscopy only, to increase ongoing pregnancy rates should be performed. (Level A)
- In infertile women with AFS/ASRM stage I/II endometriosis, CO_2 laser vaporization of endometriosis can be performed, instead of monopolar electrocoagulation, since laser vaporization is associated with higher cumulative spontaneous pregnancy rates. (Level A)
- In infertile women with ovarian endometrioma undergoing surgery, excision of the endometrioma capsule, instead of drainage and electrocoagulation of the endometrioma wall should be performed, to increase spontaneous pregnancy rates. (Level A)
- In infertile women with AFS/ASRM stage III/IV endometriosis, operative laparoscopy, instead of expectant management can be performed, to increase spontaneous pregnancy rates. (Level B)
- In infertile women with AFS/ASRM stage I/II endometriosis, clinicians may perform intrauterine insemination with controlled ovarian stimulation, instead of expectant management, as it increases live birth rates (Level B)
- The use of assisted reproductive technologies, especially if tubal function is compromised or if there is male factor infertility, and/or other treatments have failed, should be attempted. (Level B)

The management options (Table 13.2) of choice include surgery or *in vitro* fertilization and embryo transfer (IVF-ET). Suppression of ovary using medical treatment in case of minimal and mild endometriosis does not improve fecundity. In case of minimal to mild endometriosis operative laparoscopy with removal of implants either by excision or by ablation improves fertility than diagnostic laparoscopy.[21,22] The woman should be counseled regarding the possibility of reduced ovarian function after surgery and the loss of the ovary.[18] IVF should be considered in cases of a history of endometriosis that involve compromised tubal function, male factor, and/or other treatment failures. IVF following ET improves pregnancy rates more compared to surgery alone. Surgery for advance disease follows principal to restore pelvic anatomy with operative laparoscopy may enhance fertility.[23]

Incidental Findings of Endometriosis

Incidental finding of asymptomatic endometriosis at the time of surgery do not routinely require surgical excision and ablation, since the natural course of the disease is not clear. However, in case of any incidental finding of endometriosis, the woman should be fully informed and counseled.

ADENOMYOSIS (TABLE 13.3)

Adenomyosis may be defined as the benign invasion of endometrium into the myometrium, producing a diffusely enlarged uterus which microscopically exhibits ectopic non-neoplastic, endometrium. The ectopic endometrial tissue appears to induce hypertrophy and hyperplasia of the surrounding myometrium, which results in a diffusely enlarged uterus (often termed "globular" enlargement) analogous to the concentric enlargement of the pregnant uterus. However, some women have only small areas of diffuse disease that are only apparent by microscopy, whereas others develop nodules (termed adenomyomas), which clinically resemble leiomyometrial glands and stroma surrounded by the hypertrophic and hyperplastic myometrium.[24]

The incidence of endometriosis is estimated to be between 6 and 10% of all women and 35 and 50% of women with pelvic pain and infertility.[25]

Table 13.3 Postulated etiologies of adenomyosis

- Extra tissues in the uterine wall present before birth that grow during adulthood
- Invasive growth of endometrial cells into the uterine muscle due to an incision made in the uterus during surgery (such as cesarean section, myomectomy or uterine curetting)
- Stem cells in the uterine muscle wall
- Uterine inflammation that occurs after childbirth, which may break the usual boundaries of the cells that line the uterus

Pathophysiology

Inner myometrial layers underlying the endometrium have been termed the junctional zone (JZ) and appear to be a distinct anatomical structure, despite the lack of histological distinction on light optic microscopy. This portion of the myometrium presents a number of specific characteristics, such as the endometrium is of Müllerian origin, while the outer myometrium is of non-Müllerian, mesenchymal derivation; it has structural and functional differences with the outer myometrium and functional similarities with the endometrium in that it undergoes cycle-dependent changes in response to the rise and fall of ovarian steroid hormones. In normally menstruating women, uterine peristaltic activity, originates exclusively from the JZ, while the outer myometrium remains quiescent. Adenomyosis is characterised primarily by disruption of the inner myometrial architecture and function, with secondary infiltration of endometrial elements into the myometrium.

Risk Factors

Age

About 70-80% of women undergoing hysterectomy for adenomyosis are in their fourth and fifth decade of life and are multiparous. However, newer reports using MRI criteria for diagnosis suggest that the disease may cause dysmenorrhea and chronic pelvic pain in adolescents and women of younger reproductive age than previously appreciated.[26]

Multiparity

A high percentage of women with adenomyosis are multiparous. Pregnancy might facilitate the formation of adenomyosis by allowing adenomyotic foci to be included in the myometrium due to the invasive nature of the trophoblast on the extension of the myometrial fibers. In addition, adenomyotic tissue may have a higher ratio of estrogen receptors and the hormonal milieu of pregnancy may favor the development of islands of ectopic endometrium.[27]

Prior Uterine Surgery

An increased risk of adenomyosis has been found in association with prior induced abortion and cesarean delivery, myomectomy, D&E and D&C.

Tamoxifen Treatment

Tamoxifen has been described as inducing adenomyosis in postmenopausal women treated for breast cancer, because of its estrogen-agonistic effect on endometrium.[28]

Clinical Features

- Dysmenorrhea
- Heavy menstrual bleeding
- Prolonged bleeding cycles
- Chronic pelvic pain
- Severe and increasing abdominal pain throughout the month
- Back pain
- Dyspareunia
- A pelvic exam that reveals an enlarged, tender, boggy uterus.

Adenomyosis and Infertility

For successful conception, junctional zone (JZ) contractions at the time of implantation should be minimal. Excessive JZ contractions have been shown to reduce implantation rates in both spontaneous and stimulated cycles. Women with endometriosis and adenomyosis show a significant increase in JZ contractions and a disruption in the pattern of contractility which is associated with reduced fertility.

Diagnosis

Adenomyosis has been an elusive diagnosis until recently due to the need for a histological confirmation on the hysterectomy specimen. The imaging diagnosis of adenomyosis is usually made by means of transvaginal ultrasonography or magnetic resonance imaging.

Transvaginal Ultrasonography

Transvaginal ultrasonography (TAUS) have a sensitivity of 80–86%, a specificity of 50–96% and an overall accuracy of 68–86% in diagonizing adenomyosis (Table 13.4).[27]

Magnetic Resonance Imaging (Table 13.5)

The accuracy of MRI for diagnosing adenomyosis is high. Its sensitivity and specificity are 80–100%, with an overall accuracy of 85–90.5%.[29] Although it is more expensive than ultrasonography, MRI can be employed in cases with indeterminate sonographic results for adenomyosis or in patients who are undergoing uterine-sparing surgery for leiomyomas. The uterine zonal anatomy is best seen on T2-weighted images. It is advisable to perform MRI for the diagnosis of adenomyosis after menstruation, as menstrual contractions waves can mimic abnormal JZ thickening.

Diagnostic Hysteroscopy

It does not provide pathognomonic signs for adenomyosis, although the presence of an irregular endometrium with endometrial defects,

Table 13.4 Gross ultrasonographic features of adenomyosis

- Irregular myometrial cystic spaces predominantly involving the posterior uterine wall
- Enlarged uterus with a widened posterior wall
- Eccentric endometrial cavity
- Loss of the junctional zone
- Decreased uterine echogenicity without lobulations, contour abnormality, or mass effects
- Heterogeneity in the myometrium
- Echogenic linear striations of heterotopic endometrium extending into the inner myometrium

Table 13.5 MRI findings of adenomyosis[29]

- Adenomyosis can be diagnosed with a high degree of accuracy when the junctional zone thickness is 12 mm or greater. A maximum thickness of 8 mm or less usually excludes the disease. When the maximum junctional zone diameter is 8–12 mm, secondary findings, such as high signal-intensity foci on T1- or T2-weighted images, are necessary to make the diagnosis.
- The bright foci seen in the myometrium on T2-weighted images suggest islands of heterotopic endometrial tissue, cystic dilation of heterotopic glands or hemorrhage.
- Linear striations of decreased signal intensity can be seen radiating out from the endometrium into the myometrium on T2-weighted images. These striations are the direct invasion of the basal endometrium into the myometrium. When the striations blend or become indistinct, pseudowidening of the endometrium is seen.
- Focal adenomyosis, as opposed to diffuse adenomyosis, is seen as a localized, low–signal-intensity mass within the myometrium.
- MRI can be used to distinguish a focal adenomyoma from a leiomyoma. Adenomyomas lack distinct borders and any mass effect on T2-weighted and contrast-enhanced T1-weighted MRI scans.

altered vascularization and cystic hemorrhagic lesions can be possibly associated with the entity.

Treatment

Medical Treatment

A constant feature of medical therapy for adenomyosis is that, over the years, it has mimicked that which has been applied to endometriosis. At present, medical therapy of adenomyosis can be attempted for symptomatic relief from dysmenorrhoea and menorrhagia, in women who wish to become pregnant and in premenopausal women. Medical therapies as in endometriosis include OCPs, progesterone therapy, Gestrinone, Mifepristone and GnRH agonists in a dose similar to that used in endometriosis.

Levonorgestrel-releasing Intrauterine System

Following insertion of the system there is a decidualization of the endometrium and this is followed by atrophic changes that produce a marked reduction in menstrual blood loss. Through absorption within the myometrium, the progestin also acts directly on the adenomyotic foci. In addition, downregulation of estrogen receptors, in both glandular and stromal endometrial layers, occurs shortly after placement of the device and persists for at least the first year of use. Adenomyotic deposits are then reduced in size, uterine contractility improves and the uterine size decreases. The LNG-IUS positive effect on dysmenorrhea is probably mediated through a reduction of prostaglandin production within the endometrium; reduction in the size and activity of adenomyotic tissue may also account for the improvement in dysmenorrhea.

Novel Approaches

Danazol-loaded intrauterine devices: A Japanese company has developed a danazol-loaded intrauterine device containing 300–400 mg danazol. The overall shape of the device is that of a copper-T IUD, although it is much thicker in the anteroposterior diameter. Because of this characteristic, cervical dilatation may be needed for proper insertion and intrauterine placement. Serum levels of danazol remain below the detection threshold and therefore none of the systemic side-effects associated with oral danazol should be expected.

Inhibitors of Angiogenesis

Angiogenesis is altered in heterotopic uterine mucosa in case of endometriosis and adenomyosis. Pentoxiphylline—an inhibitor of enzyme phosphodiesterase, is being tried at a dose of 800 mg/day. Similarly, dopamine and its agonists, such as cabergoline, promote endocytosis of VEGF receptor-2 (VEGFR-2) in endothelial cells, is being evaluated in animal models.

Surgical and Interventional Procedures

Endometrial Ablation

Superficial submucous adenomyosis with depth of penetration < 2.5 cm can be treated by transcervical endometrial coagulation or resection. MRI or high-resolution ultrasound may be appropriate preoperative screening tools to determine the depth of adenomyosis and to select patients for endometrial ablation. It can be performed using an yttrium aluminum garnet (YAG) laser, roller ball resection, or global ablation techniques. The likelihood of recurrent symptoms and hysterectomy is correlated with the depth of penetration of the adenomyotic disease.

Myometrial/Adenomyoma Excision and Myometrial Reduction

Focal excision of adenomyosis can be performed if the location of foci can be determined. However, unlike myomectomy, it is difficult to expose the lesions, define margins and determine the extent of disease and thus, the efficacy of excision remains low at 50%.[30] If a large proportion of the myometrium is removed the wedge defect created is repaired by metroplasty.

Uterine Artery Embolization

Uterine artery embolization may be an alternative option for patients who do not wish to have hysterectomy and/or who wish to preserve their fertility. Patients contemplating pregnancy should be informed that the effects of the procedure on fertility are uncertain. Resolution of menorrhagia occurs in 50–60% of patients at a mean follow-up of 5 years. Resolution of dysmenorrhea is reported in 40% of patients. 40% of patients require subsequent treatments because of treatment failure or recurrent symptoms.[31]

Magnetic Resonance-guided Focused Ultrasound

Focused ultrasound surgery delivers a concentrated quantity of ultrasound energy to deep tissue areas without thermal effects to surrounding tissue. The underlying process in adenomyosis is smooth muscle hyperplasia and thus, magnetic resonance-guided focused ultrasound (MRgFUS) treatment is ideal to target such lesions. Although few reports show encouraging results for the use of MRgFUS to treat adenomyosis, additional studies into the safety and efficacy of MRgFUS for women with adenomyosis are necessary.[32]

Hysterectomy

For more than a century hysterectomy has been a therapeutic strategy for uterine adenomyosis. For women with adenomyosis who have completed their family and do not wish to preserve uterus or have recurrent deep adenomyosis (endometrial penetration of more than 2.5 cm), hystrecyomy can be performed.

REFERENCES

1. Kennedy S, Bergqvist A, Chapron C, D'Hooghe T, Dunselman G, Greb R, Hummelshoj L, Prentice A, Saridogan, et al. ESHRE guideline for the diagnosis and treatment of endometriosis. Hum Reprod 2005;20:2698-704.
2. Practice bulletin no. 114: management of endometriosis.Obstet Gynecol. 2010 Jul;116(1):223-36. doi: 10.1097/AOG.0b013e3181e8b073.
3. Mishra VV, Gaddagi RA, Aggarwal R, Choudhary S, Sharma U, Patel U. Prevalence; Characteristics and Management of Endometriosis Amongst Infertile Women: A One Year Retrospective Study. J Clin Diagn Res. 2015;9(6):QC01-QC03. doi: 10.7860/JCDR/2015/13687.6125.
4. Bulun SE. Endometriosis. N Engl J Med. 2009;360: 268-79.
5. Management of women with endometriosis. Guidelines of the European Society of Human Reproduction and Embryology. September 2013. https://www.eshre.eu>guidelines>endometriosis.
6. Van Holsbeke C, Van Calster B, Guerriero S, Savelli L, Paladini D, Lissoni AA, Czekierdowski A, Fischerova D, Zhang J, Mestdagh G, et al. Endometriomas: their ultrasound characteristics. Ultrasound Obstet Gynecol. 2010;35:730-40.
7. Hudelist G, English J, Thomas AE, Tinelli A, Singer CF, Keckstein J. Diagnostic accuracy of transvaginal ultrasound for non-invasive diagnosis of bowel endometriosis: systematic review and meta-analysis. Ultrasound Obstet Gynecol. 2011; 37:257-63.
8. Brown J, Farquahar C. Endometriosis: an overview of Cochrane reviews. Cochrane Database Syst Rev2014;3:CD009590.
9. Vercellini P, Trespidi L, Colombo A, Vendola N, Marchini M, Crosignani PG. A gonadotropin-releasing hormone agonist versus a low-dose oral contraceptive for pelvic pain associated with endometriosis. Fertil Steril. 1993;60:75-9.
10. Vercellini P, Barbara G, Somigliana E, Bianchi S, Abbiati A, Fedele L. Comparison of contraceptive ring and patch for the treatment of symptomatic endometriosis. Fertil Steril. 2010;93:2150-61.
11. Katayama H, Katayama T, Uematsu K, et al. Effect of dienogest administration on angiogenesis and hemodynamics in a rat endometrial autograft model. Hum Reprod. 2010;25:2851-8.

12. Strowitzki T, Marr J, Gerlinger C, Faustmann T, Seitz C. Dienogest is as effective as leuprolide acetate in treating the painful symptoms of endometriosis: a 24-week, randomized, multicentre, open-label trial. Hum Reprod. 2010;25:633-41.
13. Behamondes L, Petta CA, Fernandes A, Monteiro I. Use of levonogesterol releasing intrauterine system in women with endometriosis, chronic pelvic pain and dysmenorrhea. Contraception. 2007;75(6 Suppl):S134-9.
14. Petta CA, Ferriani RA, Abrao MS, Hassan D, Rosa E, Silva JC, Podgaec S, Bahamondes L. Randomized clinical trial of a levonorgestrel-releasing intrauterine system and a depot GnRH analogue for the treatment of chronic pelvic pain in women with endometriosis. Hum Reprod. 2005;20:1993-8.
15. Gestrinone Italian Study Group Gestrinone versus a gonadotropin-releasing hormone agonist for the treatment of pelvic pain associated with endometriosis: a multicenter, randomized, double-blind study. Gestrinone Italian Study Group. Fertil Steril 1996;66:911-9.
16. Jacobson TZ, Duffy JM, Barlow D, Koninckx PR, Garry R. Laparoscopic surgery for pelvic pain associated with endometriosis. Cochrane Database Syst Rev. 2009:CD001300.
17. Gelbaya TA, Gordts S, D'Hooghe TM, Gergolet M, Nardo LG. Management of endometrioma prior to IVF: compliance with ESHRE guidelines. Reprod Biomed Online. 2010;21:325-30.
18. Dunselman GA, Vermeulen N, Becker C, Calhaz-Jorge C, D'Hooghe T, De Bie B, Heikinheimo O, Horne AW, Kiesel L, Nap A, et al. ESHRE guideline: management of women with endometriosis. Human Reproduction. 2014;29:400-12.
19. Saleh A, Tulandi T. Reoperation after laparoscopic treatment of ovarian endometriomas by excision and by fenestration. Fertil Steril. 1999;72:322-4.
20. Schenken RS, Asch RH, Williams RF, Hodgen GD. Etiology of infertility in monkeys with endometriosis: luteinized unruptured follicles, luteal phase defects, pelvic adhesions and spontaneous abortions. Fertil Steril. 1984;41:122-30.
21. Marcoux S, Maheux R, Bérubé S. Laparoscopic surgery in infertile women with minimal or mild endometriosis. Canadian Collaborative Group on Endometriosis. N Engl J Med. 1997;337(4):217-22.
22. Practice Committee of the American Society for Reproductive Medicine (ASRM). Treatment of pelvic pain associated with endometriosis. Fertil Steril. 2006;86(5):S18-27.
23. Parazzini F. Ablation of lesions or no treatment in minimal-mild endometriosis in infertile women: a randomized trial. Gruppo Italian per lo Studio dell'Endometriosi. Hum Reprod. 1999;14(5):1332-4.
24. Benagiano G, Brosens I. History of adenomyosis. Best Pract Res Clin Obstet Gynaecol. 2006;20:449-63.
25. Kunz G, Beil D, Huppert P, et al. Adenomyosis in endometriosis–prevalence and impact on fertility. Evidence from magnetic resonance imaging. Hum. Reprod. 2005;20:2309-16.
26. Parker J D, Leondires M, Sinaii N, et al. Persistence of dysmenorrhea and nonmenstrual pain after optimal endometriosis surgery may indicate adenomyosis. Fertil Steril. 2006;86:711-5.
27. Weiss G, Maseelall P, Schott LL, et al. Adenomyosis a variant, not a disease? Evidence from hysterectomized menopausal women in the Study of Women's Health Across the Nation (SWAN) Fertil Steril. 2009;91:201-6.
28. McCluggage WG, Desai V, Manek S. Tamoxifen-associated postmenopausal adenomyosis exhibits stromal fibrosis, glandular dilatation and epithelial metaplasias. Histopathology. 2000;37(4): 340-6.
29. Mansouri R, Santos XM, Bercaw-Pratt JL, Dietrich JE. Regression of adenomyosis on magnetic resonance imaging after a course of hormonal suppression in adolescents: A case series. J Pediatr Adolesc Gynecol. 2014;29.
30. Adenomyosis: review of the literature. Garcia L, Isaacson K. J Minim Invasive Gynecol. 2011;18(4):428-37.
31. Uterine artery embolisation for treating adenomyosis. Interventional procedure guidance. NICE guidelines. Published: 16 December 2013
32. Al Hilli MM, Stewart EA Semin. Magnetic resonance-guided focused ultrasound surgery. Reprod Med. 2010;28(3):242-9.

14
Chronic Pelvic Pain

Preeti Singh, Neelam Yadav, Rini Pachori

INTRODUCTION

Chronic pelvic pain (CPP) is defined as pain in pelvic region that persists for greater than 6 months duration, causing functional disability and requiring treatment.[1] Chronic pelvic pain is common and difficult problem encountered by health practitioner. Due to its complex nature and multifactorial development, it is incorporated into educational curriculum of health professionals. Chronic pelvic pain accounts for 20% of all the appointment in secondary care. The condition causes heavy economic and social burden. CPP accounts for 1 in 10 OPD visits, 15–40% laparoscopies, 12% hysterectomies, 11% patients had reported limited routine activity, in 11.9% it affected sexual life, 15.8% took medication for pain, 3.9% wasted at least 24 hours of work per month.[2] According to World Health Organization (WHO) prevalence of noncyclical pelvic pain in India is 5.2%.[3]

Pelvis is not only the concern for gynecologist but many nongynecological causes also contribute towards CPP. One should not overlook these nongynecological causes like irritable bowel syndrome, inflammatory bowel disease, interstitial cystitis, abdominal wall and pelvic floor myofascial syndrome and pelvic neuropathy (Table 14.1) which are hereby responsible for inconclusive laparoscopy in 60–80% of patients presenting with chronic pelvic pain.[4] Patients with CPP often notice anxiety and depression in their behavior. Thus, its management requires a multidisciplinary approach involving gynecologist, urologist, gastroenterologist, psychologist, neurologist, physiotherapist. These patients generally do not respond to effective medical and surgical therapy.

PATHOPHYSIOLOGY

Pain by definition is product of brain, spinal cord and peripheral nervous system. Pain is mediated via peripheral and central nervous system and accordingly its therapy is decided. The peripheral nerves like A, delta and C fibers mediate this pain sensation, nerve uses substance-P, calcitonin gene-related peptide, L-glutamate as neurotransmitter. Release of chemicals such as potassium, bradykinin, arachidonic acid is a source of pain sensation. The painful stimuli travel to spinal cord through dorsal root which contains the nuclei of sensory nerves from both soma and viscera from where signal passes to spinothalamic tract which is mediated via N-methyl-D-aspartate (NMDA) receptors. A process of winding up develop when stimuli through the sensory nerves become very intense, generating a great deal of electrical activity in this receptor.[5] This may damage some of the inhibitory impulses which are being generated

Table 14.1 Cause of chronic pelvic pain

Gynecological	Urological	Gastrointestinal	Musculoskeletal	Psychological
Endometriosis	Interstitial cystitis	Inflammatory bowel disease	Myofascial pain trigger points	Depression
Chronic pelvic infection	Overactive bladder	Irritable bowel syndrome	Pelvic floor myalgia and spasm	Physical or sexual abuse
Adenomyosis	Urethral syndrome	Constipation	Nerve entrapment syndromes	Sleep disturbance
Pelvic adhesions	Bladder stone	Chronic appendicitis	Mechanical low back pain	Psychological stress
Endosalpingiosis	Chronic UTI		Disc disease	Substance abuse
Ovarian cysts			Hernias	
Residual ovary syndrome				
Ovarian remnant syndrome				
Post-hysterectomy pain				
Pelvic congestion syndrome				
Fibroids				
Vulvodynia				

in response to pain thereby exacerbating the painful response. Continuous painful stimulus is responsible for neuroplasticity resulting into alteration of neuronal signal in spinal cord which causes phenomenon like allodynia (pain resulting from non-noxious stimulus) and hyperalgesia (painful sensation of abnormal severity following noxious stimulation) (Fig. 14.1).

Different theories have been postulated for explaining chronic pelvic pain.

Cartesian theory: Pain is proportional to amount of tissue damage.

Gate control theory: This model suggests that nociceptive signals from peripheral tissues travel through spinal cord to higher centers and these higher centers modulate the signals via altering spinal cord neurotransmitter, interneuron activity and transmission of nociceptive signals from the periphery. Deterioration of these regulatory processes accounts for the chronic pain states by allowing too many peripheral signals through spinal cord gate.

Neuromatrix theory: Sensitization of spinal cord interneurons that have become pain amplifier, also adjacent organ may join the chorus when nociception has been emanating from an organ for prolonged period. Chronic pain state is maintained via plasticity of nervous system and alteration of signal processing.[6]

ETIOLOGY

Symptoms

Presence of following symptoms, (systemwise) clinches the involvement of that particular system:

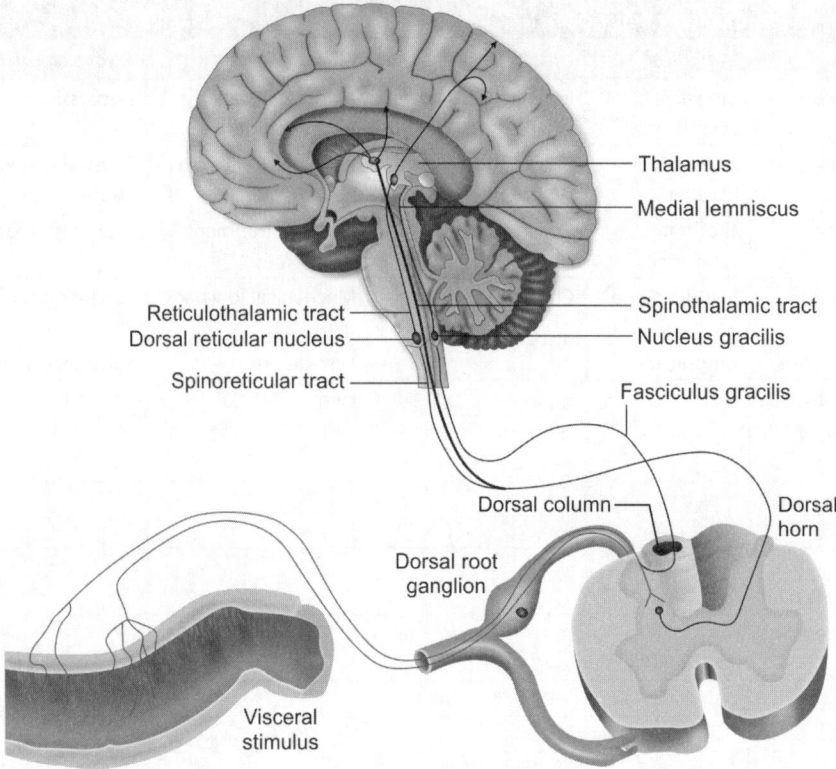

Fig. 14.1 Pain pathway

Gynecological

- Dyspareunia
- Dysmenorrhea
- Abnormal vaginal bleeding
- Abnormal vaginal discharge
- Subfertility
- Sexual dysfunction.

Gastrointestinal

- Constipation
- Diarrhea
- Flatulence
- Hematochezia
- Pain relief with bowel movement.

Urological

- Frequency
- Urgency
- Dysuria
- Nocturia
- Hesitancy
- Hematuria.

Psychological

- Depression
- Anxiety
- Panic
- Suicidal ideation
- Past and current
- Sexual trauma.

GYNECOLOGICAL CAUSES

Endometriosis

Endometriosis by definition is characterized by presence of endometrial glands and stroma outside endometrial cavity. There is altered genetic and environmental interaction leading to the condition. The incidence of endometriosis in the general population is 1-7%.[7] The prevalence of endometriosis is more than 30% in women undergoing laparoscopy for chronic pelvic pain.[8] Risk factors for endometriosis are nonmodifiable like age at menarche, frequent menses and modifiable protective factors like oral contraceptive use. Many times the severity of endometriosis does not match with the severity of the pain.[9] Around 45% of women with endometriosis are asymptomatic. Laparoscopy is the best modality to diagnose endometriosis, ultrasound is one of the modality to diagnose endometrioma, but has lower sensitivity and specificity. Endometriosis-associated CPP may be managed with hormonal preparations such as an estrogen–progestin combination, a progestin alone, danazol, or a gonadotropin-releasing hormone (GnRH) agonist, with or without nonsteroidal anti-inflammatory drugs. In a randomized controlled trial laparoscopic adhesiolysis, ablation, endometrioma drainage, laser treatment, uterine nerve transaction are better than expectant management. Finally, if fertility is not desired, and when conservative, medical, surgical therapy fails, hysterectomy with or without oophorectomy may be considered.[10] It has been observed that even after hysterectomy also there are high chances of recurrences of endometriosis, i.e. 3%.

Endosalpingiosis

Endosalpingiosis first described by Sampson[11] in 1927, is the presence of fallopian tube-like ciliated epithelium in ectopic locations. Theories behind its genesis are coelomic metaplasia and implantation of tubal epithelium tissues. Endosalpingiosis was an incidental finding in 7.9% of the women with pelvic pain, 7.3% of those without pelvic pain, 11.7% of those with infertility. Endosalpingiosis has only minor role in pelvic pain and is an incidental finding associated with other pelvic problems.

Adenomyosis

Adenomyosis is defined as endometrial glands and stroma present deep within the myometrium. The exact etiology and pathogenesis of condition is not known. The reported incidence of adenomyosis ranges from 5% to 70%.[12] Most cases occur in parous women in the fourth and fifth decades of life.[13] Symptoms include pelvic pain, dysmenorrhea, menorrhagia. The sensitivity and specificity of ultrasound is 52-89% and 50-99% respectively. MRI is an important diagnostic tool having sensitivity and specificity of 86-100% respectively. Medical therapy includes danazol and GnRH agonist. Surgical therapy includes hysteroscopic resection of endometrium involving 3 mm of myometrium and finally hysterectomy is gold standard treatment once the female has completed her family.

Adhesions

Intraperitoneal adhesions are caused mainly by previous surgery and to a lesser extent by endometriosis and abdominal and pelvic inflammation or infections.[14] The financial impact of adhesions is enormous.[15] Around 25-50% of women present with CPP, but their role as a cause of CPP remains controversial.[16] Diamond and Freeman reviewed four uncontrolled, cohort studies involving 269 women and 4 men and found rates of 69-82% for relief or reduction of chronic pain after adhesiolysis. Adhesiolysis of minor adhesions has insignificant role in pain reduction, but adhesiolysis of major adhesions involving intestinal tracts results in significant reduction in pain. Although adhesions may contribute to pelvic pain but putative treatment, i.e. repeat surgical intervention is one of the contributory factor for pain syndrome by causing repeat surgical trauma, disappointment from lack of pain relief, psychological feeling of being ill. Therefore, only major adhesion should be lysed minor adhesion should be left without lysis.

Pelvic Inflammatory Disease

Chronic pelvic pain is sequelae of pelvic inflammatory disease (PID) and has been reported to occur in 18-33% of women after an episode of PID, regardless of mode of antibiotic therapy.[17] The predisposing factors for PID are low socioeconomic status, illiteracy, early age at marriage, poor hygiene. Pelvic inflammatory disease is caused by ascending infection from microorganism colonizing the endocervix to endometrium and fallopian tubes. It is a clinical diagnosis presenting as pelvic pain, cervical motion tenderness and adnexal mass or tenderness and fever. Evaluation of both vaginal and endocervical secretions is important in work-up of patient with PID. The wet mount of vaginal secretion shows increase polymorphonuclear leukocytes. Endometrial biopsy shows the evidence of endometritis, ultrasound and other imaging modality used to diagnose tubo-ovarian abscess and laparoscopy is used to confirm salpingitis.[18] Syndromic approach is being followed for the management of PID. Empirical treatment with broad spectrum antibiotics which covers *N. gonorrhoeae, C. trachomatis, M. genitalium*, gram-negative facultative bacteria, anaerobes and streptococci. An outpatient regimen of oral cefoxitin and doxycycline as effective as inpatient parenteral regimens of same antimicrobials.

Pelvic Congestion Syndrome

Dilated pelvic veins have been seen in many women with CPP. Symptoms may include a dull aching pain as well as menstrual disorders. Vulval varicosities may be associated with pelvic venous congestion. Pelvic venography, Doppler ultrasonography, and MRI have been used to diagnose pelvic congestion syndrome. Hormonal suppression, percutaneous embolization, surgeries such as ovarian vein ligation, hysterectomy, salpingoophorectomy are some of the treatment options.

Residual Ovary and Ovarian Remnant Syndrome

This is characterized by persistent pelvic mass leading to recurrent pelvic pain after hysterectomy. In an attempt to perform oophorectomy due to difficult dissection, there is residual ovarian cortical tissue left behind which results in this syndrome. This is characterized by recurrent pelvic pain or persistent pelvic mass after hysterectomy. One study reported an incidence of residual ovary syndrome (ROS) of 2.8% (73 cases) after 2561 hysterectomies with preservation of one or both ovaries over a 20-year period.[19] Confinement of ovary within postoperative adhesions, rupture or leakage of cyst, attachment of ovary to sigmoid colon and vaginal apex are some of the reasons causing pain. The follicle stimulating hormone (FSH) stimulation results in growth of ovarian fragments which help in complete removal of ovarian tissue. When performing oophorectomy best is to open the pararectal space and completely skeletonize the infundibulopelvic ligament. In a cohort study of 119 women presenting with CPP who had previously undergone oophorectomy, ovarian remnants were found in 18%.[20] Diagnosis can be made by ultrasound after 5–10 days of clomiphene citrate therapy, FSH and estradiol assay in premenopausal range helps in clinching the diagnosis. High dose progestins, oral contraceptives, GnRH agonist are helpful medical therapy. Removal of residual ovary is definitive treatment.

UROLOGICAL CAUSES

Interstitial cystitis: More common in female of 40–60 years. The symptoms include suprapubic pain, increased day and night time frequency in the absence of proven infection or other obvious pathology with typical cystoscopic and histological features during bladder hydrodistension. The prevalence of interstitial cystitis is 38%. Exact etiology is not known but some of the contributory factors leading to above condition are infection, immunological deficiencies, lymphatic or vascular obstruction, glycosaminoglycan layer deficiency, toxic urogenous substances, neural factors and mast cell disorder. Symptoms include pain in pelvic region, urgency, frequency, nocturia. Tenderness on physical examination, i.e. suprapubic pain on pelvic examination is seen. Cystoscopy, laparoscopy, hydrodistension of bladder are performed in each patient. In cystoscopy, one can see glomerulation, submucosal hemorrhage, terminal hematuria. Hydrodistension at the time of cystoscopy is therapeutic modality in 20–30% patients and its effect lasts for 3–6 months. Instillation of potassium chloride is a sensitive diagnostic modality and will assess response to pentosan polysulfate. Pentosan polysulfate helps in repairing bladder permeability.

GASTROINTESTINAL CAUSES

Irritable Bowel Syndrome

It affects 15% of adults, more common in women. Irritable bowel syndrome (IBS) present as abdominal pain, bloating, disturbed bowel habits. It has got multifactorial etiology like altered bowel motility, visceral hypersensitivity, psychological factors. Symptoms suggesting IBS are seen in 50–80% of women presenting with chronic pelvic pain. *Rome II criteria for diagnosis of IBS*:[21]

- Pain or discomfort relieved after defecation
- Association of onset of pain and discomfort with change in stool frequency
- Association of onset of pain and discomfort with change in stool appearance.

Other associated symptoms are abnormal stool frequency, abnormal stool form, abnormal stool passage, passage of mucus. Patients over 45 years with symptoms and signs like rectal bleeding, anemia, weight loss, family history of colorectal cancer should undergo colonoscopy, sigmoidoscopy with flexible instrument. Those below 40 years without any family history should undergo sigmoidoscopy with flexible instruments. Treatment with dietary manipulation such as avoiding lactose, fructose and sorbitol is beneficial. Caffeinated products, carbonated drinks, all these gas producing substances should be avoided. If pain is predominant symptom then antispasmodic agent or tricyclic compounds may be helpful, constipated patient benefit from high dietary fibers intake and osmotic laxatives, diarrhea is managed by loperamide. GnRH agonist also has beneficial in condition unresponsive to other treatment modality. As the condition has psychological issue as well psychological therapy

with medical therapy improves the clinical response to the therapy.

MUSCULOSKELETAL PROBLEMS

Myofascial Pain

Myofascial pain is one of the most common causes of somatic pain accounting for 30% of diagnosis. These patients have numerous trigger points, hyper-reactive areas within a tight band of skeletal muscles or within its fascia. This may present as weakness and restricted mobility of affected muscles. The pain occurs due to entrapment of genitofemoral and ilioinguinal nerve most commonly after pfannenstiel incision and may get exacerbated premenstrually, fingertip pressure on trigger point result in local and referred pain, jump sign positive after palpation with fingertips or cotton swab. Massage therapy, myofascial release, pelvic floor exercises, nonsteroidal anti-inflammatory drug (NSAID), gabapentin, pregablin, low dose tricyclic antidepressant (TCA) and benzodiazepine are useful pharmacological therapy, injection of trigger point with 3 mL of 0.25% bupivacaine, lidocaine patch, acupuncture are some of the effective treatment options.

Fibromyalgia

Myofascial pain syndrome characterized by diffuse pain, fatigue and nonrestorative sleep. Commonly results from central nervous system sensitization that result in abnormal perception of pain. Education, environment changes, (balanced diet, adequate sleep), pharmacological treatment NSAID, low dose TCA, selective serotonin reuptake inhibitor (SSRI), anti-convulsant, benzodiazepine improves sleep, counseling, cognitive behavioral therapy are some of the important management options.

Low Back Pain

It is caused by gynecological, vascular, neurological, psychogenic, or spondylogenic pathology. Pain occurs after trauma, exertion, fatigue.

Diagnosis is aided by thorough examination of muscles, vertebral joints, discs. Investigations like plain films, MRI without contrast are crucial to arrive at the appropriate diagnosis.

PSYCHOLOGICAL FACTORS

Stout and Steege found that 59% of 294 women seeking evaluation at pelvic pain clinic scored in depressed range on the center for epidemiological Studies Depression Scale at the time of their initial visit. In Reiter's study of 106 women with CPP, 48% had a history of major psychosexual trauma (molestation, incest, rape) compared with 6.5% of 92% pain free control subjects presenting for annual routine gynecological examination ($p < 0.001$). Women presenting with chronic pelvic pain reports a high rates of marital distress and sexual dysfunction like dyspareunia. Cognitive behavioral therapy is an useful adjunct in treating chronic pelvic pain. When psychological factor get attached to pain it may take the form of syndrome called pelvic pain syndrome called chronic pain syndrome—duration of 6 months or more, significantly impaired function at home or work, incomplete relief with most treatments, signs of depression such as early awakening weight loss or anorexia, altered family roles.

HISTORY

Detailed chronological history of the problem with special consideration for aggravating and relieving factors as well as results of previous attempts at treatment is very important. It is very crucial to note what are aggravating factors according to patient, her insight into condition and fears associated with it.

One should elicit symptoms which points towards the involvement of particular system gastrointestinal system, urinary tract, musculoskeletal system and pelvic floor musculature (Table 14.2). The clinician should inquire about the current impact of pain on the patient's quality of life and the amount of medication used; these factors; followed over time can be used as indicators of response to treatment.

Table 14.2 Functional pelvic pain scale instructions

Function	No pain	Some pain	Moderate pain	Severe pain	Cannot function acute pain
Bladder					
Bowel					
Intercourse					
Walking					
Running					
Lifting					
Working					
Sleeping					

A detailed questionnaire can be given to the patient before her visit to facilitate history taking and make it more through and efficient. The pain questionnaire designed by the International Pelvic Pain Society is a useful resource and will allow data collection through a centralized database in future.

During the initial interview it is important to convey interest, to listen with attention and validate the patient's experience. When the patient feels that her experience of the pain is believed and that clinician will do his or her best to help her, a good relationship is established which leads to better compliance with proposed treatment plan.

- Detailed chronological history.
- Pattern of pain—onset, location, duration, characteristics, radiation, temporal association, severity, pattern during activities, relation to position changes and association to bodily functions.
- Aggravating and relieving factor.
- Results of previous treatment.
- Association with other problems-psychological and bladder, bowel symptoms, affect of movement and posture on pain.
- Past or present sexual assault.
- Intimate partner violence.
- Daily pain diary for 2–3 menstrual cycles.
- Drugs used previously whether it helped or not.

EXAMINATION

The physical examination of a patient with CPP is very different from a routine gynecological examination. It may be necessary sometimes to defer the examination to the second visit because of time or patient's distress after recounting her history. It is important to convey to the patient that she will control the timing of examination and any time feels uncomfortable she can terminate the examination. If the pain is intermittent, it is advisable to examine the patient when she is in pain. The aim of examination is look for pathological conditions, but also to reproduce the patient's usual pain to help identify physical contributes. The examinee should elicit feedback from the patient preferably using a numerical scale to determine whether the pain is the same or different from her usual chronic pain, documenting the score for each tender area. The examinee should tell the patient about what is being looked for and what pelvic structures are appearing painful. The following sequence of examination needs to be followed.

- *General physical:* Gait, posture
- *Back*: Evaluation of spine, paraspinous muscles, sacroiliac joints, scoliosis, trigger point and pelvic asymmetry.
- Abdominal
  - *Inspection:* Enlargement of abdomen, distortion or tethering of overlying skin.
  - *Palpation:* Looking for focal tenderness by finger tip examination, trigger point (focus of hyperirritability in muscles and its fascia causing increased sensitivity). Carnett test—the area of abdominal tenderness is palpated while the patient voluntarily contracts her abdominal muscles by raising her head or legs. An increase in the pain indicates a myofascial origin, whereas a decrease indicates an intraperitoneal disorder.
  - *Lumbosacral area:* Sacroiliac joint or pubic symphysis tenderness.
  - *Pelvic examination:* External review of vulva and vestibule, cotton swab test to detect area of sensitivity, single digit palpation of cervix, uterus, adnexa, bimanual examination to assess pelvic structure size shape and mobility of pelvic structure.

INVESTIGATIONS

- *Screening for infection: Chlamydia, gonorrhoea*, other sexually transmitted disease (STD).
- *Transvaginal ultrasonography (TVS) and magnetic resonance imaging (MRI):* To diagnose adenomyosis, endometrioma, fibroids. MRI has sensitivity of 69% and specificity of 75% in detecting biopsy confirmed endometriosis. TVS is useful in evaluating pelvic masses and adenomyosis and better than transabdominal scan (TAS).
- *Diagnostic laparoscopy:* Gold standard in diagnosing endometriosis and adhesions, laparoscopic pain mapping is a technique involving conscious sedation and local analgesia that is used to identify sources of chronic pelvic pain by putting traction on the pelvic tissues and probing them.
- *Blood studies:*
  - Leukocyte counts and ESR raised in chronic pelvic inflammatory disease.
  - CA-125 confirms DIE (deeply infiltrative endometriosis).
  - AMH-fertility counseling for women under going surgical extirpation for their disease.
  - FSH, estradiol levels-ovarian remnant disease (if medicated).
- *Anesthetic blocks:* 1–5 mL of 1% lidocaine or 0.5% bupivacaine blocks pain from entrapped segmental nerve or abdominal wall trigger point. Both diagnostic and therapeutic, transvaginal uterosacral block (If pain is relieved then pain is of uterine origin).
- *Psychological tests and interviews:* To measure general psychopathology and personality factors.
- *Urological:* Cystoscopy, urine routine microscopy.
- *Gastroenterological:* Colonoscopy, barium enema, sigmoidoscopy.

TREATMENT

The approach to women with chronic pelvic pain is therapeutic, optimistic, supportive, and sympathetic. There are two approaches to the treatment of chronic pelvic pain (CPP). First is to treat the pain as a diagnosis and second is to treat the disorders that cause or contribute to the pain.[4] Pharmacologic treatment of pain is based on the knowledge that different profiles and mechanisms for transmission of pain information are involved.[22]

Analgesics

These include acetylsalicylic acid, nonsteroidal anti-inflammatory drugs (NSAIDs), acetaminophen, narcotics, and medicinal marijuana. The therapy directed to peripheral nerve uses prostaglandin inhibitors like NSAID and acetylsalicylic acid and disruptor of sodium channel such as carbamazepine. NSAIDs have been studied extensively in randomized controlled trials (RCTs) for dysmenorrhea and have proven efficacious.[23] Mefenemic acid is commonly used NSAID with starting dose of 500 mg OD to maximum of 500 mg TDS. Empiric use of NSAIDs is among the first-line treatments recommended in most publications.[24] Opioid narcotics are dangerous as they cause narcotic bowel syndrome and opioid induced hyperalgesia. Relief of moderate to severe chronic pain involves around-the-clock use of sustained release opioids, the dose individually tailored according to response, with assessment of safety, compliance, and misuse. Close and regular follow-up is necessary to avoid misuse of opioid. The commonly used opioid is tramadol in the dose of 100 mg OD to maximum up to 100 mg TDS.

Antidepressants and Neuroleptics

Tricyclic antidepressants such as amitriptyline, nortriptyline and desipramine are being effective in treating chronic pelvic pain. Amitriptyline starting from 5 mg in evening increasing up to 25 mg. Newer generation neurotransmitter reuptake inhibitors duloxetine and desvenlafaxine are also useful, duloxetin is started as 30 mg in morning increasing to 60 mg. Neuroleptics such as gabapentin, pregabalin, lamotrigine employed when symptoms are neuropathic in nature. Pregabalin is started as 25 mg in the night and increased to 75 mg BD. Some studies on tricyclic antidepressants in women with CPP and normal results of laparoscopy have reported a decreased intensity and duration of pain.[25] Neuroleptics like gabapentin inhibits excessive stimulation of secondary neurons in spinal cord. Therapy directed at central processes of central inhibition include use of opiates that acts on dorsal horn of spinal cord and agent that increases the inhibition of serotonin uptake thereby increasing its availability (paroxetine and amitriptyline).

Neurolytic Therapy

Injecting neurotoxic chemicals (phenol or alcohol) or using energy (heat, cold, or laser) in doses sufficient to destroy neural tissue.

Anxiolytics

In one study alprazolam, triazolobenzodiazepine has immense analgesic effect in patients with chronic pain of malignant origin and concomitant mood changes and anxiety. They also potentiates narcotic agents. Alprazolam in the dose of 0.25 mg at bed time to be given.

Hormonal Medications

Oral contraceptive (OC) effective in reducing dysmenorrhea and cyclic symptoms associated with pain. Various low-dose OCs have proven successful in studies of the initial management of dysmenorrhea[26] continuous monophasic treatment should be in the first-line in most regimens.[27]

Progestin only formulations induces decidualization of endometrium and endometriotic tissue. In one study, 12 month trial with medroxyprogesterone acetate (MPA) depot 150 mg every 3 months has equivalent efficacy as that of GnRH agonists.[28] Oral MPA 50 mg daily dose is effective in reducing pain scores, but benefits are not sustained and risk of exacerbating depressive symptoms present but levonorgestrel intrauterine system (LNG-IUS) does not have this side effect. Thus, LNG-IUS has beneficial effect in moderate to severe dysmenorrhea.

Danazol

Synthetic androgen prevents ovarian steroidogenesis and pulsatile release of gonadotrophins. At a dose of 400–800 mg/day, danazol is effective for CPP; it should be given for a minimum of 3 months before other medical options are considered.[29]

GnRH agonists-induces hypoestrogenic states by inhibiting ovarian steroidogenesis. Examples are goserelin, leuprolide, buserelin, nafarelin and tryptorelin. The suppression is more with monthly depot preparation. Empiric use of a GnRH agonist was evaluated in an RCT involving 100 women with noncyclic pain and clinically suspected endometriosis.[30] After 12 weeks of therapy with depot leuprolide acetate (3.75 mg/month) the treatment group showed a significant reduction in pain scores, dysmenorrhea, and tenderness. Useful in case of ovarian remnant syndrome or residual ovary syndrome and DIE. Patients with no obvious endometriosis also responded to GnRH agonists. Prolonged use causes vasomotor symptoms and osteopenia and therefore add back therapy is recommended if used beyond 6 months.[31]

Surgical Therapy

Surgical therapy utilizes two basic principles:
1. Removing pelvic organs-hysterectomy
2. Treating the visible disease while leaving the pelvic organ in place, e.g. adhesiolysis, endometriotic lesion ablations, etc.

In USA, 12% of hysterectomies are performed primarily for pelvic pain. 6.1% for endometriosis or adenomyosis and 5.1% for pelvic inflammatory disease. The pelvic pain of uterine origin is 78% relieved after hysterectomy. In a prospective observational study of private practices in Maine, Carlson and associates reported that at a 1 year follow up satisfaction with the outcome of surgical treatment is much higher than satisfaction with outcome of medical treatment. Steege and Stout reported that 15 of 20 patients without CPS who were undergoing laser laparoscopic adhesiolysis had good relief of pain at follow-up of 6–12 months after surgery, however, if chronic pain syndrome is present only 4 out of 10 patients with equivalent adhesive disease found relief. Excision of endometriotic lesion is superior to ablation but there is insufficient evidence to support that one is superior to other. Presacral neurectomy act as an adjunct to laparoscopic endometriosis excision there is greater improvement in dysmenorrhea and duspareunia. Zullo et al. investigated it with double masked randomized trial and demonstrated a 20% difference in pain improvement when presacral neurectomy was added to endometriosis excision. Removal of ovarian remnant by detailed dissection of peritoneum surrounding the mass. Adhesiolysis may be facilitated by laser, electrosurgical, or sharp scissors dissection. Adhesion barriers to prevent reformation of adhesions should be considered. Laparoscopic adhesiolysis reduces pain perception in 60–90% of patients.[32]

Many women with chronic pelvic pain found to have appendicopathy and many women with chronic appendicopathy are found to have gynecologic disorders when undergoing laparoscopic appendectomy.[33] Around 20% of women with endometriosis has appendiceal disease. Laparoscopic appendectomy is advantageous in women with chronic pelvic pain.

Presacral neurectomy (PSN) and laparoscopic uterine nerve ablation (LUNA), can be technically demanding but continue to have a role in the management of CPP.[34] A recent randomized, double-blind trial of conservative laparoscopic surgery with adjunctive PSN or LUNA in women with severe dysmenorrhea caused by endometriosis demonstrated more pronounced and prolonged pain relief with PSN than with LUNA.[35]

Psychological and Alternative Treatment

Cognitive behavioral and biofeedback therapy useful in reducing automatic responses to painful stimuli. Psychotherapy is indicated for women who have pronounced depression, sexual difficulties, indications of past trauma. Relaxation technique, stress management, marital counseling, sexual counseling, hypnosis and other psychotherapeutic approaches increases CNS descending inhibition of peripheral pain signals. Meditation, yoga, acupuncture has adjunctive role in the management of chronic pelvic pain.

Manual soft tissue release is essential to reduce pelvic floor resting tone and tension. Acupuncture may also be helpful.

FOLLOW-UP

Patients with chronic pelvic pain are followed up with pain grading questionnaire which include the quantitative estimation of the amount of pain patient got relieved after medical and surgical treatment. Patients undergoing surgical interventions are followed up with medical management till the specified period of time and should turn up if any side effect of prolonged drug intake.

RECOMMENDATIONS

- Thorough history-taking and complete physical evaluation should be done for patient with chronic pelvic pain (III-B).
- Clinical measurement of pain level should be done at each visit (II-B)
- Owing to high prevalence of psychological factor attached to it the patient should be routinely screened for chronic pain syndrome (II-2A).
- Patient assisted laparoscopy is gaining importance now a days (II-B).
- Opioid can be considered for pain control under adequate supervision (II-3B).
- Hormonal treatment of chronic pelvic pain should be studied extensively and should be first-line treatment for CPP (I-II2A).
- Adjuvant medication like antibiotic and antidepressant are supportive help in specific situation (II-3B).

Level of Evidence

- *I:* Evidence obtained from at least one properly designed randomized controlled trial.
- *II-1:* Evidence from well-designed controlled trials without randomization.
- *II-2:* Evidence from well-designed cohort (prospective or retrospective) or case-control studies, preferably from more than one center or research group.
- *II-3:* Evidence from comparisons between times or places with or without the intervention.
- *III:* Opinions of respected authorities, based on clinical experience, descriptive studies, or reports of expert committees.

Classification of Recommendations

- There is good evidence to support the recommendation for use of a diagnostic test, treatment, or intervention.
- There is fair evidence to support the recommendation for use of a diagnostic test; treatment, or intervention.
- There is insufficient evidence to support the recommendation for use of a diagnostic test, treatment, or intervention.
- There is fair evidence not to support the recommendation for a diagnostic test, treatment, or intervention.
- There is good evidence not to support the recommendation for use of a diagnostic test, treatment, or intervention.

REFERENCES

1. ACOG Committee on Practice Bulletins. ACOG Practice Bulletin No. 51. Chronic pelvic pain. Obstet Gynecol. 2004;103:589-605.
2. Mathias SD, Kupperman M, Liberman RF, Lipschultz RC, Steege JF. Chronic pelvic pain: prevalence, health-related quality of life, and economic correlates. Obstet Gynecol. 1996;87: 321-7.

3. Thongkrajai P, Pengsaa P, Lulitanond V. An epidemiological survey of female reproductive health status: gynecological complaints and sexually-transmitted diseases. Southeast Asian J Trop Med Public Health. 1999;30:287-95.
4. Howard FM.Chronic pelvic pain. Obstet Gynecol. 2003;101:594-611.
5. Constandil L, Pelissier T, Soto- Myoano R, Mondaca M, Saez H, Laurido C, et al. Interleukin-1 beta increases spinal cord wind up activity in normal but not in monoarthiritic rats. Neurosci Lett. 2003;342:139-42.
6. Melzack R. From the gate to the neuromatrix. Pain. 1999;82(Suppl 6):121.
7. Barbierie RL. Etiology and epidemiology of endometriosis. Am J Obstet Gynecol. 1990;162:565.
8. Howard FM. The role of laparoscopy in chronic pelvic pain: promise and pitfalls. Obstet Gynecol Surv. 1993;48:357-87.
9. Cramer DW, Missmer SA. The epidemiology of endometriosis. Ann NY Acad Sci. 2002;955:11-22.
10. The Society of Obstetricians and Gynaecologists of Canada. SOGC Practice Guidelines on Hysterectomy. J Obstet Gynaecol Can. 2002;109(1):1-12.
11. Sampson JA. Peritoneal endometriosis due to the menstrual dissemination of endometrial tissue into the peritoneal cavity. Am J Obstet Gynecol. 1927;14:422.
12. Nikkanen V, Punnonen R. Clinical significance of adenomyosis. Ann Chir Gynaecol. 1980;69:278-80.
13. Bird CC, McElin TW, Manalo-Estrella P. The elusive adenomyosis of the uterus revisited. Am J Obstet Gynecol. 1972;112:582-93.
14. Peters AA, Trimbos-Kemper GC, Admiraal C, Trimbos JB, Hermans J. A randomized clinical trial on the benefit of adhesiolysis in patients with intraperitoneal adhesions and chronic pelvic pain. Br J Obstet Gynaecol. 1992;99:59-62.
15. Diamond MP, Freeman ML. Clinical implications of postsurgical adhesions. Hum Reprod Update. 2001;7:567-76.
16. Howard FM. Chronic pelvic pain. Obstet Gynecol. 2003;101:594-611.
17. Steege JF, Stout AL. Resolution of chronic pelvic pain after laparoscopic lysis of adhesions. Am J Obstet Gynecol. 1991;165:278-81.
18. Gupta A, McCarthy S. Pelvic varices as a cause of pelvic pain: MRI appearance. Magn Reson Imaging. 1994;12:679-81.
19. Dekel A, Efrat Z, Orieto R, Levy T, Dicker D, Gal R, et al. The residual ovary syndrome: a 20 year experience. Eur J Obstet Gynecol Reprod Biol. 1996;68:159-64.
20. Abu-Rafeh B, Vilos GA, Misra M. Frequency and laparoscopic management of ovarian remnant syndrome. J Am Assoc Gynecol Laparosc. 2003;10:33-7.
21. Drossman DA. The functional gastrointestinal disorders and the Rome II process. Gut. 1999;45(Suppl 2):1-5.
22. Reiter RC. A profile of women with chronic pelvic pain. Clin Obstet Gynecol. 1990;33:130-6
23. Roy S. A double-blind comparison of a propionic acid derivative (ibuprofen) and a fenamate (mefenamic acid) in the treatment of dysmenorrhea. Obstet Gynecol. 1983;61:628-32.
24. Milburn A, Reiter RC, Rhomberg AT. Multidisciplinary approach to chronic pelvic pain. Obstet Gynecol Clin North Am. 1993;20:643-61.
25. Walker EA, Sullivan MD, Stenchever MA. Use of antidepressants in the management of women with chronic pelvic pain. Obstet Gynecol Clin North Am. 1993;20:743-51.
26. Gambone JC, Mittman BS, Munro MG, Scialli AR, Winkel CA. Chronic Pelvic Pain/Endometriosis Working Group. Consensus statement for the management of chronic pelvic pain and endometriosis: proceedings of an expert-panel consensus process. Fertil Steril. 2002;78:961-72.
27. Moore J, Kennedy S, Prentice A. Modern combined oral contraceptives for pain associated with endometriosis (Cochrane review). In: The Cochrane Library, Issue 2. Chichester (England): Wiley, 2004.
28. Stones RW, Mountfield J. Interventions for treating chronic pelvic pain in women (Cochrane review). In: The Cochrane Library, Issue 2. Chichester (England): Wiley, 2004.
29. Reiter RC. A profile of women with chronic pelvic pain. Clin Obstet Gynecol. 1990;33:130-6.
30. Surrey ES, Judd HL. Reduction of vasomotor symptoms and bone mineral density loss with combined norethindrone and long-acting gonadotropin releasing hormone agonist therapy of symptomatic endometriosis: a prospective randomized trial. J Clin Endocrinol Meta. 1992;75: 558-63.
31. Gelbaya TA, El-Halwagy HE. Focus on primary care: chronic pelvic pain in women. Obstet Gynecol Surv. 2001;56:757-64.

32. Riedel HH, Emmert C. Pelviscopy within the scope of differential gynecologic-surgical diagnosis. Endometriosis—chronic appendicitis. Zentralbl Chir. 1998;123(Suppl 4):50-2.
33. Croce E, Olmi S, Azzola M, Russo R. Laparoscopic appendectomy and minilaparoscopic approach: a retrospective review after 8-years' experience. JSLS. 1999;3:285-92.
34. Malinak LR. Surgical treatment and adjunctive therapy of endometriosis. Int J Gynaecol Obstet. 1993;40:543-7.
35. Zullo F, Palomba S, Zupi E, Russo T, Morelli M. Effectiveness of presacral neurectomy in women with severe dysmenorrhea caused by endometriosis who were treated with laparoscopic conservative surgery: a 1-year prospective, randomized, double-blind controlled trial. Am J Obstet Gynecol. 2003;189:5-10.

15

Ectopic Pregnancy

Sangeeta Bhasin, Reena Rani

INTRODUCTION

When the fertilized ovum implants in an area other than the endometrial lining of the uterine cavity it is called an ectopic pregnancy (EP).

Although, over the years, the incidence of ectopic pregnancy has increased and may be as high as 4% in women undergoing assisted reproduction,[1] morbidity and mortality associated with tubal rupture has decreased. This has been made possible by the development of high resolution transvaginal sonography (TVS) and radioimmunoassay for β subunit of human chorionic gonadotropin, a placental hormone (β-hCG). This, along with widespread use of laparoscopy leads to an early, more accurate diagnosis and better treatment of ectopic pregnancy.

CLASSIFICATION

Ninety-five percent of ectopic pregnancies are implanted in the fallopian tubes (Fig. 15.1).[2] Of these, most are ampullary implantations. The

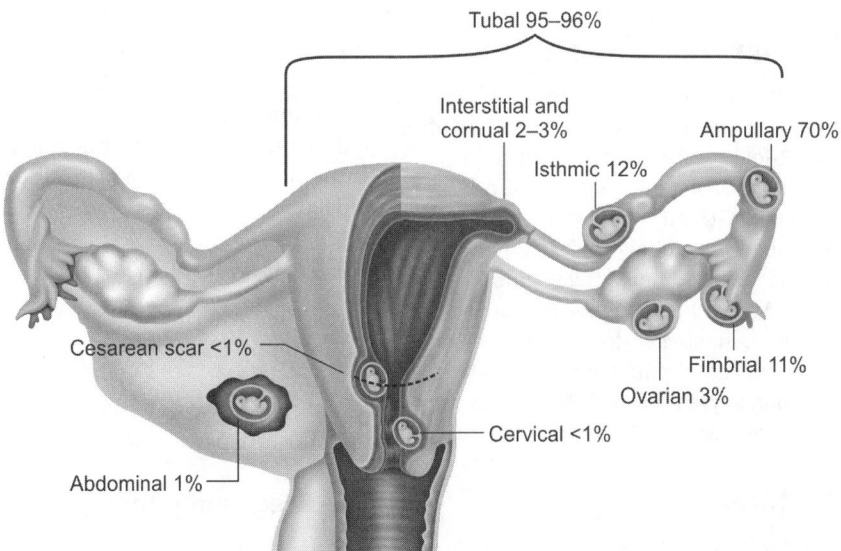

Fig. 15.1 Classification of ectopic pregnancy

Table 15.1 Risk factors for ectopic pregnancy
- Previous ectopic pregnancy
- Previous tubal corrective surgery
- Tubal sterilization
- Pelvic infections *Chlamydia, Gonorrhoea* or other sexually transmitted infections (STIs)
- Genital tuberculosis
- Pregnancy through assisted reproductive techniques (ARTs)
- Current use of intrauterine device
- History of medical or surgical abortion
- History of infertility
- Smoking
- In utero exposure to diethylstilbestrol.

remaining 5% implant in the ovary, peritoneal cavity or within the cervix.

RISK FACTORS

The fertilized ovum is transported through the fallopian tube by a combination of smooth muscle contractions and ciliary beatings. Any condition which damages tubal integrity and impairs these functions is a risk factor for ectopic pregnancy (Table 15.1).

SEQUELAE OF ECTOPIC PREGNANCY

Tubal Damage

Evaluation of tubal patency by hysterosalpingography following conservative management of EP shows a 12-fold increased risk of subsequent ipsilateral tubal obstruction if the initial β-hCG level is > 5000 mIU/mL though there is no association between tubal obstruction and size of ectopic mass.[3] Interestingly, multidose methotrexate (MDM) has a higher potential for tubal damage than single dose methotrexate (SDM) (ipsilateral tubal patency rate of 57% in MDM in comparison to 84% in SDM) though the mechanism is not clear.[4]

Tubal Rupture

The risk of tubal rupture is more after ovulation induction, when initial serum β-hCG level is > 10,000 mIU/mL and when there is no history of having used any contraception ever. The risk is also more in an acute EP as compared to a chronic EP. An *Acute EP* is associated with a healthy growing trophoblast and presents with a high β-hCG level leading to an early diagnosis. A *chronic EP* has an abnormal trophoblast and demonstrates a negative or static β-hCG in which repeated small hemorrhages or tubal abortion leads to an inflammatory response with formation of a pelvic mass.

Mortality

Severe hemorrhage resulting from tubal rupture is the main cause of mortality associated with ectopic pregnancy.

DIAGNOSIS

History and Examination

- The classic symptoms of amenorrhea, irregular bleeding per vaginum and lower abdominal pain in a woman of reproductive age group with a history of syncope, or hypotension is a strong pointer towards ectopic pregnancy (Table 15.2).
- Presence of risk factors for ectopic pregnancy.
- High index of suspicion will help make an early diagnosis.
- Nonspecific history makes it difficult to differentiate from other gynecological, gastrointestinal and urological conditions like salpingitis, abortion, corpus luteum rupture, adnexal torsion, appendicitis or urinary tract infection.

INVESTIGATIONS

- Urine pregnancy test
- Sonography-Transvaginal/Transabdominal
- Laboratory tests: β-hCG level, hemogram
- Culdocentesis
- Diagnostic laparoscopy.

Urine Pregnancy Test

Urine pregnancy test (UPT) is the first investigation in the diagnostic work-up of a

Table 15.2 Clinical presentation of ectopic pregnancy

Symptoms	Signs
• Amenorrhea, • Irregular bleeding per vaginum • Lower abdominal pain • Syncope • Right shoulder pain • Rarely nausea, vomiting and diarrhea • Vague non specific symptoms	*Unruptured ectopic pregnancy* • Vitals stable • Mild abdominal tenderness +/- • Palpable adnexal mass +/- *Ruptured ectopic pregnancy* • Pallor, tachycardia, hypotension, cold clammy skin • P/A—rebound tenderness, guarding, rigidity, distension and presence of shifting dullness. • P/V—cervical motion tenderness, bulky to normal size uterus, forniceal fullness/palpable, tender adnexal mass, fullness in cul-de-sac

patient of suspected ectopic pregnancy. It is a one-step test detecting intact and free β-hCG isoforms in the urine of pregnant women to diagnose pregnancy. The sensitivity and specificity of the urine test for diagnosing ectopic pregnancy is 97% and 83% respectively.[5] It is a cheap and easily performed test.

Sonography

With a positive UPT, the next step is to ascertain the location of the pregnancy.

TVS is the recommended imaging modality in suspected ectopic pregnancy. It is better than transabdominal ultrasound (TAS) with a sensitivity of 88–90% as compared to 77–80% for TAS.

Ultrasound Findings of Tubal Ectopic Pregnancy

Endometrial cavity

- A trilaminar endometrial pattern representing two adjacent edematous proliferative phase endometrial layers has a specificity of 94% for ectopic pregnancy but a sensitivity of 38% only.[6]

- Pseudogestational sac—this is a one layer intracavitary fluid collection caused by decidual sloughing. It typically lies in the midline within the endometrial cavity, contiguous with the endometrial stripe in contrast to a normal gestation sac which is eccentrically located.

- Decidual cyst—this is an anechoic area within the endometrium, often at the endometrial-myometrial junction and represents early decidual breakdown.

Adnexa

- An extrauterine yolk sac or embryo can be seen in only 15–20% cases.
- Presence of a 'Halo' or tubal ring encircled by a thin hypoechoic area caused by subserosal edema has a sensitivity of 95% and positive predictive value (PPV) of 92% for ectopic pregnancy.[7]
- Any adnexal mass except a simple cyst could be an ectopic pregnancy. Differentiating an ectopic from a corpus luteal cyst is important.
  - The corpus luteum is found within the parenchyma of the ovary unlike an ectopic pregnancy.
  - The corpus luteum wall is less echogenic than the tubal halo and the endometrium.
  - A spongiform lace like pattern inside the corpus luteum is characteristic of hemorrhage.
  - On transvaginal color Doppler, vascularity in the periphery of the complex mass due to placental blood flow–called the 'ring of fire'–is classical of ectopic pregnancy.
  - Gentle palpation of the adnexal mass between the vaginal probe and the examiners abdominal hand during scanning will detect a mass that moves separately from the ovary.[8]

Cul-de-sac

TVS can detect fluid as little as 50 mL in the pouch of Douglas. Blood in the paracolic gutters and Morrison's pouch indicates hemoperitoneum of at least 400–700 mL.[9]

Laboratory Tests

Serum Beta Subunit of Human Chorionic Gonadotropin (β-hCG)

A combination of serum β-hCG levels and ultrasound can be used to confirm the diagnosis of ectopic pregnancy. Absence of an intrauterine gestation sac on TVS at an hCG level of 1500 mIU/mL (the discriminatory level) or on TAS at an hCG level of 6500 mIU/mL suggests an incomplete abortion, a resolving complete abortion or an ectopic pregnancy.

Serial measurements of serum β-hCG gain importance when the ultrasound is nondiagnostic.

In a viable intrauterine pregnancy, the blood level of β-hCG should increase by at least 53–66% every 48 hours. If such doubling does not occur, this suggests that the pregnancy may not be viable or could be an ectopic pregnancy though there is no single pattern to characterize ectopic pregnancy (Approximately half may have decreasing β-hCG values, whereas the other half have increasing values). In such a situation, uterine curettage showing absence of trophoblastic villi may help make the diagnosis of EP. The procedure, however, is usually not followed for fear of iatrogenic rupture of the ectopic pregnancy.

Hemogram

A decrease in haemoglobin or hematocrit over a period of time is a valuable indicator of continuing blood loss and will help in diagnosing ruptured ectopics. Varying degree of leukocytosis up to 30,000/cu mm may also be seen.

Serum Progesterone Level

Theoretically, a single serum progesterone value > 25 ng/mL is indicative of a normal viable pregnancy and reasonably excludes ectopic pregnancy. A value < 5 ng/mL indicates an abnormal pregnancy, such as an impending abortion or an ectopic pregnancy. However, progesterone levels are neither necessary to do nor useful as it is not confirmative.

Culdocentesis

Aspiration of nonclotting blood or fragments of an old clot from the cul-de-sac of Douglas through a 16 or 18 gauge spinal needle can be used as a bedside diagnostic test for identifying intraperitoneal bleeding. However, it is not a confirmatory sign for ectopic pregnancy as it will be positive in other causes of intraperitoneal bleeding also. It has largely been replaced by diagnostic transvaginal sonography in modern times.

Diagnostic Laparoscopy

Laparoscopy is the gold standard for the diagnosis of ectopic pregnancy as it allows assessment of intraperitoneal bleeding as well as visualization of the affected and unaffected adnexa. However, with sensitive diagnostic modalities available now, EP is diagnosed much before surgery.

Endometrial Curettage

When the ultrasound is nondiagnostic and β-hCG below the discriminatory zone, endometrial curettage may help us to differentiate between an intrauterine and ectopic pregnancy. It also plays a role in the management of heterotopic pregnancy and to confirm intrauterine pregnancy when a laparoscopy/laparotomy performed for EP turns out to be negative. It has sometimes also been done to minimize bleeding per vaginum by curetting off the decidual cast as an adjunct to surgical treatment.

MANAGEMENT

Management of tubal ectopic pregnancy can be *conservative (expectant or medical)* or *surgical* depending upon hemodynamic status of the patient, size of the adnexal mass and serum β-hCG values.

EXPECTANT MANAGEMENT

This involves a period of extended observation in some select cases of *tubal ectopics* till the time that the ectopic pregnancy resolves spontaneously.

An ideal candidate for expectant management would be:[2]
- Clinically stable patient with no evidence of intraperitoneal bleeding or rupture on TVS.
- Initial serum β-hCG levels <1000 mIU/mL with falling values on follow-up.
- Ectopic mass< 3.5 cm in diameter.
- Should understand the potential complication of rupture and the importance of compliance and follow-up.

Follow-up is by weekly transvaginal scan to see reduction in size of ectopic mass and twice weekly measurement of serum β-hCG to document a fall to less than 50% of initial value in 7 days. Thereafter, weekly β-hCG and TVS are done till the level is reduced to less than 20 mIU/mL.

Expectant management should be abandoned if serum β-hCG level rises or plateaues or if the patient becomes symptomatic despite falling hCG values.

MEDICAL MANAGEMENT

Methotrexate is the drug of choice in the medical management of ectopic pregnancy. It acts as a folic acid antagonist which inhibits DNA synthesis in actively dividing cells including trophoblastic cells. It can be given as oral tablets, intravenous or intramuscular injections or can be injected into the ectopic pregnancy sac.

Other agents used for injection into the ectopic mass are hyperosmolar glucose, potassium chloride, mifepristone and prostaglandin F2α.

Indications

Inclusion criteria for successful medical management are:
- Hemodynamically stable asymptomatic patient.
- Patient motivated enough to be compliant with surveillance.
- Unruptured tubal pregnancy, persistent trophoblast after salpingotomy.
- *Predictors of success:* Serum β-hCG level < 5000 mIU/mL (this is the best prognostic indicator of success of treatment with Mtx. Success rate was found to be 92% when β-hCG was < 5000 mIU/mL and 68% with β-hCG levels >15000 mIU/mL), ectopic mass diameter < 3.5 cm and absence of fetal cardiac activity.[10] Presence of an extrauterine yolk sac and rapidly rising hCG levels both before and during methotrexate therapy may foretell an increased risk of failure.[11]

Contraindications

Absolute contraindications to methotrexate include:
- Hemodynamically unstable patient
- Presence of severe persistent abdominal pain/evidence of significant hemoperitoneum >300 mL
- Intrauterine pregnancy/heterotopic pregnancy
- Breast feeding
- Clinically significant hepatic/renal/hematological impairment
- Active peptic ulcer disease/pulmonary disease
- Immunodeficiency/blood dyscrasias/current use of steroids
- Known hypersensitivity to methotrexate.

Relative contraindications
- Patient not motivated enough for follow-up
- Initial serum β-hCG level >5000 mIU/mL
- Size of ectopic mass >3.5 cm
- Presence of fetal cardiac activity.

Pretreatment Counseling

Before starting methotrexate, counsel the woman about:
- The treatment options available to her and explain what is best for her
- Failure rate of medical management and the subsequent need for surgery (10%)
- Length of follow-up required (6–8 weeks) and the possible need for repeat doses (15%)

- Possible side effects
- Take a written informed consent.

Dosage Regimes of Methotrexate

Three dosage regimes have been described associated with an overall success rate of 90%.
1. Multiple dose regime
2. Single dose regime
3. Hybrid double dose regime.

Multiple-dose Regime

Multiple dose methotrexate treatment protocol are given in Table 15.3.

Table 15.3 Multiple-dose methotrexate (mtx) treatment protocol
Pretreatment: CBC, LFT, KFT, BG, serum β-hCG
Day 1: Measure β-hCG, give Mtx 1mg/kg IM
Day 2: Folinic acid rescue 0.1 mg/kg IM
Day 3: Measure β-hCG ; If decrease between day 1 and day 3 β-hCG value is <15%, give second dose of Mtx 1mg/kg If decrease between day 1 and day 3 β-hCG value is > 15%, stop treatment and start surveillance
Day 4: Folinic acid rescue 0.1 mg/kg IM
Day 5: Measure β-hCG; If decrease between day 3 and day 5 β-hCG value is <15%, give third dose Mtx 1 mg/kg If decrease between day 3 and day 5 β-hCG value is > 15%, stop treatment and start surveillance
Day 6: Folinic acid rescue 0.1 mg/kg IM
Day 7: Measure β-hCG; If decrease between day 5 and day 7 β-hCG value is <15%, give fourth and last dose of methotrexate If decrease between day 5 and day 7 β-hCG value is > 15%, stop treatment and start surveillance
Day 8: Folinic acid rescue 0.1 mg/kg
Surveillance: Weekly β-hCG levels till they fall below 15 mIU/mL which usually takes about 35 days

Abbreviations: CBC, complete blood count; LFT, liver function test; KFT, kidney function test; BG, blood group; hCG, human chorionic gonadotropin; IM, intramuscular

Single-dose Regime (Table 15.4)

This is actually a misnomer as the regimen has the provision for additional doses of methotrexate if response to single dose is inadequate.

Hybrid Regime (Table 15.5)

In order to balance the convenience of the single dose regime and efficacy of the multiple dose regime, a hybrid two dose protocol has been developed.[12]

Table 15.4 Single-dose methotrexate (Mtx) treatment protocol
Measure β-hCG, CBC, LFT, KFT, BG on day 1
Administer Mtx 50 mg/m² on day 1
Measure β-hCG on day 4 and day 7
If level of β-hCG drops by 15% between day 4 and day 7, monitor β-hCG weekly till level falls below 15 mIU/mL
If levels do not drop by 15% between day 4 and day 7(seen in 20% of treated women) or if fetal cardiac activity still present on day 7, give second dose of Mtx on day 7 (new day 1)
Measure β-hCG on new day 4 and day 7
If β-hCG levels do not decrease or fetal cardiac activity persists after three doses of methotrexate or if signs of hemodynamic instability appear, plan for surgical treatment

Abbreviations: CBC, complete blood count; LFT, liver function test; hCG, human chorionic gonadotropin; KFT, kidney function test; BG, blood group

β-hCG value on day 4 may be higher than value on day 1.

Table 15.5 Hybrid two-dose protocol
Administer 2 equal doses of methotrexate 50 mg/m² each on day 1 and day 4 without folinic acid rescue
Follow-up is as in single dose protocol
If β-hCG values do not fall by 15% between day 4 and day 7, another dose of methotrexate may be given

Single vs Multiple-dose Regimes

- Success rates for single dose and multiple dose regimens is similar (89% and 93% respectively).[13]
- Single dose regimen is less expensive, needs less intensive monitoring and does not require folinic acid rescue.
- Side effects are more and patient satisfaction less with multiple dose regimens.
- There is no difference in the rate of future tubal patency, intrauterine pregnancy or recurrent ectopic pregnancy.

Side Effects

Drug-related

These are seen in about 30% of patients treated but are usually self-limited. They include nausea and vomiting, transient liver dysfunction (12%), mucosal ulceration (stomatitis 6%, gastriris 1%), dermatitis and conjunctivitis. Rarely, bone marrow depression, transient drug-induced pneumonitis and anaphylactic reactions may occur.

Separation Pain

About 60–70% women complain of mild abdominal pain, which is relieved by simple analgesics, 2–7 days after receiving methotrexate. This could be due to tubal miscarriage or tubal distension from hematoma formation. Occasionally however, in about 20% women, pain may be severe enough to warrant hemodynamic assessment along with TVS to rule out intraperitoneal bleed from a tubal miscarriage or a tubal rupture where in surgery may be indicated.

Post-therapy Monitoring

- Weekly β-hCG should be done till a level < 15 mIU/mL is reached.
- *TVS:* Serial scans for ectopic mass dimensions do not provide any benefit as the persistent mass may be due to a resolving hematoma rather than trophoblastic tissue. Ultrasound should therefore, be reserved for suspected rupture only.
- To avoid folic acid containing supplements (can competitively reduce methotrexate binding to dihydrofolate reductase), NSAIDs (can reduce renal blood flow and delay drug excretion), alcohol (can predispose to concurrent hepatic enzyme elevation), sunlight (can provoke methotrexate related dermatitis), sexual activity/vaginal examination (can cause rupture).
- To use effective contraception for 2 months after follow-up is complete and at least 3 months after last injection of methotrexate (to avoid the risk of teratogenicity).

Subsequent Reproductive Performance

- There is no evidence of adverse effect of methotrexate on ovarian function or future pregnancy
- Incidence of recurrent ectopic pregnancy is 15% which rises to 30% after 2 ectopics.[14]
- Risk of recurrence is same after medical and surgical treatment.
- Subsequent intrauterine pregnancy rate is 58–89%.

SURGICAL MANAGEMENT

Surgical treatment in ectopic pregnancy is reserved for
- The hemodynamically unstable patient
- Failure of medical management
- Patient not suitable for medical management.

Laparoscopy is the gold standard surgical treatment for ectopic pregnancy in a patient who is hemodynamically stable. In a hemodynamically unstable patient, laparotomy is generally preferred, after resuscitation.

Hajenius and associates[15] performed a Cochrane Database review on comparison of laparotomy with laparoscopy, and found that laparoscopy was associated with shorter operative time, lesser blood loss, lesser requirement for analgesia and shorter hospital stay. No significant difference was found in the overall tubal patency or the subsequent uterine pregnancy rate between the two.

Tubal surgery can be conservative or radical. It is called *conservative* when the tube is salvaged like in salpingostomy, salpingotomy and fimbrial expression of the ectopic pregnancy and *Radical* when the tube is removed like in salpingectomy.

Anti-D immunoglobulin should be given to all nonsensitized Rh-negative women undergoing surgical management of EP.

Salpingostomy

The procedure involves giving a 10–15 mm linear incision using unipolar needle cautery on the antimesenteric border of the affected tube over the pregnancy and meticulous extrusion of the products through the incision. Hemostasis can be ensured with needlepoint electrocoagulation or laser. The incision is left unsutured, to heal by secondary intention.

This procedure is preferred for a small pregnancy <2 cm in length and located in the distal third of the fallopian tube. It can be performed laparoscopically or by laparotomy. When compared with salpingectomy, though the rate of subsequent intrauterine pregnancy is similar, the rate of subsequent ectopic pregnancy is higher. Also, the risk of persistent trophoblast is more with salpingostomy. Laparoscopic salpingostomy has a higher rate (1 in 12) of persistent trophoblastic disease than laparotomic salpingostomy.[16]

The procedure of salpingostomy should therefore, be reserved for the hemodynamically stable woman who is desirous of preserving fertility and has a diseased contralateral fallopian tube.

Salpingotomy

It is essentially the same procedure as salpingostomy except that the incision is closed with delayed-absorbable suture.

Salpingectomy

It involves complete removal of the fallopian tube, including a wedge of the cornua, so that the interstitial portion of the tube is also removed thereby minimizing the rare occurrence of pregnancy in the tubal stump. The procedure is recommended for recurrent ectopic in the same tube, extensively damaged tube, presence of uncontrolled bleeding, in a woman who has completed child bearing.

Persistent Trophoblast

Incomplete removal may lead to persistence of trophoblastic tissue in 5–20% of linear salpingostomies, open or laparoscopic. This can be identified by rising serum β-hCG levels and recurrence of symptoms. Hence, it is recommended to obtain weekly β-hCG measurements after linear salpingostomy. The standard treatment is 50 mg/m² single dose Mtx.

Risk factors for persistent ectopic pregnancy are small ectopic pregnancies (<2 cm diameter), early gestation (<6 weeks), and high concentrations of β-hCG (>3,000 IU/L) preoperatively.

In high-risk cases, a single prophylactic dose of Mtx (1 mg/m²) can be administered postoperatively. Graczykowski and Mishell showed that the rate of persistent ectopic pregnancy came down from 14.5% without Mtx prophylaxis to 1.9% after using Mtx prophylaxis (Table 15.6).[17]

NONTUBAL ECTOPIC PREGNANCY

Interstitial Pregnancy

Interstitial pregnancy is a rare condition when the pregnancy develops in the interstitial portion of the fallopian tube. It accounts for 2–4% of all tubal pregnancies. It is sometimes erroneously referred to as a cornual pregnancy, a term which should be reserved for conceptions that develop in the horns of uteri with mullerian anomalies.

Ipsilateral salpingectomy, where the interstitial portion of the tube has been inadvertently left behind, is a specific risk factor associated with interstitial pregnancy. Since the pregnancy is located in a relatively well covered and protected part of the fallopian tube with a greater capacity to distend and grow, it typically

Table 15.6 Representative reproductive performance in 3198 women following primary treatment for ectopic pregnancy[18]

Management	Successful treatment (%)	Tubal patency (%)	Subsequent pregnancy (%)	
			Uterine	Ectopic
Salpingostomy	93	76	58	12
Methotrexate				
Single-dose	87	81	61	8
Variable dose	93	75	52	8
Expectant	68	76	57	13

presents at a more advanced gestation (8–12 week of gestational age). Also, because of the nearness to the uterine and ovarian vessels, rupture can cause brisk hemorrhage which may be associated with profound shock and a maternal mortality rate as high as 2.5%.

Transvaginal sonography findings of interstitial pregnancy are:[19]
- Empty uterine cavity
- Products of conception/gestation sac located in the interstitial portion of the tube surrounded by a continuous rim of myometrium
- Interstitial line sign (thin echogenic line extending from a central uterine cavity echo to the periphery of the interstitial sac)

Management

If diagnosed early, conservative medical management with methotrexate can be done. The standard surgical treatment of interstitial pregnancy includes cornual resection and repair of defect by laparotomy/laparoscopy. These women will need careful observation in their next pregnancy with consideration for elective cesarean section.

OVARIAN PREGNANCY

Implantation of pregnancy in the ovary is rare occurring in <3% of all ectopic pregnancies. IVF-ET and current use of intrauterine contraceptive device are specific risk factors associated with ovarian pregnancy (OP). The clinical presentation is similar to tubal pregnancy though OP patients are less likely to present with vaginal bleeding. This is attributed to the increased vascularity of ovarian tissue which leads to good embryonic development and high β-hCG levels resulting in a well-maintained endometrium which does not bleed easily.

Ultrasound findings in ovarian pregnancy[19]
- Empty uterine cavity
- Cystic structure with a wide echogenic ring on or within the ovary, generally seen surrounded by ovarian cortex and separate from the corpus luteum

Spiegelberg criteria for diagnosis of ovarian pregnancy includes:
- A well-preserved corpus luteum can be identified in the wall of the gestational sac
- The tube, including the fimbria ovarica, is intact and is clearly separate from the ovary
- The gestational sac definitely occupies the normal position of the ovary
- The sac is connected to the uterus by the utero-ovarian ligament
- Ovarian tissue is unquestionably demonstrated in the wall of the sac

The classical treatment for OP is surgical. Early cases can be managed by ovarian wedge resection or cystectomy. With larger lesions, ovariectomy is performed either laparoscopically or by laparotomy. Methotrexate has also been used successfully to treat unruptured ovarian pregnancies.

CERVICAL PREGNANCY

Rarely, a pregnancy may get implanted in the cervical canal below the level of the internal os. The higher the implantation in the cervical canal, the more it grows and higher its tendency to hemorrhage. Previous history of dilatation and curettage is a risk factor for cervical pregnancy.

Painless vaginal bleeding is the most common symptom (90%). It is associated with abdominal pain in only 25% patients. On examination, a distended, thin-walled cervix with a partially dilated external os topped by a slightly enlarged uterine fundus are common findings.

Ultrasound findings of cervical pregnancy are:[19]
- Empty uterine cavity
- Barrel-shaped cervix
- Products of conception/gestation sac below the level of the internal cervical os
- Negative sliding organ sign

Rubin criteria for the diagnosis of cervical pregnancy include:
- Cervical glands must be opposite the placental attachment
- Placental attachment to the cervix must be situated below the entrance of the uterine vessels or below the peritoneal reflection of the anterior and posterior surfaces of the uterus
- Fetal elements must be absent from the corpus uteri

Management

Medical Management

Systemic methotrexate (as given in tubal gestation) is the first-line therapy in the stable woman. Local methotrexate injection directly into the gestation sac along with ultrasound-guided fetal intracardiac injection of 2 mL potassium chloride to induce fetal death has also been used. Uterine artery embolization before or after Mtx may be used to limit bleeding.

Curettage and Tamponade

Before curettage, uterine artery embolization, local Mtx injection into the gestation sac, bilateral ligation of descending cervical branches of the uterine artery by placement of hemostatic cervical sutures at 3 and 9 o'clock position or by placing an encircling heavy silk ligature around the cervix above the pregnancy can all be used to limit bleeding. Following curettage, a Foleys catheter can be inserted into the cervical canal and the 30 mL catheter bulb inflated. The vagina is packed tightly with gauze to further tamponade bleeding.

Abdominal hysterectomy is the last option of management if massive hemorrhage occurs.

ABDOMINAL PREGNANCY

An abdominal pregnancy is the rarest and the most serious type of extrauterine gestation.

It is *primary* when the implantation occurs directly in the peritoneal cavity exclusive of tubal, ovarian or intraligamentary implantations and *secondary* when it follows early tubal rupture or abortion. Most abdominal pregnancies are secondary.

Studdiford criteria for primary abdominal pregnancy
- Both tubes and ovaries must be in normal condition with no evidence of recent or remote injury
- No evidence of uteroperitoneal fistula should be found
- The pregnancy must be related exclusively to the peritoneal surface and be early enough to eliminate the possibility that it is a secondary implantation following a primary implantation in the tube

Ultrasound findings in abdominal pregnancy[19]
- Empty uterine cavity
- No evidence of a dilated fallopian tube or complex adnexal mass
- Gestation sac surrounded by loops of bowel and separated by peritoneum
- Wide mobility similar to fluctuation of the sac

Clinical Presentation

History of recurrent abdominal discomfort, fetal movement beneath the abdominal wall, and the presence of fetal movements high in the upper abdomen. Catastrophic hemorrhage can result from separation of the placenta later in pregnancy.

Management

Clinical management depends on the gestational age at diagnosis. Conservative management, even though it carries a risk for sudden and life-threatening hemorrhage, can be followed if diagnosis is made in advanced gestation. It includes waiting until fetal viability with in-hospital observation.

The principal surgical objective is delivery of the fetus and careful assessment of placental implantation without provoking hemorrhage. Preoperative angiographic embolization can be used to reduce intraoperative hemorrhage.

Most clinicians believe the best treatment is to clamp the cord and leave the placenta in situ but to allow retroperitoneal drainage if possible. The placenta can be removed after complete cessation of function is demonstrated by quantitative β-hCG titers. The placenta should be removed during laparotomy only if it is accessible and if its removal can be accomplished without excessive blood loss.

PREVIOUS SCAR PREGNANCY

Implantation of an otherwise normal pregnancy into a prior cesarean scar has also been reported. Pain and bleeding are most common symptoms (60%). About 40% of women are asymptomatic. The diagnosis is made during routine sonographic examination. Ultrasound findings are:[19]

- Empty uterine cavity
- Products of conception/gestation sac located anteriorly at the level of the internal os covering the presumed site of the previous lower segment cesarean section scar
- Negative sliding organ sign
- Evidence of peritrophoblastic flow on color Doppler examination.

Management is gestational-age dependent and includes methotrexate treatment, curettage, hysteroscopic resection, uterine-preserving resection by laparotomy or laparoscopy, a combination of these, or hysterectomy.

REFERENCES

1. Fernandez H, Gervaise A. Ectopic pregnancies after infertility treatment: modern diagnosis and therapeutic strategy. Hum Reprod Update. 2004;10: 503-13.
2. Cunninghm FG, Leveno KJ, Bloom SL. Williams Obstetrics, 23rd edn.
3. Elito J, Han KK, Camano L. Values of β-hCG as a risk factor for tubal obstruction after tubal pregnancy. Acta Obstet Gynecol Scand. 2005;84:864.
4. Guven ES, Dilbaz S, Dilbaz B, Ozdemir DS, Akdag D. Comparison of the effect of single dose and multiple dose methotrexate therapy on tubal patency. Fertil Steril. 2007;88:1288.
5. Mazouz S, Lee JK, Fernandez H. Evaluation of a urinary test as a diagnostic tool of a nonprogressive pregnancy. Fertil Steril. 2011;95(2):783-6.
6. Hammoud AO, Hammoud I, Bujold E. The role of sonographic endometrial patterns and endometrial thickness in the differential diagnosis of ectopic pregnancy. Am J of Obstet Gynecol. 2005; 192:1350.
7. Burry KA, Thurmond AS, Suby Long TD. Transvaginal ultrasonographic findings in surgically verified ectopic pregnancy. Am J Obstet Gynecol. 1993;168:1796.
8. Levine D. Ectopic pregnancy. Radiology. 2007; 245(2):385.
9. Rose JS. Ultrasound in abdominal trauma. Emerg Med Clin North Am. 2004;22(3):581.
10. Lipscomb GH, McCord ML, Stovall TG. Predictors of success of methotrexate treatment in women with tubal ectopic pregnancies. N Engl J Med. 1999;341:1974.
11. American Society for Reproductive Medicine: Medical treatment of Ectopic pregnancy. Fertil Steril 2008;90(5 Suppl):5206.
12. Barnhart K, Hummel AC, Sammel MD. Use of '2-dose' regimen of methotrexate to treat ectopic pregnancy. Fertil Steril. 2007;87(2):250.
13. Alleyassin A, Khademi A, Aghahosseini M. Comparison of success rates in the medical management of ectopic pregnancy with single dose and multiple dose administrations of methotrexate: a prospective, randomized clinical trial. Fertil Steril 2006;85(6):1661.

14. Juneau C Bates. Reproductive outcomes after medical and surgical management of ectopic pregnancy. Clinical Obstetrics & Gynecology. 2012; 55(2):455-60.
15. Hajenius PJ, Mol F, Mol BW. Intervention for tubal ectopic pregnancy. Cochrane Database Syst Rev. 2007;24:CD000324.
16. Mol F, Mol BW, Ankum WM. Current evidence on surgery, systemic methotrexate and expectant management in the treatment of tubal ectopic pregnancy: asystematic review and meta-analysis. Hum Reprod Update. 2008a;14(4):309.
17. Graczykowski JW, Mishell DR Jr. Methotrexate prophylaxis for persistent ectopic pregnancy after conservative treatment by salpingostomy. Obstet Gynecol. 1997;89:118.
18. Buster JE, Krotz S. Reproductive performance after ectopic pregnancy. Sem Reprod Med. 2007;25:131.
19. Kirk E, Bottomley C, Bourne T. Diagnosing ectopic pregnancy and current concepts in the management of pregnancy of unknown location. Human Reproduction Update. 2014;20(2):250-61.

16
Amenorrhea

Deepti Goswami

INTRODUCTION

Amenorrhea refers to absence of menstruation. The incidence of amenorrhea is about 3-4% in women of reproductive age group in absence of pregnancy and lactation. Amenorrhea results due to a malfunctioning hypothalamic-pituitary-ovarian axis or due to a defect in the end organ, i.e. the uterus and its outflow tract. Amenorrhea is essentially a symptom and may occur due to any of the several possible underlying causes. It is often described as "Primary" or "Secondary" depending on the clinical presentation. Some causes are unique to each of the two categories; however, there are conditions that can lead to primary as well as secondary amenorrhea. In this chapter, the two categories are discussed separately for the sake of clarity.

PRIMARY AMENORRHEA

Primary amenorrhea refers to absence of onset of menstruation by 13 years of age (when secondary sexual characteristics are absent) or by 15 years of age (when secondary sexual characteristics are present).

Causes

Genetic or anatomic abnormalities are the most common causes of primary amenorrhea. However, all causes of secondary amenorrhea can also present as primary amenorrhea.

The common causes of primary amenorrhea include:
- Chromosomal abnormalities (most common being Turner syndrome)—45%
- Physiologic delay of puberty—20%
- Müllerian agenesis (Mayer-Rokitansky-Küster-Hauser syndrome)—15%
- Transverse vaginal septum or imperforate hymen—5%
- Absent hypothalamic production of GnRH—5%
- Anorexia nervosa—2%
- Hypopituitarism—2%.

Approach to Diagnosis

A detailed history and physical examination help in guiding further investigations.[1-3] The first step in evaluation includes assessment for (a) secondary sexual characteristics and (b) patent vagina.

History

- Symptom of cyclical abdominal pain gradually worsening over a period of time is suggestive of imperforate hymen or transverse vaginal septum causing genital tract obstruction that leads to collection of blood in vagina

and uterus causing pain. Such a patient may also experience difficulty in voiding or acute retention of urine due to distended vagina or uterus
- Age at which patient's mother and sisters attained menarche
- Stature as compared to parents and siblings
- Childhood growth and development
- Symptoms of headache, hearing loss, visual disturbances
- Fatigue, polyuria or polydipsia
- Galactorrhea
- Symptoms of virilization
- Rare cases of Kallmann syndrome will have anosmia
- Eating disorder (anorexia nervosa)
- Poor nutrition (malabsorption) and chronic illness (tuberculosis, renal disease)
- Trauma (to head), surgery (ovarian/pituitary), radiation and chemotherapy (for childhood cancers) and medications (drugs that cause hyperprolactinemia)
- In rare cases of androgen insensitivity syndrome (AIS) there may be a history of surgery for inguinal hernia in childhood
- Girls with well-developed secondary sexual characters and patent vagina sexual history should always be asked about sexual exposure to rule out the possibility of pregnancy.

Examination

- *General physical examination:*
  - Height, weight and body mass index (BMI)
  - Short stature is suggestive of Turner syndrome while girls with androgen insensitivity syndrome and hypogonadotropic hypogonadism are tall.
  - Girls with anorexia nervosa and poor nutrition will be cachexic (BMI <18 kg/m²).
  - Stigmata of Turner syndrome
- *Assessment of secondary sexual characters:*
  - *Tanner staging for breast:* Breasts are well developed in mullerian agenesis and AIS and poorly developed in Turner syndrome
  - Galactorrhea
  - Tanner staging for pubic hair-pubic and axillary hair are absent in AIS
  - Signs of virilization—these are seen in cases of partial AIS, certain cases of congenital adrenal hyperplasia and androgen secreting ovarian tumors
- *Neurological findings:*
  - Visual field—affected in pituitary tumors
  - Sense of smell—affected in Kallmann syndrome
  - Optic fundus—intracranial tumors may cause changes
- *Abdominal examination:*
  - Presence of a mass arising out of pelvis is suggestive of hematometra/hematocolpos. Pregnancy should be ruled out
  - Palpation of inguinal areas—may detect hernia or swelling due to presence of gonads (testis) in case of AIS
- *Pelvic examination*
  Local and per rectal examination:
  - Bulging bluish membrane at introitus with hematocolpos, hematometra suggests imperforate hymen
  - Absence of a patent vagina suggests mullerian agenesis or AIS
  - Transverse vaginal septum will present with hematocolpos, hematometra and short vaginal length
  - Rare cases of ovarian tumors may be detected
  - Pregnancy should be ruled out if there is no obvious developmental defect.

Investigations

Investigations are planned keeping in mind the history and examination findings.

Primary Amenorrhea with Absent Vagina

- In the patient with findings suggestive of developmental defects of genital tract the first-line investigation involves ultrasonography.

Magnetic resonance imaging (MRI) is often used for a more accurate assessment.
- In girls who lack a uterus differential diagnosis include mullerian agenesis or AIS. There is absence of pubic and axillary hair in girls with AIS while those with mullerian agenesis have well developed sexual hairs. Karyotype settles the diagnosis.
- In mullerian agenesis patient is screened for
  - Renal defect (horseshoe kidney, low lying kidney) that are present in 15% of cases and
  - Skeletal abnormalities in dorsolumbar spine that is present in 5-12% of cases.

Primary amenorrhea with normal reproductive tract and poor secondary sexual characteristics:
- This indicates an ovarian or pituitary hypothalamic defect. Serum levels of follicular stimulating hormone (FSH), luteinizing hormone (LH), thyroid stimulating hormone (TSH), and prolactin are assessed.
- Elevated FSH (>25 U/L) and LH (hypergonadotropic hypogonadism) indicate ovarian dysfunction. Karytype will help diagnose Turner's syndrome (45, XO), Swyer syndrome (46, XY) or primary ovarian insufficiency (normal karyotype-46, XX).
- Low FSH and LH levels (hypogonadotropic hypogonadism) indicate pituitary or hypothalamic dysfunction. This is mostly due to constitutional delay of growth and puberty. A detailed family history may help detect this etiology, as it is often familial. Assessment of bone age is done. MRI of the brain helps rule out pituitary lesions.
- *Serum TSH and prolactin:* Severe hypothyroidism may cause primary amenorrhea. Hyperprolactinemia interferes with pulsatile GnRH secretion and suppresses secretion of gonadotropins causing primary amenorrhea.
- In presence of hyperandrogenism, assessment of serum testosterone, dehydroepiandrosterone sulphate (DHEAS) and 17-hydroxyprogesterone will help detect androgen-secreting ovarian tumor or rare forms of congenital adrenal hyperplasia.

Management

Management depends on the underlying cause of primary amenorrhea.

Constitutional Delay of Puberty[4]

There may be a history of delayed puberty in mother or sister. There are no neurological abnormalities. Many of these girls will attain pubertal growth and menarche after a few years of waiting. Lack of increase in gonadotropin levels over several years would indicate pituitary or hypothalamic dysfunction.

Hypogonadotropic Hypogonadism

- MRI of brain is done. If pituitary defects are detected other hormones secreted by pituitary are also assessed.
- Anorexia and hypothyroidism are treatable.
- An obvious tumor on MRI may require surgical removal.
- In girls with poor sexual characteristics, pubertal induction is done with low incremental doses of estrogens.[5] After 1-2 years of therapy cyclical estrogen-progesterones or combined oral contraceptive pills are given as hormone replacement therapy (HRT).
- When pregnancy is desired ovulation induction may be done by administration of gonadotropins (FSH and LH) or gonadotropin releasing hormone administered in a pulsatile manner via a subcutaneous pump.

Turner Syndrome

- They have associated health problems like growth failure, cardiovascular disease (coarctation of aorta), renal problem, hypertension, sensorineural deafness, celiac disease, thyroiditis and learning disabilities.[6,7]
- Growth hormone therapy, though expensive, helps in attaining a greater height.

- Pubertal induction is done in the same way as described in the previous section. HRT is continued until the age of 50 years.
- Periodic monitoring for the above stated health problems is required.
- Pregnancy is possible through donated oocytes. Their pregnancy is monitored closely in view of the associated cardiovascular problems.

Karyotypically normal primary ovarian insufficiency:
- Most of the cases are idiopathic. Some of the underlying causes include genetic mutations, fragile X permutation, 47 XXX.[8-10] Autoimmune disorders particularly of thyroid may coexist.[11]
- Management involves hormone replacement therapy and infertility treatment later on. Psychological counseling is required. Ovarian biopsy and assessment for anti-ovarian antibodies are not required. Pubertal induction followed by estrogen and progesterone replacement is required to maintain optimal bone health.
- Regular monitoring of thyroid functions is needed.
- Pregnancy is possible through oocyte donation.
- Prognosis for return of spontaneous ovarian function is poor.[12]

Surgical Intervention

Surgery is required in patients with congenital anatomic lesions or Y chromosome material.
- An imperforate membrane obstructing the lower vagina requires a simple incision to relieve the retained blood. All aseptic precautions should be taken and no instrument should be inserted inside the genital tract since the collected blood is a rich culture medium for bacteria and infection may be introduced with the instrument.
- Transverse vaginal septum needs surgical excision followed by regular vaginal dilation to prevent adhesion formation and re-stenosis of vagina.
- Vaginal absence requires the construction of an artificial vagina that can be achieved by nonsurgical method by consistent use of serial dilators or by surgical means. Surgical methods for vaginoplasty include:
  - *McIndoe vaginoplasty*: A space is dissected between urethra and rectum which is then lined with split thickness skin graft mounted on a mould. Mould is left in situ for 7–10 days initially and this is followed by regular dilation to maintain patency of this neovagina.
  - *William's vulvovaginoplasty*: It is surgically much less invasive and involves dissection on perineum by a U-shaped incision and then suturing of labia majora. This creates a short vagina that eventually expands with sexual intercourse.
  - *Laparoscopic Vecchietti procedure*: A laparoscopic technique where neovagina is created by upward traction on an acrylic olive placed in vaginal pouch. Threads are inserted into peritoneal cavity laparoscopically and then attached to traction device through abdominal wall. Traction device and olive are removed in 7–10 days. Vaginal dilators and intercourse are required for maintenance of neovagina.
  - *Davydov vaginoplasty*: This involves dissection of rectovesical space and mobilization of peritoneum. The peritoneum is attachment to introitus. The vault is closed with purse string suture or by suturing large bowel serosa. A mould left in situ for one week. Mc call's culdoplasty is done to prevent prolapsed. The procedure can be done laparoscopically.
  - *Intestinal vaginoplasty*: Rectovesical space is dissected and a loop of colon or ileum is created. The caudal end of intestinal segment is anastomosed to the perineum. Blood supply maintained through pedicle of bowel.
- *Uterine transplant*: The first case of successful pregnancy after uterine transplant was reported in year 2015. This involved a 36-year-old woman with mullerian agenesis

who received a uterus transplant from a postmenopausal woman aged 61 years in 2013. The recipient became pregnant one year after the transplantation, after her first single embryo transfer. She was kept on immunosuppressants throughout pregnancy. A live baby boy (1.77 kg) was born via cesarean section done preterm for abnormal fetal heart in September 2014.[13]
- In patients with Y chromosome as in AIS and Swyer syndrome, gonadectomy is needed to prevent the development of gonadal neoplasia (usually gonadoblastoma).[14,15]
- Androgen secreting tumor of ovary or adrenal will require surgical removal.
- In rare cases of partial androgen insensitivity syndrome, congenital adrenal hyperplasia or rare enzymatic disorders patients present with virilization at puberty. They require surgical correction of clitromegaly.

SECONDARY AMENORRHEA

Secondary amenorrhea is diagnosed when a woman who has previously menstruated presents with absence of menstruation for 6 months or for a duration equivalent to three normal menstrual cycles.

Causes

First and foremost pregnancy should be excluded in any woman presenting with secondary amenorrhea.

The common causes of secondary amenorrhea are:
- Ovarian disease—40%
- Hypothalamic dysfunction—35%
- Pituitary disease—19%
- Uterine disease—5%
- Other—1%.

History

- Duration of amenorrhea and preceding menstrual history.
- Contraceptive history—a woman may present with amenorrhea due to nonresumption of menstrual cycles following discontinuation of depot medroxyprogesterone acetate.
- Any symptoms suggestive of hyperandrogenism—acne, hirsutism, deepening of voice.
- Recent change in weight-loss or gain, excessive physical exercise, eating habits, recent stressful events or major illness.
- Symptoms suggestive of hypothalamic-pituitary disease—headaches and visual field defects (tumors), polyuria and polydipsia (diabetes insipidus).
- Patients with estrogen deficiency may complain of hot flashes, vaginal dryness and poor sleep.
- Inquiry about presence of breast secretions.
- Intake of drugs known to cause menstrual irregularity or amenorrhea—antipsychotic drugs, danazol/androgenic drugs, high-doses of progesterones; also enquire about recent treatment with cytotoxic agents.
- History of severe obstetrical bleeding in previous pregnancy. This leads to postpartum pituitary necrosis and hypogonadotropic hypogonadism (Sheehan's syndrome). They should also be asked about failed lactation and loss of pubic and axillary hair.
- History of endometrial curettage—a vigorous curettage done after abortion or postpartum damages the basal layer of endometrium causing scarring and loss of menstrual function (Asherman's syndrome).
- History of tuberculosis in self or history of exposure to tuberculosis—genital tract tuberculosis is a common cause of secondary amenorrhea and infertility in our population.
- Past history of surgery on uterus or ovaries, chronic diseases.

Examination

- Pregnancy should always be ruled out by clinical examination and where required by urine pregnancy test.
- Height and weight, body mass index (BMI): Excessive (>30 kg/m^2) as well as low BMI (<18 kg/m^2) can disrupt menstrual function. Excessive BMI is seen in women with polycystic ovarian syndrome (PCOS)

and causes anovulation that can lead to oligomenorrhea or amenorrhea.
- Skin—for evidence of hyperandrogenism—hirsutism, acne and acanthosis nigricans. Severity of hirsutism is assessed by Ferriman-Gallwey score. Striae may be seen in Cushing's syndrome.
- Breast—galactorrhea.
- Signs of systemic illness—particularly tuberculosis.
- In cases suspected to have intracranial lesions, neurological examination for visual field defects.
- Abdomen—masses, tenderness.
- Examination of vaginal mucosa may show signs of estrogen deficiency.

Investigations

- Pregnancy should always be ruled out where required by urine pregnancy test.
- Once the pregnancy is ruled out tests done are:
  - Progesterone challenge test
  - Serum level of TSH and prolactin.
- *Progesterone challenge test*: Medroxyprogesterone acetate 10 mg is given once or twice a day for 5–10 days. If the patient has withdrawal bleed after cessation of drug, it indicates anovulation as in PCOS. Absence of withdrawal bleed indicates an outflow tract abnormality or hypoestrogenic state. The two conditions are distinguished on the basis of *estrogen/progesterone challenge test.*
- *Estrogen/progesterone challenge test* involves sequential administration of estrogen (conjugated equine estrogen 0.625 mg or equivalent doses of other estrogen preparation) and medroxyprogesterone acetate (10 mg) so as to mimic normal physiology. Occurrence of a withdrawal bleed indicates a pituitary/hypothalamic or ovarian cause. Failure to bleed indicates a defect in outflow tract.
- The *Gonadotropin levels* help distinguish between hypogonadotropic hypogonadism, and hypergonadotropic hypogonadism which have different etiologies.
- Normal or low FSH or LH levels indicate a pituitary or hypothalamic abnormality (hypogonadotropic hypogonadism). MRI may reveal a pituitary tumor, empty sella syndrome or Sheehan syndrome.
- Elevated FSH and LH levels (hypergonadotropic hypogonadism) suggest primary ovarian insufficiency. They are further investigated with karyotype and tests for thyroid and adrenal autoimmunity. Ovarian biopsy and antiovarian antibody testing are not recommended.
- Where suspected, genital tract tuberculosis is ruled out by endometrial aspiration biopsy.
- Women presenting with sudden onset and rapid progression of hyperandrogenic symptoms are advised tests for serum levels of testosterone and other androgens.
  - Significantly-elevated testosterone) levels indicate a possible androgen-secreting tumor (ovarian or adrenal). Raised DHEAS level is suggestive of adrenal cause. USG will help detect androgen secreting ovarian tumors.
  - Elevated levels of 17-hydroxyprogesterone are diagnostic of adult-onset congenital adrenal hyperplasia.
  - Patients are screened for Cushing's syndrome when characteristic signs and symptoms are present (e.g. striae, buffalo hump, significant central obesity, easy bruising, hypertension, and proximal muscle weakness). The test used is the dexamethasone suppression test.

Management of Secondary Amenorrhea

Management of patients with amenorrhea involves correcting any underlying disorder—weight loss, hypothyroidism or hyperprolactinemia, treatment for anovulation associated with PCOS and replacement of cyclical estrogen-progesterone in women with estrogen deficiency (hypergonadotropic or hypogonadotropic).

Hyperprolactinemia

- Rule out use of medications which may cause hyperprolactinemia. A prolactin level more than 100 ng/mL suggests a prolactinoma, and MRI should be performed.
- Microadenomas (smaller than 10 mm) do not require surgery.
- Macroadenomas may be treated with dopamine agonists or removed with trans-sphenoidal resection or craniotomy, if necessary.
- Dopamine agonists (bromocriptine, cabergoline) are the mainstay of treatment. Bromocriptine is started in a dose of 2.5 mg at bed time to minimize side effects (orthostatic hypotension, nausea, headache, fainting). The dose is slowly increased up to 7.5 mg or 10 mg/day. Resumption of menstrual function indicates normalization of prolactin levels. Cabergoline is superior in effectiveness and tolerability. Cabergoline is started in a dose of 0.25 mg/day once a week, then twice a week and further up to 3 mg weekly as required.

Secondary Amenorrhea with Normal Gonadotropin Levels

Causes include outflow tract obstruction and chronic anovulation as is seen in PCOS.

- *Polycystic ovary syndrome (PCOS)*: It is the most common cause of chronic anovulation. Resistance to insulin is an essential causative factor. *Serum insulin measurement is not required for diagnosis or management.* To diagnose PCOS, any 2 of 3 criteria (Rotterdam criteria) should be present:[16]
  - Oligomenorrhea/amenorrhea
  - Signs of androgen excess
  - Presence of polycystic ovaries on ultrasound (≥12 follicles—2–9 mm in size, increased ovarian volume ≥10 mL).
- Management of PCOS:
  - It is essential to provide regular menstrual flow to protect against endometrial hyperplasia by cyclical progesterones (at least 12 days per month) or combined oral contraceptive pills.
  - The primary treatment for PCOS in obese women is weight loss through diet and exercise. Weight loss decreases insulin resistance, lowers androgen levels and normalize menses.[17]
  - Metformin can reduce insulin resistance and improve ovulatory function. Gastrointestinal side effects are common.
  - Hirsutism is treated with antiandrogens—most common being spironolactone and cyproterone acetate.
  - Infertility due to PCOS is managed with ovulation induction with clomiphene or gonadotropins.
  - Glucose tolerance test is also done and women with abnormal results are treated.
- *Asherman's syndrome*: This condition is characterized by occurrence of intrauterine adhesions usually following dilatation and curettage done after abortion or postpartum. Other causes include uterine infection, like genital tuberculosis and schistosomiasis.
  - Endometrial biopsy, hysterosalpingography and hysteroscopy help in diagnosis.
  - Management involves hysteroscopic lysis of intrauterine adhesions. Further treatment with estrogen and progestogen may stimulate regrowth of the endometrium. Prognosis is usually poor in cases of tuberculosis.

Secondary Amenorrhea with Low Gonadotropin Levels

These women have low serum FSH and LH levels due to hypothalamic or pituitary dysfunction.

- *Hypothalamic amenorrhea*: The condition is often caused by excessive weight loss, exercise, or stress which affect gonadotropin-releasing hormone (GnRH) secretion.[18]
  - Treatment involves restoration of normal weight in women with eating disorders (anorexia nervosa, bulimia nervosa). Psychological counseling is required.

- Those indulging in excessive athletic activity or exercise are advised to increase their caloric intake or limit their athletic training.
- Adequate calcium and vitamin D intake are recommended for these patients.
- *Sheehan syndrome* occurs due to pituitary necrosis following massive obstetric hemorrhage:
  - Hormone replacement with estrogen-progesterone is required.
  - Levels of other hormones secreted by anterior pituitary (TSH and ACTH) are also assessed. If deficient, thyroid hormone and corticosteroid replacement is also required.
  - Pregnancy can be achieved with ovulation induction with exogenous gonadotropins (both FSH and LH).[19]

Secondary Amenorrhea with Raised Gonadotropin Levels

These women have primary ovarian insufficiency characterized by amenorrhea, hypoestrogenism, and increased gonadotropin levels (FSH >25 IU/L) occurring before 40 years of age. Women with primary ovarian insufficiency have an increased risk of osteoporosis due to hypoestrogenism.
- Treatment involves estrogen—progesterone replacement continued till the normal age of menopause, i.e. 50 years of age.
- The condition can be associated with autoimmune endocrine disorders such as hypothyroidism and Addison's disease. Periodic screening is required for these disorders.[20]
- Though cases of spontaneous conception are reported for women with POI, these are very rare. Even on serial biochemical assessment, only a few woman show spontaneous decline in FSH levels which is not associated with ovulation or menstruation.[12]
- Pregnancy is possible through donor oocyte and *in vitro* fertilization.

KEY POINTS

- Amenorrhea is symptom of an underlying disorder.
- The underlying disorder could be a structural defect in genital tract or a functional defect of ovary, pituitary or hypothalamus. Thyroid disorder and adrenal disorder can also disrupt normal menstrual function.
- Amenorrhea can be primary or secondary.
- Systematic approach to diagnosis is essential.
- Pregnancy should always be ruled out.
- The investigations are directed to find the underlying cause of amenorrhea.
- Management involves correcting the underlying structural or hormonal defect. This may involve long-term hormonal replacement in some cases.
- Surgical intervention is required to correct the genital tract defect and for gonadectomy in women with XY karyotype.
- Prognosis will depend on the underlying cause.

REFERENCES

1. Fritz MA. Amenorrhea. In: Fritz MA, Speroff L (Eds). Clinical Gynecological Endocrinology and Infertility, 8th edition, Philadelphia: Lippincott Williams & Wilkins, 2010.
2. Edmonds DK. Primary amenorrhea. In: Studd J (Ed). Progress in Obstetrics and Gynaecology. Churchill Livingstone. 1993;10:281-96.
3. Master-Hunter T, Heiman DL. Amenorrhea: evaluation and treatment. Am Fam Physician. 2006;73:1374-82.
4. Houk CP, Lee PA. Early, precocious and delayed female pubertal development. In: Lavin N (Ed). Manual of Endocrinology and Metabolism, 4th edition. Lippincott Williams & Wilkins, New Delhi; 2009. pp. 144-263.
5. Styne DM, Grumbach MM. Puberty: ontogeny, neuroendocrinology, physiology, and disorders. In: Kronenberg HM, Melmed S, Polonsky KS, Larsen PR (Eds). Williams Textbook of Endocrinology, 11th edition. Saunders Elsevier, Philadelphia; 2008. pp. 969-1166.
6. Conway GS, Band M, Doyle J, Davies MC. How do you monitor the patient with Turner's syndrome

in adulthood? Clin Endocrinol (Oxf). 2010;73: 696-9.
7. Davenport ML. Approach to the patient with Turner syndrome. J Clin Endocrinol Metab. 2010;95: 1487-95.
8. Goswami D, Conway GS. Premature ovarian failure. Horm Res. 2007;68:196-202.
9. Goswami D, Conway GS. Premature ovarian failure. Hum Reprod Update. 2005;11:391-410.
10. Goswami R, Goswami D, Kabra M, Gupta N, Dubey S, Dadhwal V. Prevalence of the triple X syndrome in phenotypically normal women with premature ovarian failure and its association with autoimmune thyroid disorders. Fertil Steril. 2003; 80:1052-4.
11. Goswami R, Marwaha RK, Goswami D, Gupta N, Ray D, Tomar N, Singh S. Prevalence of thyroid autoimmunity in sporadic idiopathic hypoparathyroidism in comparison to type 1 diabetes and premature ovarian failure. J Clin Endocrinol Metab. 2006;91:4256-9.
12. Goswami D, Arif A, Saxena A, Batra S. Idiopathic primary ovarian insufficiency: a study of serial hormonal profiles to assess ovarian follicular activity. Hum Reprod. 2011;26:2218-25.
13. Brännström M, Johannesson L, Bokström H, et al. Livebirth after uterus transplantation. Lancet. 2015;385:607-16.
14. Michala L, Goswami D, Creighton SM, Conway GS. Swyer syndrome: presentation and outcomes. BJOG. 2008;115:737-41.
15. Berglund A, Johannsen TH, Stochholm K, et al. Incidence, prevalence, diagnostic delay, and clinical presentation of female 46,XY disorders of sex development. J Clin Endocrinol Metab. 2016 Sep 7:jc20162248. PubMed PMID: 27603905.
16. Rotterdam ESHRE/ASRM-Sponsored PCOS Consensus Workshop Group. Revised 2003 consensus on diagnostic criteria and long-term health risks related to polycystic ovary syndrome. Fertil Steril. 2004;81:19-25.
17. RCOG Green top guideline. Polycystic Ovary Syndrome, Long-Term Consequences (Green-top 33), 2007. *www.rcog.org.uk*.
18. Silveira LF, Latronico AC. Approach to the patient with hypogonadotropic hypogonadism. J Clin Endocrinol Metab. 2013;98:1781-8.
19. Kriplani A, Goswami D, Agarwal N, Bhatla N, Ammini AC. Twin pregnancy following gonadotrophin therapy in a patient with Sheehan's syndrome. Int J Gynaecol Obstet. 2000;71:59-63.
20. ESHRE Guideline Group on POI, Webber L, Davies M, Anderson R, et al. ESHRE Guideline: management of women with premature ovarian insufficiency. Hum Reprod. 2016;31(5): 926-37.

17

Polycystic Ovary Syndrome

Madhavi M Gupta

INTRODUCTION

The polycystic ovary syndrome (PCOS) is the most common endocrine disorder of women in the reproductive age group globally. The prevalence is 6–10% when using the diagnostic criteria defined by the National Institute of Health (NIH) while on applying the Rotterdam criteria may be twice as high[1] (Table 17.1). Depending on which criteria are used for diagnosing the condition the worldwide prevalence ranges from 4% to 21%.[2,3]

The disorder is manifested clinically as ovulatory dysfunction, hyperandrogenism, and polycystic ovarian morphology (PCOM) on ultrasound. Cutaneous manifestation of androgen excess (hirsutism) adversely effects the social interaction and quality of life of the woman and polycystic ovary syndrome is the most common cause of anovular infertility. Hirsutism is seen more commonly in the Indian subcontinent than in women of East-Asian origin. Also seen more in Caucasian women. Hyperandrogenism may also present as acne or alopecia. The condition affects various aspects of a woman's health right through menarche to well past her reproductive years.

Table 17.1 Diagnostic criteria for polycystic ovary syndrome (PCOS)

NIH 1990[4]	Rotterdam 2003[5,6] (ESHRE/ASRM)	AE-PCOS Society 2006[7,8]
• Chronic anovulation* • Clinical and/or biochemical signs of hyperandrogenism (with exclusion of other etiologies, e.g. congenital adrenal hyperplasia)	• Oligo- and/or anovulation • Clinical and/or biochemical signs of hyperandrogenism • Polycystic ovaries#	• Clinical and/or biochemical signs of hyperandrogenism • Ovarian dysfunction* (Oligo-anovulation and/or polycystic ovarian morphology)#
Both criteria needed for diagnosis	Two of three criteria needed for diagnosis	Both criteria needed for diagnosis
Two combinations to meet criteria for PCOS	Four combinations to meet criteria for PCOS	Three combinations to meet criteria for PCOS

*Ovulatory dysfunction: unpredictable menses at >35 days or occur less than 8 times per year. May also be present with apparent eumenorrhea and hyperandrogenism
#Polycystic ovarian morphology (PCOM): ≥12 antral follicles (2–9 mm in diameter) in either ovary, an ovarian volume of >10 mL in one or both the ovaries.
Abbreviations: NIH, National Institute of Health; ESHRE/ASRM, European Society for Human Reproduction and Embryology/American Society for Reproductive Medicine; AE-PCOS, Androgen Excess-polycystic Ovarian Syndrome Society

PATHOPHYSIOLOGY

It is a complex, polygenic disorder where the etiology is generally poorly understood. Environmental influences (those contributing to obesity)[9] also play a role. There is impaired ovarian steroidogenesis along with faulty follicular development. The pathophysiology involves a diminished negative feedback response of the hypothalamus to the circulating steroids. Consequently, there is an excess of luteinizing hormone (LH) and deficient follicle-stimulating hormone (FSH) secretion. This leads to increased ovarian androgen production, ovulatory dysfunction, and disordered insulin action in a variety of target tissues. The compensatory hyperinsulinemia leads to increased androgen production, both, ovarian and adrenal and enhanced bioavailability of androgens mediated via lower levels of sex hormone-binding globulin (SHBG).

CLINICAL FEATURES

PCOS has a broad spectrum of clinical manifestations and associated morbidities. There are significant cardiometabolic abnormalities and enhanced risk of coronary artery disease. Obesity is seen commonly, with 50–80% of women being obese.[9] Nearly a third of the women (30–35%) with PCOS have impaired glucose tolerance and 8–10% have type 2 diabetes mellitus. A family history of diabetes, age and adiposity contribute to the risk.[10,11]

There is atherogenic dyslipidemia with elevated low-density lipoprotein (LDL), cholesterol and triglycerides and lower high-density lipoprotein (HDL) levels than women who are not affected by this condition.[12]

There is a 2.7 times increased risk of endometrial cancer in these in comparison to women without polycystic ovary syndrome. The estimated lifetime risk in the women affected with the syndrome is up to 9%.[13] The contributory risk factors include obesity, insulin resistance and chronic anovulation. During pregnancy these women are at higher risk of complications like gestational diabetes (prevalence is twice as high compared to control women), pre-eclampsia, fetal macrosomia and perinatal mortality.[14] Their is a higher prevalence of obstructive sleep apnea (OSA) in women with PCOS.[15] Androgen levels and insulin resistance positively correlate with obstructive sleep apnoea in PCOS. Also women with PCOS are more prone to emotional distress (e.g. anxiety and depression).[16]

Symptoms
• Menstrual irregularity
• Hirsutism
• Acne
• Alopecia
• Obesity
• Anxiety
• Depression
• Snoring/day time sleepiness

DIAGNOSIS

Diagnosis of polycystic ovary syndrome requires a careful history and clinical examination. It should be supplemented with standardized laboratory investigations including both biochemical parameters and ovarian imaging.

Diagnosing PCOS entails three components:
1. Establishing hyperandrogenism (clinical-hirsutism, acne and lab parameters).
2. Establishing ovulatory dysfunction-unpredictable menses at >35 days or occur less than 8 times per year. In the presence of hyperandrogenism regular cycles at 21-35 days does not always correspond to normal ovulatory function. May also be present in 15-40% of women with regular menses and hyperandrogenism.
3. Establishing polycystic ovarian morphology (PCOM) on ultrasound.

Diagnosis in adolescence may be tricky as there is overlap of findings with those of normal puberty. Hence, in adolescence both ovulatory dysfunction inappropriate for the developmental stage and hyperandrogenism (increased free testosterone and moderate to severe hirsutism) are required.

MANAGEMENT

Investigations

Free testosterone (T)—more sensitive than the measurement of total testosterone. But assays for the free form are inaccurate. Equilibrium dialysis technique is recommended.[17]
- Calculated free testosterone from measurement of total testosterone alongwith sex hormone-binding globulin.[18]
- Significance of estimating other androgens is uncertain. Dehydroepiandrosterone sulfate (DHEAS) levels are high in ~30–35%[19] but does not contribute to the diagnosis significantly. In most women both, free and total T are also increased. Isolated increase in DHEAS has no proven clinical meaning.[20]
- Anti-mullerian hormone and serum 17-hydroxyprogesterone—useful investigations in establishing a diagnosis of PCOS.[17]
- *Imaging:* Polycystic ovarian morphology on ultrasound scan (USS). Transvaginal ultrasound (transducer with a frequency of ≥8 MHz) is the standard mode of evaluation. Transabdominal USS may be employed in young girls or in women who are not willing due to cultural reasons but is less sensitive. On USS it is important to look for the ovarian morphology and count the number of antral follicles. PCOM is presently defined as ≥12 antral follicles (2–9 mm in diameter) in either ovary, an ovarian volume of >10 mL in one or both the ovaries.[6] Higher antral follicle count (≥25) has been recommended by some for increasing the specificity.[21]
- *Others:* To confirm anovulation—serum progesterone level during the suspected midluteal phase (days 21 to 22) of the cycle. If lower than 3–4 ng/mL presume that the cycle is oligo-anovulatory.[22]
- Screening for cardiometabolic risk factors- measurement of blood pressure, BMI, and waist circumference to be done at each visit. Fasting lipid levels to be done every two years (earlier if the woman has gained weight).
- Screening for impaired glucose tolerance and type 2 diabetes mellitus using the 2-hour oral glucose-tolerance test and repeated every 1–5 years depending on the patient characteristics. Glycosylated hemoglobin (HbA_{1c}) levels are an acceptable alternative.
- Screen for anxiety, depression and obstructive sleep apnea.
- In case of persistent abnormal uterine bleeding or prolonged amenorrhea to be evaluated for endometrial hyperplasia.

Treatment

Treatment is decided by patient priorities, the success and risks associated with the several modalities and desire to conceive.

Treatment is targeted at hirsutism, menstrual irregularity with the associated risk of endometrial hyperplasia and infertility.

Lifestyle modification and weight loss are the first-line of management. The underlying disorder is not reversed but even a 5–10% weight loss brings down the androgen levels, reduces the cardiometabolic risk factors and also contributes in improving the menstrual function.

Hirsutism

Hirsutism is dealt in detail in Chapter 18 but its prudent to mention the role of combined oral contraceptive (COC) here.
- COC is considered to be the first-line agents.[23] The COCs suppress the gonadotropin secretion and the increased ovarian steroidogenesis. Sex hormone-binding globulin (SHBG) production in the liver is increased by the estrogen component thus, decreasing the bioavailable androgen. New terminal hair growth is reduced but these changes may take up to 6 months to be clinically visible. Low dose ethinyl estradiol (up to 30 μg) with a progestin having antiandrogenic potential or low androgenic properties can be used.
- Apart from reducing the hair growth COCs lead to improvement in acne, regular withdrawal bleed thus, preventing endometrial hyperplasia and also provide effective contraception.
- There is an increased risk of venous thromboembolism (VTE) with the use of COC

especially those containing third and fourth generation progestins. When prescribing, medical eligibility criteria (WHO/UK) to be considered carefully.

An insulin sensitizer. Lowers the insulin levels and leads to ~20 to 25% reduction in serum testosterone levels. Recommended in women with PCOS having impaired glucose tolerance or type 2 diabetes mellitus as second line after lifestyle modification.[23,25]

Dose: 500 mg daily with meals, gradually increasing to 1000 mg twice a day with meals.

Other Options

- Progestin-only contraceptive pills
- Levonorgestrel-releasing intrauterine device.

Both provide effective endometrial protection and reliable contraception.

Infertility

Clomiphene citrate is the first-line agent for ovulation induction in women with polycystic ovarian syndrome. Some women may require exogenous gonadotropins or assisted reproductive techniques.[26]

Clinical Implications in Perimenopause

The associated metabolic syndrome and increased cardiovascular risk has long-term consequences. During the perimenopause there is weight gain and both, the visceral fat tissue and the total body fat increases which further aggravates the already increased cardiovascular risk in women with PCOS is not certain. Most available evidence suggests that the long-term consequences in women with PCOS seem to be lower than expected.[27] But keeping the complex and heterogeneous nature of PCOS in consideration a complete periodical cardiometabolic and gynecologic evaluation is called for in the event of weight gain and a diagnosis of PCOS.

KEY POINTS

- Correct diagnosis is mandatory as it has long-term implications even beyond the reproductive life.
- Race and ethnicity affects the phenotype.
- Diagnosis is difficult in the perimenarcheal and perimenopausal period, and is exacerbated by obesity.
- Laboratory investigations need to be standardized.
- Hyperandrogenism identifies women at risk for coexisting metabolic conditions.
- Lifestyle modification and weight loss are the first-line of management.
- Even as little as 5–10% weight loss reduces the cardiometabolic risk.

REFERENCES

1. McCartney CR, Marshall JC. Clinical practice. Polycystic ovary syndrome. N Engl J Med. 2016; 375(1):54-64.
2. Boyle JA, Cunningham J, O'Dea K, Dunbar T, Norman RJ. Prevalence of polycystic ovary syndrome in a sample of Indigenous women in Darwin, Australia. Med J Aust. 2012;196:62-6.
3. Ma YM, Li R, Qiao J, Zhang XW, Wang SY, Zhang QF, et al. Characteristics of abnormal menstrual cycle and polycystic ovary syndrome in community and hospital populations. Chin Med J (Engl). 2010;123:2185-9.
4. Zawadzki JK, Dunaif A. Diagnostic criteria for polycystic ovary syndrome; towards a rational approach. In: Dunaif A, Givens JR, Haseltine F, Merriam G (Eds). Polycystic ovary syndrome. Boston: Blackwell Scientific; 1992.
5. Rotterdam ESHRE/ASRM-Sponsored PCOS Consensus Workshop Group. Revised 2003 consensus on diagnostic criteria and long-term health risks related to polycystic ovary syndrome. Fertil Steril. 2004;81:19-25.
6. Rotterdam ESHRE/ASRM-Sponsored PCOS Consensus Workshop Group. Revised 2003 consensus on diagnostic criteria and long-term health risks related to polycystic ovary syndrome (PCOS). Hum Reprod. 2004;19:41-7.
7. Azziz R, Carmina E, Dewailly D, Diamanti-Kandarakis E, Escobar- Morreale HF, Futterweit

W, et al. Positions statement: criteria for defining polycystic ovary syndrome as a predominantly hyperandrogenic syndrome: an Androgen Excess Society guideline. J Clin Endocrinol Metab. 2006;91: 4237-45.
8. Azziz R, Carmina E, Dewailly D, Diamanti-Kandarakis E, Escobar- Morreale HF, Futterweit W, et al. The Androgen Excess and PCOS Society criteria for the polycystic ovary syndrome: the complete task force report Fertil Steril. 2009;91:456-88.
9. Dumesic DA, Oberfield SE, Stener-Victorin E, Marshall JC, Laven JS, Legro RS. Scientific statement on the diagnostic criteria, epidemiology, pathophysiology, and molecular genetics of polycystic ovary syndrome. Endocr Rev. 2015;36: 487-525.
10. Ehrmann DA, Barnes RB, Rosenfield RL, Cavaghan MK, Imperial J. Prevalence of impaired glucose tolerance and diabetes in women with polycystic ovary syndrome. Diabetes Care. 1999;22: 141-6.
11. Legro RS, Kunselman AR, Dodson WC, Dunaif A. Prevalence and predictors of risk for type 2 diabetes mellitus and impaired glucose tolerance in polycystic ovary syndrome: a prospective, controlled study in 254 affected women. J Clin Endocrinol Metab. 1999;84:165-9.
12. Wild RA, Rizzo M, Clifton S, Carmina E. Lipid levels in polycystic ovary syndrome: systematic review and meta-analysis. Fertil Steril. 2011;95(3): 1073-9.e1.
13. Dumesic DA, Lobo RA. Cancer risk and PCOS. Steroids. 2013;78:782-5.
14. Boomsma CM, Eijkemans MJ, Hughes EG, Visser GH, Fauser BC, Macklon NS. A meta-analysis of pregnancy outcomes in women with polycystic ovary syndrome. Hum Reprod Update. 2006;12:673-83.
15. Tasali E, Van Cauter E, Ehrmann DA. Polycystic ovary syndrome and obstructive sleep apnea. Sleep Med Clin. 2008;3:37-46.
16. Veltman-Verhulst SM, Boivin J, Eijkemans MJ, Fauser BJ. Emotional distress is a common risk in women with polycystic ovary syndrome: a systematic review and meta-analysis of 28 studies. Hum Reprod Update. 2012;18:638-51.
17. Goodman NF, Cobin RH, Futterweit W, Glueck JS, Legro RS, Carmina E. American Association of Clinical Endocrinologists, American College of Endocrinology, Androgen Excess and PCOS Society disease state clinical review: guide to the best practices in the evaluation and treatment of polycystic ovary syndrome--part 1. Endocr Pract. 2015;21(11):1291-300.
18. Rosner W, Auchus RJ, Azziz R, Sluss PM, Raff H. Position statement: utility, limitations, and pitfalls in measuring testosterone: an Endocrine Society position statement. J Clin Endocrinol Metab. 2007; 92:405-13.
19. Carmina E. Ovarian and adrenal hyperandrogenism. Ann N Y Acad Sci. 2006;1092:130-7.
20. Goodarzi MO, Carmina E, Azziz R. DHEA, DHEAS and PCOS. J Steroid Biochem Mol Biol. 2015;145:213-25.
21. Dewailly D, Lujan ME, Carmina E, et al. Definition and significance of polycystic ovarian morphology: a task force report from the Androgen Excess and Polycystic Ovary Syndrome Society. Hum Reprod Update. 2014;20:334-52.
22. Legro RS, Barnhart HX, Schlaff WD, et al. Clomiphene, metformin, or both for infertility in the polycystic ovary syndrome. N Engl J Med. 2007;356(6):551-66.
23. Legro RS, Arslanian SA, Ehrmann DA, et al. Diagnosis and treatment of polycystic ovary syndrome: an Endocrine Society Clinical Practice guideline. J Clin Endocrinol Metab. 2013;98:4565-92.
24. Swiglo BA, Cosma M, Flynn DN, et al. Antiandrogens for the treatment of hirsutism: a systematic review and metaanalyses of randomized controlled trials. J Clin Endocrinol Metab. 2008;93:1153-60.
25. Conway G, Dewailly D, Diamanti-Kandarakis E, et al. The polycystic ovary syndrome: a position statement from the European Society of Endocrinology. Eur J Endocrinol. 2014;171:1-29.
26. Perales-Puchalt A, Legro RS. Ovulation induction in women with polycystic ovary syndrome. Steroids. 2013;78:767-72.
27. Lenart-Lipińska M, Matyjaszek-Matuszek B, Woźniakowska E, Solski J, Tarach JS, Paszkowski T. Polycystic ovary syndrome: clinical implication in perimenopause. Prz Menopauzalny. 2014; 13(6):348-51.

18

Hirsutism

Madhavi M Gupta

INTRODUCTION

Hirsutism in women is defined as male-pattern distribution of increased terminal (coarse) hair.[1] Race and ethnicity significantly influence the severity of hirsutism. It is seen more commonly in the Indian subcontinent and those from the Mediterranean countries than in women of East Asian or northern European descent.

Clinical assessment mandates a careful history with detailing which includes the time of onset, progression, how frequently she has to resort to hair removal and the extent to which it negatively impacts the woman's daily life. Cutaneous manifestation of androgen excess (hirsutism) adversely effects the social interaction and quality of life of the woman. Depending on the severity, it can have a significant psychological impact leading to impaired quality of life and depressive symptoms in many women.[2]

The Ferriman-Gallwey chart (Fig. 18.1) is used universally to assess the severity and distribution of the excess body hair.[3] Each of the nine androgen-sensitive areas are graded visually on a scale of 0–4 obtaining a final score. A score of ≥8 is considered subnormal.

ANDROGEN BIOSYNTHESIS, TRANSPORT AND METABOLISM IN WOMEN

The circulating testosterone in normal premenopausal women is sourced equally from the ovaries

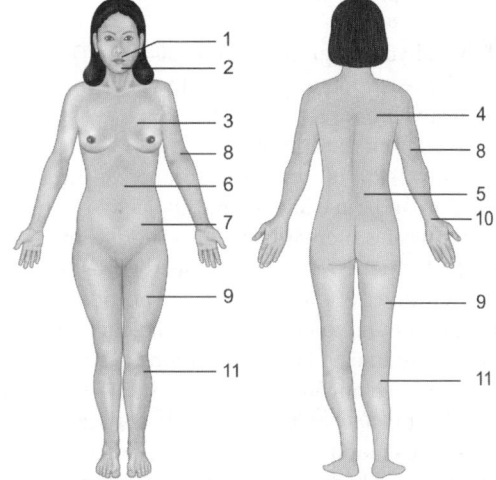

Fig. 18.1 The hirsutism scoring scale designed by Ferriman and Gallwey. The body is divided into 11 zones as illustrated, and each zone is scored 0–4 giving a maximum score of 44. Ferriman and Gallwey excluded the lower arm and leg, and defined hirsutism as a score of > 8

and the adrenals.[4,5] Almost 50% of the circulating testosterone is synthesized *de novo* from cholesterol in the adrenal cortex and the ovary (Flow chart 18.1). The rest of it is produced as a result of metabolism of androgen precursors in peripheral tissues like skin and the adipose tissue.

The androgens most abundant in the circulation, dehydroepiandrosterone (DHEA)

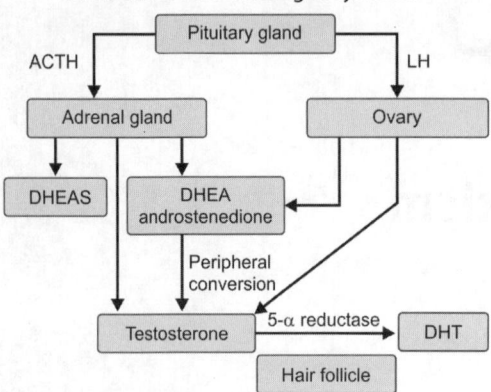

Flow chart 18.1 Androgen synthesis

Abbreviations: ACTH, adrenocorticotropic hormon; LH, luteinizing hormone; DHEAS, dehydroepiandrosterone sulfate; DHT, dehydrotestosterone

and dehydroepiandrosterone sulfate (DHEAS) are the least potent. Whereas the concentration of testosterone is low. DHEAS is exclusively sourced from the adrenals.

Only ~1% of the testosterone is the free fraction and bioavailable and the active form in target tissues. Remainder of it is bound majorly to sex hormone-binding globulin (SHBG) (~80%) and around 19% to albumin.[6] A portion of the fraction bound to albumin is also bioactive form of testosterone which differs among tissues.[7]

Serum concentration of SHBG has a significant effect on the bioactivity and hence the cutaneous manifestations of androgen excess. In hirsutism, skin is the testosterone target tissue. Androgen receptors are located at basal cells and glandular cells of sebaceous glands, in the outer root sheath of hair follicles. 5-α reductase is responsible for converting testosterone to the more potent dihydrotestosterone (DHT).

CAUSES OF HIRSUTISM

The causes are listed in Table 18.1.
Why does hirsutism happen?
- Increased serum androgens.
- Decreased levels of SHBG—increased free testosterone.
- Increased responsiveness of target organ to normal circulating androgens.
- Increased activity of 5-α reductase.

Table 18.1 Causes of hirsutism

Ovarian	Adrenal	Idiopathic
Polycystic ovary syndrome (PCOS) (>80%)	Congenital adrenal hyperplasia [classical 1%; nonclassical (late-onset) 3%]	With raised androgens (5%)
Hyperthecosis	Cushing syndrome (<1%)	Without raised androgens (7%)
Ovarian tumors (sex cord stromal tumors; Sertoli–Leydig cell tumors; adrenal-like tumors of the ovary) (<1%)	Adrenal tumors (adenoma; carcinoma) (<1%)	

Source: Adapted from Franks S. The investigation and management of hirsutism. J Fam Plann Reprod Health Care. 2012;38:182-6.

The most common and significant cause of hirsutism is polycystic ovary syndrome (PCOS). Hirsutism in PCOS has also been discussed in the section on PCOS. More than three-fourths of the women who have no menstrual irregularity but are hirsute have polycystic ovaries. Earlier this group would have been labeled as 'idiopathic hirsutism'.[3,8]

Serum testosterone and even luteinizing hormone (LH) is high in these women. Hirsutism is more commonly seen in women who are overweight or obese in comparison to those who are lean.[9] Hyperinsulinemia due to insulin resistance causes increased ovarian and adrenal steroidogenesis. It also increases the bioavailability of androgens mediated via lowered levels of sex hormone-binding globulin (SHBG).

Ovarian Hyperthecosis

Not seen commonly. Androgen-secreting theca-interstitial cells are present in the entire ovarian stroma apart from the antral follicles. May continue to secrete higher amount of androgens post-menopausally due to elevated LH levels.[10]

Nonclassical (Late-onset) Congenital Adrenal Hyperplasia

The most common adrenal cause due to the deficiency of 21-hydroxylase enzyme.[11] Polycystic ovarian morphology is also found in many. A 17-hydroxy progesterone (17-OHP) level of <200 ng/dL done in the morning in the follicular phase rules out the enzyme deficiency. To confirm the non-classical variant 17-OHP levels prior to and after stimulation with synthetic adrenocorticotropic hormone (ACTH) are estimated.

INVESTIGATIONS

Hormonal Assays

- Serum total testosterone and free testosterone concentration
- Serum DHEAS
- 17-OH progesterone
- Thyroid function tests
- Serum prolactin level.

Imaging

- Ultrasound of the abdomen and pelvis
- Adrenal CT
- If no underlying cause can be identified, the condition is considered idiopathic.

Decision to investigate can be guided by the duration and severity of hirsutism and the menstrual history as in Table 18.2.

Women who have clinically severe hirsutism, very high levels of serum testosterone (>2x the normal range for the laboratory), or those with a short history of progression of symptoms need to undergo extensive evaluation.

Aims of management:
- To remove excess hair
- To suppress or neutralize the action of androgen
- To remove the source of excess androgen.

Best results are achieved by a combination of treatments including pharmacological and mechanical hair removal treatments. The target should be to reduce the frequency of mechanically removing unwanted hair.

Table 18.2 Investigations decision

Diagnosis	Investigation/test
Mild, chronic hirsutism, regular cycles	No tests? (or testosterone, pelvic ultrasonography)
Moderate hirsutism with or without cycle disturbance	Testosterone, LH, FSH, ultrasonography
Severe hirsutism, short history, testosterone >5 nmol/L	DHEAS, 17-OHP, dexamethasone suppression test, 24-hour urine free cortisol, ovarian and/or adrenal imaging (ultrasound or MRI)

Source: Adapted from Franks S. The investigation and management of hirsutism. J Fam Plann Reprod Health Care. 2012;38:182-6.
Abbreviations: DHEAS, dehydroepiandrosterone sulfate; FSH, follicle-stimulating hormone; LH, luteinizing hormone; 17-OHP,17-hydroxyprogesterone

TREATMENT OPTIONS

- Mechanical hair removal—shaving, waxing, depilatory creams, laser, electrolysis
- Topical suppression of hair growth—eflornithine
- Suppression of androgen secretion and/or action:
  - Combined oral contraceptives (COCs)
  - Antiandrogens—cyproterone acetate, spironolactone, flutamide
  - 5-α reductase inhibitors—finasteride.

Combined Oral Contraceptives

Combined oral contraceptives (COCs) are considered to be the first-line agents. The COCs suppress the gonadotropin secretion and the increased ovarian steroidogenesis. SHBG production in the liver is increased by the estrogen component thus, decreasing the bioavailable androgen. New terminal hair growth is reduced but these changes may take up to 6 months to be clinically visible. Low dose ethinyl estradiol (upto 30 μg) with a progestin having antiandrogenic potential or low androgenic properties can be used.

- Directly or indirectly COCs can decrease adrenal DHEAS production.
- Contraceptive progestins inhibit 5-α reductase activity in skin.
- There is an increased risk of venous thromboembolism (VTE) with the use of COC especially those containing third and fourth generation progestins and also those containing cyproterone acetate. When prescribing, medical eligibility criteria (WHO/UK) to be considered carefully.

Antiandrogens

Cyproterone Acetate

- Derivative of 17OHP, inhibits gonadotropin secretion.
- Competitive androgen receptor antagonist.
- Enhances metabolic clearance by inducing hepatic enzymes.
- A progestin which also has strong antiandrogenic action.
- Combined formulation of cyproterone with ethinyl estradiol—GINETTE 35, KRIMSON, DIANE 35
- *Side effects*: Nausea, fatigue, weight gain, loss of libido, headaches, mastalgia.

Spironolactone (Aldactone)

- Antialdosterone, antiandrogenic compound
- Inhibits ovarian and adrenal androgen biosynthesis
- Competes for androgen receptors in hair follicle
- Inhibits 5-α reductase activity
- Dosage—100–200 mg/day for 6 months
- Side effects—fatigue, menstrual irregularities, urticaria, hyperkalaemia.

Flutamide (Cytomid)

- Nonsteroidal androgen receptor antagonist
- Weak inhibitor of testosterone biosynthesis
- Dosage—50 mg bid or tid
- Side effects—dry skin, hepatotoxicity, decreased libido, breast tenderness
- Should be combined with contraceptive
- Causes severe hepatotoxicity hence not preferred.

5-α Reductase Inhibitors

Finasteride (Finara, Finast)
- Inhibits 5 alpha reductase enzyme
- Blocks conversion of testosterone to DHT
- Used in treatment of benign prostatic hyperplasia
- Dosage—2.5–5 mg daily
- To be used with a highly effective contraceptive.

Eflornithine (13.9% Cream)

- US-FDA approved.
- It inhibits ornithine decarboxylase (ODC), an enzyme responsible for catalyzing the rate-limiting step for follicular polyamine synthesis, which is necessary for hair growth.
- Improvement is gradual, occurring over a period of 4–8 weeks or longer.
- Must be used continuously as hair growth reverts to the pretreatment stage ~8 weeks after stopping.
- Treatment should be discontinued if there is no noticeable improvement after 4 months.
- Adverse reactions—skin irritation.
- Best suited for patients with mild facial hirsutism.

KEY POINTS

- Hirsutism is a common benign condition but with severe psychological morbidity at times.
- Investigations have to be ordered judiciously as most cases need only a few tests.

- Best results are achieved by a combination of treatments including pharmacological and mechanical hair removal treatments.

REFERENCES

1. Ferriman D, Gallwey JD. Clinical assessment of body hair growth in women. J Clin Endocrinol Metab. 1961;21:1440-7.
2. Jones GL, Hall JM, Balen AH, et al. Health-related quality of life measurement in women with polycystic ovary syndrome: a systematic review. Hum Reprod Update. 2008;14:15-25.
3. Franks S. Polycystic ovary syndrome. N Engl J Med. 1995;333:853-61.
4. Kirschner MA, Bardin CW. Androgen production and metabolism in normal and virilized women. Metab Clin Exp. 1972;21:667-88.
5. Gilling-Smith C, Franks S. Hirsutism and virilization. Gynaecology, 3rd edn. In: Shaw RW, Soutter WP, Stanton SL (Eds). London, UK: Churchill Livingstone; 2003.pp.387-99.
6. Pardridge WM. Serum bioavailability of sex steroid hormones. Clin Endocrinol Metab. 1986;15:259-78.
7. Taieb J, Mathian B, Millot F, Patricot MC, Mathieu E, Queyrel N, et al. Testosterone measured by 10 immunoassays and by isotope-dilution gas chromatography-mass spectrometry in sera from 116 men, women, and children. Clinical chemistry. 2003;49(8):1381-95.
8. Adams J, Polson DW, Franks S. Prevalence of polycystic ovaries in women with anovulation and idiopathic hirsutism. Br Med J (Clin Res Ed). 1986;293:355-9.
9. Kiddy DS, Sharp PS, White DM, et al. Differences in clinical and endocrine features between obese and non-obese subjects with polycystic ovary syndrome: an analysis of 263 consecutive cases. Clin Endocrinol (Oxf). 1990;32:213-20.
10. Franks S. The investigation and management of hirsutism. J Fam Plann Reprod Health Care. 2012;38:182-6.
11. Koulouri O, Conway GS. Management of hirsutism. BMJ. 2009;338:b847.

19
Female Infertility

Renu Tanwar, Shristi

INTRODUCTION

Infertility is failure to achieve a pregnancy after 12 months of unprotected sexual intercourse with the same partner. Approximately 80–85% of normal couple will achieve conception within one year.[1] It affects approximately 10–15% of couples in the reproductive age group.[2]

World Health Organization (WHO) estimates that 60–80 million couple worldwide suffer from infertility.[3] Infertility varies from regions of world from 0.8–12%.[4] In India, prevalence is 3.6–16.8%, varying in different regions.[1] There *has been an upward trend in seeking infertility care* due to decline in natural fertility with female age, higher exposure to different environmental toxins and also to life style factors such as smoking and obesity. Infertility is a complex disorder with significant medical, psychosocial, and economic problems.

Initial counseling of infertile couple between 20 and 30 years of age is important as this will enhance their chance of conception and will dispel myths about unproven practices. *An earlier infertility evaluation is required in women who is aged 35 years and older*, having menstrual irregularities, persistent sexual dysfunction, history of pelvic inflammatory disease, previous history of cancer chemotherapy or with male factor issues.

CAUSES OF INFERTILITY

Ovulatory

- *Ovulatory dysfunction:* It may be identified in 15% of cases but accounts for 40% of female factor infertility.[5] Initial diagnosis may include anovulation or oligo-ovulation. The common causes include polycystic ovary syndrome, thyroid disorders, hyperprolactinemia, excessive psychological or physical stress, ovarian insufficiency and obesity. Women having regular cycles with premenstrual molimina do not need any test to confirm ovulation.
- *Age-related infertility:* The cause is multifactorial. There is decrease in number of oocytes and the rate of miscarriage and chromosomal abnormalities increase with maternal age. Fertility decreases at 32 years of age with an increase in the rate of decline after 37 years of age.[6] Irregular cyclic changes exist as the first clinical sign of ovarian aging. There is dysregulation of pulse generator in the hypothalamus due to a progressive lack of neuroendocrine control from other brain parts, resulting in changes in the regular GnRH pulse pattern. The first sign of this change is the early elevation of follicle stimulating hormone.

Tubal Factor

Accounts for 25–35% of cases of infertility.[7]

Noninfectious causes: Tubal endometriosis, salpingitis isthmica nodosa, tubal polyp, debri, tubal spasm.

Infectious causes: Pelvic inflammatory disease (PID) caused by chlamydiae, *Neisseria gonorrhoeae, M. hominis, U. urealyticum.* Most important cause in developing countries is tuberculosis.

Unexplained

It is characterized by normal parameters of ovulation, patent fallopian tube, normal semen analysis. Approximately 15% of patients may not have an identifiable cause[8] of infertility.

Uterine Factor

Anomalies of mullerian fusion, Asherman syndrome and fibroids may result in the inability of implantation or growth of the pregnancy.[9] Accounts for nearly 15% of couple seeking treatment. Women having mullerian fusion abnormalities resulting in a uterine septum or bicornuate uterus are largely associated with recurrent miscarriage rather than the ability to conceive.

Endometrial Factor

Hormonal, immune and biochemical factors may result in a hostile endometrial environment. Endometrial polyps and submucous fibroid may interfere with implantation. Luteal phase defect is a failure to develop a fully mature secretory endometrium during implantation window. The luteal phase defect is not a documented cause of infertility and hence is no longer a routine evaluation for infertility. It accounts for 4% of infertility.[10]

Cervical Factor

The history of cervical infections, surgery or cryotherapy may cause damage to the cervical glands. The lack of mucus result in the inability of the sperm to survive the harsh vaginal acidity and cannot make the assent to the uterus. Other cervical factors could be cervical stenosis or antisperm antibodies.[11]

Peritoneal Factors

Main causes include endometriosis and pelvic or adnexnal adhesions. Mechanism include anatomic distortion from adhesions or fibrosis and presence of inflammatory mediators.

Hormonal Causes

Include thyroid, pituitary, prolactin and hypothalamic disorders.

CLINICAL PRESENTATIONS

Primary infertility: Patients who have never conceived.

Secondary infertility: Patients with previous conception. Their could be various clinical presentations as shown Table 19.1.

DIAGNOSIS

A preconception evaluation should include a detailed history and examination as shown in Table 19.2. Make a record of prior infertility treatment as this will save time and resources.

Table 19.1 Clinical presentations

Cervical factors	Dysmenorrhea, dyspareunia, discharge PV, H/O cryosurgery
Endometrial factor	Premenstrual spotting, heavy menstrual bleeding
Uterine factor	Müllerian anomalies—nonspecific
Peritoneal factor	Pain, incapacitating dysmenorrhea, dyspareunia, previous abdominal surgeries
Ovulatory factor	PCOS: Anovulation, obesity, acanthosis nigricans, irregular menses
Unexplained factor	Nil

Table 19.2 History and examination[12]

History	Physical examination
• Duration of infertility • Menstrual history • Pregnancy history • Previous methods of contraception • Coital frequency and sexual dysfunction • Past surgery (procedures, indications) • Previous hospitalizations (illnesses or injuries) • Pelvic inflammatory disease (sexually transmitted infections) • Thyroid disease, galactorrhea, hirsutism • Abnormal pap smears • Current medications and allergies • Family history • Occupation and exposure to known environmental hazards • Use of tobacco, alcohol or illicit drugs	• Weight, body mass index (BMI), blood pressure, and pulse • Thyroid enlargement and presence of any nodules or tenderness • Breast secretions and their character • Signs of androgen excess • Vaginal or cervical abnormality, secretions, or discharge • Pelvic or abdominal tenderness, organ enlargement, or masses • Uterine size, shape, position, and mobility • Adnexal masses or tenderness • Cul-de-sac masses, tenderness, or nodularity

INVESTIGATIONS

Evaluation of ovarian factors-includes an evaluation of regularity of ovulation and assessment of ovarian reserve.

Ovarian reserve can be recommended to all women with infertility, but is important in women older than 35 years, or have history of unexplained infertility, ovarian surgery, chemotherapy or pelvic radiation, family history of early menopause. Diminished poor response to gonadotropins or are planning treatment with assisted reproductive technology. Oocyte quality is difficult to ascertain through ovarian reserve testing.

Ovarian Reserve Tests

Following tests are done on Day 2 of the menstrual cycle (baseline estimation) for ovarian reserve estimation
- FSH
- LH
- TSH (if anovulatory cycles)
- AMH levels
- Serum estradiol and prolactin levels
- Antral follicle count.

Post-coital test (for cervical factor)—It is very subjective, has poor reproducibility, inconvenient to patient and hence is no longer recommended for routine evaluation.

Serial basal body temperature measurements are no longer used for evaluating ovulatory function.

Urinary LH determination can identify midcycle LH surge that predicts ovulation by 1–2 days but may yield false positive and false negative results (Not recommended).

Serum progesterone determination >3 ng/mL provides presumptive but reliable evidence of ovulation if obtained approx 1 week before the expected onset of next menses.

Routine Tests

Hemogram, urine examination and culture, montoux, ESR, Chest X-ray, premenstrual EB for histopathology, acid fast bacilli (AFB) stain and culture, polymerase chain reaction (PCR) in endometrial sample for AFB nuclear fragments. Husband's semen analysis report is routine before counseling the couple.

It is prudent to do HIV, HBsAg, HCV, VDRL and blood group typing in both partners in the beginning of workup.

Evaluation of uterine, tubal and peritoneal factors is necessary to assess for gamete transport, fertilization and embryo implantation (Fig. 19.3).

USG for any uterine and adnexal pathology.

Table 19.3 Diagnostic potential of investigation[13]

	Uterine cavity	Tubal patency	Peritoneal cavity	Advantages	Disadvantages
HSG	+++	+++	+	Define size and shape, Müllerian anomalies of uterine cavity	No tubo-ovarian proximity evaluation
Saline instillation sonography	++++	+	-	Size, depth of uterine tumors, cavity conformation, less pain, lower cost and is office procedure	Assess tubal patency but not tubal anatomy, no tubo-ovarian proximity evaluation, poor for intrauterine adhesions
Hysteroscopy	++++	-	-	Gold standard for uterine cavity evaluation, corrective surgery possible, adjunctive procedure with laparoscopy	Expensive, invasive unable to evaluate tubal anatomy
Laparoscopy	-	++++	++++	Best to identify and correct uterotubal ovarian and peritoneal factors, tubal patency assessed	Expensive, invasive unable to evaluate intrauterine anatomy

MRI or 3D USG is helpful in identifying both fibroids and the type of mullerian anomaly found on hysteron-salpingogram.

Treatment modalities for infertility include: As this disease is associated with stress and anxiety so couple counseling is mandatory after the baseline evaluation of both partners. Male partner evaluation is mandatory and equally important.

- *Lifestyle considerations:*
  - Weight reduction: In obese anovulatory infertile women, a loss of 5-10% of body weight had been discovered to be enough to restore reproductive functions in 55-100% of women within 6 months.[14]
  - No specific dietary supplement has been proven to enhance fertility but research remains active in this field.
  - Tobacco smoking increases risk of miscarriage and should be avoided.[15]
  - Caffeine consumption (1-2 cups) coffee/day has no negative effect on fertility.
  - Heavy alcohol consumption should be avoided.
- Ovulation induction using clomiphene with or without gonadotropins with intrauterine insemination (IUI) for anovulatory cycles, cervical factor and unexplained infertility.
- Metformin use in polycystic ovary syndrome (PCOS) should be restricted to women with glucose intolerance and the routine use of this drug in ovulation induction is not recommended.[16]
- Medical therapy—with GnRH analogs and Dienogest for endometriomas of the ovary lead to decrease in size but are rarely completely treated and has no effect on the adhesions associated with endometriosis.[17]
- *Surgical intervention*: Uterine fibroids may be treated by myomectomy or by laparoscopy depending on the location of the fibroid. Submucous fibroids and endometrial polyps may be removed by operative hysteroscopy. Laparoscopic cystectomy should be done for endometrioma >4 cm.
- *In vitro fertilization (IVF)*: In vitro fertilization results in the highest chances of pregnancy for the couple whose infertility is the result of pelvic adhesions or blocked fallopian tubes, moderate to severe endometriosis or in cases of unexplained infertility. IVF can also be done with donor oocytes to treat women with age-related ovarian dysfunction, ovarian failure or surgically removed ovaries.
- Oocytes or embryos obtained from a donor is indicated for patients with medical or surgical

menopause or genetic disorders that may impact offspring. Oocyte donors must be physically and mentally healthy and without major genetic diseases in the family and preferably be within 21–34 years of age.
- Preimplantation genetic testing-includes procedures involving the removal of polar bodies from oocytes, blastomeres from cleavage-stage embryos, and trophectoderm cells from day 5–6 embryos to test for mutations in gene sequence or for chromosome number prior to embryo transfer.
- Fertility cryopreservation—Oocyte cryopreservation has become more prevalent in the last decade for fertility preservation in women facing cancer treatment as well as those planning to electively defer childbearing.
- *Oocyte nuclear transfer:* Research continues in assisted reproductive technology (ART) among women who are carriers for mitochondrial disorders, a diverse group of maternally-derived mutations resulting in progressive and life-threatening diseases.

REFERENCES

1. Padubidri VG, Daftary SN. Shaw's Textbook of Gynaecology, 15th edn, Elsevier 2008.
2. JLH Evers, JA Collins. Assessment of efficacy of varicocele repair for male subfertility. 2003;361(9372):1849-52.
3. Infecundity, infertility, and childlessness in developing countries. DHS Comparative Reports No. 9. Calverton, Maryland, USA: ORC Macro and the World Health Organization; 2004.
4. Sciarra J. Infertility: an international health problem. Int J Gynaecol Obstet. 1994;46:155-63. [PubMed]
5. Jirge PR. Poor ovarian reserve. J Hum Reprod Sci. 2016;9:63-9.
6. Amanvermez R, Tosun M. An update on ovarian aging and ovarian reserve tests. Int J Fertil Steril. 2016;9(4):411-5.
7. Berek SJ. Berek and Novak's Textbook of Gynecology. Wolters Kluwer. 15th ed pg 1157.
8. De Groot LJ, Chrousos G, Dungan K, Grossman A, et al. Evaluation of Infertility, Ovulation Induction and Assisted Reproduction. Endotext (Internet pubmed)
9. A Magos. Reprod Biomed Online. 2002;4 (Suppl 3): 46-51.
10. Coutifaris C, Myers ER, Guzick DS, Diamond MP, Carson SA, Legro RS, et al. NICHD National Cooperative Reproductive Medicine Network. Histological dating of timed endometrial biopsy tissue is not related to fertility status. Fertil Steril. 2004;82(5):1264-72.
11. McNight K, McKenzie JL. Evaluation of Infertility, Ovulation Induction and Assisted Reproduction. Endotext [Internet Pubmed].
12. *http://www. fertstert. org/article/S0015-0282(12)00586-9/fulltext*
13. Paul B. Marshburn. Counseling and Diagnostic Evaluation for the Infertile Couple. Reprod Endocrinol. 2015;42 (1):1-14.
14. Arain F, Arif N, Halepota H. Frequency and outcome of treatment in polycystic ovaries related infertility. Pak J Med Sci. 2015;31(3):694-9.
15. Winter E, Wang J, et al. Early pregnancy loss following assisted reproductive technology treatment. Hum Reprod. 2002;17:3220-3.
16. Consensus on infertility treatment related to polycystic ovary syndrome. Hum Reprod. 2008;23 (3):462-77.
17. Witz CA, Burns WN. Endometriosis and infertility: is there a cause and effect relationship. Gynecol Obstet Invest. 2002;53(1):2-11.

20
Ovarian Stimulation Protocols in *In Vitro* Fertilization and Ovarian Hyperstimulation Syndrome

Anjali Tempe, Komal Rastogi, Deepali Dhingra

INTRODUCTION

The incidence of infertility is 7–13% in reproductive age group.[1] About one-tenth of all infertility patients will ultimately require assisted reproductive techniques (ART). For successful *in vitro* fertilization (IVF) cycles the choice of stimulation protocol has to be appropriate. The ideal ovarian stimulation protocol for *in vitro* fertilization should decrease the side effects, risks and costs of drugs and should have a low cancellation rate. Numerous regimens have been described to fulfil the needs of patients who range from low, intermediate and high responders. These regimens range from no stimulation (natural cycles) and minimal stimulation (sequential treatment with clomiphene citrate and exogenous gonadotropins) to aggressive stimulation [gonadotropin-releasing hormone (GnRH) agonist or antagonist in combination with exogenous gonadotropins].

GnRH AGONIST DOWN-REGULATION AND GONADOTROPIN STIMULATION: THE 'LONG' PROTOCOL

Similar to native GnRH, GnRH agonists are decapeptides but modified at two amino acid residues, which increases half-life of the compound as well as its receptor binding affinities.[2] GnRH agonists suppress gonadotropin secretion by the pituitary and prevent premature LH surge during gonadotropin stimulation in IVF cycles. GnRH agonists initially upregulate pituitary GnRH receptors, leading to flare response of increased gonadotropin secretion followed by receptor desensitization suppressing pituitary gonadotropins over a period of 10–14 days.[3]

Leuprolide acetate is the most commonly used GnRH agonist administered by subcutaneous route, triptorelin is administered subcutaneously; buserelin and nafarelin administered intranasally there are other preparations commercially available.

GnRH agonist is started on day 21 (luteal phase) of the previous cycle. This diminishes the flare effect of GnRH agonists and suppresses endogenous follicle-stimulating hormone (FSH) secretion. Treatment with leuprolide acetate begins with 1 mg or 0.5 mg daily for approximately 10 days or until onset of menses, starting from day 21 of previous cycle (Fig. 20.1), decreasing to 0.5 mg or 0.2 mg daily until human chorionic gonadotropin (hCG) is administered, as a trigger.

Gonadotropins are started from day 2 of next cycle after confirming pituitary down regulation by serum estradiol levels (<30–40 pg/mL) and pelvic ultrasound (no follicles >10 mm in

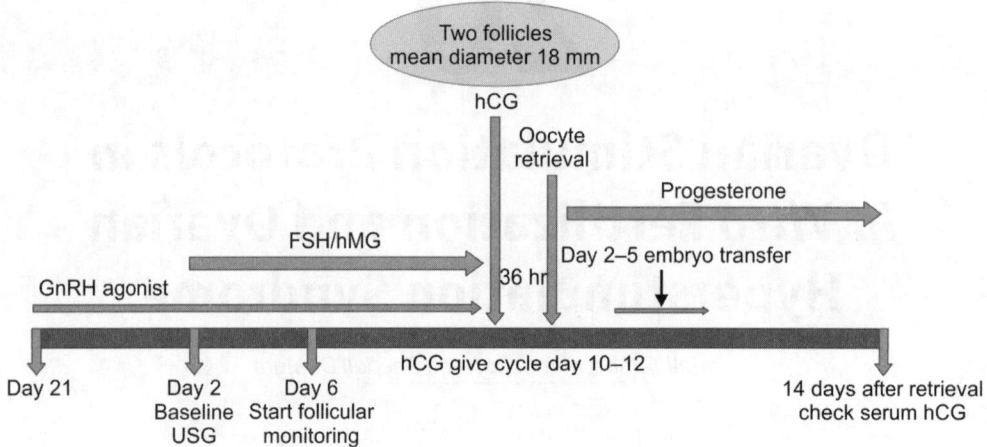

Fig. 20.1 Gonadotropin-releasing hormone agonist protocol
Abbreviations: hCG, human chorionic gonadotropin; GnRH, gonadotropin-releasing hormone; FSH, follicle-stimulating hormone; hMG, human menopausal gonadotropin; USG, ultrasonography

diameter). The starting doses of gonadotropins range between 150 and 300 IU of recombinant FSH, urinary FSH, or urinary menotropins (hMG). Any of the "step-up" or "step-down" protocol can be used. Response is monitored with transvaginal ultrasonography and serial measurements of serum estradiol. The first estradiol levels are obtained after 3–5 days of stimulation. Thereafter, sonography and serum estradiol concentrations are obtained every 1–3 days and gonadotropins dosages are adjusted. Stimulation continues until at least two follicles measure 17–18 mm diameter and others typically measure 14–16 mm. Endometrial thickness is also monitored simultaneously using transvaginal ultrasound. A final stage of follicular maturation is attained by trigger in the form of injection hCG 10,000 IU intramuscular (IM). The equivalent dose of recombinant hCG is 250 µg.

Greater cycle flexibility, better oocyte yield and quality and increased pregnancy rates are few advantages of using long agonist protocol. However, longer treatment duration, ovarian cyst formation, menopausal symptoms and greater requirement of gonadotropin ampoules and hence, increased cost of treatment preclude its universal use.

GnRH AGONIST 'FLARE' AND GONADOTROPIN STIMULATION PROTOCOL

The "short" or "flare" protocol uses both the initial flare response to a GnRH agonist and pituitary suppression following its long-term use. 1 mg of leuprolide acetate is administered daily for three days from day 2 to 4 of the menstrual cycle following which the dose is reduced to half. Gonadotropin stimulation (225–450 IU daily) begins on day 3 of the cycle (Fig. 20.1). The dose of gonadotropins is adjusted depending upon ovarian response and indications for hCG administration are same as that of long protocol. Due to late corpus luteum rescue, this regimen may cause significant increase in serum progesterone and androgen levels and thus affecting oocyte quality and pregnancy rates.

The "OC Microdose GnRH agonist flare" (Fig. 20.2) protocol involves suppression with an oral contraceptive pill for 14–21 days; followed by microdose of leuprolide acetate (40 µg BD) starting 3 days after the last pill or from day 2 after confirming pituitary downregulation. High-dose gonadotropins are started from

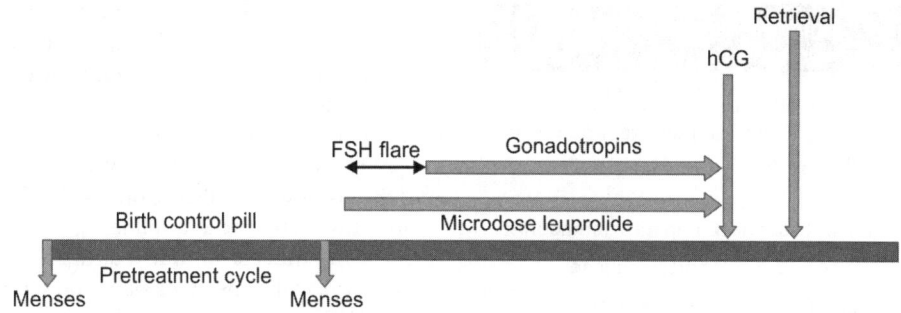

Fig. 20.2 Microdose GnRH agonist flare protocol
Abbreviations: hCG, human chorionic gonadotropin; FSH, follicle-stimulating hormone

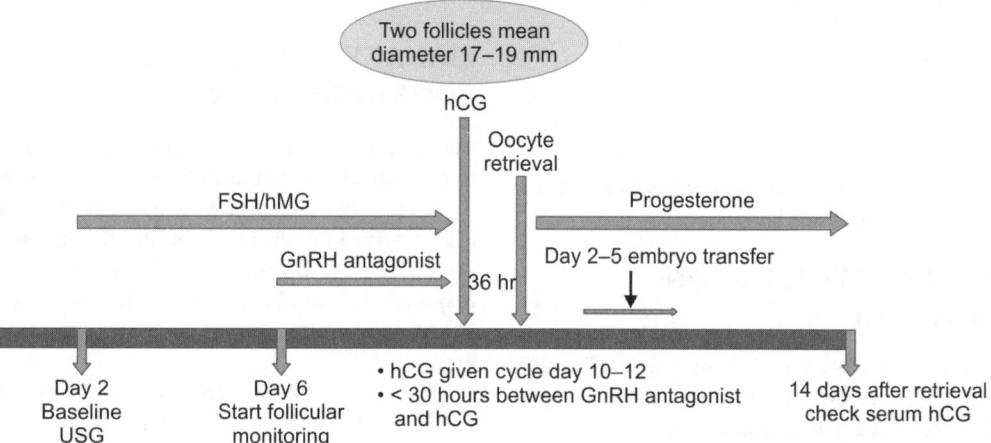

Fig. 20.3 Gonadotropin-releasing hormone (GnRH) antagonist protocol
Abbreviations: hCG, human chorionic gonadotropin; GnRH, gonadotropin-releasing hormone; FSH, follicle-stimulating hormone; hMG, human menopausal gonadotropin; USG, ultrasonography

day 3 of leuprolide therapy. This protocol does not cause rise in serum progesterone and androgen and may be useful in poor responders by causing increased endogenous FSH release.

GnRH ANTAGONIST AND GONADOTROPIN STIMULATION PROTOCOL

GnRH antagonists are decapeptides developed by modifying native GnRH at six positions. GnRH antagonists competitively inhibit GnRH receptors at pituitary and lead to immediate suppression of FSH and LH. Cetrorelix and ganirelix are the two preparations commercially available and administered in a dose of 0.25 mg daily subcutaneously. They can also be given as 3 mg single dose which will prevent an LH surge for 96 hours.

The treatment protocol (Fig. 20.3) may be fixed which involves starting antagonist after 5–6 days of gonadotropin stimulation regardless of follicular response[4] or flexible, i.e. starting antagonist when the lead follicle reaches 13–14 mm in diameter.[5] Fixed protocol was found to be associated with higher pregnancy rates when compared to flexible protocol in one meta-analysis involving four randomized trials, however, true superiority of one approach over the other remains to be determined.[6] GnRH antagonist protocol lowers duration of stimulation, reduces rates of ovarian hyperstimulation syndrome and decreases gonadotropin requirement thus reducing cost of treatment (Table 20.1).

Table 20.1 Comparison between GnRH agonist and antagonist protocol

GnRH agonist	GnRH antagonist
Lengthy downregulation phase with initial flare effect	Immediate suppression
Receptor desensitization	Competitive antagonist
Time consuming	Shorter regimen
Increased dose of gonadotropin required, more expensive	Lesser dose of gonadotropin required, less expensive
Inconvenient due to more number of injections	Lesser injections
Increased risk of OHSS	Less risk of OHSS
GnRH agonist cannot be used as trigger	GnRH agonist can be used as trigger in patients at high risk for OHSS

Abbreviations: OHSS, ovarian hyperstimulation; GnRH, gonadotropin-releasing hormone

MINIMAL STIMULATION PROTOCOL

Minimal stimulation (MS) protocol usually refers to stimulation protocols that yield fewer oocytes. This protocol involves use of clomiphene citrate or letrozole early in the cycle followed by low doses of gonadotropins. The MS protocol was less expensive (in terms of total gonadotropins used) and improved both clinical pregnancy rate and live birth rates, compared to the high dose protocol.[11]

MANAGEMENT OPTIONS FOR HIGH RESPONDERS

Patients with retrieval of more than 15 oocytes or estradiol levels >3000 pg/mL are considered as high responders and are at risk for OHSS. The management options are:
- Use of low dose gonadotropins (100–150 IU/day)
- Dual suppression with oral contraceptive pills – One pill daily for 21 days and a GnRH agonist (1 mg leuprolide SC daily starting 1 week before discontinuation of oral contraceptive pills).
- *Coasting:* GnRH agonist treatment continues without further gonadotropin stimulation for 1–3 days and hCG is given after estradiol levels moderate.
- Reducing the dose of hCG
- Cryopreservation of all embryos
- Triggering with GnRH agonist—Single bolus injection of 0.5 mg leuprolide
- Delaying transfer until five days after oocyte retrieval, while observing signs and symptoms of OHSS
- Minimal stimulation protocols
- *In vitro* maturation of oocytes.

MANAGEMENT OPTIONS FOR POOR RESPONDERS

According to 'The Bologna criteria' poor response to ovarian stimulation is defined as the presence of at least two of the following three features: (1) advanced maternal age or any risk factor for poor ovarian response; (2) previous poor ovarian response; (3) an abnormal ovarian reserve test. The management options for poor responders are:
- *Microdose GnRH agonist flare protocol:* Demirol and Gurgan[7] in their study demonstrated the efficacy of microdose flare-up protocol by improving oocyte yield in poor responders. Surrey et al also reported similar findings.
- *Luteal phase GnRH antagonist:* Late luteal phase administration of GnRH antagonist induces luteolysis and secures a synchronous cohort of recruitable follicles which improves stimulation results in poor responders.
- *GnRH Antagonist/Letrozole Protocols:* Adjunctive clomiphene or letrozole in IVF stimulation protocols in poor responders improves oocyte yield, decreases the rate of cycle cancelation and reduces the cost of treatment. These benefits have been demonstrated in various studies.[9]
- *Luteal phase estradiol supplementation:* This protocol involves administration of 4 mg per day of estradiol valerate from day 21 of previous cycle and stopping on

menstrual cycle day 3. Various studies have demonstrated an improvement in the number of oocytes retrieved, increased number of good quality embryos and decreased cycle cancelation rate.[10]

- *Dehydroepiandrosterone supplementation:* DHEA in a dose of 25 mg TDS three months prior to IVF cycle may have beneficial effects on ovarian reserve in poor responders undergoing ART.
- *Mild stimulation protocols:* According to various studies mild stimulation protocols (clomiphene citrate/gonadotropin/ antagonist) were found to be patient friendly and more cost effective and than conventional IVF as it involves less dose of gonadotropin and duration of stimulation without any difference in pregnancy rates.[11]
- *Androgens:* Transdermal testosterone pretreatment may improve ovarian sensitivity to FSH and may be of benefit for poor responders undergoing IVF cycle.

To conclude long agonist protocols are used in 40–50% and antagonist protocols are used in 40–60% of all women undergoing IVF. The antagonists protocols are beneficial for patients with poor ovarian reserve and for prevention of ovarian hyperstimulation syndrome (OHSS) in high responders.

OVARIAN HYPERSTIMULATION SYNDROME

Introduction

Ovarian hyperstimulation syndrome (OHSS) is a rare, iatrogenic complication of assisted reproductive techniques and it occurs mostly in association with exogenous gonadotropins and rarely seen with clomiphene citrate and natural cycle.[12] After stimulation with gonadotropins, OHSS mostly develops few days after oocyte retrieval. The whole pathophysiology revolves around increased vascular permeability leading to abdominal distension, enlarged ovaries, and ascites. Mild OHSS, which is common, occurs in about 20–33% in ART cycles.[13,14] Severe OHSS which is associated with extreme morbidity has been reported in 1–2% of ART cycles.[13,15] As OHSS is preventable condition, clinicians involved in prescribing ovarian stimulation drugs should be well-versed with risk factors and strategies to minimize fatalities.

Pathophysiology of Ovarian Hyperstimulation Syndrome

The main pathophysiologic mechanism of OHSS is thought to be release of vasoactive peptides from granulosa cells of hyperstimulated ovaries which results in enhanced vascular permeability and fluid shift from intravascular to extravascular compartments.[16] Vasoactive substances, notably vascular endothelial growth factor (VEGF) has been implicated as trigger for increased vascular permeability.[17] Human chorionic gonadotropin (hCG) has been implicated to increase in expression of VEGF in granulosa cells.

Risk Factors

These include age < 35 years, low body mass index, presence of polycystic ovaries, pregnancy, high serum E2 (more than 4000 pg/mL) in assisted reproductive technology (ART) cycle or more than 1700 pg/mL in ovulation induction, hCG use in luteal phase and gonadotropin-releasing hormone (GnRH) agonist long protocol.[18] High anti-Müllerian hormone (AMH) is also correlated with the higher incidence of OHSS.

Clinical Presentation and Classification

Ovarian hyperstimulation syndrome (OHSS) presents with continuum of symptoms and signs backed by typical history, ultrasonography and laboratory parameters (Table 20.2). Typically patient presents with abdominal bloating and distension within 24 hours of hCG trigger and becomes more severe 7–9 days later if conception occurs.

Investigations and Monitoring in a Case of Ovarian Hyperstimulation Syndrome

- Complete blood count
- Kidney function test
- Liver function test
- Serum electrolytes
- Coagulation profile [activated partial thromboplastin time (APTT) and international normalized ratio]
- Chest X-ray, if breathlessness is present
- Body weight and abdominal circumference
- Ultrasound measurement of fluid
- Input-output charting
- Pregnancy test.

Table 20.2 History of OHSS
• Timing of symptoms relative to trigger
• Which trigger (hCG or GnRH agonist)
• Estradiol (E2) levels on the day of trigger
• Number of oocytes retrieved
• Number of embryos transferred
• Prior polycystic appearance of ovaries
Signs and Symptoms
• Abdominal bloating and ascites
• Nausea and vomiting
• Breathlessness
• Reduced urine output
• Rapid weight gain
• Edema (pedal, vulval and sacral)
• Pleural effusion, pneumonia, pulmonary edema

The above mentioned investigations should be done at least once and would be followed-up on a daily basis or less frequently according to the severity of the disease till the disease process settles down (Table 20.3).

Outpatient Management of OHSS

Mild and moderate OHSS can be managed on outpatient basis.[18] Abdominal discomfort can be treated with acetaminophen with or without a narcotic agent. Nonsteroidal anti-inflammatory drugs (NSAIDs) should be avoided, as they may affect renal function. Paracentesis of ascitic fluid may be carried out on outpatient basis under ultrasound guidance.[19] Women should be advised to drink plenty of fluids and refrain from exercise and sexual activity. A woman is assessed every 2–3 days and investigation repeated if required and provided emergency contact number to report if symptoms worsen.

Inpatient Management of OHSS

Women who are unable to maintain hydration, worsening ascites, shortness of breath, rising hematocrit, development of oliguria or develops critical OHSS should be admitted in hospital for IV hydration and observation or in intensive care units in an event of critical OHSS. Body weight, abdominal girth, and fluid intake and output should be monitored daily, along with full blood count, hematocrit, serum electrolytes, and osmolality and liver function tests.

Table 20.3 Classification of OHSS on basis of severity[6]			
Mild	*Moderate*	*Severe*	*Critical*
Bloating, abdominal discomfort, nausea, size of ovaries <5 cm	Vomiting, abdominal pain, WBC <10,000/mm³ size of ovaries >5 cm	Massive ascites, hydrothorax, oliguria, creatinine 1–1.5 mg%, creatinine clearance, >50 mL/min, hepatic dysfunction, anasarca, HCT >45%, WBC >15,000/mm³ enlarged ovaries with size 5–12 cm	Tense ascites, hypoxemia, pericardial effusion, creatinine>1.5 mg%, creatinine clearance <50 mL/min, renal failure, thromboembolic phenomenon, ARDS, HCT >55%, WBC >25,000/mm³ enlarged ovaries with size >12 cm

Abbreviations: HCT, hematocrit; ARDS, acute respiratory distress syndrome

Fluid Management

Women are encouraged to drink according to thirst. Intravenous hydration can be maintained with crystalloid solution (100–150 mL/hr).[20] Diuretics should be avoided as it has been associated with further depletion of depleted intravascular volume. If the dehydration persists colloids, i.e. human albumin solution 25% may be used in doses of 50–100 g, infused slowly over 4 hours and can be repeated if further dehydration persists.[21] Strict fluid intake and output charting is mandatory.

Symptomatic Relief

Pain relief can be provided with acetaminophen or opioids if required. NSAIDs are to be avoided as they compromise renal function.[22]

Paracentesis

Severe abdominal distension and pain, breathlessness and if oliguria persists despite fluid replacement some cases may respond to paracentesis.[23] Paracentesis is carried out under ultrasound guidance which can be performed abdominally or vaginally.[19]

Thromboembolic Complications

Thrombus formation is the most life-threatening complication of severe OHSS. The incidence of thrombosis lies between 0.7% and 10% of cases of OHSS.[19] Those admitted with OHSS should be started with LMWH prophylaxis and its duration should be individualized as per presence of risk factors.

Surgical Management

Adnexal torsion, ectopic pregnancy and rupture of ovarian cyst are indications of surgical management.

Ovarian Hyperstimulation Syndrome Preventive Strategies

As a clinician involved in application of stimulation protocols one must balance between desire to achieve successful pregnancy and minimizing risk of OHSS. One of the most initial steps to decrease the risk of OHSS is to identify women prone to have OHSS. Secondly choosing appropriate stimulation protocols for these women and lastly taking appropriate strategies during stimulation protocol if there is a suspicion of OHSS.

- Metformin decreases the risk of OHSS in patients with polycystic ovaries.[24,25] Metformin is started 8 weeks prior to planned stimulation cycle to be effective in prevention of OHSS.[26]
- Incidence of OHSS is not affected by use of urinary vs recombinant gonadotropins.
- Use of gonadotropin-releasing hormone (GnRH) agonists trigger instead of hCG. GnRH agonist trigger has been shown to reduce not only OHSS but also reduced live birth rates.[27] Live birth rates was not affected if embryos are frozen and used in next frozen embryo cycle.[28]
- Instead of human chorionic gonadotropin, use of progesterone as luteal phase support.[29]
- Cabergoline has been shown to decrease the incidence of moderate OHSS in high risk women and has no adverse effect on the pregnancy rate.[30] Cabergoline can be started as 0.5 mg from the day of hCG trigger and continued for up to 8 days.[31]
- *Coasting:* It involves withholding the dose of gonadotropins and maintaining suppression of pituitary with an antagonist or gonadotropin releasing hormone agonist. Coasting may decrease the risk of OHSS but coasting more than 3 days and serum estradiol not falling calls for cycle cancelation.[32]
- Use of GnRH antagonists protocols instead of agonist protocol in women at high risk of OHSS. In a Cochrane review when compared with long GnRH agonist protocols, there is reduction of OHSS without impact on live birth rates.[33]
- A gonadotropin-releasing hormone (GnRH) antagonist cycle with a GnRH agonist trigger as a final oocyte maturation is recommended for donor cycles.
- Use of plasma expander such as hydroxyethyl starch (HES) prophylactically in women with high risk factors.[34]

COUNSELING

Women and their partners are counseled that management of OHSS is mostly supportive and spontaneous resolution occurs in most patients and in an event of conception the clinical course may be prolonged.

REFERENCES

1. Templeton A, Fraser C, Thompson B. Infertility-epidemiology and referral practice. Hum Reprod. 1991;6:1391-4.
2. Ortmann O, Weiss JM, Diedrich K. Gonadotrophin-releasing hormone (GnRH) and GnRH agonists: mechanisms of action. Reprod Biomed Online 2002;5:1-7.
3. Tarlatzis BC, Fauser BC, Kolibianakis EM, et al. GnRH antagonists in ovarian stimulation for IVF. Hum Reprod Update. 2006;12:333-40.
4. Albano C, Smitz J, Camus M, Riethmuller-Winzen H, Van Steirteghem A, Devroey P, Comparison of different doses of gonadotropin-releasing hormone antagonist Cetrorelix during controlled ovarian hyperstimulation, Fertil Steril. 1997;67:917.
5. Ludwig M, Katalinic A, Banz C, Schroder AK, Loning M, Weiss JM, Diedrich K, Tailoring the GnRH antagonist cetrorelix acetate to individual patients' needs in ovarian stimulation for IVF: results of a prospective, randomized study, Hum Reprod. 2002;17:2842.
6. Lainas T, Zorzovilis J, Petsas G, et al. In a flexible antagonist protocol, earlier, criteria-based initiation of GnRH antagonist is associated with increased pregnancy rates in IVF. Hum Reprod. 2005;20:2426-33.
7. Demirol A, Gurgan T. Comparison of microdose flare-up and antagonist multiple-dose protocols for poor-responder patients: a randomized study. Fertil Steril. 2009;92(2):481-5.
8. Surrey ES, Bower J, Hill DM, Ramsey J, Surrey MW. Clinical and endocrine effects of a microdose GnRH agonist flare regimen administered to poor responders who are undergoing in vitro fertilization. Fertil Steril. 1988;69:419-24.
9. Jovanovic VP, Kort DH, Guarnaccia MM, Sauer MV, Lobo RA. Does the addition of clomiphene citrate or letrozole to gonadotropin treatment enhance the oocyte yield in poor responders undergoing IVF? J Assist Reprod Genet. 2011;28(11):1067-72.
10. Chang EM, Han JE, Won HJ, Kim YS, Yoon TK, Lee WS. Effect of estrogen priming through luteal phase and stimulation phase in poor responders in in vitro fertilization. J Assist Reprod Genet. 2012;29(3):225-30.
11. Karimzadeh MA, Mahayekhy M, Mohammadin F, Moghaddam FM. Comparison of mild and microdose GnRH agonist flare protocols on IVF outcome in poor responders. Arch Gynecol Obstet. 2011;283(5):1159-64.
12. Mathur R, Kailasam C, Jenkins J. Review of the evidence base strategies to prevent ovarian hyperstimulation syndrome. Hum Fertil. 2007;10: 75-85.
13. Golan A, Ron-El R, Herman A, Soffer Y, Weinraub Z, Caspi E. Ovarian hyperstimulation syndrome: an update review. Obstet Gynecol Surv. 1989;44:430-40.
14. Morris RS, Miller C, Jacobs L, Miller K. Conservative management of ovarian hyperstimulation syndrome. J Reprod Med. 1995;40:711-4.
15. Serour GI, Aboulghar M, Mansour R, Sattar MA, Amin Y, Aboulghar H. Complications of medically assisted conception in 3,500 cycles. Fertil Steril. 1998;70:638-42.
16. Goldsman MP, Pedram A, Dominguez CE, Ciuffardi I, Levin E, Asch RH. Increased capillary permeability induced by human follicular fluid: a hypothesis for an ovarian origin of the hyperstimulation syndrome. Fertil Steril. 1995;63:268-72.
17. Levin ER, Rosen GF, Cassidenti DL, et al. Role of vascular endothelial cell growth factor in Ovarian Hyperstimulation Syndrome. J Clin Invest. 1998; 102(11):1978-85.
18. Navot D, Bergh PA, Laufer N. Ovarian hyperstimulation syndrome in novel reproductive technologies: prevention and treatment. Fertil Steril. 1992;58:249-61.
19. Royal College of Obstetricians and Gynaecologists. The Management of Ovarian Hyperstimulation Syndrome. Green top guideline No 5. RCOG 2016.
20. Fluker M, Copeland J, Yuzpe A. An ounce of prevention: outpatient management of ovarian hyperstimulation syndrome. Fertil Steril. 2000;73:821-4.
21. Practice Committee of the American Society for Reproductive Medicine. Ovarian hyperstimulation syndrome. Fertil Steril. 2008;90 (Suppl 5):S188-93.
22. Balasch J, Carmona F, Llach J, Arroyo V, Jové I, Vanrell JA. Acute prerenal failure and liver dysfunction in a patient with severe ovarian hyperstimulation syndrome. Hum Reprod. 1990;5:348-51.
23. Maslovitz S, Jaffa A, Eytan O, Wolman I, Many A, Lessing JB, et al. Renal blood flow alteration

after paracentesis in women with ovarian hyperstimulation. Obstet Gynecol. 2004;104:321-6.
24. Costello MF, Chapman M, Conway U. A review and meta-analysis of randomized controlled trials on metformin co-administration during gonadotrophin ovulation induction or IVF in women with polycystic ovary syndrome. Hum Reprod. 2006;21:1387-99.
25. Palomba S, Falbo A, Carrillo L, et al. Metformin reduces risk of ovarian hyperstimulation syndrome in patients with polycystic ovary syndrome during gonadotropin-stimulated in vitro fertilization cycles: a randomized, controlled trial. Fertil Steril. 2011;96(6):1384-90.
26. Corbett S, Shmorgun D, Claman P, et al; The prevention of ovarian hyperstimulation syndrome. J Obstet Gynaecol Can. 2014;36(11):1024-36.
27. Youssef MA, Van der Veen F, Al-Inany HG, et al; Gonadotropin-releasing hormone agonist versus HCG for oocyte triggering in antagonist-assisted reproductive technology. Cochrane Database of Systematic Reviews. 2014 Oct 31;10:CD008046. DOI: 10.1002/14651858.CD008046.pub4.
28. Garcia-Velasco JA. Agonist trigger: what is the best approach? Agonist trigger with vitrification of oocytes or embryos. Fertil Steril. 2012;97:527-8.
29. Van der Linden M, Buckingham K, Farquhar C, et al; Luteal phase support for assisted reproduction cycles. Cochrane Database of Systemic Reviews. 2011 Oct 5;(10):CD009154. DOI: 10.1002/14651858.CD009154.pub2.
30. Tang H, Hunter T, Hu Y, et al; Cabergoline for preventing ovarian hyperstimulation syndrome. Cochrane Database of Systemic Reviews. 2012 Feb 15;2:CD008605. DOI: 10.1002/14651858.CD008605.pub2.
31. Alvarez C, Marti-Bonmati L, Novella-Maestre E, Sanz R, Gomez R, Fernandez-Sanchez M, et al. Dopamine agonist cabergoline reduces hemoconcentration and ascites in hyperstimulated women undergoing assisted reproduction. J Clin Endocrinol Metab. 2007;92:2931-7.
32. Mansour R, Alboulghar M, Serour G, Amin Y, Abou-Setta AM. Criteria of a successful coasting protocol for the prevention of severe ovarian hyperstimulation syndrome. Hum Reprod. 2005;20:3167-72.
33. Al-Inany HG, Youssef MA, Aboulghar M, Broekmans F, Sterrenburg M, Smit JAM, et al. Gonadotrophin-releasing hormone antagonists for assisted reproductive technology. Cochrane Database of Systematic Reviews. 2011;11(5):CD001750.
34. Youssef MA, Al-Inany HG, Evers JL, et al. Intravenous fluids for the prevention of severe ovarian hyperstimulation syndrome. Cochrane Database of Systematic Reviews. 2011;16(2):CD001302. DOI: 10.1002/14651858.CD001302.pub2.

21

Pelvic Organ Prolapse

Anoosha K Ravi, Devender Kumar

Prolapse is derived from Latin word *prolapses*, which means falling or slipping out of place of a part or viscus. Pelvic organ prolapse is prolapse of structures around the vaginal vault.[1] Epidemiologic studies indicate vaginal birth and aging as major risk factors.[2] Other factors include connective tissue disorders, chronic respiratory conditions, neuropathies and congenital anomalies like spina bifida.[3] It is often accompanied by urinary, bowel, sexual, or local/pelvic symptoms. The exact incidence is very difficult to determine as many women do not seek medical advice.

PELVIC FLOOR ANATOMY

A dynamic coordinated system including active and passive support structures maintain the integrity of pelvic floor (Table 21.1).

Active Supports: Muscles

The pelvic diaphragm is composed made up of three pairs of striated muscles (Fig. 21.1).
1. Pubococcygeus (includes puborectalis)
2. Iliococcygeus
3. Coccygeus.

It assumes the shape of a basin with urogenital hiatus situated anteriorly.

Posterior to the rectum, the paired muscles join to form *levator plate*. This acts like a trampoline, receiving and resisting sudden increases in intra-abdominal pressure. Medial fibers of pubococcygeus surrounding the rectum form puborectalis (Fig. 21.2). Normal contraction of this results in:
- Posterior curve to vagina
- Horizontal levator plate
- Acute anorectal angle.

Table 21.1 Supports of pelvic organs

Active supports	Passive supports
Muscles	**Bony pelvis**
• Levator ani	**Connective tissue**
– Pubococcygeus	Parietal fascia
– Iliococcygeus	Visceral fascia
– Coccygeus	Deep endopelvic fascia

Passive Supports: Bony Pelvis

The normal lordotic curvature of lumbar spine is a protective feature of bipedal posture. It places the posterior part of pelvic inlet about 60° above the anterior part thus, shielding the pelvic outlet from abdominal downward pressures.

Passive Supports: Connective Tissue

It includes:
- Parietal pelvic fasciae
- Visceral pelvic fasciae
- Deep endopelvic connective tissue.

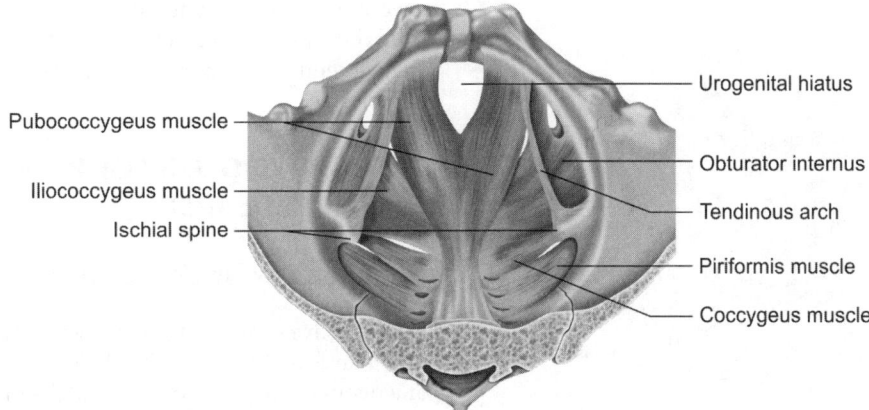

Fig. 21.1 Pelvic floor muscles

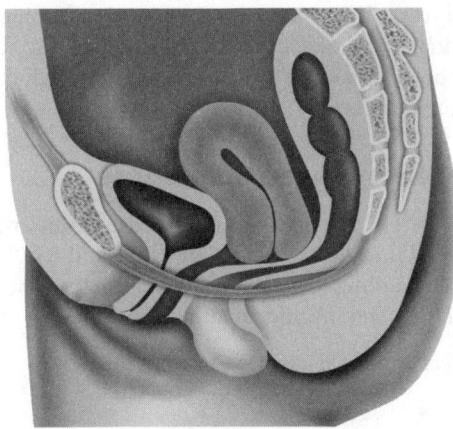

Fig. 21.2 Puborectalis muscle

Parietal Pelvic Fascia

These are dense membranes investing pelvic surface of skeletal muscles of pelvic side wall (obturator, levator ani, coccygeus and piriformis). The condensations of this fasciae form
- ATLA—arcus tendineus levator ani—inserts anteriorly to pubic rami and posteriorly to ischial spines.
- ATFP—arcus tendineus fascia pelvis—medial to ATLA, inserts anteriorly to pubic rami and posteriorly joins ATLA.

These are dense aggregations of collagen analogous to tendons and ligaments (Fig. 21.3).

Visceral Pelvic Fascia

These are loose encasements of pelvic organs including vagina, uterus, bladder and rectum. The portion of the fascia that attaches to uterus is *parametrium* and the portion of the fascia that attaches to vagina is *paracolpium*.

Deep Endopelvic Fascia

It includes:
- *Six ligaments (Fig. 21.4):*
  - Uterosacral ligaments (rectal pillar)
  - Cardinal ligaments (Mackenrodt's or lateral cervical ligament)
  - Pubocervical ligaments (bladder pillar)
- *Two septae:*
  - Pubocervical septum
  - Rectovaginal septum (Denonvillier's fascia)
- *Pericervical ring.*

Uterosacrals are strong ligaments which hold the cervix in the posterior pelvis at or just above the level of ischial spine. This maintains a flexed position of uterus with that of vagina and thus prevents prolapse.

Perineal body is very important structure and it provides strength to pelvic diaphragm as it is connected to endopelvic fasciae surrounding the outlets of pelvic viscera. Perineal body is a pyramidal structure with its base on the perineum and joins the rectovaginal septum proximally. Perineal body has insertion of bulbo-

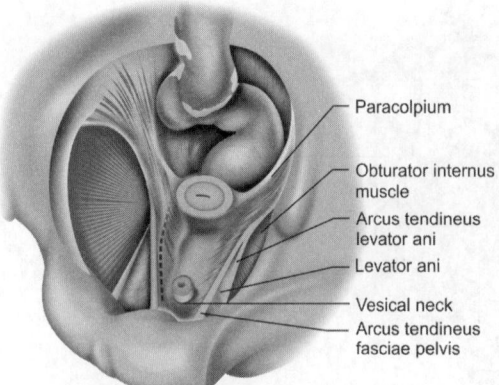

Fig. 21.3 Parietal fascia and its condensations

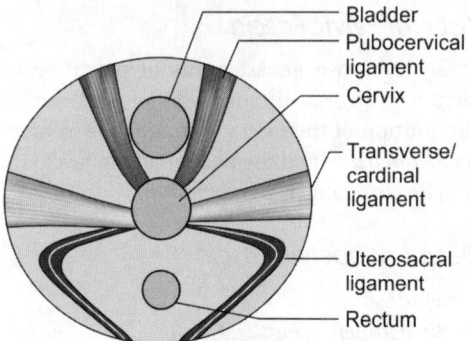

Fig. 21.4 Six ligaments of deep endopelvic fascia

cavernous muscles anteriorly, the superficial transverse perineal muscles laterally and rectovaginal septum with portion of levator ani muscle superiorly.

PATHOPHYSIOLOGY OF PELVIC ORGAN PROLAPSE

Boat in a Dry Dock Concept

Loss of active support of pelvic organs is like that of a boat in a dry dock (Fig. 21.5).[3] The water is analogous to the pelvic muscle and the moorings to the pelvic ligaments and fascia. When there is loss of pelvic floor tone, undue stress is placed of the ligaments and fascia thus, causing breaks and tears. This along with the already atrophied vaginal vault like in menopause, give way for the pelvic organs to slip downwards through the vaginal vault.

DeLancey Levels of Support

The levels of pelvic support are arbitrarily divided into three levels (Figs 21.6A and B). The understanding of this helps to localize the defect and thus, site specific repair can be done.

Level I: Proximal vaginal support

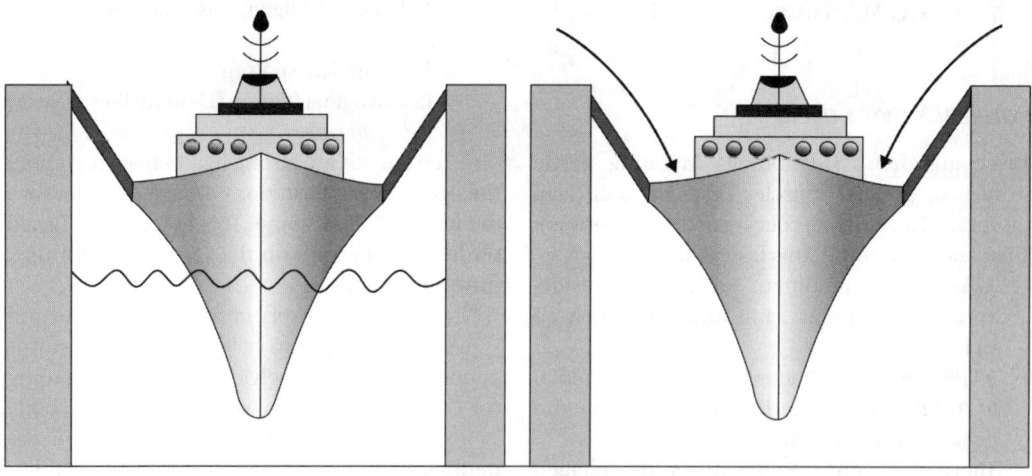

Fig. 21.5 Boat in a dry dock analogy

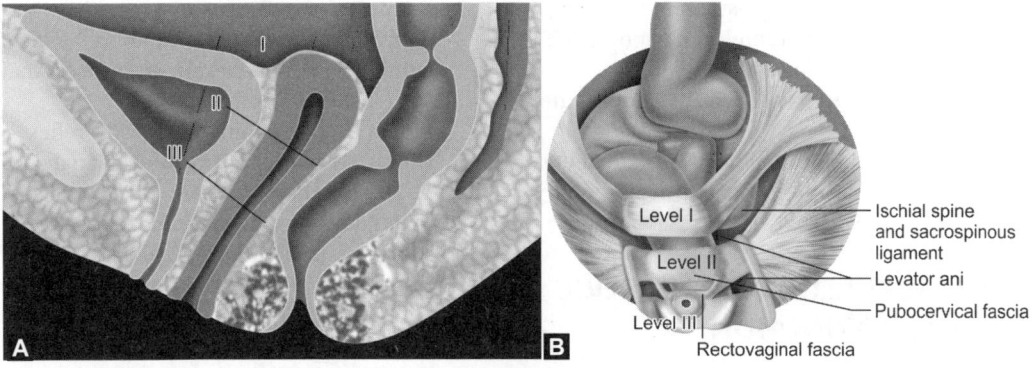

Figs 21.6A and B (A) DeLancey three levels; (B) DeLancey's biomechanical levels of support

- Proximal suspension by uterosacral-cardinal ligaments
- Damage results in uterovaginal prolapse, posthysterectomy vaginal prolapse and enterocele.

Level II: Midvaginal support
- Lateral attachment to ATFP and ATFRV
- Damage results in paravaginal and pararectal defects.

Level III: Distal vaginal support
- Distal fusion to urogenital diaphragm anteriorly and proximal perineum posteriorly
- Anterior damage results in urinary incontinence and posterior damage results in perineal body deficits.

Cystocele and rectocele are due to central defects within pubocervical and rectovaginal septa respectively.

At *tissue level*, it has been suggested that abnormal synthesis or degradation of collagen contributes to prolapse.[4] The findings in women with prolapse are:
- Increase in total collagen content in vaginal wall
- Immature collagen is more than mature collagen.

Causes of Pelvic Organ Prolapse

There are congenital and acquired causes of pelvic organ prolapse (POP). Common cause is acquired and related to menopause and obstetrics (multiparity, deliveries not attended by trained birth attendants or fundal pressure, etc.). The damage caused by multiple child births is aggravated due to menopause and/or malnutrition.

- *Predisposing factors:*
  - Connective tissue disorders, e.g Ehler—Danlos syndrome
  - Spina bifida
  - Bladder exstrophy
- *Inciting factors:*
  - Menopause
  - Multiparity (RR of 10.85)[5]
  - Malnutrition
  - Trauma/infection like polio, TB spine
  - Others
- *Promoting factors:*
  - Increased Intra-abdominal pressure (cough, constipation, etc.)
  - Obesity
  - Smoking
  - Pelvic surgeries

- *Medications*: Antiestrogenic drugs, angiotensin-converting enzyme (ACE) inhibitors causing cough
- Traction (due to cervical or endometrial polyp)
- Chronic medical illness like diabetes mellitus, chronic obstructive pulmonary disease (COPD).

CLINICAL EVALUATION OF PELVIC ORGAN DYSFUNCTION

Symptoms

Common symptoms associated with pelvic organ prolapse are following:
- Sensation of something falling out
- Pelvic discomfort like dragging sensation
- Urinary symptoms
  - Urinary incontinence
  - Frequency
  - Urgency
  - Urinary retention
- Difficulty in emptying rectum
- Sexual dysfunction
- Decubitus ulcer
- Leukorrhea—due to congestion/inflammation.

General Physical Examination

It should include an evaluation of mental status, nutritional status, body mass index, anemia and lymphadenopathy.[6]

Review of systems—with pertinent to prolapse or incontinence; in
- Neurological system[7,8]—look for
  - Gait (pyramidal gait in upper motor neuron lesion, waddling gait in proximal muscle weakness, stamping gait in sensory dysfunction, foot drop in peripheral neuropathy).
  - Spine (kyphotic, lordotic or scoliotic abnormality, lipoma or tuft of hair in spina bifida, gibbus in skeletal tuberculosis).
  - Joints—range of motion.
  - *Muscle* tone and power; hip flexion is controlled by motor segments of S2 and S3, plantar flexion is controlled by S1 and S2.
  - Deep tendon reflexes.
  - *Superficial reflexes:* Babinski reflex; fanning and dorsiflexion if corticospinal tracts are interrupted.
    Bulbocavernosus and anal wink reflex is elicited by gently stroking the perianal skin. Absence of these reflexes reflect damage of pudendal nerve, however in 10% of normal subjects it is too weak to visualize.
  - *Sensations:* Touch, cold and prick, S2-S4 dermatomes of the perineum is evaluated.
- Abdomen: Look for distension, free fluid, mass, scars, hernia.

LOCAL GENITAL EXAMINATION

Position: After emptying the bladder patient is asked to lie in dorsal lithotomy position. However, the semi-upright position would be a suitable to examine a case of prolapse. A mirror can be provided to the patient to confirm the maximum prolapse that is being observed on forceful straining. If not satisfactory, patient is to be examined in the standing position.

On *inspection*, comment on external genitalia including pubic hair, mons pubis, labia majora, clitoris, fourchette, scars, tears. Patient is asked to maximally strain or cough. If seen, prolapsed mass can be of anterior or posterior vaginal walls or cervix, individually or in combination. Note should be made of any congestion, pigmentation, hyperkeratinization and ulcers.

Decubitus ulcer should be recorded with location, dimensions, margins, edges, floor, sensations and relation to underlying structures. Sloping edges with granulation tissue is suggestive of a healing ulcer. However, edges like punched out in syphilis, undermining in tuberculosis and beaded in malignancy are abnormal.

CLASSIFICATIONS FOR PELVIC ORGAN PROLAPSE[9,10]

- Malpas classification
- Jeffcot's classification
- Shaw's classification
- Baden–Walker's classification
- DeLancey classification
- POP-Q classification

Commonly used classifications for the prolapse are:
- Shaw's classification
- Baden-Walker Halfway system
- POP-Q system.

Shaw's Classification

After reducing the prolapse, posterior vaginal wall is retracted by Sim's speculum to examine anterior vaginal wall and vice versa. Apical or superior segment can be examined with a bivalve speculum. On maximum straining, the amount of prolapse noted in each segment with hymen as reference point.[10]
- *Anterior vaginal wall:* Upper two-thirds—cystocele, lower one-third—urethrocele
- *Posterior vaginal wall:* Upper one-third—enterocele, lower two-thirds—rectocele
- *Uterine descent*
  - Descent of cervix into the vagina below the ischial spine but above hymen—**1st degree**
  - Descent of cervix up to hymen or introitus—**2nd degree**
  - Descent of cervix outside hymen or introitus—**3rd degree**.

Procidentia is when whole of the uterus is lying outside the introitus. At the stalk of the prolapsed mass, thumb placed anteriorly and 2 fingers placed posteriorly meet each other (getting over the fundus of uterus). Tube like structures suggesting ureters can be felt on either side in case of procidentia.

According to Shaw's classification, example of prolapse with all three compartment defects shown in Figure 21.7.

Baden-Walker Halfway System

After reducing prolapse, anterior, superior and posterior segments are examined individually using Sim's speculum. Points 1-6 represent urethra, bladder, uterus, cul-de-sac, rectum and perineum in order. Each point is graded from 0 to 4 on maximum straining[1]
- Grade 0—no prolapse
- Grade 1—prolapse halfway to hymen
- Grade 2—prolapse up to hymen

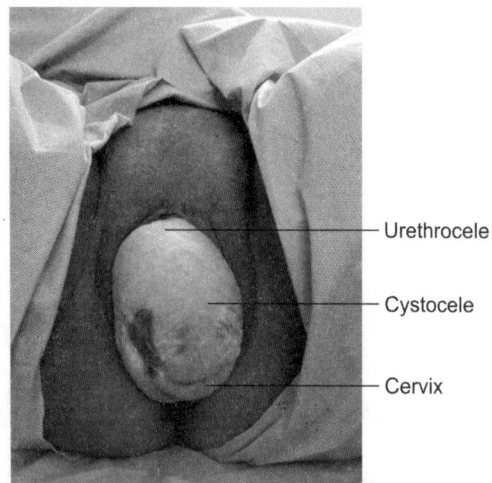

Fig. 21.7 Example of prolapse with all three compartment defects. According to Shaw's classification, it is a 3rd degree cervical descent with urethrocystocele, enterocele and rectocele with decubitus ulcer *(For color version, see Plate 4)*

- Grade 3—prolapse halfway past hymen
- Grade 4—maximum descent

When in doubt, use the greater grade. These points and their respective grades can be plotted on the pelvic organ prolapse map (Fig. 21.8).

For the same example quoted above.

Pelvic Organ Prolapse Quantification System or POP-Q

Nine measurements are used in POP-Q system (Fig. 21.9) as follows:
- A_a is a fixed point which is 3 cm from the hymen on the anterior wall (Fig. 21.10)
- A_p is a fixed point which is 3 cm from the hymen on the posterior wall (Fig. 21.12)
- B_a is the most leading point on the anterior wall from point A_a to apex (Fig. 21.11)
- B_p is the most leading point on the posterior wall from point A_p to apex (Fig. 21.13)
- C is the most distal point on the cervix (Fig. 21.11)
- D point is the posterior fornix and is omitted in hysterectomized patient. In case of cervical

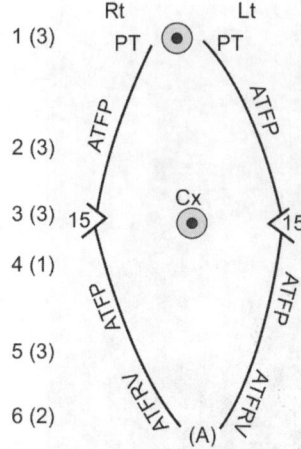

Fig. 21.8 Example for Baden-Walker Halfway classification of prolapse. It is 33/31/32 significant cystocele, rectocele and apical prolapse with enterocele with perineal attenuation to the level of external anal sphincter

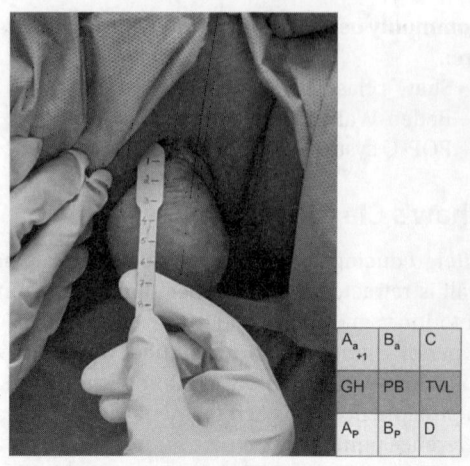

Fig. 21.10 Point A_a: fixed point 3 cm from the hymen on the anterior wall *(For color version, see Plate 4)*

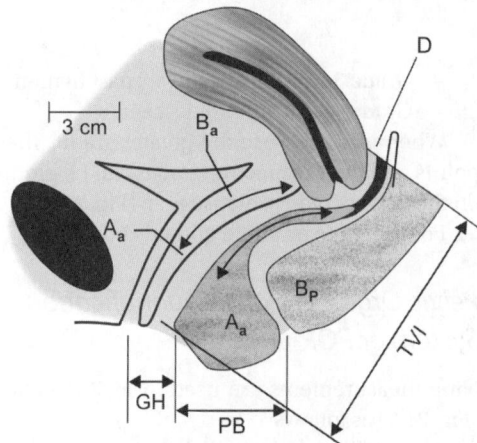

Fig. 21.9 POP-Q system
Abbreviations: TVL, total vaginal length; PB, perineal body; GH, genital hiatus

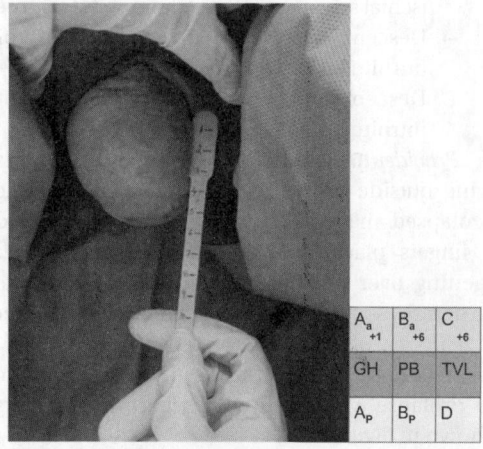

Fig. 21.11 Point B_a: most leading point on the anterior wall from point A_a to apex; Point C: most distal point on the cervix *(For color version, see Plate 4)*
Abbreviations: TVL, total vaginal length; PB, perineal body; GH, genital hiatus

elongation, point D is much higher than point C (Fig. 21.14)

All these 6 points are measured in centimeter in relation to hymen on maximum straining. It is positive when it is outside the hymen, negative when inside and 0 when it is at the hymen

- GH or genital hiatus is measured from the middle of external urethral meatus to the inferior hymenal ring. In cases of severe

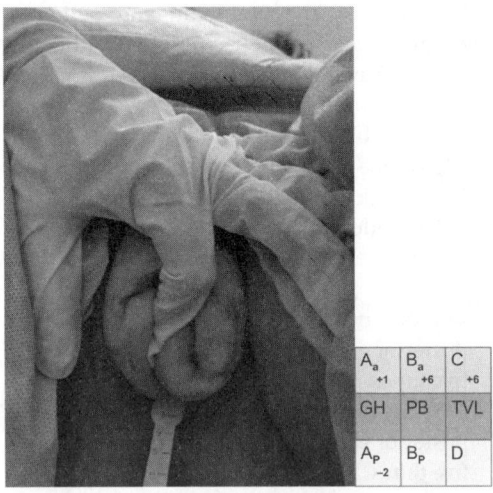

Fig. 21.12 Point A_p: fixed point 3 cm from the hymen on the posterior wall *(For color version, see Plate 4)*

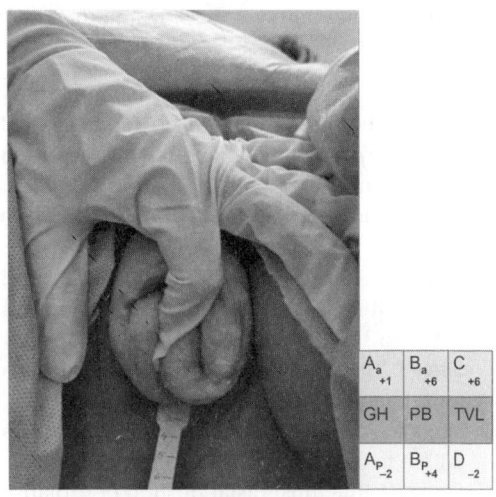

Fig. 21.14 Point D is posterior fornix *(For color version, see Plate 5)*

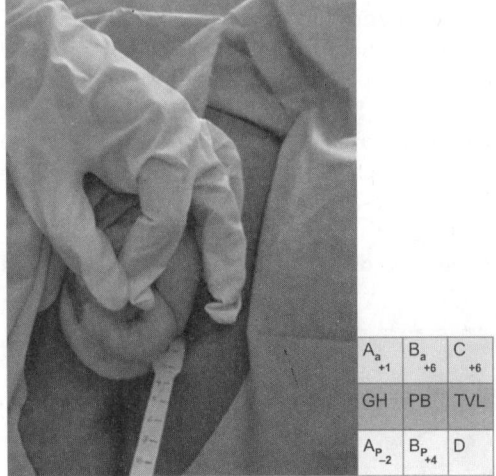

Fig. 21.13 Point B_p: most leading point on the posterior wall from point A_p to apex *(For color version, see Plate 5)*

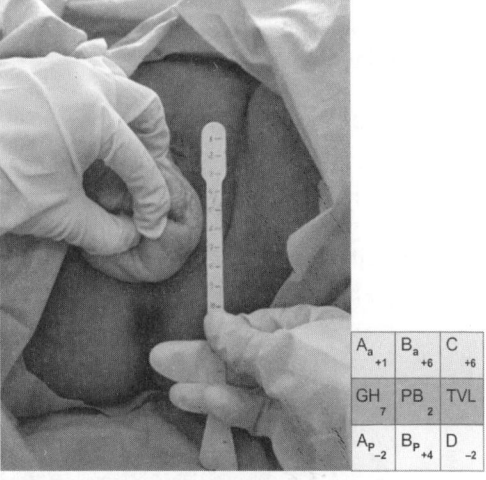

Fig. 21.15 GH measured from the middle of external urethral meatus to the inferior hymenal ring; PB measured from inferior hymenal ring to middle of anal orifice *(For color version, see Plate 5)*

prolapse, it is widened indicating perineal descent (Fig. 21.15)
- PB or perineal body is measured from inferior hymenal ring to middle of anal orifice. In cases of severe prolapse, it is thinned out (Fig. 21.15)
- TVL or total vaginal length is the only measurement among the nine which is measured in the reduced prolapse. It is the least reproducible measurement of all. It can be measured on pervaginal examination with the tip of middle finger at posterior fornix and marking the relation of hymenal ring on the gloved finger.

The order of these measurements depends on the amount on prolapse. If an obvious mass is seen lying outside the introitus, one can start with points A, B, C, D and then GH, PB and TVL (Fig. 21.16)[1,9]

Example: First reduce the prolapse and mark point A on both anterior and posterior vaginal walls 3 cm proximal to hymen. Ask the patient to strain and note these points in relation to hymen.

Staging of the prolapse based on POP-Q is as follows:
- *Stage 0*: No prolapse. Points A_a, A_p, B_a and B_p are all at -3 cm and either point C or D is between TVL cm and (TVL-2) cm
- *Stage I*: The most distal portion of prolapse is more than 1 cm above the hymen
- *Stage II*: The most distal portion of prolapse is ± 1 cm to the plane of hymen
- *Stage III*: The most distal portion of prolapse is more than 1cm below hymen but no further than 2 cm less than the TVL
- *Stage IV*: The most distal portion of prolapse is ≥ (TVL-2) cm.
  In the above said example, it is Stage III with the leading point C.

Pervaginal Examination

A bimanual examination should be made to note the direction and size of uterus and adnexa. Levator tone should be appreciated with 2 fingers on the posterior vaginal at 5 or 7 o' clock position with thumb on the perineum and patient is asked to squeeze the pelvic muscle like holding the urine or avoiding passing of gas. It is graded according to modified oxford scale:[6]
- 0/5—unable to contract
- 1/5—trace contraction, <2 seconds
- 2/5—weak contraction, ≥3 seconds
- 3/5—moderate contraction, 4–6 seconds, posterior elevation of fingers, repeated three times
- 4/5—strong contraction, 7–9 seconds, posterior elevation of fingers, repeated four to five times
- 5/5—very strong contraction, ≥10 seconds, posterior elevation of fingers, repeated four to five times.

Per-rectal Examination

Rectocele is confirmed by insinuating the finger on the anterior rectal wall towards vagina. Anal sphincter tone is graded on a scale of 0–4+.[9] With a thumb on perineum, the perineal body should be assessed for the bulk and integrity. Levator plate is a horizontal structure felt posterior to rectum which represents confluence of pelvic floor muscles.

Bidigital recto vaginal (PV and RV) examination is done to assess the thickness of

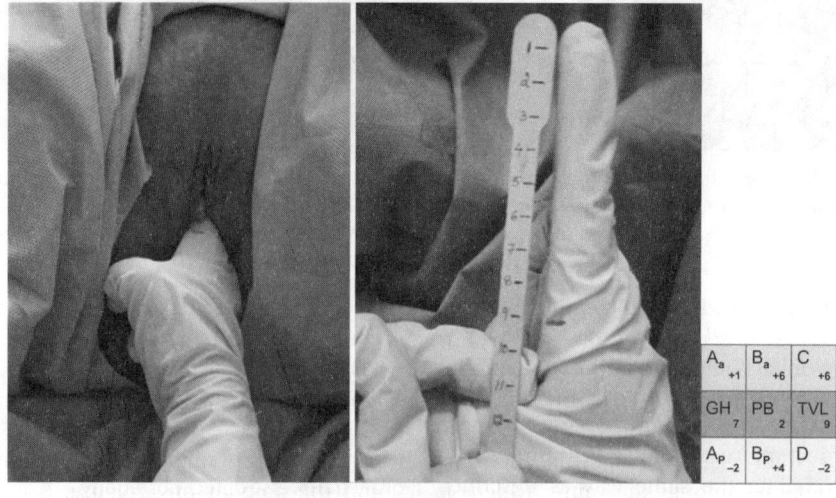

A_a +1	B_a +6	C +6
GH 7	PB 2	TVL 9
A_p -2	B_p +4	D -2

Fig. 21.16 Total vaginal length *(For color version, see Plate 6)*

rectovaginal septum. On straining if prolapsed mass is felt between the vaginal and rectal finger, it is indicative of enterocele.

EVALUATION OF BLADDER FUNCTION

In patients with complaints of urinary incontinence, any leaking of urine with straining is documented. If present, then urethral hypermobility can be tested with a well lubricated cotton swab stick inserted in the urethra up to 3 cm and asked to strain. If the angle of deflection is more than 30° from horizontal, it is indicative of loss of support at urethrovesical angle or urethral hypermobility. A protractor or a goniometer is used to measure the angle.[1,6]

In cases of severe prolapse, stress urinary incontinence can be masked due to kinking effect of the prolapse. Thus, prolapse should be reduced and patient is asked to strain with full bladder to note the leaking.

MAPPING OF TEARS

- Rugosities on the vaginal walls are indicative of the underlying attached endopelvic fascia.
- Lateral vaginal sulci are the location of junction of pubocervical and rectovaginal to the respective arcuate attachments.
- The defects in the pubocervical septum can be proximal, distal, lateral or central. To map these tears, posterior vaginal wall is retracted with Sim's speculum and the anterior prolapsed mass is reduced with ring forceps posteriorly and cranially. If on straining, bulge is noted it is indicative central or combined central and paravaginal defects. If on straining, no prolapse is noted, the defect is mostly unilateral or bilateral paravaginal which can be detected by supporting each sulci with closed ring forceps. If a bulge is seen just adjacent to the cervix in the anterior fornix, it is mostly due to apical detachment of pubocervical septum from pericervical ring.
- The defect in rectovaginal septum can be appreciated in the same way as described above. On per-rectal examination, the edge of torn septum can be felt.

These tears are mapped on the pelvic organ prolapse map which aid in the site specific repair. The most common defect is right paravaginal defect due to the predominance of left occipito anterior position of fetal head during labor.[1]

Example for mapping of tears is shown in Figure 21.17.

Investigations

- Hemoglobin, hematocrit, total leukocyte count
- Urine routine, microscopy, culture and sensitivity
- Blood sugar, urea, serum creatinine
- CXR-PA view
- Pap smear
- Other investigations should be tailored to the clinical situation:
  – If patient has abnormal uterine bleeding (AUB) then endometrial biopsy or aspiration must be done

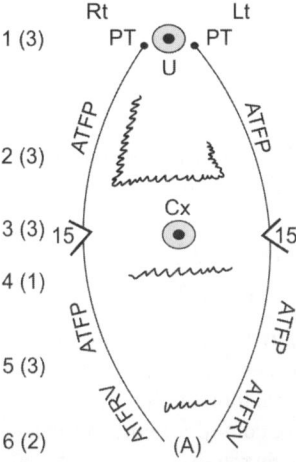

Fig. 21.17 Example for mapping of tears. In this case there is a predominant right paravaginal defect with apical transverse and proximal left paravaginal defect anteriorly. Also there is apical transverse and distal transverse defect posteriorly

- Urodynamic study may be required if urinary incontinence is not clinically defined
- Decubitus ulcer biopsy in case of non-healing ulcers
- Ultrasound KUB, IVP in case of hydronephrosis.

Management Options

Nonsurgical (mainly for minimal or mild prolapse):
- Pelvic floor exercise—Kegel exercise
- Lifestyle changes like weight loss, cessation of smoking
- Treatment of underlying conditions like chronic cough and constipation
- Hormonal therapy with estrogens for menopausal women
- Mechanical devices like pessary.

Surgical (moderate to severe prolapse): Surgical options have vaginal or abdominal approach. The type of surgical correction should be tailored to the clinical situation depending on history and physical findings and patient's wishes.

Factors which determine the type of surgery are as follows:
- Age
- Parity
- Associated complaints like stress urinary incontinence
- Associated diseases for example COPD
- Any past history of surgery.

SURGERIES FOR PELVIC ORGAN PROLAPSE

Vaginal approach:
- Manchester operation
- Anterior colporrhaphy
- Posterior colpoperineorrhaphy
- Enterocele repair
- Site specific repair
- Colpofixation
- Hysterectomy with pelvic floor repair
- Obliterative procedures like Le Fort partial colpocleisis, colpocleisis or colpectomy.

Abdominal approach:
- Colposuspension or sling surgeries
- Enterocele repair
- Site specific repair
- Hysterectomy with vault suspension.

Mesh repair is usually reserved for recurrent prolapse or failure of previous corrective surgeries.[11]

Complications of surgeries
- Immediate
  - Hemorrhage
  - Injury to bladder, rectum, bowel or ureters
- Early
  - Hematoma/hemorrhage
  - Infection
  - Mesh-related complications
- Late
  - Recurrence
  - Failure of procedure.

Preventive Measures

General

- Improvement of nutrition
- Regular bowel habits
- Avoid smoking, obesity
- Hormone replacement therapy for menopausal woman.

During Labor and Puerperium

- Allow full dilation of cervix
- Cut down second stage of labor
- Repair episiotomy and tears in layers
- Avoid expression of uterus for delivery of placenta
- Postpartum pelvic floor exercise
- Treat puerperal constipation.

During Pelvic Surgery

Abdominal
- Attach cardinal and uterosacral ligament stumps to vaginal vault
- Obliterate deep cul-de-sac by Moschcowitz sutures
- Sacrospinous fixation not recommended prophylactically (Am J Obstet Gynecol 1998)

Vaginal
- Remove redundant peritoneum
- Cardinal and uterosacral ligament attachment to vaginal vault
- McCall culdoplasty.

The failure of pelvic floor repair is associated with uncorrected enterocele or failure to recognize or treat underlying cause.

KEY POINTS

- Pelvic organ prolapse (POP) is common problem in multiparous women.
- It affects there social, psychological life especially cause bladder bowel and sexual complaints.
- Common cause for POP are menopause, multiparity with inadequate spacing and it is aggravated further due to malnutrition, anemia and increase intra-abdominal pressure due to COPD, manual labor, etc.
- Assessment of POP is clinical skill and it's essential to recognize the defects and plan the management. Causative and aggravating factors both have to be included in management plan.
- Enterocele repair and stress urinary incontinence treatment should be included in management.
- Preventive measures are always better than cure spacing of births, one or two births, delivery attended by trained birth attendants, nutritional improvements, no smoking, and change to healthy life style will reduce this disease to bare minimum.

REFERENCES

1. Zimmerman WC. Pelvic organ prolapse: Basic principles. In: Rock JA, Jones HW (Eds) TeLinde Operative Gynecology, 10th edn. New Delhi, Lippincott and Williams and Wilkins, 2008.pp.854-73.
2. Malhotra N, Kumar P, Malhotra J, Bora MN, Mittal P. Pelvic organ prolapse. Jeffcoate's Principles of Gynaecology, 8th edn, Jaypee Brothers; 2014. pp.251-68.
3. Gill EJ, Hurt WG. Pathophysiology of pelvic organ prolapse; urogynecology and pelvic floor dysfunction. Obstetrics and Gynecology Clinics of North America. 1998;25(4):757-69.
4. Ann Word R, Pathi S, Schaffer JI. Pathophysiology of pelvic organ prolapse. Obstet Gynecol Clin N Am. 2009;36:521-39.
5. Mant J, Painter R, Vessey M. Epidemiology of genital prolapse: observations from Oxford Family Planning Association study. Br J Obstet Gynaecol. 1997;104:579-85.
6. Bump RC, Cundiff GW. The clinical evaluation of pelvic floor dysfunction; urogynecology and pelvic floor dysfunction. Obstetrics and Gynecology Clinics of North America. 1998;25(4):783-804.
7. Douglas G, Nicol F, Robertson C. The nervous system. Macleod's Clinical Examination, 12th edn, 2009.pp.267-306.
8. Douglas G, Nicol F, Robertson C. The musculoskeletal system. Macleod's Clinical Examination, 12th edn; 2009.pp.355-400.
9. Gleason JK, Richter HE, Varner ER. Pelvic organ prolapse. In: Berek JS (Ed). Berek & Novak's Gynecology, 15th edn, New Delhi, Lippincott and Williams and Wilkins; 2012.pp.906-39.
10. Padubidri VG, Daftary SN. Genital prolapse. Howkins and Bourne Shaw's Textbook of Gynaecology, 14th edn, 2008.pp.298-309.
11. The American College of Obstetricians and Gynaecologists. Committee opinion, Number 513, 2011.

22

Urodynamics in Stress Urinary Incontinence

Nikhil Khattar, Ritesh Kumar Singh

INTRODUCTION

Urodynamics (UDS) is the term used to describe the testing and measurements of the function of the lower urinary tract. The lower urinary tract has two essential functions: the storage of urine at low pressure (filling phase) and the voluntary release of urine (voiding phase). Low-pressure storage is essential to protect the kidneys and for continence, whereas voluntary release allows for the elimination of urine without fear of leakage or over distension. The main quest for any urodynamic study is to know actual pressures generated by the detrusor muscle of the bladder (P_{det}) during both storage and voiding. This can be achieved only by deriving two easily calculable pressures, i.e. vesical pressure (P_{ves}) and abdominal pressure (P_{abd}).

Multichannel UDS (Fig. 22.1) is favored at present and is performed with two catheters, one in the bladder to measure the P_{ves} and one in the rectum or vagina to measure the P_{abd}. The detrusor pressure is then obtained by subtracting the abdominal pressure from the vesical pressure ($P_{ves} - P_{abd} = P_{det}$) (Fig. 22.2).

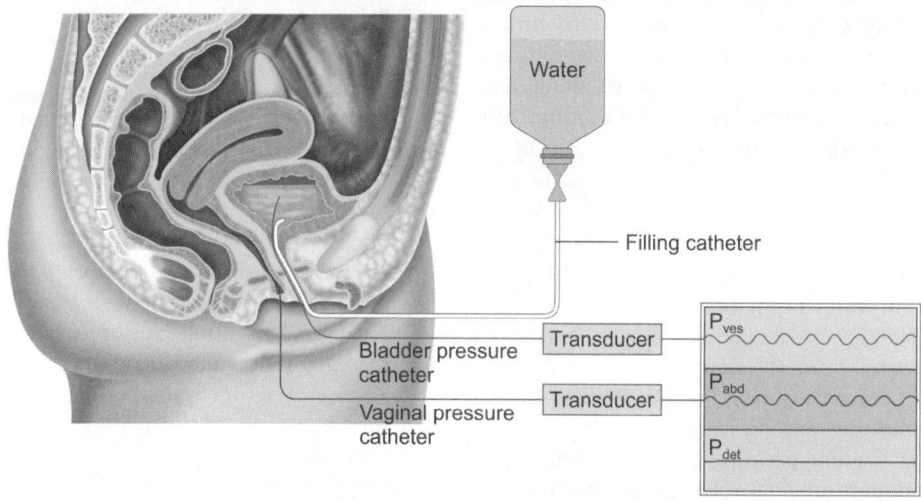

Fig. 22.1 Catheter placement and pressures

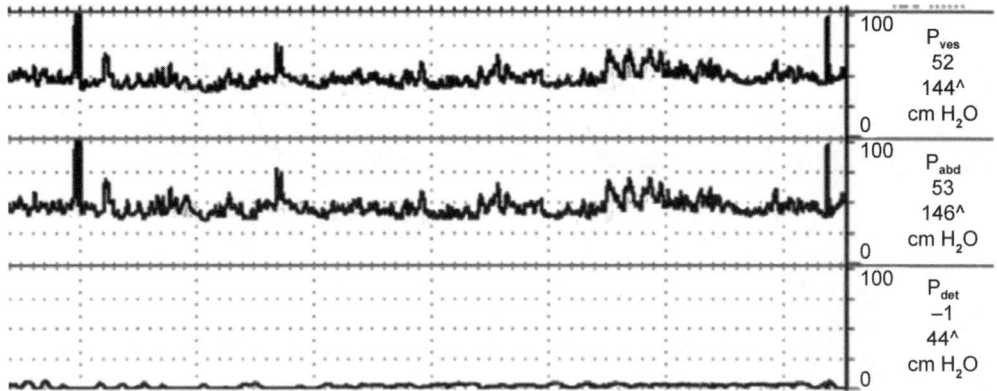

Fig. 22.2 Multichannel urodynamics

Urodynamics only supplements the clinical findings or provides objective evidence of clinical suspicion, and is not used as a diagnostic modality. It is important to remember that UDS is not done in natural sitting and hence does not always duplicate the symptoms per se. Before conducting a UDS, the clinician should have a clear understanding of what needs to be answered from the said investigation.

WHAT TO LOOK FOR IN URODYNAMICS?

In the filling phase or storage phase, one should look for sensation (decreased/normal/increased), compliance, detrusor overactivity (Fig. 22.3) and capacity. The voiding phase analyzes detrusor contractility. The term requiring specific mention is compliance, which is the relationship between change in bladder volume and change in detrusor pressure (Δ volume/Δ pressure) and is measured in mL/cm H_2O. It is difficult to define normal compliance, but values less than 20 mL/cm H_2O are considered poor compliance.[1] Normally, detrusor pressure should remain near zero during the entire filling cycle until voluntary voiding is initiated. That means baseline bladder pressure stays constant (and low) and there are no involuntary contractions.

There are few terms worth mentioning and relevant to UDS in stress incontinence as:
- *Abdominal leak point pressure:* The intravesical pressure at which urine leakage occurs because of increased abdominal pressure in the absence of a detrusor contraction.[2] It basically signifies sphincter strength.
- *Urethral pressure measurements:*
  - *Urethral pressure:* The fluid pressure needed to just open a closed urethra.
  - *Urethral pressure profile:* A graph indicating the intraluminal pressure along the length of the urethra.
  - *Urethral closure pressure profile:* The subtraction of intravesical pressure from urethral pressure.
  - *Maximum urethral pressure:* The maximum pressure of the measured profile.
  - Despite an abundant literature on urethral profilometry, its clinical relevance is controversial. Many urologists do not routinely perform urethral profilometry. The urethral pressure profile (UPP) represents the intraluminal pressure along the length of the urethra.
- *Maximum urethral closure pressure (MUCP)* is the maximum difference between the urethral pressure and the intravesical pressure. In most continent women, the

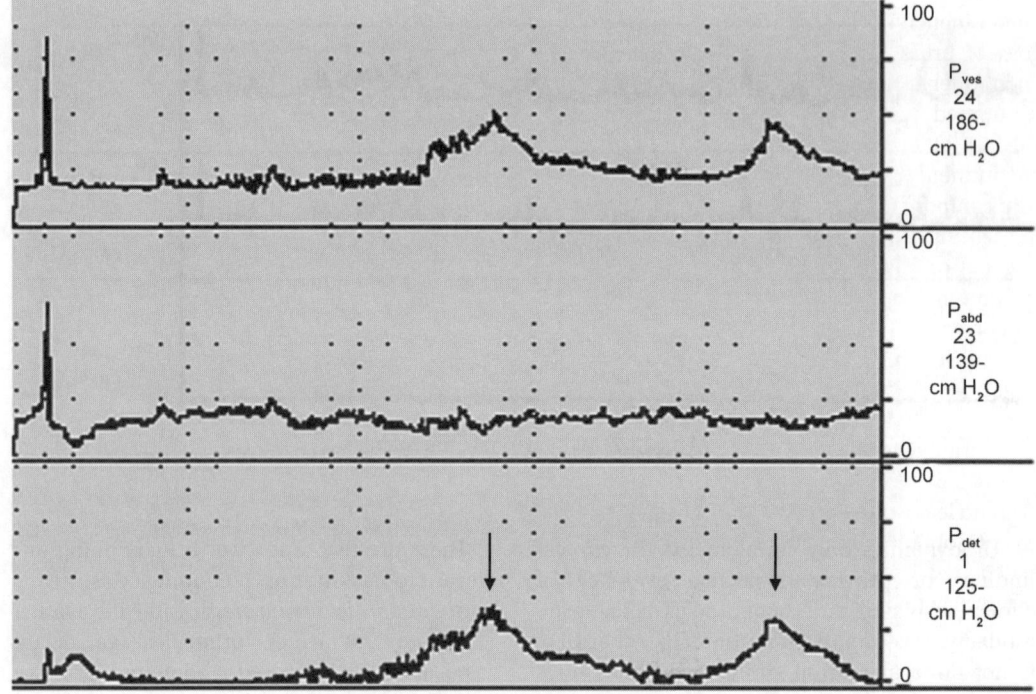

Fig. 22.3 Detrusor overactivity shown with arrows

functional urethral length is approximately 3 cm and the MUCP is 40–60 cm H_2O, but the normal values vary widely; MUCP less than 20 defines ISD; however, this definition varies depending on several factors and hence cannot be considered a standard definition.

- *Detrusor leak point pressure (DLPP)*: The lowest detrusor pressure at which urine leakage occurs in the absence of either a detrusor contraction or increased abdominal pressure.
- *Uroflowmetry and PVR (post-void residue)-* Men or women void on a machine with near full bladder and system generates values showing maximum flow rate, average time to void, total voided volume and the urine remaining following voiding in the bladder, i.e PVR.

Urinary incontinence is defined as the "complaint of involuntary loss of urine".[3] The prevalence of urinary incontinence in women older than 20 years is 25% and increases with age. Half of incontinent women experience stress incontinence alone, and 36% have mixed incontinence.[4]

Stress urinary incontinence (SUI) is defined as the "complaint of involuntary loss of urine on effort or physical exertion, or on sneezing and coughing". The diagnosis of SUI in women is based on symptoms and signs as demonstrated on the physical examination or on urodynamic observation in the absence of a detrusor contraction.[2]

Stress incontinence may also be diagnosed in the presence of other conditions, such as urinary frequency, urgency, nocturia, or voiding difficulty.[5] Other types of urinary incontinence can coexist with SUI, such as urgency urinary incontinence (UUI), mixed urinary incontinence (MUI), or nocturnal enuresis. Identifying coexisting urge incontinence in a patient with SUI is of paramount importance while managing a patient with SUI. Urgency is characterized by a strong, sudden, uncomfortable need to void. Urge incontinence is characterized by the precipitate loss of urine accompanied by urgency. Stress incontinence accompanied by urge incontinence is termed mixed incontinence. An estimated 30–65% of women with SUI present with mixed incontinence (McGuire and Savastano, 1985). The components vary in their contribution to the presenting symptom complex. In some cases, urgency or urge-related incontinence may be the predominant symptom. Any procedure intended to correct SUI will increase urethral resistance and consequently risks worsening of pre-existing urgency symptoms as detrusor begins to react in presence of increased outlet resistance.

Normal physiology mandates urethra to be competent enough to store urine in storage phase with no leak, and if there is leak it is either due to hypermobility of urethra or intrinsic sphincteric deficiency (ISD). Figure 22.4 shows analogy for urethral hypermobility (Urethral support defect).

Causes of SUI

Stress UI, the third most common type of UI in older women, results from failure of the sphincter mechanism(s) to preserve outlet closure during bladder filling. Stress UI occurs coincident with increased intra-abdominal pressure, in the absence of a bladder contraction. Leakage is either due to hypermobility of urethra (Urethral support defect) or intrinsic sphicnter deficiency (ISD).

Causes of *hypermobility* of urethra:
- Pregnancy
- Vaginal delivery,
- Pelvic surgery, and chronic abdominal straining (e.g. chronic constipation)
- Neurologic injury leading to pudendal nerve damage or muscular dystrophy.

Causes for ISD

- Previous urethral or periurethral surgery (e.g. anti-incontinence surgery, urethral diverticulectomy)[6]
- Neurologic insult may cause ISD[7]
- Pelvic radiation therapy has been associated with damage to the mucosal seal coaptation of the urethra and local neurologic damage.[6]

Risk Factors for SUI

- Prevalence of SUI is more during pregnancy and also increases with advancing gestational age.
- Vaginal and large baby deliveries increase the risk of SUI as compared to cesarean section.

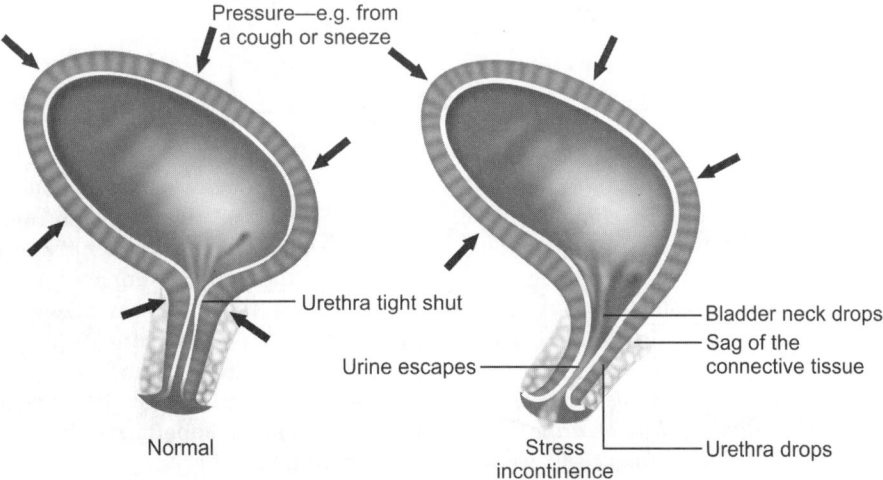

Fig. 22.4 Bladder neck and urethral descent (hypermobility)

- Caucasian women have higher prevalence of SUI as compared to Asian women.
- Multiparity has higher risk for SUI.
- Obesity (BMI > 30) is also a risk factor for SUI.

Diagnostic Evaluation

Essential to the management of SUI is an accurate diagnosis. The diagnostic evaluation includes a thorough history and physical examination supplemented by urinalysis and other appropriate laboratory studies. There are two basic factors to be evaluated: urethral hypermobility and/or ISD. The two may coexist. Hypermobility, present in the majority of women with SUI, is the rotational descent of the proximal urethra and bladder neck into the vagina, associated with increases in abdominal pressure that occur with activities such as coughing, postural changes, etc. Hypermobility can be observed visually or radiographically (videourodynamics) (Fig. 22.5). Its presence, however, does not necessarily indicate SUI; many women have urethral hypermobility without SUI. If incontinence does occur, an element of sphincter weakness is present. The second factor, ISD, also represents a significant component of incontinence in women. The prevalence of ISD is not fully known, but in the panel's expert opinion, it is present in a significant percentage of women with stress incontinence. ISD refers to a deficiency in the urethral sphincter function, which is unrelated to urethral support. The most common reasons for loss of this urethral function are prior incontinence surgery, prior pelvic surgery (radical hysterectomy, abdominoperineal resection of rectum), neurologic disorders (spina bifida), urethral mucosal atrophy and, in rare cases, radiation exposure. The result is poor urethral mucosal coaptation (pipe stem urethra) and incontinence with minimal stress activities. The selection of a surgical procedure should reflect the relative contributions of these two conditions, which as noted previously and may coexist.

Now the question arises whether UDS needs to be done or not before management of SUI patient, and its pros and cons and does it alter management plan.

Urodynamics includes noninvasive uroflowmetry followed by multichannel filling cystometry. Urodynamics is an expensive, invasive and uncomfortable investigation carrying a risk of urinary tract infections (3–5%).

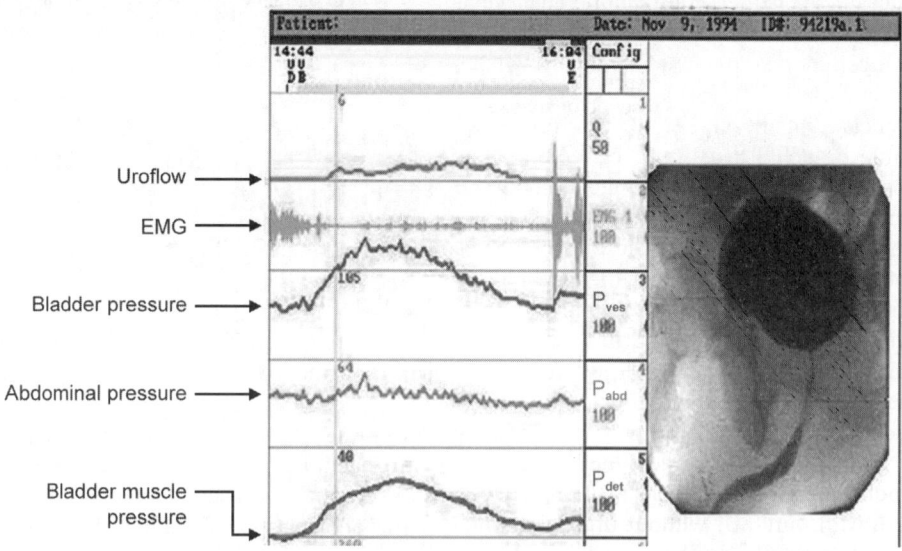

Fig. 22.5 Videourodynamics *(For color version, see Plate 6)*

Office evaluation for SUI includes focused history-taking, quality of life (QoL) questionnaires, bladder diaries, pelvic examination, cough test, uroflowmetry, measurement of post-void residual (PVR) urine volume and urine analysis. The role of urodynamics in predicting the success of surgical treatment or postoperative complications has been a matter of debate. Clinicians may be concerned that in women who do not undergo urodynamics, discordant diagnoses such as provoked detrusor overactivity (DO) and voiding dysfunction may be missed, to the detriment of a good outcome of surgery for SUI. DO is the occurrence of involuntary contractions which may be spontaneous or provoked during the filling phase of cystometry and may be seen in 20% of patients with a history of pure SUI.

What to Look for in UDS for SUI?

See for compliance, detrusor overactivity, in storage phase and detrusor contractility (normal/underactive) in voiding phase.

As explained previously the term alkaline phosphatase, placental type precursor (ALPP) can only be demonstrated in a patient with stress urinary incontinence (SUI). Conceptually, the lower the ALPP, the weaker the sphincter. There is no normal ALPP because patients without stress incontinence will not leak any physiologic abdominal pressure. ALPP lower than <60 show ISD deficiency, between 60 and 90 eqivocal, and >90 little or no ISD. Current technology does not permit a method to distinguish between ISD in the face of urethral hypermobility in women. Therefore, although these ALPP values are often used as guidelines, they should be interpreted with caution. For example, if there is no urethral hypermobility, SUI must be caused by ISD, regardless of the ALPP. Thus, an isolated measure of ALPP without considering other factors such as cystometry and urethral mobility is of limited utility in predicting success for commonly performed female SUI procedures. Women with pure SUI without urge symptoms who void normally and demonstrate SUI on physical examination, UDS will not provide much useful information. As a general rule, one should start testing at 150 mL and then every 50 mL thereafter until SUI is demonstrated. If there is no SUI demonstrated at capacity, the urethral catheter is removed and ALPP is measured via the rectal catheter (provided there is no increase in P_{det} from DO or impaired compliance).

Likewise as explained earlier MUCP less than 20 to define ISD; however, this definition has many of the same problems as ISD definitions for ALPP. Another caveat of UPP is that its measurement does not diagnose stress incontinence and SUI is not required to measure it (contrary to ALPP). MUCP in incontinent women has been shown to be lower than in continent. Figure 22.1 showing catheter placement and pressures women, but there is certainly overlap.[8] In addition, MUCP is not always indicative of the severity of incontinence.

International Continence Society standardization subcommittee concluded that the clinical utility of urethral pressure measurement is unclear. Furthermore, there are no urethral pressure measurements that

- Discriminate urethral incompetence from other disorders
- Provide a measure of the severity of the condition; and
- Provide a reliable indicator to surgical success and return to normal after surgical intervention.[9]

EVIDENCE FOR AND AGAINST URODYNAMICS

The National Institute for Health and Care Excellence (NICE) guideline recommends that urodynamics not be performed in the small group of women where pure SUI is diagnosed based on a detailed clinical history and examination. According to the Cochrane review on urinary incontinence, urodynamics does not predict surgical failure or postoperative DO. Despite this evidence, a recent survey of urologists and urogynecologists concluded that 89% would arrange urodynamics for women with SUI or stress-predominant mixed urinary incontinence (MUI). However, the majority of respondents recognized the need for further research to address this question. The objective of this review was to assess whether the performance of urodynamics altered the outcomes of cure or complications in women undergoing surgery with isolated SUI or stress-predominant MUI symptoms.

In a randomized trial comparing the efficacy of Burch procedure versus pubovaginal sling in 655 selected women with pure or predominate SUI who had fewer than 12 micturitions/day, a positive standardized stress test (volume < 300 mL), a maximum cystometric capacity of at least 200 mL, a PVR of less than 150 mL and unobstructed voiding (Q_{max} > 12 mL/sec, $P_{det}Q_{max}$ < 50 cm H_2O), UDS including ALPP, and presence of DO added little to help determine surgical outcomes with respect to efficacy or postoperative voiding dysfunction.[5] Likewise MUCP has also been used to define ISD. Certain observations or diagnoses that can coexist with SUI can only be made with the urodynamic evaluation: an overactive detrusor function (with or without incontinence), an abnormal detrusor activity during voiding (detrusor underactivity), or abnormal compliance. Abnormal urethral functions, such as a bladder outlet obstruction or dysfunctional voiding, can only be confirmed during pressure-flow studies.

The randomized controlled trial (RCT) "Value of Urodynamics prior to Stress Incontinence Surgery randomized 59 women with SUI or stress-predominant MUI to a treatment strategy with or without UDS from different centers. The clinical reduction of complaints after 12 months was in favor of the group without urodynamics. Urodynamics did not result in a lower occurrence of de novo urgency.[10] The large multicenter Value of Urodynamic Evaluation (VaLUE) study randomized 630 women planning to undergo surgery for SUI to an office evaluation or urodynamic testing. A provocative stress test was positive for all patients before randomization. After adjusting for the baseline differences between the 2 groups (duration of incontinence; Incontinence Severity Index score; and status with respect to smoking, history of nonsurgical treatment of urinary incontinence, current use of hormone-replacement therapy, and urethral mobility), the treatment success met the noninferiority for office evaluation only at the 1-year follow-up. There were no differences in adverse events outcomes. The preoperative diagnosis was more likely to change after the urodynamic evaluation but did not change the distribution of surgical treatment compared with the office evaluation only.[11] The physician's confidence in the diagnosis improved after UDS but did not correlate with the treatment success.[12]

The Trial of Mid-Urethral Slings (TOMUS) randomized 597 women with a positive urinary stress test to undergo a midurethral sling through either a retropubic or transobturator route. They all had a preoperative urodynamic evaluation blinded to the surgeon, and the urodynamic stress leakage was not required. There were no objective or subjective differences in treatment success between both groups, even when adjusted for Valsalva leak-point pressure (VLPP) or maximum urethral closure pressure at 12 or 24 months.[13,14]

In other words, urodynamics is not routinely recommended for women before surgery for a "clearly defined clinical diagnosis of stress urinary incontinence." In the prospective, randomized Stress Incontinence Surgical Treatment Efficacy (SISTER) trial comparing Burch colposuspension and pubovaginal sling, leak point pressures were not found to be predictive of surgical outcome for either procedure.[5]

CONCLUSION

Urodynamics is recommended before surgery for urinary incontinence only if (1) there is a clinical suspicion of DO, (2) there has been previous surgery for stress incontinence or anterior compartment prolapse, or (3) there are symptoms suggestive of voiding dysfunction.
- UDS asesses basically storage and voiding coordination of bladder, urethra and higher center of micturition.

- In UDS for SUI, most important is to look for is detrusor overactivity.
- Urethral hypermobility and ISD are most importment cause of SUI.
- Urodynamics are prudent when the diagnosis of stress urinary incontinence is not confirmed by other investigations or when prior surgical intervention has failed.
- The decision to perform preoperative urodynamics should be made on an individual basis and with a clear understanding of how the results will have an impact on patient counseling or treatment.
- Two recent noninferiority randomized controlled trials did not demonstrate a significant difference in objective and subjective treatment outcome following stress urinary incontinence surgery between women who had a preoperative office evaluation or urodynamic studies.

REFERENCES

1. Stöhrer M, Goepel M, Kondo A, et al. The standardization of terminology in neurogenic lower urinary tract dysfunction with suggestions for diagnostic procedures. Neurourol Urodyn. 1999;18:139-58.
2. Abrams P, Cardoza L, Fall M, et al. The standardisation of terminology in lower urinary tract function: report from the standardisation sub-committee of the International Continence Society. Neurourol Urodyn. 2002;21:167-78.
3. Haylen BT, de Ridder D, Freeman RM, et al. An International Urogynecological Association (IUGA)/Inter- national Continence Society (ICS) joint report on the terminology for female pelvic floor dysfunction. Neurourol Urodyn. 2010;29(1):4-20.
4. Hannestad YS, Rortveit G, Sandvik H, et al. A community-based epidemiological survey of female urinary incontinence: the Norwegian EPINCONT Study. J Clin Epidemiol. 2000;53(11):1150-7.
5. Nager CW, FitzGerald M, Kraus SR, et al. Urodynamic measures do not predict stress continence outcomes after surgery for stress urinary incontinence in selected women. J Urol. 2008;179:1470-4.
6. Haab F, Zimmern PE, Leach GE. Female stress urinary incontinence due to intrinsic sphincteric deficiency: recognition and management. J Urol. 1996;156:3-17.
7. Blaivas JG, Olsson CA. Stress incontinence: classification and surgical approach. J Urol. 1988;139(4):727-31.
8. Schick E, Dupont C, Bertrand PE, et al. Predictive value of maximum urethral closure pressure, urethral hypermobility and urethral incompetence in the diagnosis of clinically significant female genuine stress incontinence. J Urol. 2004;171:1871-5.
9. Lose G, Griffiths D, Hosker G, et al. Standardization of urethral pressure measurement: report from the Standardization Sub-Committee of the International Continence Society. Neurourol Urodyn. 2002;21:258-60.
10. Van Leijsen SA, Kluivers KB, Mol BW, et al. Can preoperative urodynamic investigation be omitted in women with stress urinary incontinence? A non-inferiority randomized controlled trial. Neurourol Urodyn. 2012;31(7):1118-23.
11. Nager CW, Brubaker L, Litman HJ, et al. A randomized trial of urodynamic testing before stress-incontinence surgery. N Engl J Med. 2012;366(21):1987-97.
12. Zimmern P, Litman H, Nager C, et al. Pre-operative urodynamics in women with stress urinary incontinence increases physician confidence, but does not improve outcomes. Neurourol Urodyn. 2014;33(3):302-6.
13. Richter HE, Albo ME, Zyczynski HM, et al. Retropubic versus transobturator midurethral slings for stress incontinence. N Engl J Med. 2010;362(22):2066-76.
14. Albo ME, Litman HJ, Richter HE, et al. Treatment success of retropubic and transobturator mid ure- thral slings at 24 months. J Urol. 2012;188(6):2281-7.

23

Benign Adnexal Masses

Akansha Shrivastava, Asmita M Rathore

The term adnexa is derived from the Latin word meaning "appendage." The adnexa comprises of the ovaries, fallopian tubes, and structures of the broad ligament and their pathology may lead to adnexal masses. Sometimes nongynecologic conditions may simulate adnexal masses and may be considered in their differential diagnosis.

EVALUATION OF ADNEXAL MASSES

Clinical

A thorough history is taken which includes detailed history of the presenting complaints, menstrual history, obstetric history, any bowel/bladder-related complaints followed by significant past medical/surgical history and family history. Complete examination should be performed which includes general examination, abdominal, per speculum, vaginal and rectal examination. Size, mobility, consistency and laterality of masses is determined clinically which helps to differentiate benign from malignant masses. Common clinical features are described in Table 23.1. Patient may present in one of the three ways:

1. Patient may be completely asymptomatic and mass may be diagnosed incidentally on ultrasonography (USG) or pelvic examination. These are usually small simple cystic masses.
2. Patient may present with chronic symptoms as described in Table 23.1 alongwith pelvic mass, then the first step is to findout whether the mass is gynecological or nongynecological in origin. A gynecological mass may be uterine or adnexal mass. Adnexal masses is distinguished from uterine masses on pelvic examination by following points:

Table 23.1 Common clinical features of benign adnexal masses	
Symptoms	Signs
• Asymptomatic (incidental finding on USG or pelvic examination) • Chronic abdominal/pelvic pain • Acute pain (in cases of torsion, rupture or hemorrhage) • Abdominal swelling (gradual onset, slow progression) • Nausea, vomiting and fever (in case of torsion) • Pressure symptoms— difficulty in micturition and defecation (in case of large mass) • Menstrual irregularity in hormone producing tumors	• Abdominopelvic examination—smooth, cystic, mobile, unilateral tumors, not associated with ascites • General examination—features of precocious puberty (in hormonally active functional cysts or neoplasm)

- A simple technique that differentiates uterine from adnexal mass includes sounding and measuring the depth of the uterine cavity.
- In case of uterine mass, uterus may not be felt separately.
- Movement of the mass felt per abdominally is transmitted to the cervix and vice versa in case of uterine mass.
- *Hingorani' sign*: Examination of the patient in Trendelenburg position results in upward displacement of the adnexal mass and then the examiner can elicit a grove between the uterus and the adnexal mass.

  Adnexal mass is further differentiated as ovarian or nonovarian in origin based on clinical examination and USG findings.
  - If the mass is found to be ovarian in origin then the lesion is categorized on the basis of USG characteristics as simple cyst, hemorrhagic cyst, endometrioma, mature cystic teratoma, complex cysts or benign neoplasm.
  - Nonovarian mass may be purely tubal (hematosalpinx/hydrosalpinx/pyosalpinx) or may be complex tubo-ovarian masses.

    Hematosalpinx: It may be seen in prepubertal girl as a consequence obstructive mullerian anomalies.

    Complex tubo-ovarian mass: It may be a complication of pelvic inflammatory disease (PID) in reproductive years or may be a result of tuberculosis in any age group. Another presentation of complex tubo-ovarian mass in reproductive age may be *chronic ectopic* if patient presents with positive pregnancy test.

3. Sometimes patient may come to emergency with acute abdomen, then various complications of adnexal masses such as torsion, rupture or infection are to be suspected and managed accordingly (described later).
   - Pregnancy must be excluded in reproductive age group.
   - Pap test should be done in all married women after 21 years.
   - Endometrial sampling with an endometrial biopsy or D and C is mandatory when both a pelvic mass and abnormal bleeding are present. An endometrial lesion (carcinoma or hyperplasia) may coexist with a benign mass such as a leiomyoma or hormonally active ovarian cysts.
   - After clinical work-up, patients are advised further given investigations.

Imaging

Ultrasonography

Ultrasonography is the most valuable tool for diagnosing adnexal masses, it differentiates ovarian masses from masses of other origin. Characteristics of ovarian mass such as unilocular, multilocular or cyst with solid component can be determined on USG and thus helps in discriminating benign from malignant ovarian masses *transvaginal ultrasound* is very effective and is preferred over transabdominal sonography (TAS) due to its increased sensitivity for internal architecture or anatomy of the mass and used as the first-line imaging modality in reproductive and postmenopausal women. Transabdominal ultrasound is used when an ovarian cyst is large or beyond the field of view of transvaginal sonography (TVS). Based on internal architecture ovarian cysts may be classified as:[1]

- *Simple cyst:* Simple are seen as anechoic lesion with posterior acoustic enhancement, they are unilocular with thin and smooth walls and have no solid or vascularized component. Most simple cysts are functional cysts, usually follicular cysts. They are commonly seen in premenopausal women, but can be seen in prepubertal and postmenopausal women also. Some simple cysts may turn out to be paraovarian or paratubal cyst on laparotomy.
- *Hemorrhagic ovarian cyst:* Hemorrhagic ovarian cysts are formed due to expanding hemorrhage within a corpus luteum or other functional cyst. Hemorrhagic cysts are seen

as a complex cystic mass with internal echoes but without internal blood flow.
- *Dermoid cysts:* Dermoid cysts may occur in any age group but most frequently seen in reproductive periods. They are suspected if ultrasound shows following features:
  - Hypoechoic mass with *hyperechoic nodule* (Rokitansky nodule or dermoid plug)
  - Usually unilocular (90%)
  - May contain calcifications (30%)
  - May contain hyperechoic lines caused by floating hair
  - May contain a fat-fluid level, i.e. fat floating on aqueous fluid.
- *Endometrioma:* They are seen as homogeneous and hypoechoic mass with diffuse low-level echoes (ground-glass) without any internal flow at color Doppler and without any enhancing nodules or solid masses. In 30% echogenic foci are seen within cyst, this finding makes diagnosis of endometrioma more likely.
- *Benign neoplasm:* Benign neoplasm is suspected in case of a cysts with multiple thin (<3 mm) septations, i.e. multiloculated or with a small solid nodule, but without detectable flow on Doppler USG. Irregularity or tiny areas of focal thickening of the cyst wall may be sometimes difficult to distinguish from a small solid component and thus, are indeterminate for malignancy. Cysts with these indeterminate features requires follow-up at short-interval (6–12 weeks) with USG or occasionally with magnetic resonance imaging (MRI) for further characterization.[2] Short-interval follow-up of 6-12 weeks allow sufficient time for a physiologic cyst to resolve. If the lesion persists, and continues to have indeterminate findings at USG or MRI, surgical evaluation should be considered.
  - *Serous cystadenoma* are usually thin walled (less than 3 mm) cyst, unilocular or rarely multilocular cysts. They are usually bilateral and smaller than mucinous cystadenomas.
  - *Mucinous cystadenoma* are larger in size than serous cystadenoma. On US and MRI, it presents as multilocular (honeycomb like locules) with a thin regular wall and septa without any endo- or exocytic vegetation.
  - *Ovarian cystadenofibroma* occur in the reproductive period and are usually benign and an accurate preoperative diagnosis may avoid surgical intervention. On imaging some of them are purely cystic and resemble cystadenomas while others may have complex cystic masses with a solid component and/or thick septa, thereby mimicking a malignant lesion.
- *Paraovarian cysts:* It may be difficult to decide whether such a cystic mass rises from one ovary or the other. In such cases, MRI may be done to verify the nature of such cystic masses. They can attain very large size, but usually have simple cyst characteristics.

> There is no clear consensus regarding the need for further imaging apart from transvaginal ultrasound in the presence of apparently benign disease. However, these additional imaging modalities like CT, MRI have a place in the evaluation of more complex lesions (Evidence Level 2++).

Doppler Ultrasound

It is helpful in ovarian torsion (discussed later). They may also be used in discriminating the benign from malignant. Malignant masses generally demonstrate neovascularity, with abnormal branching patterns or vessel morphology. These neovessels have lower resistance flow than native ovarian vessels.

Abdominal Radiograph

It can detect pelvic calcifications (teeth) consistent with a benign cystic teratoma, a calcified uterine fibroid, or scattered calcifications consistent with psammoma bodies of a papillary serous cystadenoma.

CT or MRI

It may be advised in case of the following:
- When a nongynecologic origin of an adnexal cyst is suspected.

- When a malignant cyst is suspected as it can detect omental metastases, peritoneal implants, pelvic or para-aortic lymph node enlargement, hepatic metastases, obstructive uropathy.
- Alternate primary cancer site, including pancreas or colon is suspected.

Tumor Markers

Tumor markers are useful aid in evaluation of ovarian masses.
- *Cancer antigen 125 (CA125):* CA 125 is raised in over 80% of cases with epithelial ovarian cancer.[3] It helps in differentiating benign from malignant ovarian mass.

  In premenopausal woman, it has a limited role (Evidence Level 2++) due to its low sensitivity as it is increased in various other causes like PID, uterine leiomyoma, pregnancy, endometriosis, adenomyosis, acute pancreatitis, liver cirrhosis.

  So, in this age group serial monitoring of CA125 is more helpful as rapidly rising levels are more likely to be associated with malignancy than high levels which remain static. But if levels of CA125 assay is more than 200 units/mL, possibility of malignancy is to be kept in mind.

  In postmenopausal woman CA125 has a sensitivity and specificity of 78% (Evidence Level 2+) in differentiating benign from malignant ovarian masses.[4] A routinely used cut-off value is 35 IU/mL. While a high value helps in ascertaining the diagnosis, a normal value does not exclude ovarian cancer due to the nonspecific nature of the test.
- *AFP, beta-hCG, LDH:* These are useful in diagnosis of germ cell tumor and are advised in prepubertal girls with suspicion of malignancy as these are the most common tumor in children and adolescents. They should be measured in premenopausal women with complex ovarian mass because of the possibility of germ cell tumors.

Since the causes and management of benign adnexal masses varies in different age group due to concern of preservation of future fertility and risk of malignancy, chapter will be further discussed in three groups (1) prepubertal (2) reproductive (3) postmenopausal, though there may be some overlap.

PREPUBERTAL AGE GROUP

Diagnosis of adnexal masses are often missed or delayed in this age group due to low level of suspicion, nonspecific abdominal symptoms which mimics more common causes such as appendicitis. Pelvic masses, very quickly becomes abdominal in location as it enlarges in this age group because of the small size of the pelvic cavity and thus, further confounding the diagnosis with other common abdominal masses occurring in children, such as Wilms' tumor or neuroblastoma. Another concern in this age group is limitation of pelvic examination as pervaginal examination is not performed due to intact hymen. Diagnosis is often made by abdominal palpation and bimanual rectoabdominal examination.

Common causes are following:
- Ovarian
  - Functional ovarian cysts
  - Germ cell tumor
- Genital tuberculosis
- Obstructive mullerian anomalies; hematometra/hematosalpinx.

Ovarian Tumors

Functional cysts: Functional ovarian cysts are the most common adnexal mass in all pediatric age groups.[5] Usually ovarian follicles are anechoic and <3 cm in diameter but sometimes they fail to involute and mature into functional cysts and corpus luteal cysts. In prepubertal girls ovarian cysts are caused due to intermittent gonadotropin production by the developing pituitary gland.[6]

Germ cell tumors: Germ cell tumors are derived from primordial germ cells of the ovaries. They are the most common ovarian neoplasm in children and adolescents and account for approximately 70% of ovarian neoplasms in children and adolescents compared to 20% of these tumors in adults and one-third of these are malignant.[7,8] Germ cell tumors are classified on the basis of histology (Table 23.2). All germ cell tumors are malignant except *gonadoblastoma, mature cystic teratomas and struma ovarii which are benign.*

Benign cystic teratomas (dermoid cysts): They are the most common neoplasm in pediatric age group and constitute 55–70% of pediatric ovarian neoplasms and are bilateral in up to 10% of cases.[9] The risk of torsion with dermoid cysts is high (15%) as compared to other ovarian tumors because of the high-fat content of dermoid cysts, allowing them to float within the abdominal and pelvic cavity.[10] As a result of this fat content dermoid cyst are frequently described as anterior in location on pelvic examination.

Gonadoblastoma: Gonadoblastomas are rare germ cell tumors found in patients with mosaic Turner's syndrome (46X/46XY karyotype), pure gonadal dysgenesis (46XY) or rarely a 46XX karyotype containing a part of the Y-chromosome. Although pure gonadoblastoma is a benign neoplasm, risk of malignant transformation is high and thus, the treatment of choice remains bilateral gonadectomy in all mosaic Turner's syndrome (46X/46XY karyotype) or 46XY patients with pure gonadal dysgenesis. In 46XX patients with mixed gonadal dysgenesis and a normal appearing ovary on one side, streak gonad is removed alongwith biopsy of the normal appearing ovary with close follow-up.[11]

Management

Conservative Management

Small unilocular thin walled cysts less than 7 cm are usually always benign and regresses in 3–6 months; thus, they do not require surgical management and patients are asked to follow-up with repeat scan after 3 months.[10] But risk of ovarian torsion in cysts larger than 5 cm must be discussed with the child's parents.

In patients with simple cysts where the treatment plan includes follow-up with serial ultrasounds, serum AFP and beta-hCG should be done if cysts persists beyond 3 months as although rare (<1%), but malignancy has been reported in these simple cysts also.[12]

In prepubertal girls with multilocular cysts, karyotyping is advised to exclude gonadoblastoma.

Surgical treatment: It is required in:
- Symptomatic cysts (although mildly symptomatic cysts presumed to be functional may be managed with analgesics) to prevent surgical complications
- Solid suspicious masses
- Enlarging masses
- Masses larger than 8 cm (even if unilocular as there is high risk of torsion).

Oophorectomy should be avoided for benign masses as preservation of ovarian tissue alongwith symptom relief is the primary goal in this age group.

Table 23.2 Classification of germ cell tumors		
Primitive GCT	Biphasic or triphasic teratoma	Monodermal teratoma and somatic type tumors

• Gonadoblastoma
• Dysgerminoma
• Yolk sac tumor
• Embryonal carcinoma
• Polyembryoma
• Nongestational choriocarcinoma
• Mixed germ cell tumor
	• Immature teratoma
	• Mature teratoma
	  – Solid
	  – Cystic
	    - Dermoid cyst
	    - Fetiform teratoma
		• Thyroid tumor (Struma ovarii)
		  – Benign
		  – Malignant
		• Carcinoid
		• Neuroectodermal tumors

Abbreviation: GCT, germ cell tumor

Laparoscopic cystectomy is the method of choice in case of unilocular cyst.

The role of laparoscopy has been more controversial in the removal of dermoid cysts than with other benign masses due to risk of spillage of the cyst contents and consequent chemical peritonitis. If inadvertent spillage occurs, meticulous peritoneal lavage is performed using large amounts of warmed fluid.

Genital Tuberculosis

Genital tuberculosis is typically seen in young women between 20 and 40 years of age, but it may also occur in girls before puberty or in postmenopausal women. It is said that bilateral pelvic masses in a virgin girl is almost always tubercular in origin. Clinical features and management of genital tuberculosis is described later in postmenopausal section.

Obstructive Mullerian Anomalies

Patients with these conditions may present as adnexal mass when menstruation starts as menstrual blood tends to collect behind the obstruction. Initially vagina fills with blood (hematocolpos), which increases gradually and in course of time the cervix, uterus (hematocervix and hematometra), and finally the tube (hematosalpinx) is filled with blood which may lead to uterine and adnexal masses. Diagnosis is suspected when patient presents with amenorrhea in the presence of secondary sexual characters, cyclic abdominal discomfort, urinary symptoms (retention of urine) and abdominopelvic mass.

- *Imperforate hymen:* It can be detected on local examination. On performing the valsalva maneuver, the membrane bulges outward and seen as convex bluish bulge. Pelvic sonography reveals presence of hematocolpos, hematometra hematosalpinx and presence of internal genitalia. The membrane is excised in cruciate manner with free drainage of collected blood. The edges subsequently heal rapidly.

- *Transverse vaginal septum:* The most common site for the occurrence of a transverse septum is the junction of the upper and middle third of the vagina. Transverse septum reveals presence of a short vagina, and absence of bulging on Valsalva maneuver.
Treatment consists of surgical excision of the septum.

REPRODUCTIVE AGE

In reproductive age group, PID and pregnancy-related problems dominate the etiology though neoplasms have to be kept in mind. Common causes are enumerated in Table 23.3.

Ovarian Tumor

Ovarian masses are divided into functional and neoplastic and neoplastic masses may be benign or malignant. Approximately 60–70% of ovarian

Table 23.3 Common causes in reproductive age group

Gynecologic origin		

• Ovarian
  – Functional
    - Follicular cysts
    - Corpus luteum cysts
    - Theca lutein cyst
  – Neoplastic
    - Cystadenomas (serous/mucinous)
    - Fibroma
    - Brenner tumor
    - Teratoma
	• Tubal
	  – Pyosalpinx
	  – Hydrosalpinx
	  – Hematosalpinx
		• Others
		  – Endometrioma
		  – Tubo-ovarian abscess
		  – Ectopic pregnancy
		  – Leiomyoma
		  – Paraovarian cyst

Nongynecologic		
• Appendiceal abscess • Pelvic kidney • Diverticulosis • Peritoneal inclusion cyst • Feces in rectosigmoid		

tumors are encountered during the reproductive years and most (80–85%) of them are benign in this age group.[13] The chance that a primary ovarian tumor is malignant in a woman of less than 45 years is less than 1 in 15, but this risk increases with the advancing age.[10] Thus, the approach of management of ovarian masses in a perimenopausal woman becomes similar to postmenopausal woman.

Functional Ovarian Cysts

Include follicular cysts, corpus luteum cysts, and theca lutein cysts. They are essentially benign and usually do not cause symptoms or require surgical management.

- *Follicular cysts:* The most common functional cyst is the follicular cyst and is seldom larger than 8 cm. Cysts less than 3 cm are normal follicles during reproductive age group. Thus, cystic follicle is defined as a follicular cyst only when its diameter is greater than 3 cm. These cysts are usually found incidentally during pelvic examination or lower abdominal ultrasound done for other reasons. Sometimes they may rupture, resulting in acute abdomen. They usually resolve in 4–8 weeks.
- *Corpus luteum cysts* are less common than follicular cysts. They may rupture, leading to a hemoperitoneum and may require surgical management. Cyst rupture generally occurs on day 20–26 and may occur after exercise or intercourse. Patients on anticoagulation are at particular risk.
- *Theca lutein* cysts are the least common of functional ovarian cysts. They are usually bilateral, multicystic and regress spontaneously. They may grow to quite large (up to 30 cm) and may be found with the following conditions: molar pregnancies, choriocarcinoma, clomiphene citrate and GnRH analogs therapy.
- *Hemorrhagic cysts* may be formed due to bleeding into the corpus luteal cysts. Patient may present with mild pain and are managed conservatively with analgesics. They typically resolve within 8 weeks. In women of reproductive age, cysts ≤5 cm: do not need follow-up while cysts >5 cm: are asked to follow-up with repeat scan at 6–12 weeks.[1]

Since women in early postmenopause may occasionally ovulate and develop complex cysts with the appearance of a classic hemorrhagic cyst and patients are asked to follow-up with repeat scan at 6–12 weeks. Late postmenopausal women should never have a hemorrhagic cyst, any cyst with such an appearance should be considered neoplastic and surgical evaluation should be considered.[1]

Benign Ovarian Tumors

Epithelial tumors

- *Serous cystadenomas:* Serous tumors are generally benign; 5–10% have borderline malignant potential and 20–25% are malignant.[10] Serous cystadenomas occur in 3rd–5th decades of life and risk of malignancy increases with the advancing age.
- *Mucinous ovarian tumors:* Mucinous tumors are multiloculated cysts and contains mucoid material within the cystic loculations. Benign mucinous tumors typically have a lobulated and smooth surface. They may grow to very large size filling the abdominal cavity. They are usually unilateral but may be bilateral in up to 10% of cases and 5–10% of them are malignant.[10]

Pseudomyxoma peritonei: Sometimes mucinous tumor may rupture leading to spread of abundant mucoid or gelatinous material within the pelvis and abdominal cavity surrounded by fibrous tissue leading to extensive visceral adhesions. They may also occur with appendiceal mucinous neoplasm.

- *Brenner tumors:* It is an essentially benign and rare (1–2%) solid fibroepithelial tumor. Small to moderate in size, the tumor is generally seen in peri- or postmenopausal women and may causes postmenopausal bleeding. Sometimes, it may be associated with ascites and hydrothorax (*Meigs syndrome*).

Benign cystic teratoma (dermoid cysts): Dermoid cysts have a wider range of age distribution, but most of them occur in reproductive years.

Fibromas: Ovarian fibroma comprises about 3% of ovarian neoplasms and less than 1% of them are malignant. They are benign sex cord stromal tumor and has no particular age incidence. The tumors are often accompanied by ascites and sometimes with hydrothorax. The triad of an ovarian fibroma with ascites and hydrothorax (usually right-sided) is known as *Meigs syndrome*. Meigs syndrome can occur with other solid ovarian tumors such as granulosa cell tumor and Brenner tumor.

> Ascites is not associated with benign tumors, but Brenner tumor and fibromas are the exception.

Management of Ovarian Masses

Conservative Management (Evidence Level 4)

Women with asymptomatic simple cystic structures of less than 50 mm are more likely to be physiological and almost always resolve within 3 menstrual cycles.[14,15]

- Simple cysts 30–50 mm in diameter do not require follow-up.
- Simple cysts 50–70 mm require yearly follow-up with USG.
- Cysts more than 70 mm in diameter should be considered for either further imaging (MRI) or surgical intervention due to difficulties in examining the entire cyst adequately at time of ultrasound.[16]

Surgical Management

It is warranted in the following cases[15] (Evidence Level 4):
- Larger cysts (>8 cm) as they are prone for torsion/rupture.
- Cysts that persist or increase in size after several cycles as they are less likely to be functional.
- Symptomatic cysts (although mildly symptomatic masses suspected to be functional should be managed with analgesics rather than surgery to avoid the development of adhesions that may impair subsequent fertility).
- Severe pain or the suspicion of rupture or torsion.

- Mature cystic teratomas (dermoid cysts) have been shown to grow over time increasing the risk of pain and ovarian accidents.
- On ultrasonography, large cysts and those that have multiloculations, septa, papillae, and increased blood flow is suspicious of neoplasia and exploratory laparotomy is warranted in such cases.

Role of aspiration: Aspiration of ovarian cysts is not recommended as it is less effective and is associated with a high rate of recurrence (Evidence Level 2++). Ultrasonographic or CT-directed aspiration procedures should not be used in women in whom there is a suspicion of malignancy.[13]

Laparoscopy: The laparoscopic approach is preferred over laprotomy for ovarian masses presumed to be benign as it is associated with lower postoperative morbidity and shorter recovery (Evidence Level 1++).[17-19]

Endometriomas ("Chocolate" Cysts)

Approximately 10–15% of reproductive-aged women have endometriosis.[20] Women with endometriosis may develop ovarian endometrioma which may enlarge to 6–8 cm size and may be suspected when a mass does not resolve with observation. In women of any age, probable endometriomas require initial 6–12 week follow-up to rule out a hemorrhagic cyst.[1] About 1% of endometriomas are believed to undergo malignant transformation, usually endometrioid or clear cell carcinoma.[21] So, until surgically removed, endometriomas require follow-up with ultrasound on a yearly basis to ensure the change in cyst size or internal architecture (for example, new development of a solid element).[1] Rapid cyst growth or development of a significant solid component with flow at Doppler USG should raise concern for malignancy.

Inflammatory Masses

Inflammatory masses can be sequelae of PID or genital tuberculosis. They may be in the form of hydrosalpinx, pyosalpinx, tubo-ovarian cysts or tubo-ovarian abscess (TOA). In tubo-ovarian cyst, there is communication between hydrosalpinx and follicular cyst of the ovary, while in TOA ovarian abscess communicates with pyosalpinx.

Clinical Features

Patients commonly presents as chronic pelvic pain, dysmenorrhea, dyspareunia, dysuria, urinary frequency and rectal discomfort. Occasionally, fever with the symptoms of pelvic peritonitis may develop. Pervaginal examination may reveal fixed and retroverted uterus, adnexal or cervical motion tenderness, enlarged masses adherent to the cul-de-sac or lateral to uterus and are usually bilateral adnexa is indurated with immobilized pelvic structures (*frozen pelvis*).

Diagnosis

Ultrasonography: Often, the tubal contour cannot be clearly delineated, and therefore, ultrasonography simply shows a dilated, tortuous structure in the adnexal region. A hydrosalpinx is generally anechoic, whereas a pyosalpinx may have increased echoes within the fluid and thus is hyperechoic. Fluid may also be seen in the cul-de-sac. TOA are seen as complex cystic, thick walled, irregular mass in adnexa or POD, can be multiloculated with septations or solid components leading to varied echotexture.

CT scan: In case of TOA shows spherical/tubular structure with low attenuation center along with thick walls and septations. Internal gas bubbles or air fluid levels if present are pathognomonic of inflammatory masses. Free fluid may be present.

Treatment

TOA is treated with parental antibiotic regimen and 75% of the patients generally responds to antimicrobial therapy. Failure of medical therapy may require USG/CT-guided percutaneous drainage or surgical exploration. Trocar drainage with or without placement of drain is successful in almost 90% of the cases.[22]

Suspected inflammatory mass not resolving on antibiotics may be tubercular in nature.

Chronic Ectopic Pregnancies

Chronic ectopic pregnancy is to be suspected in any women of reproductive age positive pregnancy test and adnexal mass. Clinical features, diagnosis and management is described in respective chapter of this book.

Leiomyomas

Pedunculated or broad ligament fibroids often mimic adnexal masses. Common symptoms include chronic pelvic pain, dysmenorrhea/dyspareunia. Acute pain may result from torsion of a pedunculated leiomyoma or infarction and degeneration. Urinary symptoms include frequency due to extrinsic pressure on the bladder. Partial ureteral obstruction may be caused by pressure from large tumors at the pelvic brim. Bowel disturbances such as constipation due to rectosigmoid compression or intestinal obstruction. Venous stasis of the lower extremities and possible thrombophlebitis secondary to pelvic compression and polycythemia (broad ligament fibroids) are less common.

Abdominopelvic examination may reveal adnexal mass separate from uterus, firm in consistency and nontender.

Ultrasound helps in ascertaining the diagnosis and shows well-defined mass with hypoechoic contents. Ultrasonography or an intravenous pyelogram may be appropriate to demonstrate ureteral deviation, compression, or dilation in the presence of large and laterally located fibroids. Such findings may be indication for surgical intervention for otherwise asymptomatic leiomyomas. Laparoscopic myomectomy is the procedure of choice in expert hand.

Paraovarian Cysts

Parovarian cysts are extraperitoneal cysts lying in the broad ligament adjacent to the ovary, below the fallopian tube. They are generally seen in younger women. Small parovarian cysts are extremely common and may be an incidental finding during laparotomy performed for other reasons. They sometimes form a cyst as large as 15–30 cm in diameter. They usually unilocular, and contains clear fluid. Its wall is smooth, thin and translucent. Unlike the ovarian cyst, the wall of a parovarian cyst frequently contains smooth muscle as do the mesonephric tubules. Parovarian cyst is clinically diagnosed as an ovarian cyst and identified as a broad ligament cyst on laparotomy. Histological identification of the muscle in a cyst establishes the correct diagnosis.

POSTMENOPAUSAL AGE GROUP

Benign adnexal masses in a postmenopausal women are mostly ovarian in origin, although inflammatory masses also come in differential diagnosis and common causes are enumerated in Table 23.4.

Ovarian Tumor

Main concern of the ovarian masses in this age group is the risk of malignancy which increases with age. About 30% of the ovarian neoplasms are malignant in postmenopausal women whereas the frequency is 7% in premenopausal women.[23] So it is important to timely diagnose and differentiate a benign from malignant ovarian mass and to proceed accordingly.

Table 23.4 Common causes in postmenopausal women

Ovarian masses
- Benign ovarian tumors
  - Serous cystadenoma
  - Mucinous cystadenoma
  - Brenner tumor
  - Mature cystic teratoma
  - Fibroma
  - Thecomas
- Functional ovarian cysts

Inflammatory masses
- Gynecologic—Tubercular masses
- Nongynecologic—Diverticulitis

Ovarian cysts are observed in 5–17% of cases of postmenopausal women.[24-26] The risk of malignancy is low (1%) in small unilocular cysts whereas large, complex cysts in postmenopausal women have the risk of malignancy in 6–39% of the cases[27,28] and thus predicting the approach of management accordingly as described below:

Risk of malignancy index
The risk of malignancy index (RMI) was first described by Jacobs in 1990 and since then used to predict ovarian malignancy. It is calculated using ultrasound characteristics, menopausal status and levels of CA125. It is used in both premenopausal and postmenopausal women, but its sensitivity is less in premenopausal women as CA125 is increased in various benign causes as described above. The NICE guideline on ovarian cancer recommends that RMI score should be calculated and used for further management in women with suspected ovarian malignancy[29] (Evidence Level 1+). RMI score with a threshold of 200 predicts the likelihood of ovarian cancer with sensitivity of 78% and specificity of 87% and helps in planning further management (Evidence Level 1++). CT of the abdomen and pelvis should

Table 23.5 Calculation of the risk of malignancy index

RMI = U x M x CA-125	Ultrasounds characteristics (U) U = 0 (for an ultrasound score of 0) U = 1 (for an ultrasound score of 1) U = 3 (for an ultrasound score of 2–5)	Menopausal status (M)	CA-125 level
	Bilateral lesions	Premenopausal : M=1	U per mL
	Evidence of metastasis	Postmenopausal: M=3	
	Evidence of solid areas		
	Multilocular cysts		
	Presence of ascites		

be performed for all postmenopausal women with ovarian cysts who have a RMI score greater than or equal to 200 (Table 23.5).[30]

Management of Ovarian Cysts

Conservative management: A simple, unilateral, unilocular ovarian cysts less than 5 cm in diameter and asymptomatic cysts generally have a low risk of malignancy. In the presence of normal serum CA125 levels, these cysts can be managed conservatively, with a repeat evaluation in 4–6 months (Evidence Level 2-).[30]

Surgical management: Suspicious or persistent complex adnexal mass or if a woman is symptomatic, further surgical evaluation is necessary.

Role of laparoscopy in postmenopausal ovarian cysts: Women with a RMI of less than 200 (i.e. at low risk of malignancy) can be considered for laparoscopic management by a surgeon with suitable experience.[29,31] Laparoscopic management of ovarian cysts in postmenopausal women comprises of bilateral salpingo-oophorectomy rather than cystectomy and patients should be counseled preoperatively that procedure may be converted into full staging laparotomy if evidence of ovarian malignancies is found (Evidence Level 1-).

All ovarian cysts that are suspicious of malignancy in a postmenopausal woman, as indicated by a RMI greater than or equal to 200, clinical assessment, CT findings, or findings at laparoscopy, require a full laparotomy and staging procedure (Evidence Level 4).[30]

Inflammatory Masses

Adnexal masses in postmenopausal women suspected to be inflammatory are usually tubercular in origin rather than the complication of PID.

Genital Tuberculosis

It may be suspected on following signs and symptoms.

Clinical features: Patient may be completely asymptomatic or may present with other features such as evening rise low grade fever, malaise, anorexia, vague abdominopelvic pain, vaginal discharge or sometimes as postmenopausal bleeding. Occasionally patient may present with abdominal lump which is a result of encysted ascites, matted intestinal loops, pyometra and tubo-ovarian abscess. Abdominal examination may reveal a "doughy" sensation due to tubercle formation on the intestines and peritoneum. Adnexal mass may be palpated which may vary in size and consistency and may result from thickened edematous tubes, pyosalpinges, matted intestine, omentum and pelvic organs or a tubo-ovarian abscess. These masses are fixed, irregular in shape and usually bilateral. Enlarged and tender uterus may be felt indicating pyometra as a result of stenosed cervix. Ascites may be present in advanced cases.

Diagnosis: It may be difficult as abdominal mass along with ascites in this age group mimics ovarian malignancy. CA125 is raised in tuberculosis also further confounding the diagnosis. Routine laboratory studies may show raised ESR or lymphocytosis. Chest X-ray may show features of active or old healed tubercular infection. Endometrial histology/culture may help in establishing diagnosis. PCR testing of the endometrial tissue/menstrual blood can also be done. Laparoscopy with peritoneal biopsy can be performed if diagnosis remains uncertain.

Management: Antitubercular therapy (ATT) remains the mainstay of therapy.

Acute diverticulitis: Acute diverticulitis is a condition in which there is inflammation of a diverticulum or outpouching of the wall of the colon, usually involving the sigmoid. Diverticulitis typically affects postmenopausal women but can occur in women in their 30s and 40s.

Clinical Features

Patients presents with severe, left lower quadrant pain often associated with fever, chills, and constipation. Past history of symptoms of irritable bowel (bloating, constipation, and diarrhea) may be revealed. Abdominopelvic examination may reveal a poorly defined, mobile, doughy inflammatory mass in the left lower quadrant, often associated with tenderness. Bowel sounds are sluggish and may be absent if peritonitis is present.

Diagnosis and Management

Leukocytosis is frequently is associated. CT scan reveals swollen edematous bowel and differentiates it from abscess. Initial management includes broad-spectrum intravenous antibiotics alongwith IV fluids and restriction of oral intake. Presence of diverticular abscess requires surgical intervention.

COMPLICATIONS OF ADNEXAL MASSES

Torsion

It can occur in any age group, but is more likely in prepubertal girls because ovarian ligament becomes elongated due to abdominal location of ovarian tumors in this age group and thus predisposing to torsion. Cysts larger than 8 cm, are prone to rupture. A benign cystic teratoma is the most common neoplasm to undergo torsion.

Clinical features: Patients typically presents with the sudden, severe, sharp/stabbing unilateral lower abdominal pain that worsens intermittently over many hours. The pain is usually localized over the affected side but may radiated to the back, pelvis, or thigh. Fever, nausea and vomiting is usually present in cases of torsion.

On examination, the abdomen is tender, and localized rebound tenderness can be noted in the lower quadrants. The most important sign is the presence of a large pelvic mass on physical examination. Mild temperature elevation and leukocytosis may accompany the infarction. The diagnosis must be suspected in any woman with acute pain and unilateral adnexal mass.

Diagnosis: On ultrasonography—enlarged ovaries as a result of blocked venous and lymphatic drainage is the most common sonographic finding. Due to ovarian edema and venous congestion small follicles are displaced peripherally and seen as multiple peripheral cysts within the ovary. Irregular echogenic areas may also be seen within the ovary due to stromal edema and/or hemorrhage.

Color Doppler is the *method of choice* for the diagnosis of adnexal torsion. The most common finding is little or no intraovarian venous flow, absence of arterial flow is less common and occurs in prolonged state and is a poor prognostic sign. Twisted vascular pedicle may be seen as whirlpool (*Whirlpool sign*). A positive Whirlpool sign is most definitive sign of ovarian torsion. Sometimes in cases of intermittent torsion or dual supply from both the ovarian and uterine arteries, vascularity may not be disturbed and thus normal vascularity does not exclude torsion.

Management: Primary management in any age group is surgical. Both laparoscopy/laparotomy can be performed depending upon the skill of surgeon. Procedure includes detorsion with ovarian cystectomy, if a cyst is present. Oophorectomy should be avoided as ovarian function frequently resumes even in ovaries appearing to be nonviable.

Rupture

Functional ovarian cysts (e.g. follicle, corpus luteum) rupture more readily compared to other benign or malignant masses. Nonmalignant neoplasms such as cystic teratomas (dermoid cysts) or cystadenomas or inflammatory ovarian masses, such as endometriomas, can also rupture.

Clinical features: There is sudden onset of pain and is usually generalized in whole abdomen. Presence of syncope and dizziness or syncope indicates hemoperitoneum. Patient may be pale depending on the amount of hemoperitoneum. Abdomen may be distended and tender due to peritonitis. On pelvic examination, mass may be found if the cyst is leaking and not completely ruptured.

As these presentation simulate ruptured ectopic, pregnancy tests must be done to rule out ectopic.

Diagnosis: Complete blood count, ultrasound or culdocentesis are used for confirm the diagnosis. The culdocentesis is helpful in determining the cause of peritonitis.
- Fresh blood—corpus luteum, chocolate color old blood—endometrioma
- Oily sebaceous fluid—benign teratoma
- Purulent fluid—tubo-ovarian abscess.

Management: Surgical exploration is indicated if cyst rupture leads to hemoperitoneum (corpus luteum) or chemical peritonitis (endometrioma, benign cyst teratoma), which could impair future fertility. Orthostasis, anemia, or hematocrit of the culdocentesis fluid of greater than 16% suggests hemoperitoneum and usually requires surgical treatment by laparoscopy or laparotomy. Patients who are not orthostatic or anemic and who have a small amount of blood in the cul-de-sac fluid (culdocentesis fluid hematocrit less than 16%) can often be observed in the hospital, without surgical intervention, or even discharged home from the emergency room after observation.

Infection

Ovarian cysts may get infected in the course of PID or following puerperium as a part of ascending infection. Patient may present with fever or peritonitis in advanced cases. Sometimes tubo-ovarian abscess may rupture leading to generalized peritonitis and septicemia and is a life-threatening condition. Broad spectrum antibiotics are started along with fluid resuscitation. Immediate surgery is required which consists of drainage of the pelvic abscess and copious irrigation of the abdominal cavity.

KEY POINTS

- The adnexa comprises of the ovaries, fallopian tubes, and structures of the broad ligament and their pathology may lead to adnexal masses.
- Functional cysts are common during reproductive age group. They are usually asymptomatic and regresses with time.
- Genital tuberculosis is the common differential diagnosis of adnexal masses in all age groups and bilateral adnexal masses in a virgin girl is almost always tubercular.
- Benign cysts are simple, cystic, mobile and generally unilateral and not associated with ascites.
- Transvaginal ultrasound is highly sensitive for internal architecture or anatomy of the mass and used as the first-line imaging modality for adnexal masses.
- CA125 is a sensitive marker for epithelial ovarian cancers in postmenopausal women, but is less reliable in premenopausal women. A routinely used cut-off value is 35 IU/mL in postmenopausal women.
- AFP, bhCG, LDH are advised in prepubertal girls to rule out germ cell tumor as these are the most common tumors in children and adolescents.
- Of all germ cell tumors gonadoblastoma, mature cystic teratomas and struma ovarii are benign and rest all are malignant.
- In prepubertal girls with multilocular cysts, karyotyping is advised to exclude gonadoblastoma.
- Dermoid cysts constitute 55–70% of pediatric ovarian neoplasms and are bilateral in up to 10% of cases.
- Ovarian tumors in reproductive age group is generally benign but risk of malignancy increases with the advancing age.
- Pregnancy must be excluded in reproductive age group in women with pelvic mass.
- Suspected inflammatory mass not resolving on antibiotics may be tubercular in nature and must be investigated.
- RMI score with a threshold of 200 predicts the likelihood of ovarian cancer with sensitivity of 78% and specificity of 87%. CT of the abdomen and pelvis should be performed for all postmenopausal women with ovarian cysts who have a RMI score greater than or equal to 200.
- Not all cysts in postmenopausal women needs surgical management. A simple, unilateral, unilocular ovarian cysts less than 5 cm in

diameter have low risk of malignancy and in the presence of normal serum CA125 levels, these cysts can be managed conservatively, with a repeat evaluation in 4-6 months (Evidence Level 2-).
- Laparoscopic cystectomy is the method of choice in case of simple cyst in any age group.

REFERENCES

1. Deborah Levine, et al. Management of asymptomatic ovarian and other adnexal cysts imaged at US: Society of Radiologists in Ultrasound Consensus Conference Statement. 2010;256:943-54.
2. American College of Radiology. ACR Appropriateness Criteria: clinically suspected adnexal masses. http://www.acr.org/Secondary Main MenuCategories/quality_safety/app_criteria/ pdf/ExpertPanelonWomensImaging/Suspected AdnexalMassesDoc11.aspx. Accessed September. 2009.
3. Zorn KK, Tian C, McGuire WP, Hoskins WJ, Markman M, Muggia FM, et al. The prognostic value of pretreatment CA 125 in patients with advanced ovarian carcinoma: a Gynecologic Oncology Group study. Cancer. 2009;115:1028-35.
4. Myers ER, Bastian LA, Havrilesky LJ, Kulasingam SL, Terplan MS, Cline KE, et al. Management of adnexal mass. Evid Rep Technol Assess (Full Rep). 2006;130:1-145.
5. Cassandra M Kelleher, Allan M. Goldstein. Adnexal Masses in children and adolescent. Clinical Obstetrics and Gynecology. 2015;58:76-92.
6. Brandt ML, Helmrath MA. Ovarian cysts in infants and children. Semin Pediatr Surg. 2005;14:78-85.
7. Breen JL, Maxson WS. Ovarian tumors in children and adolescents. Clin Obstet Gynecol. 1977; 20:607-23.
8. Berek JS, Hacker NF. Practical Gynecologic oncology, 3rd edn. Philadelphia: Lippincott Williams & Wilkins; 2000.pp.3-38.
9. Choudhary S, Fasih N, Mc Innes M, et al. Imaging of ovarian teratomas: appearances and complications. J Med Imaging Radiat Oncol. 2009;53:480-8.
10. Paulla J Adams Hillard. Benign diseases of the female reproductive tract. Berek, Novak's Gynecology, 15th edn. Wolters Kluwer: Lippincott Williams & Wilkins; 2012.pp.374-437.
11. Esin S, Baser E, Kucukozkan T, et al. Ovarian gonadoblastoma with dysgerminoma in a 15 year-old girl with 46, XX karyotype: case report and review of the literature. Arch Gynecol Obstet. 2012;285:447-51.
12. Valentin L, Ameye L, Franchi D, et al. Risk of malignancy in unilocular cysts: a study of 1148 adnexal masses classified as unilocular cysts at transvaginal ultrasound and review of the literature. Ultrasound Obstet Gynecol. 2013;41:80-9.
13. Cannistra SA. Cancer of ovary. N Engl J Med. 2004; 351:2519-29.
14. MacKenna A, Fabres C, Alam V, Morales V. Clinical management of functional ovarian cysts: a prospective and randomized study. Hum Reprod. 2000;15:2567-9.
15. Royal College of Obstetricians and Gynaecologists. Management of suspected ovarian masses in premenopausal women. RCOG Green-top Guideline No. 62;2011.
16. Levine D, Brown DL, Andreotti RF, Benacerraf B, Benson CB, Brewster WR, et al. Management of asymptomatic ovarian and other adnexal cysts imaged at US: Society of Radiologists in Ultrasound Consensus Conference Statement. Radiology. 2010;256:943-54.
17. Mais V, Ajossa S, Mallarini G, Guerriero S, Oggiano MP, Melis GB. No recurrence of mature ovarian teratomas after laparoscopic cystectomy. BJOG. 2003;110:624-6.
18. Panici PB, Muzii L, Palaia I, Manci N, Bellati F, Plotti F, et al. Minilaparotomy versus laparoscopy in the treatment of benign adnexal cysts: a randomized clinical study. Eur J Obstet Gynecol Reprod Biol. 2007;133:218-22.
19. Fanfani F, Fagotti A, Ercoli A, Bifulco G, Longo R, Mancuso S, et al. A prospective randomised study of laparoscopy and minilaparotomy in the management of benign adnexal masses. Hum Reprod. 2004;19:2367-71.
20. Thomas M.D'Hooghe. Endometriosis. Berek & Novak's Gynecology, 15th edn. Wolters Kluwer: Lippincott Williams & Wilkins; 2012.pp.505-56.
21. Kawaguchi R, Tsuji Y, Haruta S, et al. Clinicopathologic features of ovarian cancer in patients with ovarian endometrioma. J Obstet Gynaecol. 2008;34(5):872-7.
22. Varghese J C, O' Neill M J, Gervais D A, Boland G W, Mueller P R. Transvaginal catheter drainage of tuboovarian abscess using the trocar method: technique and literature review. AJR Am J Roentgenol. 2001;177:139-44.

23. Jonathan S Berek, Teri A Longacre. Ovarian, Fallopian tube and Peritoneal Cancer. Berek & Novak's Gynecology, 15th edn. Wolters Kluwer: Lippincott Williams & Wilkins; 2012.pp.1350-425.
24. Greenlee RT, Kessel B, Williams CR, Riley TL, Ragard LR, Hartge P, et al. Prevalence, incidence, and natural history of simple ovarian cysts among women >55 years old in a large cancer screening trial. Am J Obstet Gynecol. 2010;202:373.e1-9.
25. Zalud I, Busse R, Kurjak BF. Asymptomatic simple ovarian cyst in postmenopausal women: syndrome of 'visible ovary'. Donald School J Ultrasound Obstet Gynecol. 2013;7:182-6.
26. Healy DL, Bell R, Robertson DM, Jobling T, Oehler MK, Edwards A, et al. Ovarian status in healthy postmenopausal women. Menopause. 2008;15:1109-14.
27. Modesitt SC, Pavlik EJ, Ueland FR, et al. Risk of malignancy in unilocular ovarian cystic tumors less than 10 centimeters in diameter. Obstet Gynecol. 2003;102:594-9.
28. Hilger WS, Magrina JF, Magtibay PM. Laparoscopic management of the adnexal mass. Clin Obstet Gynecol. 2006;49:535-48.
29. National Institute for Health and Care Excellence. Ovarian cancer: The recognition and initial management of ovarian cancer. NICE clinical guideline 122. Manchester: NICE; 2011.
30. Royal College of Obstetricians and Gynaecologists. The Management of Ovarian Cysts in Postmenopausal Women. RCOG Green-top Guideline No.34; 2016.
31. Scottish Intercollegiate Guidelines Network. Management of epithelial ovarian cancer. SIGN publication no. 135. Edinburgh: SIGN; 2013.

SECTION 3

Malignant Gynecological Diseases

Chapters

- Premalignant Lesions of Female Lower Genital Tract
- Gestational Trophoblastic Neoplasia
- Vulval Cancer
- Vaginal Cancer
- Carcinoma Cervix
- Endometrial Carcinoma
- Ovarian Cancer
- Borderline Ovarian Tumors
- Introduction to Radiotherapy and Chemotherapy
- Chemotherapy in Gestational Trophoblastic Neoplasia
- Chemoradiotherapy in Carcinoma Vulva
- Chemoradiotherapy in Carcinoma Vagina
- Chemoradiotherapy in Carcinoma Cervix
- Chemoradiotherapy in Carcinoma Endometrium
- Chemotherapy in Ovarian Cancer

SECTION 3

Malignant Gynecological Diseases

24

Premalignant Lesions of Female Lower Genital Tract

Poonam Sachdeva, Akanksha Sharma

Genital tract cancers are associated with high morbidity and mortality in women. Detection of preinvasive lesions is very crucial in preventing such cancers. Among genital tract cancers, cancer of cervix is the most common.

Premalignant lesions of lower genital tract can be picked up in routine screening. Early diagnosis of cancer in preinvasive state has better prognosis and advance-stage morbidity is prevented. Its cheaper as compared to cancer treatment in the long run.

CERVICAL INTRAEPITHELIAL NEOPLASIA

Introduction

Cervical intraepithelial neoplasia (CIN) is a premalignant transformation and abnormal changes in squamous cells on the surface of cervix. The concept of CIN was introduced in 1968 when epithelial changes with appearance of invasive cancer were identified, but they were actually limited to epithelium and if left untreated, could progress to invasive cancer of cervix.[1,2]

Dysplasia is a potentially reversible change characterized by an increase in mitotic rate, atypical cytological features and abnormal organization. In CIN, a part or full thickness of squamous epithelium is replaced by dysplastic cells.

If the dysplastic cells are limited to lower-third, it is called as CIN1. If it involves middle and upper third of epithelium, it is termed as CIN2 and 3 respectively (Fig. 24.1). Most of the CIN1 and 2 lesions regress spontaneously; however, CIN3 may progress to frank cancer if left untreated in which 4% reach the invasive stage by 1 year, 11% by 3 years, 22% by 5 years and 30% by 10 years.[2] CIN is now replaced with low-grade squamous intraepithelial lesion (LSIL) and high-grade squamous intraepithelial lesion (HSIL).

Anatomy of Cervix

The cervix is the lower fibromuscular portion of the uterus. It is cylindrical or conical in shape and measures 3–4 cm in length and 2.5 cm in diameter (Fig. 24.2).

The cervix varies in size and shape depending on the woman's age, parity and hormonal status. The cervix is made up of columnar epithelium lining the endocervical canal and squamous epithelium lining the ectocervix. The point at which they meet is called as squamocolumnar junction.[2,3]

Squamocolumnar Junction

The location of the squamocolumnar junction in relation to the external os is variable (Figs 24.3A to E) and it depends upon a number of factors such as age, hormonal status, birth trauma and certain physiological conditions such as pregnancy.

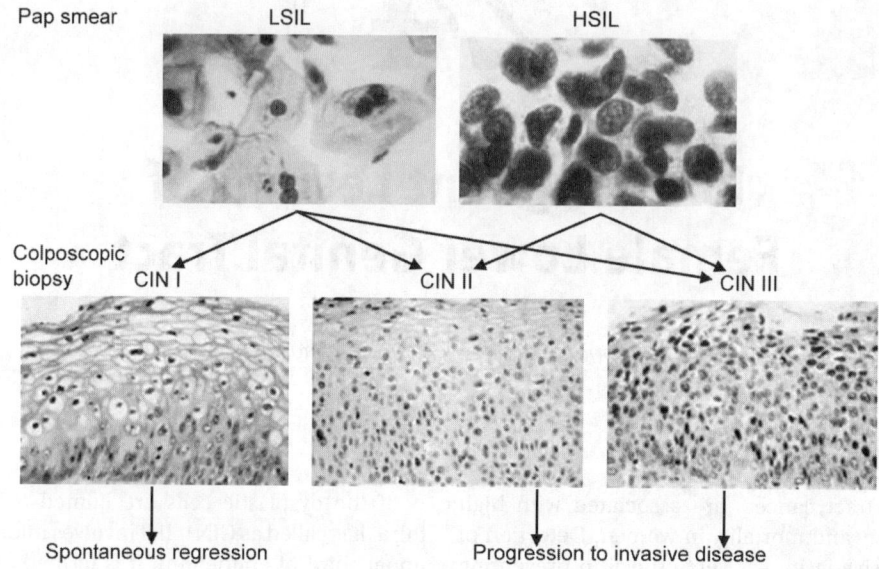

Fig. 24.1 Abnormal cytology and histopathology *(For color version, see Plate 7)*

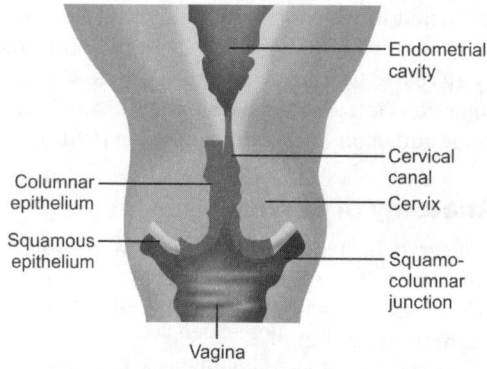

Fig. 24.2 Anatomy of cervix

The squamocolumnar junction visible during childhood, after puberty and early reproductive period is referred to as the original squamocolumnar junction, as this represents the junction between the columnar epithelium and the 'original' squamous epithelium. During childhood, the original squamocolumnar junction is located at or very close to the external os. After puberty and during the reproductive period, the female genital organs grow under the influence of estrogen and the endocervical canal elongates. This leads to the eversion of the columnar epithelium on to the ectocervix. This is called as ectropion or ectopy.[3]

The physiological replacement of the columnar epithelium by a newly formed squamous epithelium is called as squamous metaplasia. The vaginal environment is acidic during the reproductive years and during pregnancy. The irritation of exposed columnar epithelium by the acidic environment leads to the appearance of sub-columnar reserve cells. These cells proliferate causing reserve cell hyperplasia and form the metaplastic squamous epithelium.[3]

Transformation Zone

The region of the cervix where the columnar epithelium has been replaced by the new metaplastic squamous epithelium is referred to as the transformation zone. It corresponds to an area of cervix bound by the original squamocolumnar junction at the distal end and proximally by the furthest extent that squamous

Etiology

Human Papillomavirus Infection

Human papillomavirus (HPV) is a nonenveloped deoxyribonucleic acid (DNA) viruses with approximately 100 serotypes, of which 15–20 are oncogenic.[4,5] HPV is commonly associated with cervical cancer (HPV-16 in 50–60% and HPV-18 in 10–12%). Nononcogenic HPV serotypes-6 and 11 contribute to 90% of benign genital infections.[6]

Etiopathogenesis of cancer cervix is well-explained in Figure 24.5 in association with HPV infection.

Diagnosis of CIN

Diagnosis of CIN is a histopathological diagnosis that is obtained by performing a biopsy from suspicious areas of the cervix. If there is no obvious growth on cervix to target the biopsy, patient has to undergo various screening tests which are as follows:

Visual Inspection with Acetic Acid (VIA)

It is performed by applying dilute (3–5%) acetic acid to the cervix. The acetic acid dehydrates the abnormal areas which have increased nuclear material and protein. Abnormal tissue temporarily appears white when exposed to acetic acid. The cervix is viewed with the naked eye to identify color changes (Fig. 24.6A).

The advantages are that it is simple, easy-to-learn approach, not expensive and the test results are available immediately and as such the issue of follow-up is out of the question. It only requires a single visit. However, there is a need for developing standard training methods and quality assurance measures.[3]

Visual Inspection with Lugol's Iodine

Also known as Schiller's test, uses Lugol's iodine instead of acetic acid and it is also based on color changes. Normal cells which contain glycogen take up iodine and turn mahogany brown whereas abnormal areas remain unstained (Fig. 24.6B).

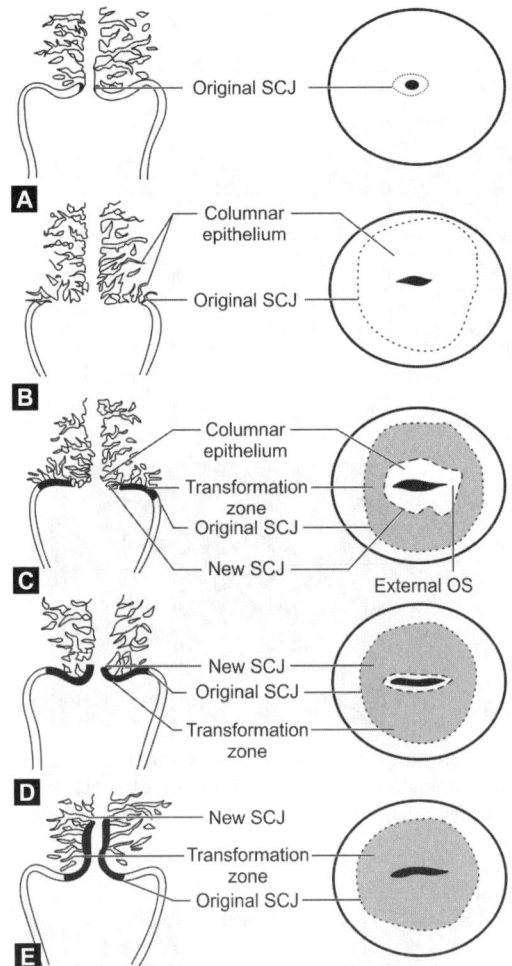

Figs 24.3A to E Squamocolumnar junction. Location of the squamocolumnar junction (SCJ) and transformation zone: (A) Before menarche; (B) After puberty and at early reproductive age; (C) In a woman in her 30s; (D) In a perimenopausal woman; (E) In a postmenopausal woman

metaplasia has occurred.[3] In most cases, CIN is believed to originate in transformation zone at advancing squamocolumnar junction (Figs 24.4A to C). The anterior lip of cervix is twice as likely to develop CIN as the posterior lip and it occurs rarely in lateral angles.[2]

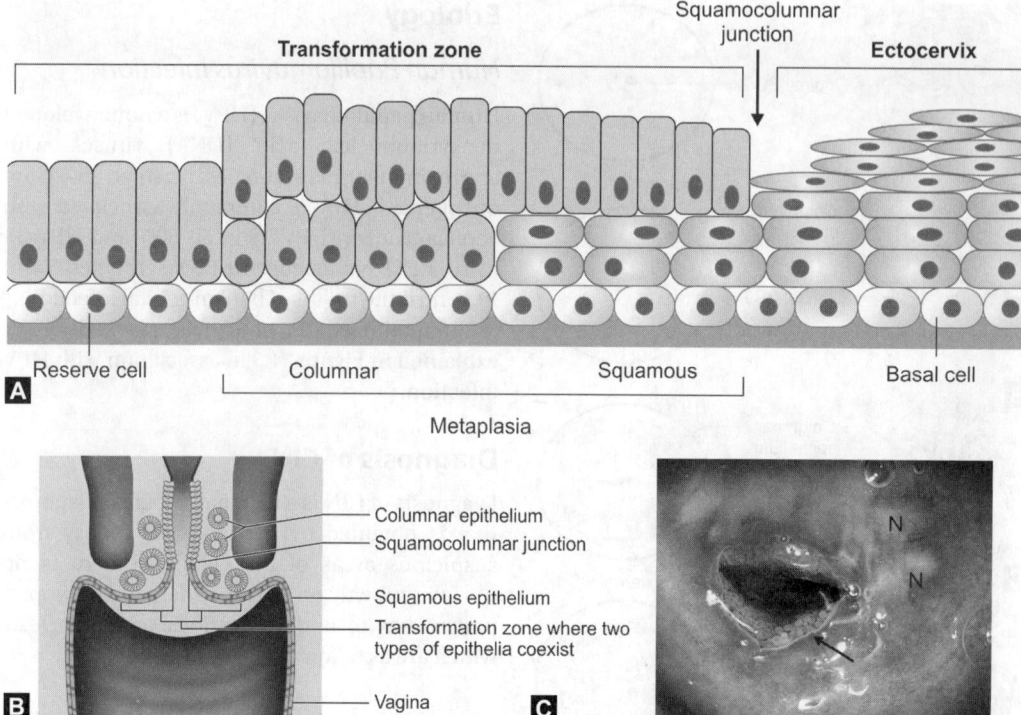

Figs 24.4A to C (A) Schematic display of histology; (B) Longitudinal view to understand the location; (C) Colposcopic view of normal cervix. Normal or typical transformation zone: Tongues of metaplastic epithelium shown as arrow, gland openings, nabothian follicles (N), islands of columnar epithelium *(For color version, see Plate 7)*

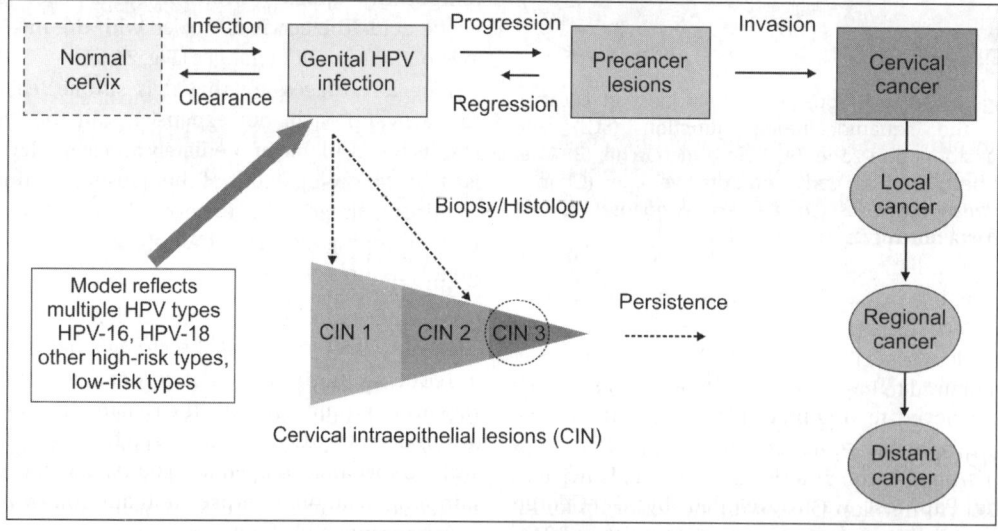

Fig. 24.5 Etiopathogenesis of cervical cancer

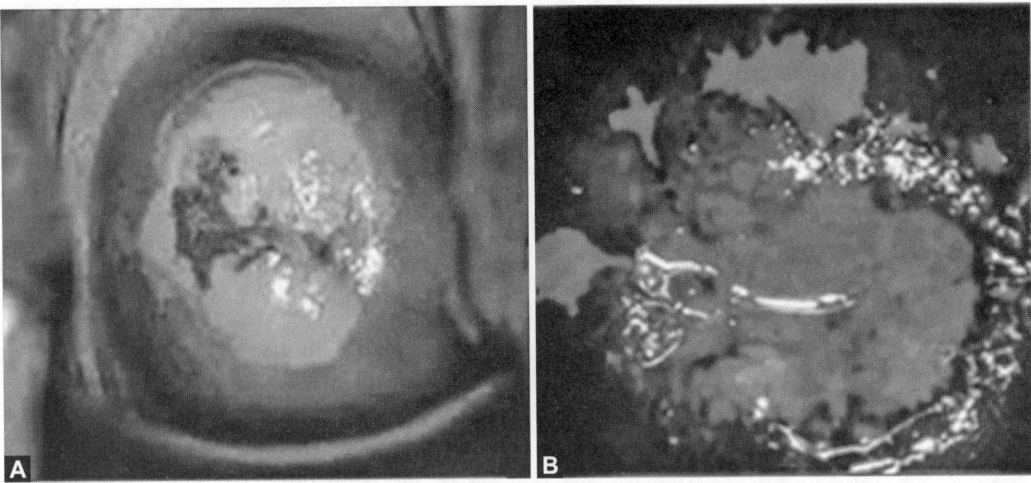

Figs 24.6A and B VIA (A) VILI; (B) Positive cervix *(For color version, see Plate 8)*

Iodine negative areas are seen in columnar epithelium, immature metaplasia, atrophy, inflammation, HPV infection, CIN and cancer.

Biopsy should be targeted at acetowhite or iodine negative areas (Table 24.1). Ideal biopsy is loop biopsy, however in the absence of facility, multiple punch biopsy or a knife biopsy can also be done. Various studies have proven that pickup rate of disease is higher with loop biopsy as compared to punch biopsy.

"See and treat" approach (for CIN) in one sitting is possible with VIA and VILI if one is equipped with setup of large loop excision of transformation zone (LLETZ) which has loops of all sizes and electrosurgical unit. Though it may prove to be an overtreatment (around 7.8%) as many of them have benign lesions but it is a feasible approach in rural setup on patients not expected to come back for follow-up.

In Indian scenario test with VIA and VILI for screening of cancer cervix and pickup of pre-invasive disease is proving to be highly sensitive but less specific and very cost effective as compared to Pap smear.

Paps Smear

The Pap test was developed by Dr George Papanicolaou, an American anatomist in 1944.

Table 24.1 Visual inspection with acetic acid test results

VIA category	Clinical findings
Test-negative	No acetowhite lesions or faint acetowhite lesions; polyp, cervicitis, inflammation, nabothian cysts.
Test-positive	Sharp, distinct, well-defined, dense (opaque/dull or oyster white) acetowhite areas—with or without raised margins touching the squamocolumnar junction (SCJ); leukoplakia and warts.
Suspicious for cancer	Clinically visible ulcerative, cauliflower-like growth or ulcer, oozing or bleeding on touch.

Pap test is used primarily as a tool for screening healthy women for preinvasive cervical cancer (CIN) and early invasive cancer. Screening for cervical cancer using Paps test was successful in reducing the incidence of cervical cancer by 79% and mortality by 70%. The sensitivity of Pap test in detecting CIN 2 or 3 ranged from 47–62% and the specificity ranged from 60–95%. Errors of sampling, fixation, interpretation and follow-up may be responsible for missed cases.[2]

Colposcopy

Colposcopy was introduced by Hinselmann in 1927. The purpose of colposcopy is to detect abnormal areas so that selective biopsy can be done. It is not done routinely in all patients. Only patients with positive cervical cytology for malignant cells or suspicious cells with normal looking cervix need colposcopy (Fig. 24.7).

Indications of Colposcopy

- Abnormal Pap smear of cervix
- Abnormal areas on vagina and vulva
- To detect abnormal areas for biopsy
- Precise conservative treatment with cone biopsy and laser
- To follow-up cases on conservative treatment.

Abnormal Colposcopic Findings

It includes acetowhite epithelium, mosaics, punctation and abnormal vessels.

Acetowhite epithelium: The epithelium which turns white after application of dilute (3–5%) acetic acid is known as acetowhite epithelium. The acetic acid coagulates the proteins of nucleus and cytoplasm and makes them opaque and white. It does not penetrate beneath the outer one-third of normal mature glycogen producing epithelium which has very small nuclei and a large amount of glycogen. These areas appear as pink on colposcopy. Dysplastic cells contain large nuclei with abnormally large amounts of chromatin and appear acetowhite (Fig. 24.8).

Flat acetowhite epithelium: It occurs in areas of immature metaplasia and CIN 1 which appears slowly and disappears fast.

Dense acetowhite epithelium: It appears fast and lasts longer and may indicate CIN 2, CIN 3 and invasive lesions.

Punctation

It refers to dilated capillaries terminating on the surface of epithelium. Normally, the capillary regresses whereas in CIN, the capillary persists and are more prominent (Fig. 24.9).

Fine punctation: The finer the punctation, the more likely the lesion is of low grade, e.g. inflammation, metaplasia

Coarse punctation: The coarser the punctation, the more likely the lesion is of severe grade, e.g. high grade CIN.

Mosaic

Terminal capillaries surrounding the acetowhite epithelium crowded together are called mosaic as they appear similar to mosaic tile. They arise

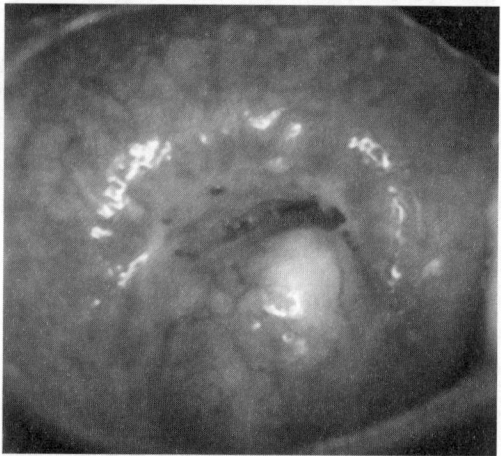

Fig. 24.7 Colposcopic of normal cervix
(For color version, see Plate 8)

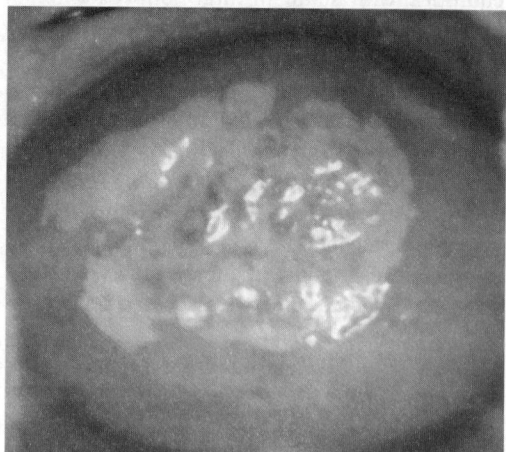

Fig. 24.8 Colposcopic of acetowhite cervix
(For color version, see Plate 8)

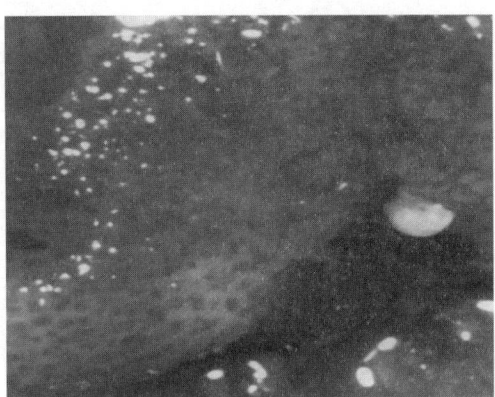

Fig. 24.9 Colposcopic showing punctations *(For color version, see Plate 8)*

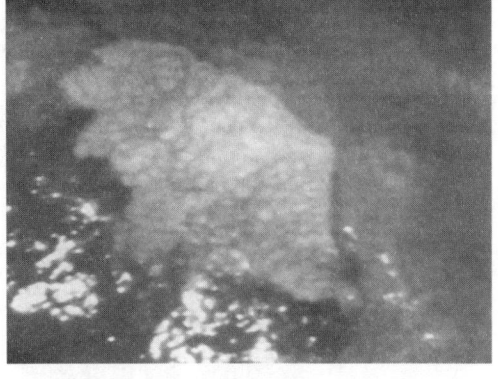

Fig. 24.10 Colposcopic picture showing coarse mosaic pattern *(For color version, see Plate 8)*

from coalescence of many terminal punctate vessels.

Fine mosaic: The smoother and finer the mosaic, the more likely the lesion is of low grade or metaplasia.

Coarse mosaic: The coarser and wider the mosaic, the more likely the lesion is of high grade or invasive cancer (Fig. 24.10).

Abnormal Vessels

Atypical vessels run parallel to the surface of epithelium (Fig. 24.11) and are of irregular caliber and branching. They appear like wide hairpins, commas, cork-screws or spaghetti-like forms (Figs 24.12A and B). They are indicative of invasive cancer but can also be seen in high grade CIN and rarely, inflammation.

Presumptive diagnosis of CIN is made as per Reid colposcopy index (RCI) given in Table 24.2 but final diagnosis is made on histopathological report of directed biopsy.

COLPOSCOPIC-DIRECTED BIOPSY

Patients with abnormal colposcopy are subjected to biopsy which is sent for histopathological diagnosis to confirm or rule out cervical intraepitheliac neoplasia (CIN).

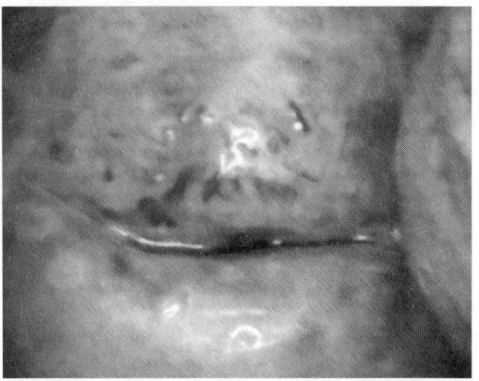

Fig. 24.11 Abnormal vessels on colposcopy of cervix *(For color version, see Plate 9)*

Methods of Biopsy

- Punch biopsy
- Wedge biopsy
- Loop biopsy
- Cone biopsy.

Instruments Used

- Punch biopsy forceps
- Endocervical curette
- Cervical hook
- Endocervical speculum
- Lateral wall retractor (or condom covered speculum with cut tip).

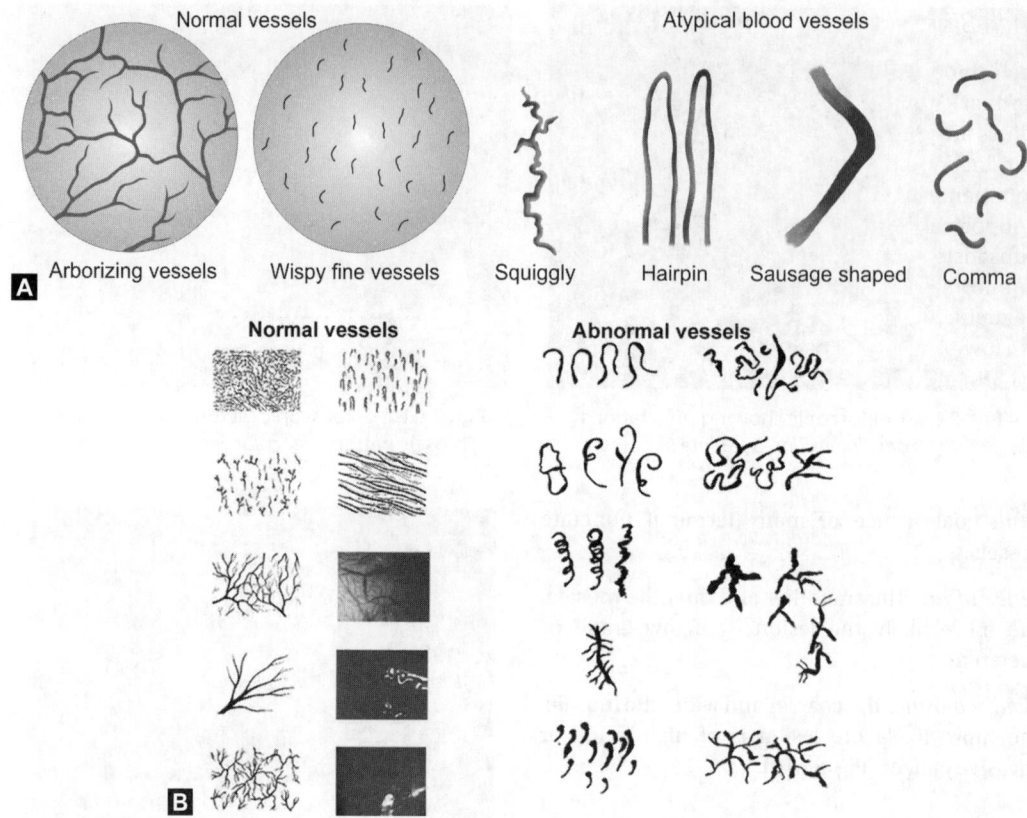

Figs 24.12A and B Normal and abnormal vessel pattern on colposcopy *(For color version, see Plate 9)*

Table 24.2 Reid colposcopic index			
Signs	Zero point (0)	One point (1)	Two points (2)
Margin	Indistinct acetowhitening feathered flocculated angular condylomatous	Regular smooth straight	Rolled, pealing internal demarcations
Color	Shiny, snow white, transparent	Intermediate shiny gray	Dull, oyster white
Vessels	Fine caliber, fine mosaic, poorly formed patterns	Absent	Well-defined, coarse punctuations or coarse mosaic
Iodine staining	Positive stain, negative uptake of lesions scoring <2/6 on above 3 categories	Partial uptake by a lesion	Negative stain by a lesion scoring 3/6 or more on above 3 categories
0–2 → likely to be CIN I 3–4 → overlapping CIN I or CIN II 5–8 → likely to be CIN II or III			

Punch Biopsy

Punch biopsy should be taken at squamocolumnar junction or wherever colposcopy findings are abnormal.

Endocervical curettage (ECC) is recommended when:
- Abnormal Pap smear and colposcopy is unsatisfactory.
- Abnormal Pap smear in a previously treated patient.
- In low-grade squamous intraepithelial lesions (LSIL), if colposcopy shows no lesion.
- Those at risk for recurrence.

ECC is contraindicated in pregnant women.

Wedge Biopsy

Taking out a wedge of tissue involving abnormal and part of normal tissue by knife or cautery is called wedge biopsy.

Loop Biopsy

The concept of loop biopsy and large loop excision of transformation zone. Large loop excision of transformation zone (LLETZ) was introduced to treat CIN but these days loop biopsy is considered superior to punch biopsy for diagnosis of CIN since the depth of tissue is more around 5 mm as compared to 2-3 mm in punch biopsy. Details of the procedure are given in management part.

Cone Biopsy

It can be both diagnostic as well as therapeutic.

Indications:
- Area of abnormality is large or its inner margin has receded in endocervical canal.
- Squamocolumnar junction is not completely visible on colposcopy.
- If there is discrepancy between cytology and colposcopy findings.

Procedure: To be done in operation theater keeping blood available. After the patient is anesthetized and put in lithotomy position, parts are cleaned and draped. Descending cervical arteries are clipped with no. 1 vicryl at 3 and 9 o'clock position. Cervix is painted with Lugol's iodine, to cover all negative area within the incision, a circumoral incision is given with knife which is deepened in cone shaped fashion (Fig. 24.13). The size of the specimen varies from 2 × 2 cm to 3 × 3 cm depending upon whether its postmenopausal small cervix or multiparous cervix with large area. Attempts should be made to include all iodine negative area within the incision line (Fig. 24.14A and B).

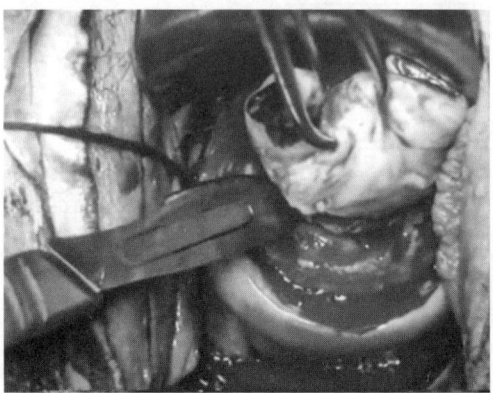

Fig. 24.13 Cone biopsy with cold knife *(For color version, see Plate 9)*

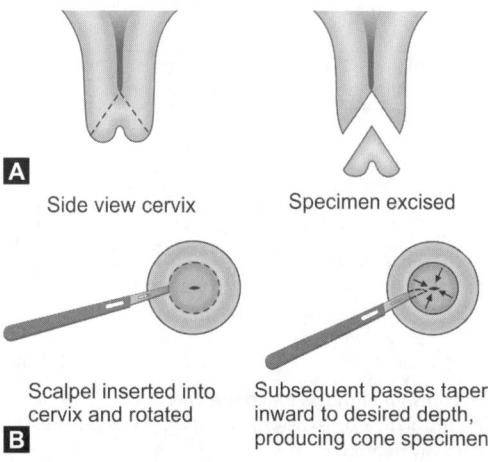

Figs 24.14A and B Procedure of cone biopsy

Complications: They include bleeding which can be severe requiring blood transfusion in 5% of operated cases. To reduce blood loss it should always be done in postmenstrual phase and descending cervical vessels should be ligated before giving incision. Other complications can be sepsis which can be prevented by judiciously selecting the case after treating cervicitis and vaginitis if it pre-exists. There can be cervical stenosis leading to hydrometra or pyometra which can be prevented by dilating the cervix before giving incision. If woman conceives following cone biopsy she has more chances of midtrimester abortion and preterm labor.

Contraindications
- Untreated cervicitis or PID
- Pregnancy
- Childbirth within past 12 weeks
- Obvious invasive cancer.

Management

Conization was the only therapeutic modality available through 1970s for treatment of CIN. Large loop excision of transformation zone (LLETZ) has revolutionised the treatment of CIN.

CIN 1

CIN 1 regresses spontaneously in 60–85% of cases and it occurs typically within a 2-year follow-up with cytology and colposcopy. Patients with CIN1 (after cytologic finding of ASC, ASC-H, LSIL) with satisfactory colposcopy may be followed with Pap testing at 6 and 12 months or HPV testing at 12 months (Flow chart 24.1). After two negative tests or single negative HPV test, routine screening can be resumed. Colposcopy and repeat cytology at 12 months or a diagnostic excisional procedure is recommended if CIN1 was preceded by high grade squamous intraepithecial lesion (HSIL) or atypical glandular epithelial cell (AGC) cytology (Flow chart 24.2).[2,7]

CIN 2 and 3

CIN 2 and 3 lesions require treatment in women >21 years old as CIN 2 progresses to CIS in 20% cases and to invasion in 5% (Flow chart 24.3). Women <21 years can be offered cytology and colposcopy at 6 month intervals, with treatment only for persistence at 24 months (Flow chart 24.4).[2,7]

Flow chart 24.1 Algorithm of ASCCP guidelines of management of CIN 1

Management of women with a histological diagnosis of cervical intraepithelial neoplasia grade 1 (CIN 1) preceded by ASC-US, ASC-H or LSIL cytology

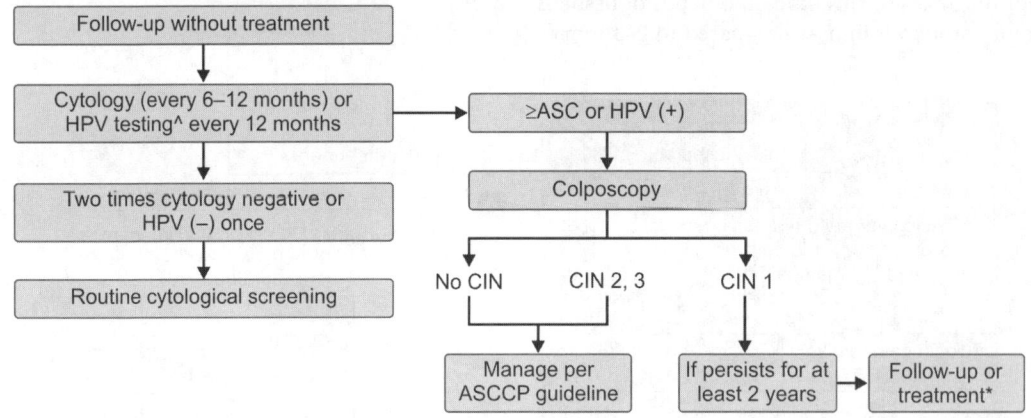

^Test only for high-risk (oncogenic) types of HPV
*Either ablative or excisional method. Excision preferred if colposcopy unsatisfactory, ECC is positive, or patient previously treated

Abbreviations: ASCCP; American Society for Colposcopy and Cervical Pathology; ASC, atypical squamous cells; HPV, human papillomavirus; US, unknown significance; HSIL, high grade squamous intraepithelial lesion; H, HSIL cannot be excluded

Flow chart 24.2 Algorithm of ASCCP guidelines of management of CIN 1
Management of women with a histological diagnosis of cervical intraepithelial neoplasia grade 1 (CIN 1) preceded by HSIL or AGC-NOS cytology

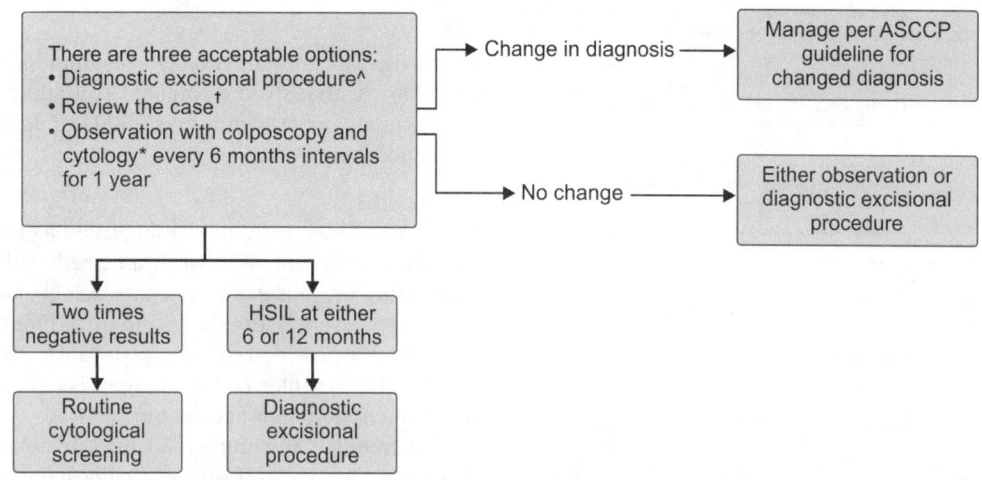

^Except in special populations
†Includes referral cytology, colposcopic findings and all biopsies
*Provided colposcopy is satisfactory and endocervical sampling is negative. If not, diagnostic excisional procedure

Abbreviations: HSIL, high grade squamous intraepithelial lesion; AGC-NOS, atypical squamous cells not otherwise specified

Flow chart 24.3 Algorithm of ASCCP guidelines of management of CIN 2 and 3
Management of women with a histological diagnosis of cervical intraepithelial neoplasia grade 2, 3 (CIN 2, 3)*

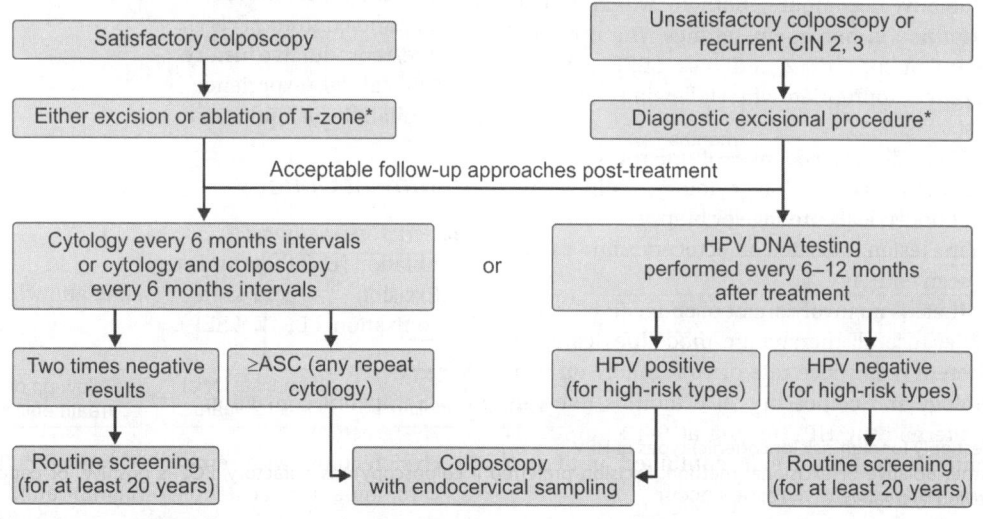

*Management options will vary in special circumstances

Abbreviations: HPV, human papillomavirus; ASC, atypical squamous cells

Flow chart 24.4 Algorithm of ASCCP guidelines of management of CIN1 in adolescent women

Management of adolescent women (20 years and younger) with a histological diagnosis of cervical intraepithelial neoplasia grade 1 (CIN 1)

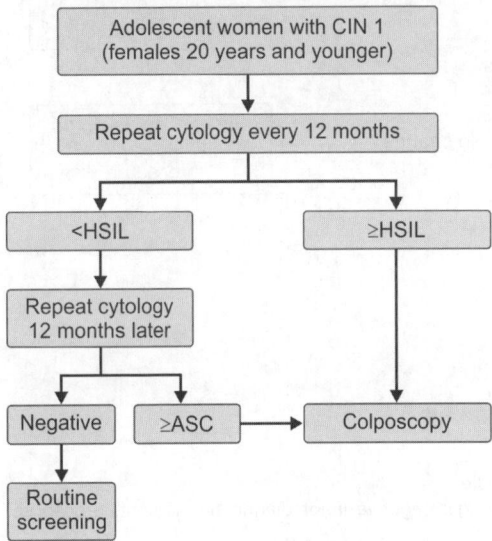

Abbreviations: HSIL, high grade squamous intraepithelial lesion; ASC, atypical squamous cells

CIN 2 and 3 can be treated by excisional or ablative techniques, both of which can be performed in outpatient settings. The preferred treatment for CIN 2 and 3 is LEEP. Ablative therapy is appropriate when following conditions exist:[2]

- There is no evidence of microinvasive or invasive cancer on cytology, colposcopy, endocervical curettage or biopsy
- The lesion is located on ectocervix and can be seen entirely
- There is no involvement of endocervix.

Because all therapeutic modalities carry an inherent recurrence rate of 10%, follow-up with cytology and colposcopy at 6 months intervals or alternatively HPV testing at 6–12 months is required. Surveillance is continued until two consecutive negative results occur.

CIN in Adolescents and Pregnancy (Flow chart 24.5)

CIN1:
Follow-up with annual cytology is recommended. Only those with HSIL or greater at 12 months and ASCUS or greater at 24 months should be referred for colposcopy.[2,7]

CIN 2 and 3
For adolescents with a histological diagnosis of CIN 2 or 3 not otherwise specified, either treatment or observation by cytology and colposcopy every 6 months for up to 24 months is acceptable provided colposcopy is satisfactory. Observation is preferred for a diagnosis of CIN 2 alone but treatment is acceptable.

Treatment is recommended for a histologic diagnosis of CIN 3 or if colposcopy is unsatisfactory. After two consecutive negative cytology tests and satisfactory colposcopic examinations, adolescents can return to routine annual cytologic screening.[2,7]

Treatment Modalities

Selection of treatment modality depends upon
- Grade of the lesion
- Size and placement of the lesion
- Size and contour of cervix
- Age/reproductive history
- Clinical skill/experience
- Availability of equipment.

Treatment Options

Conservative methods:
- Ablation (cryotherapy/laser)
- Excision (cold-knife conization/laser conization/LLETZ/LEEP).

Surgery:
- Therapeutic conization
- Hysterectomy
- Hysterectomy with removal of vaginal cuff if carcinoma *in situ* extends to vaginal vault.

Flow chart 24.5 Algorithm of ASCCP guideline of management of CIN 2, 3 in adolescent and young women

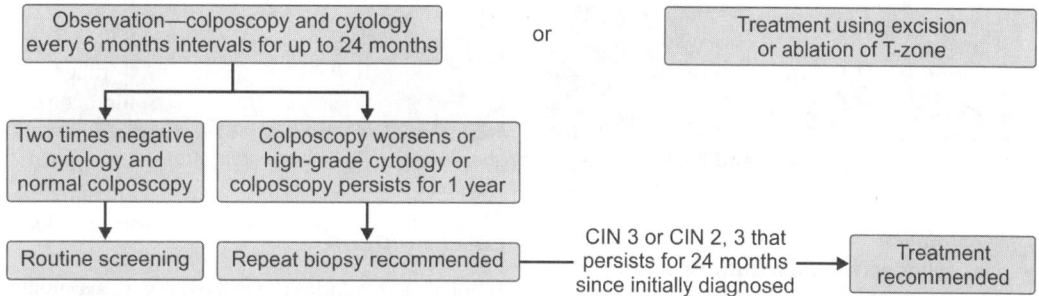

Criteria for conservative methods:
- Entire lesion should be visible within squamocolumnar junction
- No micro- or macro-invasion on biopsy
- No endocervical involvement
- No discrepancy in cytology and histology findings
- Young women desirous of pregnancy.

Cryotherapy

It destroys the cervical epithelium by crystallizing the intracellular water which causes destruction of the cell (Figs 24.15A and B).

Prerequisites
- CIN confirmed by biopsy or colposcopy
- CIN1 persisting for 2 years
- CIN 2
- Ectocervical lesion only (ECC negative)
- Small lesion (to be covered by cryoprobe)
- Negative endocervical curettage samples
- No endocervical involvement on biopsy
- No evidence of invasion
- No glandular dysplasia
- Pregnancy ruled out or at least 3 months postpartum
- Informed consent.

Contraindications:
- Evidence or suspicion of invasive disease
- Lesion extends >2 mm beyond cryoprobe
- Pregnancy
- Cervicitis and vaginitis (until treated)
- Pelvic inflammatory disease (PID) (until treated)
- Active menstruation.

Technique:
The most effective method is believed to be "freeze-thaw-freeze" in which an ice ball is formed 5–7 mm beyond the edge of the cryoprobe. The temperature needed is in the range of –20 to –30°C. Nitrous oxide (–89°C) and CO_2 (–65°C) produce temperatures below this range and are most commonly used.

Advantages:
- OPD procedure
- Requires no anesthesia
- Cheap and easily available
- No learning curve
- Electricity not required
- Takes very less time ~15 minutes
- No major complications
- No hemorrhage
- No long-term sequelae especially if future pregnancy is desired.

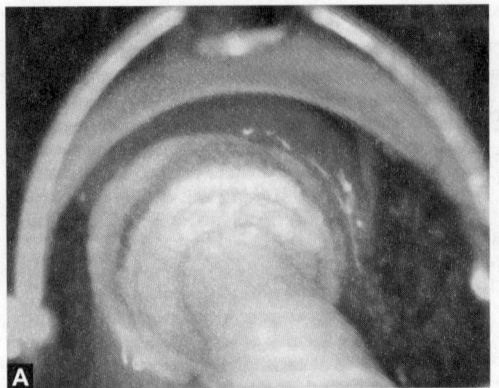 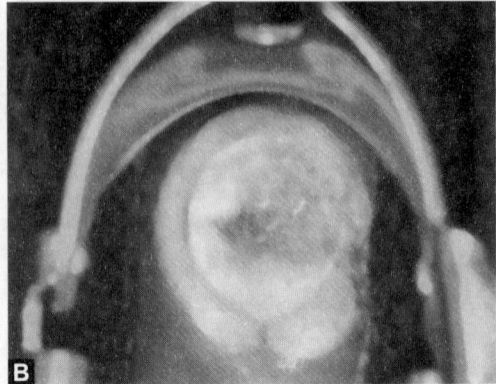

Figs 24.15A and B (A) Cryotherapy probe on cervix; (B) Frozen cervix after cryoprobe removed *(For color version, see Plate 9)*

Disadvantages:
- Gas cylinders required (nitrous or CO_2)
- Lesser effective for larger lesions (cure rates 80%)
- Tissue not available for histopathological examination
- Profuse and watery discharge.

Complications:
- Cramping, vasomotor symptoms
- Profuse watery discharge in 20%
- Slight spotting for 1–2 weeks
- PID <1%
- Necrotic plug syndrome ~3%
- Cervical stenosis—rare
- Cervical stenosis—rare.

Precautions after cryotherapy:
- Abstinence for 4 weeks or barrier
- Avoid vaginal douche or tampon for 4 weeks
- To report if any warning sign like
  - Fever >1 day
  - Severe lower abdominal pain especially with fever
  - Foul smelling or pus discharge
  - Bleeding heavier than heaviest of menstrual bleeding >2 days.

Results

The cure rate is 80–90% and is related to the grade of the lesion. The recurrence rate for CIN 1, 2, 3 is 5%, 8% and 10–15% respectively. Endocervical gland involvement has more failure rate (29%) as compared to ectocervix (9%).

Laser Ablation

It boils and explodes the cells. It is very expensive and can cause harm to personnel using it.

Indications:
- Large lesions that cannot be covered by cryoprobe
- Satellite lesions in vagina
- Lesions with extensive glandular involvement.

Advantages:
- It is an OPD procedure done under local anesthesia
  - Higher success rate (recurrence—2–10%)
  - Ability to control depth and width of destruction
  - Minimal bleeding, no infection and no postscar formation
  - Rapid healing (4 weeks)
  - Do not cause indrawal of squamo-columnar junction so repeat laser is possible for residual lesion.

Loop Electrosurgical Excision Procedure (LEEP)

The LEEP is a valuable tool in management of CIN. It offers the advantage of being diagnostic and therapeutic in the same sitting. It is an OPD procedure and can be done under local anesthesia (Figs 24.16 and 24.17).

It uses low voltage diathermy and is harmless to personnel using it which makes it more popular than laser. Besides, it takes less time and has similar success and recurrence rates as that of laser.

Principle:
If blend current of 35–55 watts with small wire loop of 0.5 mm is used, then effect is electrosurgical and thermal damage is minimal. The actual cutting is due to steam envelope developing at the interface of wire loop and tissue.

Eligibility criteria for LEEP:
- Cervical intraepithelial neoplasia (CIN) confirmed by biopsy when possible
- Lesion going into endocervical canal not >1 cm

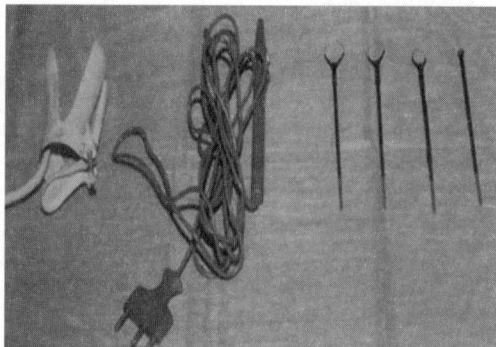

Fig. 24.16 Large loop excision of transformation zone (LLETZ)—Instruments and procedure: Insulated cuscos speculum, loops in 3 sizes (large, medium, small) and roller ball cautery *(For color version, see Plate 10)*

- No evidence of invasive cancer or glandular dysplasia
- No evidence of cervicitis, vaginitis, PID
- At least 3 months postpartum
- Informed consent.

Complications:
- Hemorrhage (1–2%)
- Cervical stenosis (1–4%)
- Recurrence rate (2–4%)
- Thermal destruction of tissue.

Post-LEEP Care:
- Routine antibiotics for 1 week (Doxycycline and metrogyl)
- Abstinence for 4 weeks
- Avoid douche or tampon for 4–6 weeks
- Condom use for 6–8 weeks.

To report if any warning sign like:
- Foul smelling discharge
- Excessive bleeding
- Fever with pain lower abdomen.

Advantages of LEEP:
- High cure rates (91–98%)
- *Tissue is available for histopathological examination*
- OPD procedure
- Fast and technically simpler
- Complications are few
- See and treat approach (overtreatment by only 7.8%).

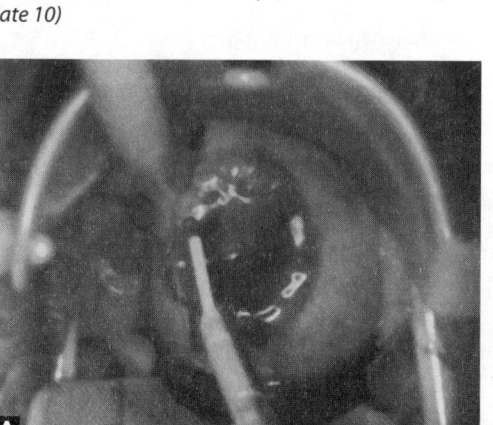
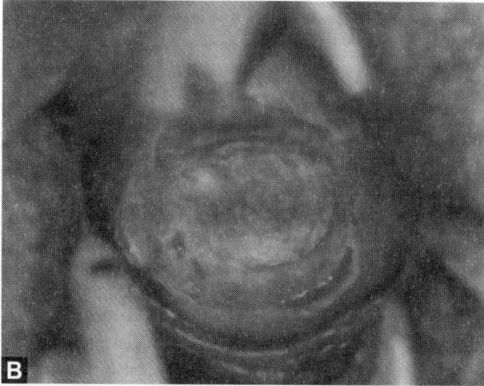

Figs 24.17A and B (A) Large loop excision of transformation zone (LLETZ); (B) Crater after large loop excision of transformation zone (LLETZ) *(For color version, see Plate 10)*

Disadvantages of LEEP:
- Requires training
- Equipment sophisticated
- Requires electricity
- Requires local anesthesia
- Thermal effect.

Conization

Indications:

- Unsatisfactory colposcopy
- Microinvasion on biopsy/colposcopy/Pap smear
- Endocervical cytology positive for CIN II/CIN III
- Uncertainty regarding presence of microinvasion or invasion following direct biopsy for CIN
- Lack of correlation between Pap smear, colposcopy and biopsy
- Adenocarcinoma *in situ* on biopsy or endocervical curettage (ECC).

Complications:

- Immediate:
  - Hemorrhage (5–10%)
  - Bladder injury
  - POD may be opened.
- Late:
  - Affect future fertility
  - Incompetent os
  - Preterm labor.

Hysterectomy

It is the treatment of last resort for recurrent high grade CIN.

Indications:
- Microinvasion
- CIN III at margins of cone specimen
- Poor compliance with follow-up in CIN III
- Other gynecological problems requiring hysterectomy like fibroids, prolapse and endometriosis.

Adenocarcinoma in situ (AIS)

Hysterectomy remains the preferred treatment for women with a histological diagnosis of AIS on a specimen from a diagnostic excisional procedure. If future fertility is desired, conservative excisional management is acceptable. If a conservative excisional procedure is performed and margins are involved or the endocervical sample shows AIS or CIN, re-excision is recommended (Flow chart 24.6). Surveillance at 6 months using a combination of cytology, colposcopy, human papilloma virus (HPV) testing and endocervical sampling is acceptable.[2]

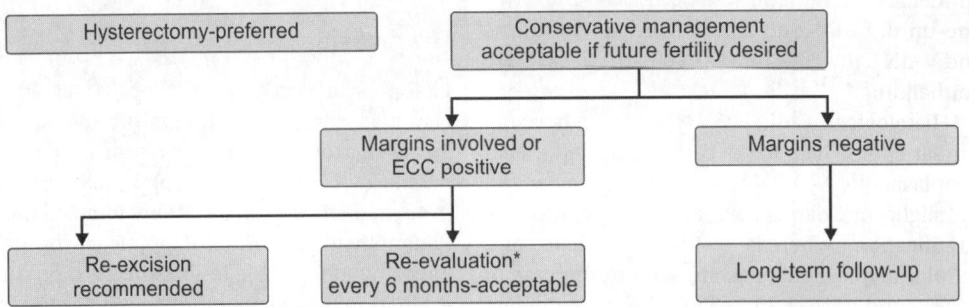

Flow chart 24.6 ASCCP algorithm of management of AIS

*Using a combination of cytology, HPV testing, and colposcopy with endocervical sampling
Abbreviations: ECC, endocervical curettage; AIS, adenocarcinoma *in situ*

VAGINAL INTRAEPITHELIAL NEOPLASIA

Introduction

Vaginal intraepithelial neoplasia (VAIN) is defined as the presence of squamous cell atypia without invasion. VAIN is a rare clinical condition, therefore its natural history as well as the potential of progression to invasive carcinoma is poorly understood[8] and there is scarce information about the effectiveness of each treatment modality.[9] However, risk factors for the development of VAIN are similar to cervical intraepithelial neoplasia (CIN). High-risk strains of human papillomavirus are implicated with HPV 16 being the most frequent subtype.[10,11]

VAIN is thought to be a precursor to malignant disease,[12] but its progression is slower than in CIN 3 lesions. VAIN is often accompanied by CIN and both share a common etiology. The lesions can extend on to vagina from CIN or they may be satellite lesions. Since vagina does not have a transformation zone, so mechanism of entry of HPV is primarily through sexual activity.

VAIN lesions are often asymptomatic, although they may present with vulvar warts or vaginal discharge due to accompanying HPV infection.[2]

Classification

VAIN is classified according to the depth of epithelial involvement. VAIN 1 involves the lower one-third, VAIN 2 involves the lower two-thirds and VAIN 3 involves more than two-thirds of the epithelium.

Histological grading of VAIN is done by using similar criteria like that of cervical intraepithelial neoplasia (CIN).[13] VAIN 1 is characterized by slight nuclear atypia and preservation of stratification whereas evident nuclear and cellular atypical changes are seen in the case of VAIN 2 and VAIN 3. In VAIN 3, there is complete loss of stratification. VAIN is also categorized as low-grade (VAIN 2 and 3) and high-grade (VAIN 3).

Epidemiology

VAIN accounts for approximately 0.4% of lower genital tract intraepithelial neoplasia.[12,14] The incidence of VAIN is expected to rise due to the more common use of cytologic screening and colposcopy.[13] VAIN is more common in patients aged more than 60 years.

Risk Factors

- History of previous abnormal Pap smear
- Genital warts
- Radiotherapy
- Immunosuppression
- History of concomitant CIN or cervical cancer.

VAIN is frequently associated with cervical intraepithelial neoplasia. Progression of VAIN to invasive form is about 5% which is significantly higher than the progression rate of patients treated for CIN. The reason for this difference could be less effective treatment and follow-up for VAIN than CIN.[13]

Screening

Since VAIN is nearly always accompanied by CIN, the Pap test is likely to be positive when VAIN is present. The vagina should be thoroughly inspected at time of colposcopic examination for CIN lesion. Women with persistent abnormal Pap tests without evident cervical pathology and those with abnormal cytology after treatment of CIN should be carefully examined for VAIN.

Diagnosis

Patients can present with postcoital spotting or unusual vaginal discharge but most of them are asymptomatic. The first sign of a possible neoplasia is usually an abnormal Pap smear from vaginal vault in a hysterectomized patient. Patients with abnormal Pap smear who do not have any identifiable lesion of cervix, on further evaluation may be found to have a disease in the vagina.

After the diagnoses by an abnormal Pap smear, it is crucial to detect lesion in the vagina but most

VAIN patients have no visible lesions. The follow-up of abnormal Pap smear needs colposcopic evaluation, so as to identify the abnormal areas for tissue biopsy. Colposcopy of vagina is much more difficult and time consuming procedure due to the length, surface area, and redundancy of the vagina. The majority of lesions (95.8%) are located in upper third of the vagina mainly at the apex and present in a multifocal manner in most of the cases (75%).[15]

Colposcopic examination and directed biopsy is the mainstay of diagnosis. VAIN 1 lesions are usually accompanied by koilocytosis indicating their HPV origin. VAIN 2 lesions have thicker acetowhite epithelium, a more raised external border and less iodine uptake. In VAIN 3, surface becomes papillary and vascular patterns of punctuations and mosaic may occur.

Treatment

There are various treatment modalities which have various success rates and associated complications.

Factors affecting choice of treatment:
- Number of the lesions
- Location of lesions
- Previous radiation therapy
- Previous VAIN treatment
- Sexual activity
- Operator experience and patient preference.

Most lesions regress after initial treatment but some may recur and progress to invasive cancer. Recurrence is more commonly seen in VAIN 3, multifocal lesions, and VAIN associated with other anogenital neoplasia.

Treatment Modalities

Ablative

Topical 5-flourourocil, or topical trichloroacetic acid.

Surgical
- Biopsy—local excision
- Loop electrosurgical excision procedure (LEEP)
- Wide local excision
- Partial or total vaginectomy.

Patients with VAIN 1 and HPV infection do not require treatment as these lesions usually regress. VAIN 2 lesions can be managed expectantly or treated by ablation. VAIN 3 lesions can be treated with laser therapy.[2]

Topical 5-FU: Topical 5-FU has provided good results with prolonged periods of remission.[16] It is considered to be an ideal treatment modality for multifocal VAIN and recurrences. Vaginal pain, burning, pruritus and ulcerations are major problems and result in noncompliance of patients.

CO_2 laser vaporization: The goal of laser vaporization is to minimize the area of tissue necrosis which is accomplished by using high wattage (20 watts) with medium beam size (1.5 mm) and moving the beam uniformly but quickly over the surface.[2] The major advantage of laser therapy is the ability to control the depth and width of destruction. Also, it is an outpatient procedure associated with minimal blood loss and suitable for multifocal lesions. Potential complications with laser therapy include bleeding and damage to the bowel or bladder.

Local excision: Local excision of the involved area is the treatment of choice when there is a single well-demarcated small lesion.[17] This procedure has remission rates of 64–67%.

LEEP: Advantage of LEEP is the presence of a histologic specimen and it can be performed as an outpatient surgical procedure. Excision consists of the vaginal mucosa and a portion of the submucosal tissue.

Wide local excision: It is found to be efficacious in treating high grade VAIN. The surgical complications of wide local excision can be severe, especially in irradiated patients, so it should be performed in experienced centers only.

Partial vaginectomy: Partial vaginectomy is the best treatment option in unifocal lesions or multifocal lesions involving the upper third of the vagina.[18] It has the advantage of providing a specimen to assess the possibility of invasive cancer and to control the resection margins.

Partial upper vaginectomy can be performed transvaginally or transabdominally.[19] It is associated with minimal postoperative pain and no vaginal irritation, but it has complications like hemorrhage, bladder or rectum injury and stenosis of vagina. Though topical chemotherapy and laser vaporization are less time consuming and can treat multifocal lesions, they have more undesired complications like vaginal irritation and they do not allow for a tissue diagnosis.

Total vaginectomy:
Total vaginectomy is not preferred because vaginal intercourse becomes impossible[20] without a graft but it may be required occasionally to treat VAIN 3 occupying most vagina. It is to accompanied by split thickness skin graft. This surgery is not recommended for VAIN.

Follow-up after Treatment

Long-term follow-up is necessary because of the high risk of residual or recurrent disease. It includes periodic clinical examinations, cytology and colposcopy at 3 months, 6 months and after 12 months for the first year and then once a year subsequently.[21]

VULVAR INTRAEPITHELIAL NEOPLASIA

Introduction

The term vulvar intraepithelial neoplasia (VIN) was introduced in the early 1980s as the generic designation for severe squamous epithelial atypia (severe dysplasia) and squamous cell carcinoma *in situ* (CIS) of the vulva. The concept was later expanded to encompass the entire spectrum of morphologic changes believed to be potential precursors of invasive vulvar squamous cell carcinoma (Fig. 24.18).[22]

In 1987, the ISSVD (International Society for Study of Vulvar Disease) and committee

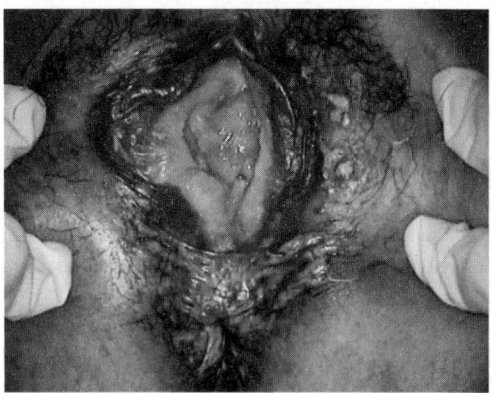

Fig. 24.18 Vulvar intraepithelial neoplasia (VIN)
(For color version, see Plate 10)

Table 24.3 ISSVD classification[24]

ISSVD classification of vulvar pathology
Non-neoplastic epithelial disorders: • Lichen sclerosis • Squamous hyperplasia • Other dermatoses
Mixed non-neoplastic and neoplastic epithelial disorders

Intraepithelial neoplasia:
• Squamous intraepithelial neoplasia
  – VIN 1
  – VIN 2
  – VIN 3
• Nonsquamous intraepithelial neoplasia
  – Paget's disease
  – Tumors of melanocytes, noninvasive

Invasive tumors

Abbreviations: ISSVD, International Society for Study of Vulvovaginal Disease; VIN, Vulvar intraepithelial neoplasia

on histological classification of vulvar tumors and dystrophies of International Society of Gynaecological Pathologists recommended the term vulvar intraepithelial neoplasia (Table 24.3).

According to these classifications, VIN lesions were graded depending on the level of involvement of the affected epidermis by cellular disarray, nuclear atypia and mitotic activity. In VIN 1 (mild dysplasia), the lowest third is involved; in VIN 2 (moderate dysplasia), the lower two-thirds and in VIN 3 (severe dysplasia), greater than two-thirds of epithelium is involved. This grading scheme parallels the grading of cervical intraepithelial neoplasia (CIN). However, the criteria used for CIN are not strictly applicable to VIN. While CIN 1 is very a common cervical lesion, VIN 1 lesions are very uncommon and caution must be exercised before making such a diagnosis.[22]

In 2004, ISSVD changed the nomenclature of VIN. It is now divided into usual type VIN and differentiated type VIN.[23]

Epidemiology

Over the last 20 years incidence of VIN has increased from 1.2 to 2.1 per 100,000 women and this increase has been especially pronounced in younger patient population due to concomitant increase in HPV infection.[24]

Etiopathogenesis

By definition, VIN is made up of neoplastic cells, confined to the boundaries of surface epithelium. The term VIN is used to denote high-grade squamous lesions and is subdivided into usual-type VIN (including warty, basaloid and mixed VIN) and differentiated-type VIN (Fig. 24.19).

Usual-type VIN is commonly associated with carcinogenic genotypes of HPV and other HPV persistence risk factors such as cigarette smoking and immunocompromised status whereas differentiated VIN usually is not associated with HPV and is more often associated with vulvar dermatologic conditions such as lichen sclerosus. It may regress spontaneously or may persist and if untreated may progress to invasive carcinoma.[23]

Treatment

The treatment of VIN 3 varies from wide excision to superficial vulvectomy. Progression occurs in only 5–10% of cases, so extensive surgery is not required. The therapeutic modalities for VIN 3 are simple excision, laser ablation and superficial

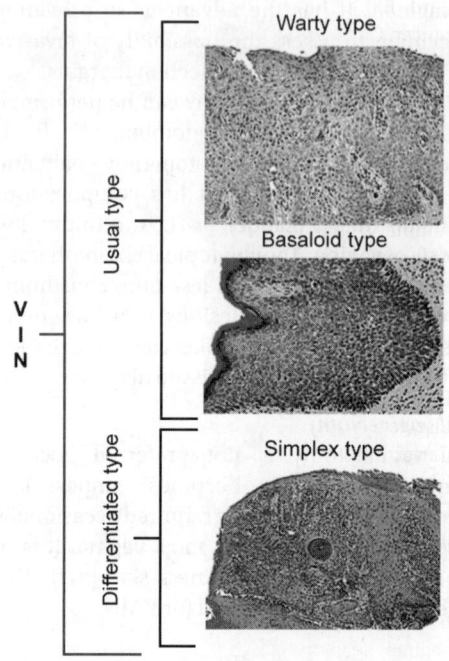

Fig. 24.19 Vulvar intraepithelial neoplasia histopathology *(For color version, see Plate 10)*

vulvectomy with or without split-thickness skin grafting.[2]

Excision of small foci of disease has excellent results and has advantage of providing a histological diagnosis. The carbon dioxide laser can be used for multifocal lesions, but it is painful, costly and does not provide a histological diagnosis. Superficial vulvectomy can be done for treating extensive disease and recurrent VIN.[2]

REFERENCES

1. Kumar V, Abbas AK, Fausto N, et al. Robbins Basic Pathology, 8th edition. Saunders Elsevier; 2007. pp.718-21.
2. Berek JS. Berek and Novak's Gynecology, 15th edition. Lippincott Williams and Wilkins; 2012. pp.574-618.
3. Sellors JW, Sankaranarayanan R. Colposcopy and Treatment of Cervical Intraepithelial Neoplasia. A Beginner's Manual. France, International Agency for Research on Cancer, World Health Organization; IARC, 2003.

4. Burd EM. Human papillomavirus and cervical cancer. Clin Microbiol Rev. 2003;16:1-17.
5. Munoz N, Bosch FX, de Sanjose S, Herrero R, Castellsague X, Shah KV, et al. Epidemiologic classification of human papillomavirus types associated with cervical cancer. N Eng J Med. 2003; 348:518-27.
6. World Health Organization. HPV IARC monograph summary. Lancet Oncol. 2005;6:204.
7. American Society for Colposcopy and Cervical Pathology. Journal of Lower Genital Tract Disease. 2013;17:1-27.
8. Bodurka DC, Frumovitz M. Malignant Diseases of the Vagina. In: Lentz GM, Lobo RA, Gershenson DM, Katz VL (Eds). Comprehensive Gynecology. Elsevier Mosby. 2012;31:703-11.
9. Carter JS, Downs LS. Vulvar and vaginal cancer. Obstet Gynecol Clin North Am. 2012;39:213-31.
10. Davies M, Mount S. Premalignant and malignant lesions of the vagina. Diagnostic histopathology. 2010;16(11):509-16.
11. Frega A, French D, Piazze J, Cerekja A, Vetrano G, Moscarini M. Prediction of persistent vaginal intraepithelial neoplasia in previously hysterectomized women by high-risk HPV DNA detection. Cancer Lett. 2007;249(2):235-41.
12. Cardosi RJ, Bomalaski JJ, Hoffman MS. Diagnosis and management of vulvar and vaginal intraepithelial neoplasia. Obstet Gynecol Clin North Am. 2001;28(4):685-702.
13. Vedat Atay, Murat Muhcu, Çalışkan AC. Treatment of vaginal intra-epithelail neoplasia. Cancer Therapy. 2007;5:19-28.
14. Gurumurthy M, Cruickshank ME. Management of vaginal intraepithelial neoplasia. J Low Genit Tract Dis. 2012;16(3):306-12.
15. Lenehan PM, Meffe F, Lickrish GM. Vaginal intraepithelial neoplasia, biologic aspects and management. Obstet Gynecol. 1986;68:333-7.
16. Petrilli ES, Townsend DE, Morrow CP, et al. Vaginal intraepithelial neoplasia, biologic aspects and treatment with topical 5-fluorouracil and the carbon dioxide laser. Am J Obstet Gynecol. 1980; 138:321-8.
17. Benedet JL, Sanders BH. Carcinoma *in situ* of the vagina. Am J Obst Gynecol. 1984;148:695-700.
18. Hoffman MS, DeCesare SL, Roberts WS, Fiorica JV, Finan MA, Cavanagh D. Upper vaginectomy for in situ and occult superficially invasive carcinoma of the vagina. Am J Obstet Gynecol. 1992;163:30-3.
19. Curtis P, Shepherd JH, Lowe DG, et al. The role of partial colpectomy in the management of persistent vaginal neoplasia after primary treatment. Br Obstet Gynaecol. 1992;99:587-9.
20. Sillman FH, Fruchter RG, Chen YS, Camilien L, Sedlis A, McTigue E. Vaginal intraepithelial neoplasia, risk factors for persistence, recurrence and invasion and its management. Am J Obstet Gynecol. 1997;176:93-9.
21. Gemmel J, Holmes MD, Duncan LD. How frequently need vaginal smears be taken after hysterectomy for cervical intraepithelial neoplasia? Br J Obstet Gynaecol. 1990;97:58-61.
22. Hart WR. Vulvar intraepithelial neoplasia: historical aspects and current status. Int J Gynecol Pathol. 2001;20:16-30.
23. Sideri M, Jones RW, Wilkinson EJ, Preti M, Heller DS, Scurry J, et al. Squamous vulvar intraepithelial neoplasia: 2004 modified terminology, ISSVD Vulvar Oncology Subcommittee. J Reprod Med. 2005;50:807-10.
24. Modesitt SC, Waters AB, Walton L, et al. Vulvar intraepithelial neoplasia III: occult cancer and the impact of margin status on recurrence. Obstet Gynecol. 1998;92(6):962-6.

25
Gestational Trophoblastic Neoplasia

Reva Tripathi, Meenoo S

INTRODUCTION

Gestational trophoblastic disease (GTD) refers to a spectrum of disorders of abnormal growth and development of the placental trophoblasts that may continue even beyond the pregnancy.

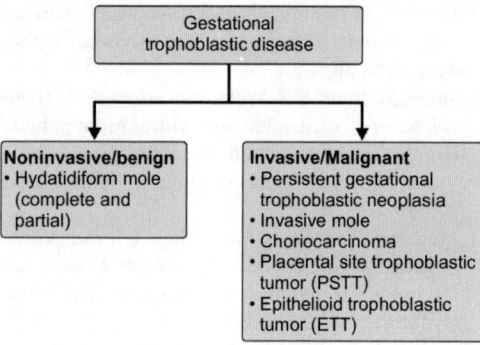

Among gestational trophoblastic disease, incidence of hydatidiform mole is 80–90% and invasive mole is 5–8% whereas choriocarcinoma and PSTT account for only 1–2%.[1] The various entities in the invasive group are collectively named as gestational trophoblastic neoplasia (GTN). The subtypes in this group have the ability to invade, metastasise and lead to death if untreated. The individual subtypes in the invasive or malignant group can be differentiated only by a histological diagnosis but that is generally not necessary as they are clubbed under clinical term GTN. Histopathological diagnosis of GTN is very rare. The incidence of GTN varies over different subcontinents, viz. it is 0.6–1.1 per 1000 pregnancies in North America and Europe while it is 2 per 1000 pregnancies in Japan[2] and 1 in 160 pregnancies in India and other middle east countries.[3]

The importance of GTN in gynecological oncology is that these are neoplasms that can be cured even despite presence of widespread metastases. A study by Seckl et al. in 2009 has reported a cure rate of >98% for this neoplasm, irrespective of metastases.[4]

This chapter will focus on GTN and not on diagnosis and management of benign GTD or hydatidiform mole. However, follow-up of hydatidiform mole is discussed for recapitulation of the readers.

FOLLOW-UP AFTER MOLAR EVACUATION

After molar evacuation, follow-up of the patient with β-hCG levels is essential to detect trophoblastic sequelae because about 15–20% of complete moles develop into GTN and about 4% of partial moles develop into GTN.[5]

It is advised to get serial serum β-hCG levels done every 1–2 weeks until three consecutive tests show normal β-hCG levels. The mean time to achieve normal β-hCG levels after molar evacuation is 7–9 weeks. Once β-hCG levels have remained normal for 3 serial tests, patient can undergo monthly or every 2 monthly serum β-hCG levels estimation for additional 6–12 months. This frequency can be modified by the discretion of the treating gynecologist depending on economical status of the patient.

Patient must be counseled about the use of contraception during every visit and compliance should be ensured. Oral contraceptives are preferred once the β-hCG levels have reverted to normal as these pills suppress LH. History of any abnormal bleeding or any other complaints especially those suggesting metastatic activity must be elicited. Pelvic examination must be done to evaluate the size of uterus and presence of any enlarged ovaries at every visit. In case of any abnormality, patient must be evaluated for persistent disease.

CLINICAL PRESENTATION

- Past history of *any* type of pregnancy
- Irregular or acyclical vaginal bleeding
- Symptoms related to metastases
  Cough breathlessness and hemoptysis—in case of lung metastases
  Headache, convulsion—in case of metastases to brain.
- Enlarged, soft uterus (Generally larger than period of amenorrhea)
- Unilateral or bilateral enlarged ovaries
- Purplish red nodule in lower third of anterior vaginal wall (Suburethral nodule) which indicates a metastatic lesion in vagina. These nodules are highly vascular and hence biopsy or any disruption to this nodule can cause torrential bleeding
- Liver enlargement due to metastasis
- Rarely, hemoperitoneum due to uterine perforation or neurological signs of raised intracranial pressure.

INVESTIGATIONS

Serum β-hCG levels must be estimated to confirm the diagnosis. USG pelvis, preferably TVS, must be done to determine local extent of disease. Doppler evaluation showing increased vascularity in the uterine cavity or in the myometrium is usually pathognomonic. Complete blood count, ABO and Rh typing, liver and kidney function tests are done as baseline investigations as patient may require chemotherapy.

Uterine curettage is not necessary for cases of GTN as most cases are managed based on clinical diagnosis and histological documentation is not required. It also increases the risks of bleeding, uterine perforation and infection and is hence not recommended.

Sometimes, in cases of GTN with extremely high β-hCG levels, false negative low levels of serum β-hCG may occur. This is explained by hook effect.

Once the patient has been diagnosed as GTN, a detailed workup for metastases should be done. The common mode of spread is hematological and the frequent sites of spread are lung, vagina, spleen, kidney, liver and brain. The symptoms and management of these metastases are discussed in detail in later part of this chapter. The following investigations must be done as a part of metastatic workup.

Chest X-ray generally follows detection of high β-hCG levels. It may have different distinct patterns in cases of metastatic GTN. Chest X-ray shows alveolar or "snow storm" pattern, discrete rounded densities or an embolic pattern suggestive of pulmonary arterial occlusion. Pleural effusion may also be present.

Computed tomography (CT) chest may be considered as there can be micrometastatic lesions in 40% of patients which would be undetectable on chest X-ray.[6] the significance of this finding is that in absence of metastases to lung; spread to other sites is unlikely. If there is no lesion found in CT chest, there is no need for further metastatic workup.

USG abdomen/MRI abdomen can be considered if there is any suspicion of metastases to liver, spleen or kidney if any symptoms are suggestive.

Computed tomography (CT) brain may be required to identify lesion in brain parenchyma. Rarely, β-hCG of CSF can be done and if the ratio of hCG levels between CSF and serum is higher than 1:60, then it is suggestive of cerebral metastases.[7] However, this is not routinely recommended in the workup because its accuracy is uncertain.

Very rarely, FDG–PET may be advised to detect the sites of metabolically active or viable metastases and hence helps in assessing the tumor resectability.[8] This can be done to detect occult lesions in cases where serum β-hCG is high but there is no lesions detectable clinically or in imaging modalities.

Staging and Prognostic Scoring

Similar to all malignancies, FIGO has advised a staging system for GTN (Table 25.1) but contrary to other malignancies, the staging does not determine type of treatment, which is primarily chemotherapy. Choice of drug and decision for use of single or multiple drugs is largely based on WHO prognostic scoring which is detailed in Table 25.2.

PERSISTENT GESTATIONAL TROPHOBLASTIC NEOPLASIA

When there is persistence of trophoblastic activity during follow-up period of mole the term

Table 25.1 FIGO anatomic staging for GTN (2000)

Stages	Extension
Stage 1	Confined to uterus
Stage 2	Spread outside uterus but confined to genital tract
Stage 3	Metastases to lung
Stage 4	Metastases to liver, spleen, gastrointestinal tract, brain

Abbreviations: FIGO, international Federation of Obstetrics and Gynecology; GTN, gestational trophoblastic neoplasia

Table 25.2 Modified WHO prognostic scoring system as adapted by FIGO for GTN (2000)

Criteria	Score 0	Score 1	Score 2	Score 4
Age (years)	≤40	>40	—	—
Antecedent pregnancy	Hydatidiform mole	Abortion	Term pregnancy	—
Interval months from index pregnancy*	<4	4–6	7–12	>13
Pretreatment β-hCG**	<10^3	10^3–<10^4	10^4–<10^5	≥10^5
Largest tumor including uterus (cm)	<3	3–4	>5	
Site of metastases***	Lungs****, pelvis	Spleen, kidney	Gastrointestinal tract, liver	Brain
Number of metastases	—	1–4	5–8	>8
Prior chemotherapy	—	—	Single drug	Two or more drugs

Low risk <6; High risk ≥7
*Interval months from index pregnancy refers to interval from antecedent pregnancy to start of chemotherapy.
**β-hCG levels at the time of diagnosis of GTN should be considered and not at the time of molar evacuation (if it was a preceding event).
***In case of metastases to multiple sites, the highest scoring organ must be taken for calculating the risk score instead of adding score for various sites. [For example, if patient has both splenic and cerebral metastases, the score is only 4 (score for brain) and it is not 5].
****Lung metastases counted only on chest X-ray not on a CT chest.
The identification of an individual patient's stage and risk score is expressed by allotting a Roman numeral to the stage and an arabic numeral to the risk score separated by a colon (e.g. I:5, IV:11, or II:9)

Abbreviations: FIGO, International Federation of Obstetrics and Gynecology; GTN, gestational trophoblastic neoplasia; WHO, World Health Organization

persistent GTN is often used. It is also sometimes referred to as post molar GTN or persistent trophoblastic disease (PTD).

The following are the main criteria for diagnosis of persistent GTN.
- Plateauing of serum β-hCG level for 4 measurements during a period of three weeks or longer (day 1, 7, 14 and 21), i.e. +/– 10%
- Rise of serum β-hCG of >10% during three consecutive measurements or longer during a period of two weeks (day 1, 7 and 14)
- The presence of metastases in addition to abnormal β-hCG levels.
- Persisting serum β-hCG levels for 6 months or more after evacuation of mole
- Histology suggesting choriocarcinoma, placental site trophoblastic tumor (PSTT) and ETT.

A rise in β-hCG following a normal regression pattern must also be considered as persistence of trophoblastic activity. The persistent GTN can also be termed as post molar GTN if this follows a molar pregnancy.

INVASIVE MOLE

It used to be called as chorioadenoma destruens. It arises when hydatidiform mole invades myometrium. The most common clinical presentation is irregular, acyclical vaginal bleeding with elevation or plateauing of serum β-hCG levels. It generally manifests within six months of antecedent pregnancy. Rarely, uterine wall may be perforated at multiple sites showing purple fungating growth leading to massive hemoperitoneum. Neoplasm may invade the pelvic blood vessels and metastasises to vagina or distant sites via direct extension or through venous channels.

On histology: There is penetration of the myometrium by the hyperplastic trophoblastic cells which retain villous structure without evidence of muscle necrosis.

CHORIOCARCINOMA

It is a highly malignant tumor arising from chorionic epithelium but is currently rarely diagnosed as patients are not subjected to tissue diagnosis.

Incidence: Choriocarcinoma affects one in 40,000 pregnancies and one in 40 hydatidiform moles in Europe and North America whereas it is 9.2 per 40,000 pregnancies in South East Asia and 3.3 per 40,000 pregnancies in Japan. When GTN develops after nonmolar pregnancy, the chances of choriocarcinoma is 1000 times more likely.[9] In a very old textbook, incidence of choriocarcinoma in India is given and it varied even in different cities of India. It was one in 4000 pregnancies in Kolkata, one in 2958 pregnancies in Chennai whereas it was one in 525 pregnancies in Kerala (Trivandrum).[10]

Naked Eye Appearance

The lesion is usually localized nodular type, red, hemorrhagic and necrotic mass in the lower genital tract. A suburethral or vaginal nodule is characteristic.

Microscopic Appearance

Anaplastic sheets of trophoblastic cells invading the uterine musculature are seen. There is extensive necrosis and hemorrhage and villus pattern is completely absent. Clusters of cytotrophoblast separated by syncytiotrophoblast forming dimorphic plexiform pattern are generally seen.

PLACENTAL SITE TROPHOBLASTIC TUMOR

Incidence: It is a very rare tumor and constitutes to 1% of all GTN.[1]

The common clinical symptom is irregular bleeding or amenorrhea. Tumor arises from the trophoblasts of the placental bed. This tumor most commonly follows a normal pregnancy. It is commonly diagnosed following curettage in a patient reporting irregular vaginal bleeding following delivery. It consists of mononuclear intermediate trophoblast cells predominantly without chorionic villi infiltrating between myometrial fibers. Syncytiotrophoblasts are absent. Its presentation ranges from self-limited neoplasm to highly aggressive metastatic tumor. It has less vascular invasion and it metastasises through lymphatics.

Marker: β-hCG levels are low and human placental lactogen (hPL) is secreted but is rarely detected in serum. Immunohistochemistry shows diffuse presence of cytokeratin and hPL with focal hCG. The cause for low hCG levels is that intermediate trophoblasts produce only minimal amount of hCG. Specifically in *treatment of these cases,* hysterectomy is the preferred as it is not responsive to chemotherapy.

EPITHELIOID TROPHOBLASTIC TUMOR

It is extremely rare. It may be misdiagnosed as squamous cell carcinoma of cervix, choriocarcinoma or PSTT. It also arises from intermediate trophoblasts but these differ from the cells that give rise to PSTT. The intermediate trophoblasts here are small and show less nuclear pleomorphism and also the cells grow in a nodular pattern when compared with PSTT which shows an infiltrative pattern. It is managed in the same way as PSTT.

METASTATIC GESTATIONAL TROPHOBLASTIC NEOPLASIA

The most common sites of metastases are lung (80%), vagina (30%), brain (10%) and liver (10%).[11] Generally fragile vessels supply these tumors. Hence, biopsy from the metastatic regions is not recommended. Cerebral and liver metastases are uncommon unless there is a metastases to lung or vagina. Therefore, if there is no metastatic lesion found on CECT chest and the patient is asymptomatic, other metastatic workup is not necessary.[12]

Various symptoms and signs of the metastatic lesions depend on the site of the lesion.

Pulmonary metastases may cause dyspnea, chest pain, cough and hemoptysis. This may be due to pulmonary artery occlusion by trophoblastic emboli. Vaginal metastases may lead to irregular vaginal bleeding or purulent vaginal discharge. They may be seen as vascular lesions in vagina especially in suburethral region or vaginal fornices. Cerebral metastases may cause nausea, vomiting, headache, seizures, slurred speech, visual problems, and hemiparesis because of increased intracranial pressure or intracranial bleeding. In case of metastases to liver, patient may have jaundice and epigastric pain.

MANAGEMENT OF GESTATIONAL TROPHOBLASTIC NEOPLASIA

Chemotherapy is the mainstay of treatment for patients with GTN. Chemotherapy is extensively used as the first line of treatment in patients with gestational trophoblastic neoplasia because of the response of these neoplasms to cytotoxic agents. The cure rate will depend upon the type of regimen used and also on the stage of the patient. Along with chemotherapy, surgery and radiation also have some role in management of selected patients. Prophylactic chemotherapy is also used by some gynecologists and it is discussed in detail in later part of this chapter.

TREATMENT OF LOW-RISK GESTATIONAL TROPHOBLASTIC NONMETASTATIC NEOPLASIA

These patients are generally given single agent chemotherapy. The commonly used chemotherapy regimen in this group is methotrexate with folinic acid or actinomycin D. In this, methotrexate folinic acid can be given over 8 days with methotrexate every alternate day (D1, 3, 5, 7) and folinic acid on the intervening days (D2, 4, 6, and 8). This regimen was first proposed by Bagshawe et al. in 1989. Methotrexate can be also given as IV bolus followed by IV infusion followed by folinic acid. Actinomycin D can be given as pulsed dose or over 5 days. The detailed regimen, dose, schedule and frequency of the chemotherapy drugs in GTN are discussed in Chemotherapy chapter of this book.

Various studies have been conducted on single agent chemotherapy comparing various regimes in patients with GTN. On comparing 8 day regime of methotrexate with IV infusion of methotrexate, there was higher remission rate in the former group.[13]

Cure rate of single agent approaches 100%. One to two cycles of maintenance chemotherapy should be given after the first normal β-hCG. The recurrence rates are <5% if two more cycles are given after normalization of β-hCG because normal or negative β-hCG indicates that the number of tumor cells is less than 10^5 and it does not mean that the disease is completely eliminated. Single agent methotrexate typically achieves complete response rate of 73% after four to five cycles whereas single agent actinomycin-D has better response rate of 100%.[14]

Even though actinomycin D has better response than methotrexate, methotrexate is preferred as a first-line agent due to its lower side effects, i.e. less nausea, less vomiting, no alopecia and no cardiotoxicity. Actinomycin D should be carefully injected as it may cause sloughing of skin when extravasated. Actinomycin is used as first line in cases of hepatic dysfunction or who have a known adverse reaction to methotrexate.

Cochrane review in 2009 has showed that pulsed actinomycin D was superior to methotrexate (level of evidence A).[15] Osborne et al. 2011 had reported that twice weekly intravenous actinomycin D showed a better response compared to weekly IM methotrexate (50 mg/m²)[16] (level of evidence A).

However, large multicenter randomized trials are yet to be conducted to establish the most appropriate regimen for these patients. We use methotrexate as the first line drug because of its safety profile and feasibility in administering it to patients.

About 3% of patients with low risk GTN and 7–10% patients with high risk GTN are known to develop drug resistance. If the patient is found to be resistant to single agent chemotherapy, then multiagent combination chemotherapy MAC regimen containing methotrexate, actinomycin D and cyclophosphamide or chlorambucil can be started. The remission rate is found to be between 65% and 75%.[17]

MANAGEMENT OF HIGH-RISK METASTATIC GTN

These high-risk patients generally need multiagent chemotherapy. The most commonly used combination chemotherapy in patients with high-risk metastatic GTN is EMACO regimen containing etoposide, actinomycin D, methotrexate, cyclophosphamide and vincristine (oncovin) because of its less toxicity when compared to other regimes. The next commonly used combination is EMACE regimen which is similar to EMACO except for vincristine which is replaced by a platinum agent (cisplatin) and cyclophosphamide is not given on day 8 instead etoposide is repeated. The detailed regimen of these various combinations is discussed later.

Some other regimens that may be used are:
- MACE—Methotrexate, actinomycin D, cisplatin and etoposide
- MFA—Methotrexate, folinic acid, actinomycin D
- CHAMOCA—Cyclophosphamide, hydroxycarbamide, doxorubicin, actinomycin D, methotrexate, melphalan and vincristine
- BEP—bleomycin, etoposide and cisplatin
- ICE—ifosfamide, carboplatin, etoposide

During this 8 day cycle, G-CSF (filgrastim) can be given between D3 and D7. Before start of next cycle, routine investigations must be done and next cycle is started only when WBCs >3000 cells/mL, granulocytes >1500/mL and platelets >1 lakh/mL.

All these multiagent chemotherapy must be given every 2 weeks for three cycles beyond negative β-hCG. The cure rate for EMACO regimen was up to 76% while cure rate of EMA/CE regimen was between 67% when used as 2nd line therapy.[18]

A study by Kim et al. has compared the effectiveness of various regimens like EMACO, CHAMOCA, MAC and MFA in patients with high risk GTN.[17] The respective remission rates were 91%, 71%, 68% and 63%.

Risk of secondary malignancies is high with etoposide and the risk ratio is 1.5 when compared to normal population. Myeloid leukemia (RR 16.6) is the most common secondary malignancy followed by breast (RR 5.8), colon cancer (RR 4.6) and melanoma.[19] EMA/CE regimen is associated with hematological toxicity, ototoxicity and peripheral neuropathy.

PROPHYLACTIC CHEMOTHERAPY

Prophylactic chemotherapy is controversial in patients of molar pregnancy but some workers have considered the following risk factors for persistent GTN.
- Maternal age >40 years
- Previous history of molar pregnancy
- Uterine size >20 weeks
- Serum β-hCG levels >100,000 IU/mL at the time of diagnosis of molar pregnancy
- Bilateral theca lutein cysts >6 cm
- Women of molar pregnancy with medical complications like hyperthyroidism as this complication occur with very high β-hCG.
- β-hCG levels fail to become normal by 7-9 weeks since evacuation of a molar pregnancy or there is elevation
- Evidence of metastasis irrespective of level of β-hCG
- Women who are noncompliant for future follow-up.

Cochrane review 2012 had concluded that prophylactic chemotherapy of single course of methotrexate and folinic acid may reduce the risk of persistent GTN in women with molar pregnancy who are at a high risk of malignant transformation; however, it also simultaneously increases drug resistance and unnecessary toxic side effects, hence this practice cannot currently be recommended.[20] The gold standard is subjecting the women to close follow-up and monitoring for diagnosis of persistent GTN. Also, prophylactic chemotherapy does not eliminate the need for follow-up.

INDICATIONS OF HYSTERECTOMY

Though the primary therapeutic modality is chemotherapy occasionally surgical intervention by way of hysterectomy could be considered in the following situations:
- Placental site trophoblastic tumor, epithelioid trophoblastic tumor as both these tumors are chemoresistant.
- In emergency conditions like rupture uterus, uncontrolled bleeding per vaginum.
- Failed chemotherapy or drug resistant chemotherapy in both low risk and high risk GTN as indicated. Patient must be individualized by the gynecologist and decision must be taken accordingly.
- Some patients who have completed their families may want hysterectomy to avoid chemotherapy or prolonged follow-up. These patients must be explained that even after hysterectomy there is still 3-10% chance for need for chemotherapy.[21]
- Localized uterine lesion resistant to chemotherapy.

EMERGENCY SITUATIONS

Emergency situations that can occur in these patients are acute abdomen, uterine perforation, rupture uterus, peritonitis, excessive bleeding per vaginum, hemoperitoneum, respiratory distress.

In all these conditions, initial measures must be taken to resuscitate the patient, i.e. airway, breathing, circulation to be maintained. Intravenous fluid replacement and blood transfusion must be done depending on patient's blood loss and vital condition. In case of uterine rupture or perforation or uncontrolled uterine bleeding, patient must be taken up for emergency hysterectomy. In these patients, after hysterectomy, chemotherapy may be required for treating metastases. In case of respiratory distress, conservative management is done. Patient can be provided positive pressure ventilation or put on mechanical ventilator. In cases of hemoptysis or respiratory distress, if there are localized pulmonary metastases, thoracotomy is preferred.

MANAGEMENT OF METASTASES AT VARIOUS SITES

Brain Metastases

Patients with cerebral metastases are at increased risk for intracerebral hemorrhage.
- Craniotomy for acute decompression can be done or surgical resection.
- Whole brain irradiation (2000–4000 cGy over 10–20 fractions) with or without chemotherapy. Brain irradiation acts as both tumoricidal and hemostatic over cerebral metastases.
- Systemic chemotherapy with combined intrathecal methotrexate 12.5 mg and high dose IV methotrexate (300–1000 mg/m^2) as part of EMACO system.

Lung Metastases

Thoracotomy with pulmonary wedge resection may be required for patients when they present with hemoptysis in spite of chemotherapy.

Liver Metastases

These patients are at increased risk of hepatic bleeding and active intervention may be required to manage hepatic rupture.
- Selective hepatic artery occlusion
- Selective chemoembolization
- Chemotherapy/radiotherapy (2000 cGy over 10 fractions)

NEWER OPTIONS IN PATIENTS WITH EMACO RESISTANCE

In recent years, there has been a reported increase in drug resistance in GTN patients in western literature and hence some alternative chemotherapeutic agents to treat GTN has been studied.[22] Wang et al. has proposed TP/TE regimen (paclitaxel, etoposide and cisplatin) for relapsed high risk GTN.[23] 5-fluorouracil containing drug regime has also found to have 100% efficacy for drug resistant GTN. Giacolone et al. had also reported that autologous bone marrow transplantation with high dose chemotherapy was found to have improved outcome in refractory GTN cases.[24] Table 25.3 shows the various treatment protocols in different stages of GTN.

FOLLOW-UP AND SURVEILLANCE

All patients must be followed with weekly serum quantitative β-hCG levels until levels are undetectable (<2 mIU/mL) for four weeks, then fortnightly for two months followed by monthly for total of one year in stage I, II and III, and this period of follow-up is extended for 24 months in stage IV disease.

History and pelvic examination should be done at every visit.

CONTRACEPTION

The patient must be advised not to conceive until one year of completion of chemotherapy. This is because the risk of abnormal pregnancy was found to be greater during the first six months following treatment compared to one year later.[25] The patients must be explained regarding the options of contraception. Oral contraceptives are safe.

ADVICE ON FUTURE PREGNANCY

The patients must be advised to report immediately if she has a missed period and first trimester ultrasound and β-hCG is a must in all these patients. Postpartum β-hCG levels should be done after 6 weeks to confirm that the levels are normalized after delivery so that occult trophoblastic disease can be ruled out and placenta must be sent for histopathology examination.

Blagden et al. (2002) from London in his study had reported 71% pregnancies were full term delivery following GTN.[26] There was no increase in the incidence of congenital anomalies in

Table 25.3 Treatment protocols for different stages of gestational trophoblastic neoplasia

Stage/risk	Initial treatment	If resistant	Follow-up*
Stage 1	• Methotrexate/Actinomycin D • Hysterectomy if patient persisting along with adjuvant single agent chemotherapy	• MAC • EMACO if MAC fails • Hysterectomy with adjuvant chemotherapy • Local uterine resection (if localized lesion and patient wants to preserve fertility)	Up to 12 months after achieving normal β-hCG levels
Stage 2 and 3 low risk	Methotrexate/Actinomycin D	• MAC or EMACO • Hysterectomy as indicated	Up to 12 months after achieving normal β-hCG levels
Stage 2 and 3 high risk	• EMACO • EMACE	• VBP • Surgery if required	Up to 12 months after achieving normal β-hCG levels
Stage 4	• EMACO • Management of metastases accordingly	• EMACE • VBP • Management of metastases accordingly	Up to 24 months after achieving normal β-hCG levels

*Contraception is mandatory until complete follow-up is over.

these patients. It remained the same as that of normal population.

QUIESCENT GESTATIONAL TROPHOBLASTIC DISEASE

This refers to persistent low levels of real β-hCG in patients with history of molar pregnancy or abortion without clinically evident disease. Normally the levels range between 50 mIU/mL and 100 mIU/mL. There is no change in the serum levels of β-hCG with any treatment neither chemotherapy nor surgery. hCG in these cases revealed absence of hyper glycosylated variant of hCG which is responsible for cytotrophoblastic invasion. On subsequent follow-up, about 25% of patients developed active trophoblastic disease after several weeks to several years.[11] Once the active disease develops there is increase in hCG-H and at this period of time, it is chemosensitive.

KEY POINTS

- Gestational trophoblastic disease (GTD) refers to a spectrum of disorders of abnormal growth and development of the placental trophoblasts that may continue even beyond the pregnancy.
- The individual subtypes in the invasive or malignant group can be differentiated only by a histological diagnosis but that is generally not necessary as they are clubbed under clinical term GTN.
- Persistent gestational trophoblastic neoplasia, invasive mole, choriocarcinoma, placental site trophoblastic tumor (PSTT) and epithelioid trophoblastic tumor (ETT) have the ability to invade and metastasis and are collectively termed as gestational trophoblastic neoplasia (GTN).

- The most common sites of metastases are lung (80%), vagina (30%), brain (10%) and liver (10%).
- If there is no metastatic lesion found on CECT chest and the patient is asymptomatic, other metastatic workup is not necessary.
- Immediately after diagnosis, patient must be assigned FIGO and modified WHO prognostic score and must be categorized into low risk or high risk.
- The commonly used chemotherapy regimen for low risk GTN are methotrexate with folinic acid or actinomycin D and their cure rate is around 100%.
- The most commonly used combination chemotherapy in patients with high risk metastatic GTN is EMACO regimen. The cure rate for EMACO regimen was up to 76%.
- Follow-up according to standard schedule is essential. Patient must be evaluated repeatedly using both clinical and investigating parameters.
- History and pelvic examination should be done at every visit of follow-up.
- The patient must be advised not to conceive until one year of completion of chemotherapy.
- The patients must be advised to report immediately if she has a missed period. First trimester ultrasound and β-hCG is a must in all these patients.
- Postpartum β-hCG levels should be done after 6 weeks to confirm that the levels are normalized after delivery.

REFERENCES

1. Miller FM, Laing FC. Gestational trophoblastic disease. *http://brighamrad.harvard.edu/cases/bwh/hcache/34/full.html* accessed on July 29, 2016.
2. Berkowitz RS, Goldstein DP. In: Berck JS. Gestational trophoblastic neoplasm. Philadelphia: Lippincott, Williams and Wilkins; 2002. pp. 1353-74.
3. Daftary SN, Padubidri VG. Trophoblastic diseases. In: Padubidri VG, Daftary SN (Eds). Shaw's Textbook of Gynaecology, 13th edition, New Delhi. Elseiver India Ltd; 2004.pp.248-59.
4. Seckl MJ, Sebire NJ, Berkowitz RS. Gestational trophoblastic disease. Lancet. 2010;376:717-29.
5. Berkowitz RS, Goldstein DP. Chorionic tumors. N Engl J Med. 1996;335 (23):1740-98.
6. Garner EIO, Garrett A, Goldstein DP, et al. Significance of chest computed tomography findings in the evaluation and treatment of persistent gestational trophoblastic neoplasia. J Reprod Med. 2004;49:112-8.
7. Bakri Y, Al-Hawashim N, Berkowitz RS. Cerebrospinal fluid/serum β-subunit human chorionic gonadotrophin ratio in patients with brain metastases of gestational trophoblastic tumor. J Reprod Med. 2000;45:94-6.
8. Dhillon T, Palmieri C, Sebire NJ, et al. "Value of whole body FDG-PET to identify the active site of gestational trophoblastic neoplasia." J Reprod Med Obstet Gynaecol. 2006;51(11):879-87.
9. Lurain JR. Gestational Trophoblastic Disease 1: Epidemiology, pathology, clinical presentation and diagnosis of gestational trophoblastic disease, and management of hydatidiform mole. Am J Obstet Gynecol. 2010;203(1):531-9.
10. JE Holland et al. (Eds). A study of choriocarcinoma its incidence and its etiopathogenesis by Dr Narayana Pai. Springer, Berlin Heidelberg, 1967.
11. Ngan YS, Kohorn EI, Cole LA, Kurman RJ, Kim SJ, Lurain JR, et al. Trophoblastic disease. Int J Obstet Gynecol. 2012;S130-6.
12. May T, Goldstein DP, Berkowitz RS. Current Chemotherapeutic Management of Patients with Gestational Trophoblastic Neoplasia; 2011, Article ID 806256, 12 pages doi:10.1155/2011/806256.
13. Growdon WB, Wolfberg AJ, Goldstein DP, et al. "Evaluating methotrexate treatment in patients with low-risk post molar gestational trophoblastic neoplasia," Gynecol Oncol. 2009;112(2):353-7.
14. Lertkhachonsuk AA, Israngura N, Wilailak S, et al. Actinomycin D versus methotrexate-folinic acid as the treatment of stage I, low-risk gestational trophoblastic neoplasia: a randomized controlled trial. Int J Gynecol Cancer. 2009; 19(5):985-8.
15. Alazzam M, Tidy J, Hancock BW, et al. First line chemotherapy in low risk gestational trophoblastic neoplasia. Cochrane Database Syst Rev. 2009;(1):CD007102.
16. Osborne RJ, Filiaci V, Schink JC, Mannel RS, Alvarez Secord A, Kelley JL, et al. Phase III trial of weekly methotrexate or pulsed dactinomycin for low-risk gestational trophoblastic neoplasia: a Gynecologic Oncology Group study. J Clin Oncol. 2011;29(7):825-31.
17. Kim SJ, Bae SN, Kim JH, Kim CT, Han KT, Lee JM. "Effects of multiagent chemotherapy and

independent risk factors in the treatment of high-risk GTT—25 years experiences of KRI-TRD." Int J Obstet Gynecol. 1998;60:S85-S96.
18. Mao Y, Wan X, Lv W, Xie X. Relapsed or refractory gestational trophoblastic neoplasia treated with the etoposide and cisplatin/etoposide, methotrexate, and actinomycin D (EP-EMA) regimen. Int J Gynaecol Obstet. 2007;98(1):44-7. Epub 2007 May 3.
19. Rustin GJS, Newlands ES, Lutz JM, et al. "Combination but not single-agent methotrexate chemotherapy for gestational trophoblastic tumors increases the incidence of second tumors," J Clin Oncol. 1996;14(10):2769-73.
20. Fu J, Fang F, Xie L, Chen H, He F, Lawrie TA, et al. Prophylactic chemotherapy for hydatidiform mole to prevent gestational trophoblastic neoplasia. Cochrane Database Syst Rev. 2012 Oct 17; 10: CD007289. doi: 10.1002/14651858.CD007289.pub2.
21. Bahar AM, El-Ashnehi MS, Senthilselvan A. Hydatidiform mole in the elderly: Hysterectomy or evacuation? Int J Gynecol Obstet. 1989;29(3):233-8.
22. Alazzam M, Tidy J, Osborne R, Coleman R, Hancock BW, Lawrie TA. Chemotherapy for resistant or recurrent gestational trophoblastic neoplasia. Cochrane Database Syst Rev. 2012 Dec 12; 12:CD008891. doi: 10.1002/14651858.CD008891.pub2.
23. Wang J, Short D, Sebire NJ, et al. "Salvage chemotherapy of relapsed or high-risk gestational trophoblastic neoplasia (GTN) with paclitaxel/cisplatin alternating with paclitaxel/etoposide (TP/TE)," Ann Oncol. 2008;19(9):1578-83.
24. Giacalone PL, Benos P, Donnadio D, et al. "High-dose chemotherapy with autologous bone marrow transplantation for refractory metastatic gestational trophoblastic disease," Gynecol Oncol. 1995;58(3):383-5.
25. Matsui H, Iitsuka Y, Suzuka K, Yamazawa K, Tanaka N, Mitsuhashi A, et al. Early pregnancy outcomes after chemotherapy for gestational trophoblastic tumor. J Reprod Med. 2004;49(7):531-4.
26. Blagden SP, Foskett MA, Fisher RA, Short D, Fuller S, Newlands ES, et al. The effect of early pregnancy following chemotherapy on disease relapse and foetal outcome in women treated for gestational trophoblastic tumours. Br J Cancer. 2002;86(1):26-30.

26

Vulval Cancer

Gauri Gandhi, Snigdha Pathak

INTRODUCTION

Vulvar cancer is uncommon representing about 4% of malignancies of the female genital tract and 0.6% of all cancers in women.[1]

It is predominantly a disease of postmenopausal women and mean age at diagnosis is about 65 years and only 15% patients are younger than 40 years.[2-4]

The incidence of *in situ* vulvar cancer is increasing worldwide, primarily because of the increasing occurrence in younger women, who account for 75% of cases of *in situ* cancer. This increase has been ascribed to the effect of increasing human papilloma virus (HPV) infection.

PATHOLOGY OF VULVAR CANCER—HISTOLOGICAL TYPES

- Squamous—92%
- Melanoma—2-4%
- Basal cell carcinoma—2-3%
- Bartholin gland carcinoma—1%
- Metastatic—1%
- Verrucous—<1%
- Sarcoma—<1%
- Appendage—rare.

Squamous Cancer

There appear to be at least two distinct etiologic entities of squamous cell carcinoma:
- *Basaloid or warty types*: Multifocal, in younger patients and related to HPV infection, vulvar intraepithelial neoplasia (VIN) and cigarette smoking.
- *Keratinizing, differentiated or simplex types*: Unifocal, in older patients and often found in areas adjacent to lichen sclerosus and squamous hyperplasia (Itch-scratch cycle is implicated as an etiologic variable for keratinizing type).

ETIOLOGY AND RISK FACTORS

Human papilloma virus and vulvar cancer: Human papilloma virus (HPV) infection is an established risk factor for basaloid or warty type of vulval cancer. This infection can lead to vulvar intraepithelial neoplasia (VIN) and invasive vulvar cancer. HPV deoxyribonucleic acid (DNA) is found in 89% of VIN 3 and up to 86% of basaloid or warty type of carcinoma vulva, although it is present in <10% of keratinizing type. HPV 16, 33 are the prevalent subtypes.

Cervical intraepithelial neoplasia (CIN) and cervical cancer are the other pathologies associated with HPV infection.

Other risk factors for vulvar cancer include lichen sclerosus, squamous hyperplasia, cigarette smoking, alcohol consumption and immunosuppression.

CLINICAL PRESENTATION

The common symptoms of vulval cancer are as follows:

Symptoms	Signs
• Vulval itching • Vulval irritation/pain • Vulval mass • Ulcerative lesion • Vulval bleeding • Discharge • Dysuria • Metastatic groin mass	• Irregular fungating mass or irregular ulcer or warty lesion or plaque-like lesion over Labia majora and minora (60%), clitoris (15%) or perineum (10%). (10% are too extensive to determine site of origin; 5% are multifocal) • Pigmentation—red/white—overlying neoplastic lesion • Tenderness +/− • Enlarged groin nodes

Though many women may have these symptoms, they may not seek timely intervention.

A careful inspection of the vulva should be part of every gynecologic examination.

Evaluation of a vulval lesion should include—size, location, extent of the lesion, whether unifocal or multifocal, appearance of background epithelium (changes suggestive of lichen sclerosus), any involvement of vagina, urethra, base of bladder or anus. Also presence of groin lymphadenopathy, size of lymph nodes palpable and fixity with skin.

CONFIRMATION OF DIAGNOSIS

Diagnosis is made by examination followed by directed biopsy.

Any suspected premalignant vulval lesion in a woman (premenopausal or postmenopausal) should be biopsied.

A biopsy should be taken under local or regional anesthesia from the interface between normal and abnormal epithelium. Either a wedge biopsy can be taken or a punch biopsy using *Keyes* punch biopsy instrument (Fig. 26.1).

Keyes Punch Biopsy[5]

After adequate local anesthesia, determine the direction of skin tension lines. Using the operator's nondominant hand, hold the skin taut for stabilization perpendicular to the tension lines. Place the Keyes punch (Fig. 26.1) against the lesion at the chosen biopsy site. Place the punch biopsy firmly against the skin and rotate with a constant firm pressure clockwise and then counterclockwise (if necessary) for penetration through the skin. Avoid a back-and-forth twisting motion or stopping the biopsy midprocedure to check the depth of the biopsy, which may result in a shredded tissue sample with rough edges. Generally there is a change in resistance of the Keyes punch on the skin once the biopsy has reached the subcutaneous fat. At this time, the Keyes punch may be removed and the operator may apply pressure using two fingers to elevate the circular tissue to assist in grasping it with forceps. Using the forceps, further elevate the core of skin and subcutaneous tissue and cut the base of the biopsied tissue with curved scissors. Place the excised specimen with the epithelial surface facing upwards on a square piece of filter paper or nonstick pad.

The biopsy should include sufficient underlying dermis to assess the depth of invasion.[6] The biopsy should be a diagnostic biopsy and should not aim to remove the whole lesion.[6]

Vulval cytology is not sufficient and diagnostic biopsies are required.[6]

Other Investigations

- To rule out surrounding vulvar dystrophies and other genital malignancies:

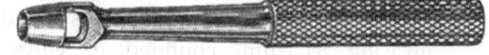

Fig. 26.1 Keyes punch

- Pap smear
- Colposcopy of cervix and vagina
- Vulvoscopy for lesions at other sites on the vulva—Toluidine Blue testing is done to localize the site of biopsy.
- In women with pre-existing vulval lesion, exfoliative cytology using scalpel scraping or Dacron swabs can also be used.

The HPV testing is not a proven screening tool for vulval cancer and does not aid diagnosis.[6] And at present, there is no evidence to support screening an unselected population for vulval cancer.[6]

- *Imaging:*
  - Ultrasound pelvis to look at the uterine cavity, myometrium, adnexa—to rule out other pelvic pathology.
  - Computed tomography (CT)/magnetic resonance imaging (MRI) scan of groin, pelvis, abdomen (epigastrium to mid-thigh, including groin) may be done to see extent of tumor and involvement of lymph nodes. Occasionally other pathology may be found.
- *Additional investigations in large and locally advanced lesions:*
  - Cystourethroscopy—to rule out bladder and urethral involvement in case of midline disease involving external urethral meatus, vestibule or clitoris
  - Intravenous pyelography (IVP)—if bladder base seems involved
  - Proctosigmoidoscopy—if anus or rectum seems involved
- Routine preoperative investigations should be done.

Staging

Revised FIGO Staging 2009 (surgico-pathological):[7]

- *Stage I*: Tumor confined to the vulva
  - *IA*: Lesions <2 cm size, confined to vulva/perineum and with stromal invasion <1 mm and no nodal metastasis.
  - *IB*: Lesions >2 cm size or with stromal invasion >1 mm, confined to vulva/perineum and no nodal metastasis.
- *Stage II*: Tumor of any size with extension to adjacent perineal structures (1/3 lower urethra, 1/3 lower vagina, anus) with negative nodes.
- *Stage III*: Tumor of any size with or without extension to adjacent perineal structures (1/3 lower urethra, 1/3 lower vagina, anus) with positive inguinofemoral lymph nodes.
  - *IIIA*:
    - 1 lymph node ≥ 5 mm or
    - 1-2 lymph nodes <5 mm
  - *IIIB*:
    - 2 or more lymph nodes ≥ 5 mm;
    - 3 or more lymph nodes <5 mm
  - *IIIC*: Positive nodes with extracapsular spread
- *Stage IV*: Tumor invades other regional (2/3 upper urethra, 2/3 upper vagina) or distant structures.
  - *IVA*: Tumor invades any of the following:
    - Upper urethral and/or vaginal mucosa, bladder mucosa, rectal mucosa or fixed to pelvic bone, or
    - Fixed or ulcerated inguinofemoral lymph nodes.
  - *IVB*: Any distant metastases including pelvic lymph nodes.

Depth of invasion is defined as the measurement of the tumor from the epithelial stromal junction of the adjacent most superficial dermal papilla to the deepest point of invasion.

ROUTES OF SPREAD

Vulvar cancer spreads by the following routes:
- Direct extension—to adjacent structures (vagina, urethra, anus)
- Lymphatic spread—to regional inguinal and femoral lymph nodes
- Hematogenous spread—to distant sites (lung, liver, bone). Usually occurs late and is rare in the absence of lymph node metastasis.

Lymphatic metastasis may occur early in the disease. ~30% women with operable disease have nodal spread.[6]

Lymphatics of vulva from each side form a rich network of anastomoses along the midline. Lymphatic drainage from the clitoris, *centrally located* tumors, anterior labia minora and perineum is *bilateral*.

When the tumor invades 1 mm or less, metastasis to the inguinal lymph nodes is extremely rare. When the invasion is greater than 1 mm, there is a significant risk of inguinal lymph node metastasis.

About 12% of tumors ≤ 2 cm in diameter have regional metastasis.[2,8]

However, for lateral tumors ≤ 2 cm in diameter or with ≤ 5 mm invasion, metastases to contralateral lymph nodes in the absence of ipsilateral nodal involvement is very rare (0 to 0.4%).[8,9]

Overall, the incidence of inguinofemoral lymph node involvement is 32%,[10,11] pelvic node involvement is 12% and pelvic node involvement in the absence of groin node involvement is 0.6%. Pelvic node involvement occurs in 16% cases with positive groin nodes, 33% cases with clinically suspicious groin nodes and 40–50% cases having 3 or more pathologically positive inguinal-femoral nodes.[3,9,12,13]

Initially, spread is usually to the inguinal lymph nodes (located between Camper's fascia and fascia lata). From these superficial groin nodes, the disease spreads to deep femoral nodes (located medially along femoral vessels). Cloquet's or Rosenmuller's node, situated beneath the inguinal ligament, is the most cephalad of the femoral node group. Metastases to femoral nodes without involvement of inguinal nodes have been reported.[14] From the inguinofemoral lymph nodes, cancer spreads to the pelvic nodes, particularly the external iliac group.

Histologic features that correlate with the occurrence of inguinal lymph node metastasis are lymph-vascular space invasion, tumor thickness, depth of stromal invasion, histologic pattern of invasion (spray and stellate versus broad and pushing) and increased amount of keratin.[15]

TREATMENT OF PRIMARY DISEASE

Surgery is the main treatment modality and has become more individualized and conservative due to the well-recognized psychosexual sequelae and the morbidity associated with groin node dissection.[16,17] The need for adequate resection margins (1 cm after tissue fixation) and groin node dissection are important basic principles. Reconstructive surgery also has a role in the management of these cancers. Radiotherapy is used in the adjuvant setting and with or without chemotherapy and surgery in advanced disease.

SURGICAL MANAGEMENT

Earlier radical vulvectomy with bilateral inguinofemoral lymphadenectomy by en bloc dissection was the standard therapy. However, the disadvantages of en bloc dissection are:
- Large loss of vulvar tissue with psychosexual sequelae
- A 50% wound breakdown rate
- High incidence of lower extremity lymphedema.

Thus, en bloc dissection has now been replaced by the *triple incision technique*. Separate incisions are given for vulvectomy and lymphadenectomy. This results in significant reduction in wound morbidity. Also, experience with a separate incision technique confirmed that metastases rarely occur in the skin bridge in patients without clinically suspicious groin nodes.[18]

Recent modifications in surgical management are:[19]
- Individualization of treatment for all patients with invasive disease
- Use of separate incisions for groin dissection to improve wound healing
- *Modified radical vulvectomy/wide radical resection*: The types of modified radical vulvectomy include anterior or posterior hemivulvectomy or lateral hemivulvectomy with clitoral sparing

- Omission of groin dissection for patients with Stage IA and no risk factors
- Omission of contralateral groin dissection in patients with lateral lesions <2 cm and negative ipsilateral nodes
- Elimination of routine pelvic lymphadenectomy if inguinofemoral nodes are negative
- Use of preoperative radiation to obviate the need for exenteration in patients with advanced disease
- Use of postoperative radiation therapy to decrease the incidence of groin recurrence in patients with multiple positive groin nodes.

Wide Local Excision

Recommendation is to resect the primary tumor with a 2 cm margin of normal tissue and to carry the dissection up to the deep perineal fascia of the urogenital diaphragm. In tumors <2 cm size, radical local excision results in 90% survival rate.

Radical Vulvectomy

This is done by two elliptical incisions on the vulva. The outer one is placed on the labiocrural folds and anteriorly brought across the mons pubis and posteriorly across the perineal body. The inner incision circumscribes the vaginal introitus and vulvar vestibule. The dissection is carried down to the deep perineal fascia. The aim should be to have a 1.5 cm surgical tumor free margin.[6] Once dissection is complete, the levator ani muscles should be approximated to prevent rectocele formation. After achieving hemostasis, the skin is sutured to vaginal mucosa by interrupted sutures.

Ultraradical Vulvectomy

When tumor involves distal urethra, vagina or anus, but is still resectable, partial resection of these structures may be done. However, if >1 cm of urethra is excised, risk of urinary incontinence is there. Partial resection of external anal sphincter combined with radical local resection of perianal tissue is associated with significant rate of fecal incontinence. Careful sphincter re-approximation and levator muscle plication are done in an effort to minimize incontinence.

Lymphadenectomy

Bilateral inguinofemoral lymphadenectomy is done by separate longitudinal incisions centered midway between the femoral artery and pubic tubercle, extending from 1 inch above to 2 inch below the inguinal ligament. The skin and subcutaneous tissue is incised. The superficial inguinal nodes lie above the cribriform fascia and associated with saphenous vein and its tributaries (superficial circumflex, superficial external pudendal and superficial epigastric), which are first identified and ligated and superficial inguinal nodes are removed. The saphenous vein is identified and ligated at its entry to the femoral vein. A segment of the saphenous vein along with the longitudinal group of lymph nodes is removed. Saphenous vein can be spared also. All lymph nodes around the saphenofemoral junction should be removed and any prominent deeper lymph node (Cloquet node) medial to the femoral vein should also be removed. This can be used as the sentinel node and sent for frozen section. If positive, extraperitoneal pelvic lymphadenectomy may be done. The alternative treatment for positive inguinofemoral nodes is postoperative radiotherapy to the pelvis and groin.

Lymphadenectomy may be omitted in Stage 1A squamous cell cancer, melanoma, basal cell carcinoma and verrucous tumor.[6]

Unilateral lymphadenectomy may be done in a "lateralized lesion" (wide excision of 1 cm beyond visible tumor edge would not impinge upon a midline structure like—clitoris, urethra, vagina, perineal body or anus),[6] which are well differentiated with no lymphovascular space involvement and negative ipsilateral inguinal lymph nodes.

Management of Pelvic Nodes

If a preoperative pelvic imaging study reveals bulky pelvic lymph nodes, resection of these nodes should be done by an extraperitoneal approach prior to radiation.

Sentinel Lymph Node Procedure

Sentinel node is the initial site of metastatic disease and histology of the sentinel node reflects histology of rest of the lymph nodes in that basin. The inguinal-femoral lymph nodes are the sentinel nodes for carcinoma vulva. They can be identified by intraoperative lymphatic mapping using lymphoscintigraphy with Tc-99 labeled nanocolloid or isosulfan blue dye. The advantage of this technique is that extensive lymphadenectomy is avoided in cases where sentinel node is negative.

When a sentinel node is identified in either groin, it should be biopsied. If biopsy negative, no further surgery is required. If biopsy positive, bilateral inguinofemoral lymphadenectomy is to be done. If sentinel lymph node is not identified, then also bilateral groin dissection should be done.[6]

Eligibility criteria[19] given by International Sentinel Node Society's expert panel for performing the sentinel node procedure is:
- Unifocal primary tumor
- <4 cm diameter
- >1 mm invasion
- Absence of obvious metastasis on clinic-radiological examination
- Absence of suspicious groin nodes.

The sentinel node technique should be limited to carefully selected patients in expert centers, ideally on research protocols. Ideally all patients undergoing sentinel lymph node biopsy should be enrolled in ongoing clinical studies like GROINSS-V II.[6]

Reconstructive Surgery[6]

It should be considered for patients where a major resection is planned and there is doubt as to whether direct closure of the wound will be possible. Reconstructive surgical options include:
- *Secondary intention*: If tension-free direct wound closure is not possible, smaller defects can be left to heal by secondary intention. Regular dressing changes and nursing care would be required.
- *Split skin grafts*: Usually taken from the buttock or thigh and rely on a healthy blood supply from the wound bed. Usually reserved for large areas where no flap options are available to provide adequate soft tissue cover. They do not have any bulk, are often tight and can cause difficulty in walking and sexual function. Also, they are unreliable following radiotherapy or in a scarred area.
- *Flaps*: They provide healthy vascularized tissue and do not rely on blood supply from the wound bed. They are thicker and can give bulk which will be useful if radiotherapy is planned in the area.
    - *Local flaps*: Rhomboid flaps, lotus petal flaps or pudendal thigh flaps. Require less dissection to raise but have a possibility of compromised blood supply in case of previous surgery to the area.
    - *Distant flaps*: Gracilis and rectus abdominis muscle flaps. They are larger with a more predictable blood supply. However, they involve a complex surgery with increased donor site morbidity.

Treatment According to Stage

- *Stage 1A*: (tumor <2 cm and stromal invasion <1 mm, no nodes)
    - Wide local excision with 1.5 cm normal tissue margin is usually sufficient
    - Lymph node dissection may be omitted because the risk of lymph node metastases is negligible; except in— poorly differentiated tumor, capillary or lymphatic space involvement or multifocal lesions.
- *Stage 1B*: (tumor >2 cm or stromal invasion >1 mm, no nodes)

Various factors have to be considered to decide surgical approach, including patient's age, size of tumor and site of lesion.
  - *Wide local excision with inguinofemoral lymphadenectomy*
    - Suitable for younger patients with well-localized, small, unifocal lesions.

- In well-lateralized well differentiated, early tumors (RCOG-<2 cm) with no capillary or lymphatic space involvement—ipsilateral inguinofemoral lymphadenectomy is done and sent for frozen section. If positive, then contralateral and pelvic node dissection is done. If negative, no further dissection or postoperative radiotherapy is needed.
- Bilateral lymph node dissection should be done in tumors involving midline structures (clitoris, labia minora, perineal body) or within 2 cm of midline.
  - Radical vulvectomy with bilateral inguinofemoral lymphadenectomy.
- *Stage II* (tumor involving adjacent perineal structures, i.e. lower 1/3 urethra, lower 1/3 vagina, anus) and
- *Stage III* (stage I or II with positive inguinofemoral lymph nodes):
  - Ultraradical vulvectomy with bilateral inguinofemoral lymphadenectomy:
    - In highly selected cases which are clearly resectable with not > 2 positive lymph nodes.
  - Radiotherapy:
    - In medically unfit patients
    - Unresectable disease
    - External beam therapy is appropriate for most cases, with more selective use of brachytherapy.
  - Preoperative chemoradiation followed by limited resection
    - Megavoltage radiotherapy regresses cancer to a point where limited resection can be done with sparing of organ function and better quality of life
    - Surgery is performed 2–6 weeks after completing radiotherapy
    - With combined radiation-surgical approach, 5-year survival rates as high as 76% are reported[20]
    - Nowadays, regarded as the "treatment of choice" for advanced vulvar cancer patients who would otherwise require some type of pelvic exenteration or stoma
- *Stage IV*: (tumor invades other regional or distant structures):
  - Ultraradical surgery—pelvic exenteration
  - Radiotherapy followed by limited resection if possible
  - Combination of chemoradiation followed by surgery
  - Fixed, unresectable groin nodes—primary chemoradiation followed by resection of residual nodes.

The tumor margin should be the same whether a radical vulvectomy or a radical local excision is performed.

If groin dissection is indicated, it should be a thorough inguinal-femoral lymphadenectomy. Superficial inguinal node dissection alone is associated with a higher risk of groin recurrence.

In advanced vulvar cancer, if surgical approach would risk sphincter damage resulting in urinary or fecal incontinence, then treatment by radiotherapy should be considered (curative/neoadjuvant).[6] However, it should be noted that surgery in the postradiation setting can be more challenging with increased morbidity and all management options with their risks and benefits should be discussed with every patient.

When vulvar cancer arises in the presence of VIN or vulvar dystrophy, treatment is according to the patient's age. Radical vulvectomy can be done in elderly patients; whereas for younger patients, radical local excision should be performed for the invasive disease and the associated intraepithelial disease should be treated appropriately. For example, topical steroid may be required for lichen sclerosus or squamous hyperplasia, whereas VIN may require superficial local excision with primary closure or laser ablation.

Postoperative Management

- Low residue diet can be started from 1st postoperative day
- Ambulation can be started from postoperative day 1 or 2
- Pneumatic calf compression or subcutaneous heparin can be given to prevent DVT; active leg movements should be encouraged

- Vulvar wound to be kept dry by frequent dressings
- Urinary catheter is removed when starts to ambulate
- In case of vulvar wound breakdown, sitz bath or whirlpool therapy followed by drying of perineum with a hair dryer is to be done.

POSTOPERATIVE COMPLICATIONS

Early Complications

- *Wound breakdown*: Groin wound infection, necrosis and breakdown is seen in about 53–85% patients having 'en bloc excision' and is reduced to about 44% (major breakdown in only 14%) with 'triple incision technique'.
- Lymphocyst formation may occur in ~40% cases. Treatment is by sterile periodic aspirations.
- Femoral nerve injury is a complication of inguinofemoral lymphadenectomy and can be prevented by avoiding dissection lateral to femoral artery. It usually resolves slowly.
- *UTI*: Treated with antibiotics
- *Thromboembolism*: DVT and pulmonary embolism may occur due to immobilization. Prophylactic low molecular weight heparin can avoid this complication in high-risk patients.
- *Osteitis pubis*: Rare. Bed rest and NSAIDs are used as treatment.

Late Complications

- *Chronic lymphedema*: In ~30% patients[2-4,21]
- Recurrent lymphadenitis or cellulitis of leg: In 10% patients. Responds to antibiotics.
- *Dyspareunia*: Due to introital stenosis. Treated by a vertical relaxing incision sutured transversely.
- Urinary and fecal incontinence.
- *Rectocele*: If levators not approximated.
- *Femoral hernia*: Uncommon.
- Pubic osteomyelitis and rectovaginal fistula are rare.
- Psychosexual complications.

ROLE OF RADIATION

Radiotherapy for vulval cancer is indicated in:
- Preoperatively in patients with advanced disease who would otherwise require pelvic exenteration; also patients with fixed, unresectable groin nodes.
- Postoperatively in patients with positive groin nodes to treat the groin and pelvic lymph nodes.
- Postoperatively in patients with close surgical margins (<5 mm) to prevent local recurrence.[22,23] There is insufficient evidence to recommend adjuvant local therapy routinely in patients with close surgical margins.[6]
- As primary therapy for young patients with small primary tumor involving clitoral and periclitoral regions in whom surgery would have adverse psychological consequences.

If clinically evident groin metastases, any extracapsular spread or ≥ 2 microscopically positive groin nodes are found—patient should receive postoperative groin and pelvic irradiation.

Teletherapy at a dose of 45–55Gy to whole pelvis, including vulva and groins is given.

ROLE OF CHEMOTHERAPY

Mostly used in the neoadjuvant setting along with radiation in advanced vulvar cancer where primary resection would have high morbidity.

Drugs used are—bleomycin, cisplatin and 5-fluorouracil.

PROGNOSIS

Overall 5-year survival rate in operable cases is 70–80%.

Prognosis depends on the following:
- *Stage of the disease*: The prognosis of patients with early stage disease is good.
- *Lymph node status*: The number of positive groin nodes is the most important prognostic factor. With negative groin nodes, the 5-year survival rate for invasive carcinoma is over 80%; for patients with positive groin nodes it

is below 50%. Patients with 3 or more positive nodes have a 2-year survival rate of only 20%. With positive pelvic nodes, survival falls further to 11%. The size of the nodal metastases, proportion of the node replaced by tumor cells and presence of extracapsular spread are important predictors of survival.
- Depth of stromal invasion and lymphvascular space involvement.
- Histologic grade of tumor.

FOLLOW-UP

After treatment completion, a long-term follow-up is needed—every 6 months for the first 5 years and annually thereafter. Aim is to detect local recurrences, recurrence in groin nodes, distant metastases or a new primary vulval tumor. Treatment related complications should be looked for. Also, surveillance for associated cervical or vaginal malignancies should be done.

RECURRENCE

Incidence is 15–35% (~30% vulval cancers will recur even after satisfactory primary treatment).

The sites are: Vulva (70%), groin (24%), pelvis (15%) and distant organs (18%).

Status of surgical margins is the most powerful predictor of recurrence, with ~50% recurrence rate with margins <8 mm.

Treatment: Depends on site and extent of recurrence
- Vulval recurrence—wide local excision or radiotherapy (combination of external beam + interstitial)
- Groin recurrence—radiotherapy or radical groin dissection
- Advanced beyond vulva—pelvic irradiation or palliative surgery or chemotherapy
- Distant recurrence; difficult to treat; poor prognosis. Chemotherapy may be used.

REFERENCES

1. Siegel R, Ward E, Brawley O, et al. Cancer statistics 2011. CA Cancer J Clin. 2011;61:212-36.
2. Rutledge F, Smith JP, Franklin EW. Carcinoma of the vulva. Am J Obstet Gynecol. 1970;106:1117-30.
3. Podratz KC, Symmonds RE, Taylor WF, et al. Carcinoma of the vulva: analysis of treatment and survival. Obstet Gynecol. 1983;61:63-74.
4. Cavanagh D, Fiorica JV, Hoffman MS, et al. Invasive carcinoma of the vulva: changing trends in surgical management. Am J Obstet Gynecol. 1990;163:1007-115.
5. Goldstein GR, Goldstein AT. Punch biopsy for the evaluation of vulvar dermatoses. J Sex Med. 2009;6:1214-7.
6. RCOG: Guidelines for the Diagnosis and Management of Vulval Carcinoma; 2014.
7. Pecorelli S. Revised FIGO staging for carcinoma of the vulva, cervix and endometrium. Int J Gynaecol Obstet. 2009;105:103-4.
8. Hacker NF, Van der Velden J. Conservative management of early vulvar cancer. Cancer. 1993;71:1673-7.
9. Gonzalez Bosquet J, Magrina JF, Magtibay PM, et al. Patterns of inguinal groin metastasis in squamous cell carcinoma of the vulva. Gynecol Oncol. 2007;105:742-6.
10. Stehman FB, Bundy BN, Dvoretsky PM, et al. Early stage I carcinoma of the vulva treated with ipsilateral superficial inguinal lymphadenectomy and modified radical hemi-vulvectomy: a prospective study of the Gynecologoc Oncology Group. Obstet Gynecol. 1992;79:490-7.
11. Levenback C, Burke TW, Morris M, et al. Potential applications of intraoperative lymphatic mapping in vulvar cancer. Gynecol oncol. 1995;59:216-20.
12. Hopkins MP, Reid CG, Vettrano I, et al. Squamous cell carcinoma of the vulva: prognostic factors influencing survival. Gynecol oncol. 1991;43:113-7.
13. Homesley HD, Bundy BN, Sedlis A, et al. Radiation therapy versus pelvic node resection for carcinoma of the vulva with positive groin nodes. Obstet Gynecol. 1986;68:733-40.
14. Chu J, Tamimi HK, Figge DC. Femoral node metastasis with negative superficial inguinal nodes in early vulvar cancer. Am J Obstet Gynecol. 1981;140:37-9.
15. Binder SW, Huang I, Fu YS, et al. Risk factors for the development of lymph node metastasis in vulvar squamous cell carcinoma. Gynecol Oncol. 1990;37:9-16.
16. Andersen BL. Predicting sexual and psychologic morbidity and improving quality of life for women with gynecologic cancer. Cancer. 1993;71:1678-90.

17. Andersen BL, Turnquist D, LaPolla J, Turner D. Sexual functioning after treatment of in-situ vulvar cancer: preliminary report. Obstet Gynecol. 1988;71:15-9.
18. Hacker NF, Leuchter RS, Berek JS, et al. Radical vulvectomy and bilateral inguinal lymphadenectomy through separate groin incisions. Obstet Gynecol. 1981;58:574-9.
19. Holschneider CH, Berek JS. Vulvar Cancer. Berek and Novak's Gynecology, 15th edition. Lippincott Williams & Wilkins; 2012.pp.1428-57.
20. Boronow RC, Hickman BT, Reagan MT, et al. Combined therapy as an alternative to exenteration for locally advanced vulvovaginal cancer. Am J Clin Oncol. 1987;10:171-81.
21. Gaarenstroom KN, Kenter GG, Trimbos JB, et al. Postoperative complications after vulvectomy and inguinofemoral lymphadenectomy using separate groin incisions. Int J Gynecol Cancer. 2003;13: 522-27.
22. Faul CM, Mirmow D, Huang Q, et al. Adjuvant radiation for vulvar carcinoma: improved local control. Int J Radiat Oncol Biol Phys. 1997;38:381-9.
23. Hoffman MS, Stickles BX. Malignancies of the Vulva. Te Linde's Operative Gynecology, 11th edition. Wolters Kluwer; 2015.pp.1141-78.

27

Vaginal Cancer

Gauri Gandhi, Snigdha Pathak

Vagina develops from lower parts of fused müllerian ducts and sinobulbar part (Fig. 27.1). It is the lower part of the female genital tract which opens in vestibule below and connected to cervix above. It primarily has stratified squamous epithelium which is nonkeratinizing. There are no secretory glands in vagina but it is kept moist by secretions from cervix and secretory glands near the opening of vagina in vestibule.

Premalignant lesion vaginal intraepithelial neoplasia (VAIN) share common etiology with cervical malignancies. It often accompanies cervical intraepithelial neoplasia (CIN), mechanism of human papilloma virus (HPV) entry through microabrasions resulting from sexual activity.

Screening: By cervical cytology. Suspect VAIN when persistent abnormal Pap without cervical lesion and abnormal Pap after CIN treatment.

Careful vaginal inspection when colposcopy done for CIN lesion; particularly upper vagina.

Diagnosis: Colposcopy and directed biopsy.

Lesions are located along vaginal ridges, ovoid, slightly raised and have surface spicules.

Treatment
- VAIN I—no treatment. Lesions are multifocal, often regress; recur when ablated.
- VAIN II—expectant management OR ablation.
- VAIN III—colposcopy directed laser vaporization therapy or ball cautery fulguration (after ruling out invasion) OR excision (upper vaginal small lesion) OR total vaginectomy with split thickness skin graft (lesion involving entire vagina).

VAGINAL CANCER

Majority of vaginal cancers are metastatic ~84%.[1] Primary vaginal cancer is uncommon—2–3% of malignant neoplasms of female genital tract. Most common histology—squamous (80%).[2]

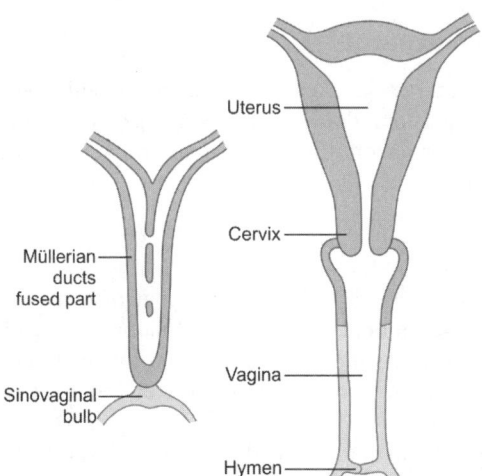

Fig. 27.1 Development of vagina

Etiology

Squamous cell cancer (SCC) of vagina is associated with high rate of infection with oncogenic strains of HPV and has many risk factors in common with SCC of cervix.[3] ~30% women with vaginal cancer have history of cervical cancer treated within last 5 years. Vaginal cancer developing 5 years after cervical cancer is considered a new primary lesion.

Three mechanisms for development of vaginal cancer after cervical cancer:
1. Residual disease after cervical cancer treatment
2. New primary vaginal cancer in a patient with increased susceptibility to lower genital tract carcinogenesis (suspect role of HPV)
3. Increased susceptibility to carcinogenesis due to radiotherapy.

Screening

It is recommended that yearly Pap smear should be done in women on follow-up for cervical/vulvar neoplasia after they have completed surveillance for cervical/vulvar cancer.

If hysterectomy was done for benign disease (without prior history of CIN2/3), Pap smear is unnecessary.

Apart from Pap smear, bimanual examination of vagina and vulva—for women at high risk.

Diagnosis

Symptoms	Signs
• Painless bleeding PV • Discharge PV • Urinary retention, bladder spasm, hematuria, increased frequency • Tenesmus, constipation, blood in stool	• Submucosal irregularities in the vagina • Ulcerative lesion Note: Most common site—upper one-third of vagina on posterior wall.

Physical examination, per-speculum examination, palpation of vagina and bimanual pelvic and rectal examination are important to rule out vaginal cancer (Important to rotate the speculum all around as posterior vaginal wall lesions may be missed).

Investigations
- Pap smear—many cases may be incidentally picked up on routine screening
- Colposcopy followed by targeted biopsy of suspicious vaginal areas.

Staging—FIGO 2009[4]
- Stage I—Carcinoma limited to vaginal wall.
- Stage II—Subvaginal tissue involved but no extension to pelvic wall
- Stage III—Extension to pelvic wall
- Stage IV—Carcinoma has extended beyond true pelvis OR involved mucosa of bladder/rectum.
  - IVA—Tumor invades bladder/rectal mucosa and/or direct extension beyond true pelvis
  - IVB—Spread to distant organs.
- Clinical staging—Cystoscopy, proctoscopy and chest/skeletal X-ray can be used for staging (if indicated).
- Tumor extending from cervix to vagina—regard as cancer cervix; tumor involving both vulva and vagina—regard as vulval cancer.

Treatment

Primary vaginal carcinoma is treated either with surgery or radiotherapy depending on lesion size, tumor location in the vagina, and stage of the disease.

Stage 1

Radiotherapy: It is the treatment of choice for most tumors especially large lesions not permitting clear surgical margins (e.g. proximity to the bladder or rectum) OR middle or distal vaginal tumors.
- Superficial, small lesions—intracavitary radiation
- Larger, thick lesions—external teletherapy (decrease tumor volume, regional node

treatment) followed by intracavitary, interstitial therapy (if lesion >0.5 cm thick; Syed interstitial implants).

Surgery: It can be done in tumors involving upper vagina.

Lesions in vaginal fornix—Wertheim hysterectomy, partial vaginectomy, and bilateral pelvic lymphadenectomy. If margins clear + negative lymph nodes—no additional treatment.

Reconstruction: Upper vagina may need to be replaced with split-thickness skin graft to re-establish normal vaginal length in case of radical surgery in a sexually active woman.

Stages 2 and 3

Radiotherapy is the primary treatment modality.

Stage 4

When advanced lesions involve only the bladder or the rectum, pelvic exenteration may be required to control the disease effectively.

Advanced or recurrent disease:
For patients who have failed primary irradiation therapy—pelvic exenteration is the treatment of choice.
- Combination chemoradiation treatment—little reported experience.
- For advanced metastatic/recurrent disease- no established anticancer drugs can be considered of proven clinical benefit, although patients are often treated with regimens used to treat cervical cancer.[5]

Sequelae

Complication rate ~10–15% for both surgery and radiotherapy:
- Bladder/bowel fistula
- Radiation cystitis, proctitis
- Rectal strictures, ulceration
- Radiation necrosis of vagina
- Vaginal fibrosis, stenosis, stricture a using vaginal dilators, resumption of sexual activity, topical estrogen can be used
- Premature menopause (ovarian damage)

Prognostic Factors

Patient prognosis depends primarily on the stage of disease, but survival is reduced among those who are older than 60 years, are symptomatic at the time of diagnosis, have lesions of the middle and lower third of the vagina, or have poorly differentiated tumors.[5]

In addition, the length of vaginal wall involvement has been found to be associated with survival and stage of disease in vaginal SCC patients.

Survival

- 5-year survival rate ~52%[2].
- Stage I disease—5-year survival—74%.

REFERENCES

1. Fu YS. Intraepithelial, invasive and metastatic neoplasms of the vagina. In: Pathology of the Uterine Cervix Vagina and Vulva, 2nd edn, Philadelphia: Saunders; 2002.pp.531.
2. Miller C, Elkas JC. Cervical and Vaginal Cancer. Berek and Novak's Gynecology, 15th edn. Lippincott Williams and Wilkins; 2012.pp.1428-57.
3. Daling JR, Madeleine MM, Schwartz SM, et al. A population-based study of squamous cell vaginal cancer: HPV and cofactors. Gynecol Oncol. 2002;84 (2):263-70.
4. FIGO Annual Report. Int J Gynecol Obstet. 2009; 105:3-4.
5. Board PA. Vaginal Cancer Treatment (PDQ®).

28
Carcinoma Cervix

Pushpa Mishra

INTRODUCTION

Carcinoma cervix is a major healthcare problem worldwide and it is preventable. Though it has significantly decreased in its incidence in the developed world, its decline is not that impressive in the developing world. Mortality from this can be reduced to minimal with the knowledge and practice of various screening techniques, vaccinations, early diagnosis, prompt and adequate management. Populations should be educated about different avoidable risk factors to decrease the disease load at its root.[1,2]

EPIDEMIOLOGY

Cervical carcinoma is the most common cancer in Indian women accounting for 22.86% of all cancers and it is the most common cause of cancer deaths in the developing countries. According to GLOBOCAN 2012, 528,000 new cases were diagnosed in 2012 and patients who died of the disease were 266,000. Seventy percent of cases are from the resource poor, developing countries. In India new cases registered were 123,000 and deaths were 67,500 in 2012. One-fifth of new cases in the world are from India.[1]

Cervical cancer is the most common cancer in India among the women with an age adjusted incidence rate of 19.4 to 43.5 per 100,000 women. Seventy percent of new cases registered in India are stage III or above. Overall 5 years survival rate observed are 63.3, 44.0, 30.3 and 5.7% for stage I, II, III and IV respectively.[1-4]

Carcinoma cervix is the third largest cause of cancer mortality in India causing nearly 10% of all cancer related deaths in the country. One woman dies of cancer cervix every 8 minutes in India.[3,4]

It is less common in the populations where circumcision is practiced in the males, i.e. Muslims and Jews.

RISK FACTORS

Sex Related[5,6]

- Younger age at intercourse (before 16 years)
- Multiple sexual partners
- Sexually transmitted diseases, human papiloma virus (HPV) infection (16 and 18 are the most common).

Pregnancy Related[5,6]

- Teenage pregnancy
- High parity
- Less inter-pregnancy interval.

Others[5-8]

- Oral contraceptive pills (OCPs)
- Certain races
- Poor perineal hygiene
- Low immune status (HIV).

Social Risks[5-8]

- Low socioeconomic strata
- Illiteracy
- Nutritional deficiencies
- Cigarette smoking.

CLASSIFICATION[9-11]

According to Site of Origin

- Ectocervix—70–80%
- Endocervix—20–30%.

According to Gross Appearance

- Occult
- Exophytic—cauliflower like growth replacing cervical tissue
- Ulcerative—produces eaten up appearance to cervix
- Infiltrative—mostly seen in endocervical growth, cervix gets expanded and becomes barrel shaped.

According to Histopathological Examination (HPE)

- *Squamous cell carcinoma (70–80%):*
  - Large cell keratinizing
  - Large cell nonkeratinizing
  - Small cell
  - Others—verrucous carcinoma
    - Papillary (transitional) carcinoma
- *Adenocarcinoma (20–27%):*
  - Endocervical
  - Endometroid
  - Clear cell
  - Mixed
  - Villoglandular papillary adenocarcinoma
  - Adenoma malignum (minimal spread)
- Adenosquamous carcinoma
- Sarcoma
- Malignant melanoma
- Neuroendocrine carcinoma
- Lymphoma.

CLINICAL PRESENTATION[9-11]

History

Patient presents in her fourth or fifth decade of life with history of few or many of risk factors listed before with common complaints of:

- Irregular bleeding per vaginum
- Postmenopausal bleeding
- Postcoital bleeding
- Discharge per vaginum (mild-to-excessive foul smelling)
- Backache
- Asymptomatic patients come with abnormal screening reports
- Late symptoms include bladder (frequency, dysuria, urgency and hematuria, incontinence in late stages) and bowel (abnormal bowel movements, bleeding prerectum, incontinence, etc.) complaints, chronic pelvic pain, edema of lower limbs, etc.
- Due to ureteric involvement pyelonephritis, hydronephrosis, renal failure are the common features.

Examination

Patients should be assessed for the following signs:
- Anemia
- Weight loss
- Lymphadenopathy
- Breast examination
- Hepatomegaly
- Pelvic examination
  Per speculum examination
  - Cervix can be normal in screen positive patients
  - Nodular lesions/cauliflower growth/punched out ulcerative growth/firm to hard expanded cervix
  - Mucopurulent discharge/blood mixed discharge/frank bleeding
  - Growth can be seen involving vagina

  Digital examination, bimanual and rectal examination
  - Cervical consistency, extent of disease/growth, uterine size, pyometra, parametrial involvement

- If the vaginal fornices are obliterated, rectal examination is the best way to assess the size of cervix and parametrial extension.

Cause of Death

- Uremia
- Hemorrhage
- Sepsis.

DIAGNOSIS

- Cervical biopsy (in obvious growth)
- Colposcopic-guided cervical biopsy with endocervical curettage in screen positive patients
- Conization may be required in inconclusive reports
- Cone is superior for the assessment of the depth of the growth than punch biopsy.

Staging[9-12]

International Federation of Gynecology and Obstetrics (FIGO) allowed certain procedures to stage the disease clinically to standardized in all parts of world.

Staging Procedures

- Physical examination—examination of lymph nodes, of vagina, bimanual and rectal examination
- Radiological procedures intravenous pyelogram (IVP), barium enema, chest X-ray, skeletal X-ray
- Others—biopsies (punch, cone, endocervical, etc.), colposcopy, hysteroscopy, cystoscopy, proctoscopy.

FIGO Staging of Carcinoma of the Cervix Uteri (2008)

Stage 1: The carcinoma is strictly confined to the cervix (extension to the corpus would be disregarded).

- *IA*: Invasive carcinoma which can be diagnosed only by microscopy, with most deep invasion ≤5 mm and largest extension 7 mm.
- *IA1*: Measured stromal invasion of ≤3.0 mm in depth and extension of ≤7 mm
- *IA2*: Measured stromal invasion of >3.0 mm and not >5.0 mm with an extension of not >7.0 mm
- *IB*: Clinically visible lesions limited to the cervix uteri or preclinical cancers greater than stage IAa
- *IB1*: Clinically visible lesion ≤4.0 cm in dimension
- *IB2*: Clinically visible lesion >4.0 cm in dimension.

Stage II: Cervical carcinoma invades beyond the uterus, but not the pelvic wall or to the lower third of the vagina.

- *IIA*: Without parametrial invasion
- *IIA1*: Clinically visible lesion ≤4.0 cm in greatest dimension.
- *IIA2*: Clinically visible lesion >4 cm in greatest dimension.
- *IIB*: With obvious parametrial invasion

Stage III: The tumor extends to the pelvic wall and/or involves lower third of the vagina and/or causes hydronephrosis or nonfunctioning kidney.

- *IIIA*: Tumor involves lower third of the vagina, with no extension to the pelvic wall.
- *IIIB*: Extension to the pelvic wall and/or hydronephrosis or nonfunctioning kidney.

Stage IV: The carcinoma has extended beyond the true pelvis or has involved the mucosa of the bladder or rectum. A bullous edema, as such, does not permit a case to be allotted to stage IV

- *IVA*: Spread of the growth to the adjacent organs.
- *IVB*: Spread to distant organs.

Other staging procedures, not allowed by FIGO are CT scan, USG scan, MRI scan, PET scan, laparoscopy, etc.

Surgicopathological staging many a times upstage the disease but it should be treated on the basis of the clinical staging done prior to surgery.[9-12]

MANAGEMENT[9-25]

Depends on the age of the patient, stage of the cancer, medical health of the patient and prognostic factors of the disease.

Prognostic Factors[9-12]

- Age of the patient—younger the patient better the prognosis
- Stage of the disease—5-year survival rate according to stage are 95-99% (1a), 78-88% (1b), 64-68% (11), 40-43% (111), 15-20% (1V).
- Tumor size—5 year survival is 90% in tumor size <2 cm where as it is 60% and 40% for <2 cm and 4 cm respectively.
- Depth of invasion—<1 cm invasion have 90% survival rate but it is low if invasion is more.
- Lymphovascular space invasion (LVSI)—it was given too much importance in the past but it is seen as a predictor of lymph node involvement. Many studies reported 90% survival when LVSI is absent.
- Lymph node status—negative lymph nodes predicts 90%, 5 year survival.
- Histopathology type.
- Recurrent disease.

TREATMENT MODALITIES

- Surgical
- Radiotherapy
- Concurrent chemoradiotherapy
- Palliative treatment.

Surgery

The stagewise treatment of a carcinoma of cervix is described in Table 28.1.

Cone Biopsy

It is done for both diagnostic and therapeutic indication. Conventional cold knife cone is desirable as margins are better evaluated with this. Excision of full transformation zone with

Table 28.1 Stagewise treatment of carcinoma cervix[9]

Stage of the disease	Fertility preservation	Standard therapy
FIGO stage IA1 SCCA (no LVSI) or AIS	Cone biopsy	Extrafascial hysterectomy
FIGO stage IA1 with LVSI	Cone Biopsy Laparoscopic lymphadenectomy	Extrafascial hysterectomy +/− lymphadenectomy
FIGO stage IA2 or occult IB1	Radical trachelectomy with lymphadenectomy (vaginal, robotic-assisted, laparoscopic, abdominal)	Modified radical hysterectomy with lymphadenectomy (robotic, laparoscopic, open); tailored adjuvant therapy
FIGO IB1-IIA	Radical trachelectomy with lymphadenectomy as outlined	Radical hysterectomy with lymphadenectomy (robotic-assisted or laproscopic for stage IB1); tailored adjuvant therapy
FIGO IB2-IVA	Radical hysterectomy with lymphadenectomy (select IB2-IIA); tailored adjuvant therapy	Chemoradiation + HDR Brachytherapy (pretreatment laparoscopic extraperitoneal lymphadenectomy as indicated clinically)
Central pelvic recurrence	No prior radiotherapy: chemoradiation	*Prior radiotherapy:* Pelvic exenteration with urinary diversion (if no hydronephrosis, negative paraaortic nodes)
FIGO IVB, persistent, and/or noncentral recurrence	Cisplatin + paclitaxel; palliative radiotherapy for pelvic bleeding and or pain secondary to bony metastases: percutaneous nephrostomies/ureteral stents	*GOG protocol 240:* Cisplatin + paclitaxel +/− bevacizumab versus topotecan + paclitaxel +/− bevacizumab

good depth of endocervical canal is therapeutic. In occult lesions cervix is stained with Lugol's iodine to delineate the lesion completely. It can be done with many technique, i.e. cold knife, Laser, LEEP.[13]

Cone biopsy is proceeded with laparoscopic lymphadenectomy for fertility preservation in stage 1a1 patients.

It is associated with hemorrhage, infection, cervical stenosis and incompetent cervix. LEEP causes shallower wound so less complications.

Extrafascial Hysterectomy

It is specimen comes with pubocervical fascia and one cm of cuff of vagina. While doing the hysterectomy clamps are not bounced over cervix so adjacent parametrium comes with the specimen.

If evidence of lymphovascular space invasion is there, pelvic lymphadenectomy should be done too for stage IA1.

Radical Trachelectomy[9-11,14,15]

In fertility sparing surgery, after laparoscopic pelvic lymphadenectomy, cervix is removed from vaginal side (can be done abdominally or laparoscopically) with upper 1–2 cm of vagina and medial part of parametrium. Prophylactic ligature is placed over the lower uterine segment.

Pregnancies are reported in several studies with average risk of abortion in first trimester, slightly increased risk in second trimester and significant prematurity in newborns. FGRs are not seen in these patients more than general population.

Follow-up is very cumbersome as typical cervical tissue is not there and atypical glandular cells from lower uterine segment raises false alarm.

Robotic radical trachelectomy is also getting popularized.

Radical Hysterectomy [9-11,18,19]

This the standard surgical procedure done for stages Ia2 to IIa. In early 12th century Wertheim started this surgery later Meigs described pelvic lymphadenectomy, hence it was called by their names.

In late 20th century and in 21st century, radical hysterectomy with pelvic lymphadenectomy is the standard treatment. Table 28.2 describes the indications of different types of extended hysterectomy.

Here in type II radical hysterectomy, specimen consist of uterus, cervix with medial half of parametrium, upper one third of vagina whereas in type III, total parametrium is removed with upper half of vagina.

Note: Type III radical hysterectomy is the standard Wertheim-Meigs radical hysterectomy.

Table 28.2 Piver-Rutledge-Smith classification of extended hysterectomy[9]		
Class	Description	Indication
1.	Extrafascial hysterectomy; pubocervical ligament is incised, allowing lateral deflection of the ureter	CIN, early stromal invasion
2.	Removal of the median half of the cardinal and uterosacral ligaments; upper third of the vagina removed	Microcarcinoma postirradiation
3.	Removal of the entire cardinal and uterosacral ligaments; upper third of the vagina removed	Stages IB and IIA lesions
4.	Removal of all periureteral tissue, superior vesical artery, and three-fourths of the vagina where preservation of the bladder is still possible	Anteriorly occurring central recurrences
5.	Removal of portions of the distal ureter and bladder	Central recurrent cancer involving portions of the distal ureter or bladder

Steps of Type III Radical Hysterectomy[9-11]

- Preoperative management starts with informed consent, bowel preparation, appropriate antibiotics and adequate blood and blood product arrangement.
- Position of patient on operative table, vary from supine (various tilts) to proper lithotomy position according to surgical team's preference.
- Bladder remains catheterized throughout the procedure.
- Per vaginal/rectal examination is done to reassess the spread of disease.
- Abdomen is opened by midline vertical incision or suprapubic transverse incision (Maylard/Cherney/Pfannenstiel).
- All peritoneal surfaces and pelvic cavity are assessed for extent of the tumor and any enlarge lymph nodes.
- Suspicious lymph node is excised and sent for frozen section.
- Pelvic lymphadenectomy is done by opening the retroperitoneum at lateral pelvic wall by opening the paravesical and pararectal spaces.
- Common iliac, external iliac and obturator chains of lymph nodes are dissected avoiding injury to genitofemoral nerve.
- Paravesical and pararectal spaces are developed by dissecting the areas lateral to bladder and rectum respectively.
- Uterovesical fold is cut and bladder is mobilized caudally exposing upper one third of vagina.
- Uterine artery is traced to its origin, ligated, divided but preserving the superior vesical artery.
- Ureter is dissected and separated from the vesicouterine ligament and traced to its entry to bladder.
- Rectum is freed from the uterosacral ligaments and ligaments are cut midway.
- The junction of upper one third and middle third of vagina is incised and an adequate length of vaginal cuff is removed with the specimen with dissected paravaginal tissues.
- Pelvic lymph node groups, removed are:
    - Obturator chains
    - Common iliac bifurcation
    - External iliac group (medial)
- During dissection for external iliac group of lymph nodes, lateral group of lymph nodes should be spared to avoid lymphedema of the lower limbs. Injury to genitofemoral nerve should be avoided.
- On palpation, if para-aortic lymph node is enlarged and frozen section biopsy comes positive for tumor metastasis, procedure should be abandoned in the favor of adjuvant chemoradiotherapy.
- In fertility-sparing surgery where ovaries are left, ovarian transposition should be done. This way ovaries can be protected from the radiotherapy.[20]
- In last 20th years laparoscopic and robotic radical hysterectomies and trachelectomies are getting popularity with increasing expertise and decreasing complications.

Nerve-sparing Radical Hysterectomy[9-11]

This approach is practiced by many researchers to improve bladder, bowel and sexual function of the patient, postsurgery. Here sympathetic (T11 to L2) and parasympathetic (S2 to S4) fibers to the above areas are preserved during surgery.

Schauta-Mitra Radical Vaginal Hysterectomy[11]

Schauta started doing vaginal hysterectomy as extended vaginal hysterectomy for cancer cervix which popularized once Mitra from India combined it with extraperitoneal pelvic lymphadenectomy.

It is nowadays done as laparoscopic-assisted radical vaginal hysterectomy.

Steps of the surgery:
- *Abdominal:*
    - Pelvic lymphadenectomy (laparoscopic or extraperitoneally)
    - Dissection of ureter and uterine artery and ligation of uterine artery

- *Vaginal*
  - A centimeter of vaginal mucosa below the cervix is dissected to take out with the specimen
  - Opening of vesicouterine space, paracervical space and dissection of the ureter
  - Opening of cul-de-sac, para rectal space and excision of paracolpos
  - Excision of parametrium
  - Excision of specimen and closure.

Complications of radical hysterectomy:[9-11,19]
- *Immediate complications* (1-2%)
  - Hemorrhage
  - Infection
  - Vaginal fistulas (urinary and rectal)
  - Ureteral injury
  - Bowel injury
  - Injury to nerves (genitofemoral and obturator)
  - Multiple blood transfusions
  - Deep vein thrombosis
  - Pulmonary embolism
- *Late complications*
  - Prolonged febrile illness
  - Bladder and bowel dysfunction (dysuria, frequency, atonia, stress urinary incontinence, constipation, stool incontinence)
  - Lymphocyst formation (may require recurrent drainage and if not treated relaparotomy may be done)
- *Chronic complications*
  - Bladder dysfunction (due to atonia, may require recurrent catheterization)
  - Recurrent lymphocyst formation and its complications
  - Ureteral strictures (may require stenting)
  - Recurrent cancer.

Pelvic Exenteration[9-11,21]

These are extensive surgeries done for stage IIB without any peritoneal extension of the disease.
- *Anterior*: It is done for tumor confined to cervix and anterior vagina. Rectal extension should be ruled out before the surgery by proctoscopy/sigmoid proctoscopy.
- *Posterior*: It is done for tumor confined to cervix and posterior vagina. Here, anterior extension should be excluded before the surgery.
- *Total*: Total exenteration is quite extensive surgery. In the presence of any peritoneal evidence of tumor, total exenteration should be abandoned as patient's survival is very bleak even with the surgery.

Sentinel Lymph Node Detection[9-11]

This is a lymph node which primarily gets the drainage of the tumor, if comes out as negative, in early cancer cervix, lymphadenectomy can be averted. It is not included in the standard management but seems promising in future.

Radiotherapy[9-11,22,23]

Surgery is preferred choice of management in early stages/nonbulky tumor of cervix and in late stages, radiotherapy is the choice of treatment, globally.

For stages IB/IIB, results are comparable in favor of both the management options depending upon the surgeon's expertise and patient's choice.

This is the mainstay of the treatment of the carcinoma cervix. This is the only modality which can be used in every stage of the tumor even in the palliation. Radiotherapy used for localized disease is brachytherapy and teletherapy for widespread disease.

Concurrent Chemoradiation[9-11]

In many randomized studies, it was found that platinum-based chemotherapy with radiation after surgery was better in preventing recurrence and treating the advanced cervical cancer.

Palliative Treatment[9-11]

- This is the treatment used for incurable advanced disease for the symptomatic relief of the patient.

- It can be given as radiotherapy (brachy or tele) and can be added with chemotherapy according to patient's response.

Comparison of surgery versus radiotherapy stage IB/IIB cancer of the cervix is mentioned in Table 28.3.

SPECIAL SCENARIOS

Carcinoma Cervix with Pregnancy[9-11,24,25]

- This is not a very uncommon case. Patients are managed according to their stage and trimester.
- First trimester with abnormal paps or AIS or very early lesion patients should be re-evaluated and cone biopsy should be done in second trimester. In first trimester there is more risk of abortion, hemorrhage and infection.
- Patients with more than 5 mm invasion should be treated with external beam radiation after counseling her for its adverse effect on pregnancy.
- In second trimester, treatment can be postponed in very early disease but many studies of chemotherapy treatment are reported without much harm to fetus.
- Late second trimester, and early third trimester patients should be optimized for baby's lung maturity and preferably delivered by cesarean section. Cancer is treated after six weeks of delivery in routine way.

Pyometra with Carcinoma Cervix[9-11]

- It is present usually in patients with advanced disease who require radiotherapy.
- It should be drained with antibiotic cover to avoid flare up of infection during radiotherapy.

Recurrence of Cervical Carcinoma[9]

- Most patients have recurrence of disease within two years. Their time with good health hardly last for a year as they start having cachexia, loss of appetite and ill health well before having demonstrable disease.
- Recurrence is called when there is at least three months of disease free period after completion of radiotherapy.
- It is not usually respond to treatment well.
- Doublet therapy with cisplatin and praclitaxel is the standard treatment.

Persistent Cervical Carcinoma[9]

If there is a tumor remains there even after treatment or reappears a new growth in the pelvis during the treatment, then it is a case of persistent disease.

Table 28.3 Comparison of surgery versus radiation for stage IB/IIB cancer of the cervix		
	Surgery	Radiation
Survival	85%	85%
Serious complications	Urologic fistuals 1–2%	Intestinal and urinary strictures and fistuals 1.4–5.3%
Vagina	Initially shortened, but may lengthen with regular intercourse	Fibrosis and possible stenosis, particularly in postmenopausal patients
Ovaries	Can be conserved	Destroyed
Chronic effects	Bladder atony in 3%	Radiation fibrosis of bladder and bowel in 6–8%
Applicability	Best candidates are younger than 65 years of age, <200 lb, and in good health	All patients are potential candidates
Surgical morality	1%	1% (from pulmonary embolism during intracavitary therapy)

New Cancer Cervix[9]

If a patient comes with a new growth of cancer cervix after 10 years of dieses free period then this is called new cancer cervix.

Prevention of Cancer Cervix[9-11]

Public awareness and health education should be promoted extensively across the population.
- *Things to be avoided:*
  - Early marriage
  - Unsafe sex, i.e. promiscuity, poor sexual hygiene
  - Multiple pregnancy, early pregnancy
  - Smoking
- *Things to be practised:*
  - Safe sex
  - Using barrier contraception
  - Screening for cancer cervix
  - Vaccination.

Screening[2,9-11]

Carcinoma cervix is the only cancer for which causative microbe is known and best screening modalities are there. This is the cancer which is fully preventable, if desired.

Screening Modalities

- Paps smear—conventional pap smear
- Liquid-based cytology
- HPV screening
- Colposcopy
  In resource poor settings, following modalities are quite promising
- Visual inspection using acetic acid (VIA)
- Visual inspection using Lugol's iodine (VILI)
   American College of Obstetricians and Gynaecologists Recommendations for Screening of the Cervix, 2009.
- Women from age 21 to 29 should be screened every 2 years using either the standard Pap or liquid-based cytology.
- Women 30 years or older who have had three consecutive negative cervical cytology test results may be screened once every 3 years with either standard Pap or liquid-based cytology.
- Co-testing using combination of cytology plus HPV DNA testing is appropriate for women older than 30 years. Any woman 30 years or older at low risk who had negative cytology and HPV DNA testing can be rescreened at 3-year intervals.
- Cervical cancer screening can be discontinued between the ages of 65 and 70 years in women who have had three or more negative consecutive test results and no abnormal test results in the past 10 years.
- Cervical cancer screening is not recommended in women before 21 years of age.
- Women with certain risk factors may need more frequent screening, including those with HIV; those who are immunosuppressed; those exposed to DES *in utero*; and those who have been treated for CIN II, CIN III, or cervical cancer.

Note: Early CIN progresses to higher ones in years, therefore despite low sensitivity of pap smear, *consecutive three negative pap reports patient has less than 1% risk of high grade CINs.

Vaccination[2,9,10,26-28]

In the last two decades, various HPV vaccines are developed and extensive trials are done. Finally, gardasil and cervarix were approved by FDA in 2006 for the prevention of HPV infection and so carcinoma cervix (Ca Cx).

Table 28.4 Human papilloma virus vaccines		
Name of vaccine	Gardasil	Cervarix
Type	Tetravalent	Bivalent
HPV types	6, 11, 16, 18	16, 18
Dose schedule	0, 2, 6	0, 1–2, 6
Age group	9–26	9–25
Population	Males and females	Females
Prevention	Ca Cx, AIS, vulvar lesions CIN, IN, VAIN, anogenital warts	Ca Cx, CIN, AIS
Efficacy to prevent Ca Cx	95–97.2%	99–100%
Years of protection	8.5 years	9 years

Note: A nonvalent gardasil vaccine is also developed but more studies are required.

More than 150 types of HPVs are known and they are divided in high risk, low risk and possible high risk types. HPV type 16 and 18 are high risk and most prevalent cause of higher CINs therefore targeted for vaccination. Type 6 and 11 are responsible for majority of anogenital warts. Table 28.4 describes the 2 HPV vaccines which are commonly used.

REFERENCES

1. IARC [Internet]. Globocan 2008, IARC, 2010. World Cancer Factsheet. Available from: *http://globocan.iarc.fr/factsheets/population/factsheet.asp?uno=900.*
2. NCCN Clinical Practice Guidelines in oncology (NCCN Guidelines) Version 1. 2016, NCCN.org.
3. National Cancer Registry Program (NCRP, ICMR). Consolidated report of population based cancer registries 2004-2005. Bangalore: NCRP; 2008.
4. National Cancer Registry Programme (NCRP, ICMR). The trends in cancer incidence rates: 1982-2005. Bengaluru: NCRP; 2009.
5. Wang SS, Carreon JD, Gomez, Devesa SS. Cervical cancer incidenceamong 6 asian ethnic groups in the United States, 1996 through 2004. Cancer. 2010;116:949-56.
6. Singh GK, Azuine RE, Siahpush M. Global inequalities in cervical cancer incidence and mortality are linked to deprivation, low socioeconomic status, and human development. Int J MCH and AIDS. 2012;1:17-30.
7. International Collaboration of Epidemiological Studies of Cervical Cancer. Comparison of risk factors for invasive squamous cell carcinoma and adenocarcinoma of the cervix: collaborative reanalysis of individual data of 8,097 women with squamous cell carcinoma and 1,374 women with adenocarcinoma from 12 epidemiological studies. Int J Cancer. 2007;120:885-91.
8. Dugue PA, Rebolj M, Garred P, et al. Immunosuppression and cervical cancer. Expert Rev Anticancer Ther. 2013;13:29-42. *http://www.ncbi.nim.gov/pubmed/23259425.*
9. Di Saia PJ, Creasman WT, et al. Clinical Gynecologic Oncology, 8th edition, (Indian Edition). 2012;2:51-119.
10. Jonathan S. Berek, Berek and Novak's Gynecology, 15th edition (Indian Edition). 2011;1304-39.
11. Jones III HW, Rock JA. Te Linde's Operative Gynaecology, 11th edition (Indian edition) 2015; 1192-251.
12. Gold MA. Tian C, Whitney CW, et al. Surgical versus radiographic determination of para-aortic lymph node metastasis before chemoradiation for locally advanced cervical carcinoma: a Gynecologic Oncology Group Study. Cancer. 2008;112:1954-63.
13. Greenspan DL, Faubion M, Coonrod DV, et al. Compliance after loop electrosurgical excision procedure or cold knife cold biopsy. Obstet Gynecol. 2007;110:675-80.
14. Ramirez PT, Pareja R, Rendon GJ, et al. Management of low risk early stage cervical cancer: should conisation, simple trachelectomy, or simple hysterectomy replace radical surgery as the new standard of care? Gynecol Oncol. 2014;132: 254-9.
15. Raju SK, Papadopoulos AJ, Montalto SA, et al. Fertility-sparing surgery for early cervical cancer-approach to less radical surgery. Int J Gynecol Cancer. 2012;22:311-7.
16. Journal of the National Comprehensive Cancer Network. JNCCN December. 2010.
17. Bipat S, Glas AS, Velden J, et al. Computed tomography and magnetic resonance imaging in staging of uterine cervical carcinoma: a systemic review. Gynecol Oncol. 2003;91:59.
18. Webb M, Symmonds R. Wertheim hysterectomy: a reappraisal. Obstet Gynecol. 1979;54:140-5.
19. Hatch KD, Parham G, Shingleton HM, et al. Ureteral strictures and fistulae following radical hysterectomy. Gynecol Oncol. 1984;19:17-23.
20. Feeny DD, Moore DH, Loo KY, et al. The fate of the ovaries after radical hysterectomy and ovarian transposition. Gynecol Oncol. 1995;56:3.
21. Maggioni A, Roviglione G, Landoni F, et al. Pelvic exenteration: ten year experience at the European Institute of Oncology of in Milan. Gynecol Oncol. 2009;114:64-8.
22. Monk BJ, Sill MW, McMeekins DS, et al. Phase III trial of four cisplatin-containing doublet combinations in stage IVb, recurrent, or persistent cervical carcinoma: a Gynecological Oncological Group study. J Clin Oncol. 2009;29: 4649-55.
23. Rose PG, Bundy BN, Watkins AB, et al. Concurrent cisplatin-based radiotherapy and chemotherapy for locally advanced cervical cancer. N Engl J Med. 1999;340:1144-53.

24. Sood AK, Sorosky JI, Mayr N, et al. Cervical Cancer diagnosed shortly after pregnancy: prognostic variables and delivery routes. Obstet Gynecol. 2009; 95:832-8.
25. Bader AA, Petru E, Winter R. Long-term follow-up after neoadjuvant chemotherapy for high risk cervical cancer during pregnancy. Gynecol Oncol, 2007;105:269-72.
26. Ault KA. Effect of prophylactic human papillomavirus L1 virus like-particle vaccine on risk of cervical intraepithelial neoplasia grade 2, grade 3 and adenocarcinoma in situ: a combined analysis of four randomised clinical trials. Lancet. 2007;369:1861-8.
27. Quadrivalent vaccine against human papillomavirus to prevent high-grade cervical lesions. N Engl J Med. 2007;356:1915-27. http://www.ncbi.nlm.gov/pubmed/17494925.
28. Chan JK, Berek JS. Impact of the human papilloma vaccine on cervical cancer. J Clin Oncol. 2007;25: 2975-82.

29

Endometrial Carcinoma

Yedla Manikya Mala, Bhoomika Tantuway, Karishma Bhatia

INTRODUCTION

Endometrial cancer is one of the important causes of postmenopausal bleeding. The new cases of endometrial cancer were reported to be about 25 per 100,000 women per year leading to a mortality rate of 4–5 per 100,000 women per year.[1] After breast, lung and colorectal cancer, uterine cancer holds the fourth position among most common cancer in women.[2] In India the incidence is reported as 4.3 per 100,000 women per year.[3]

CLINICAL PRESENTATION

- Endometrial cancer is more common in the postmenopausal age group, i.e. 55–65 years age. Median age at diagnosis is about 62 years[2]
- However, 20% present before menopause out of whom 5% present before the age of 40 years.
- There are two types of ndometrial cacer (Table 29.1).

The histopathological classification is as follows:[17]

Malignant epithelial tumor	Malignant mesenchymal/stromal tumor
Pure endometrioid	Uterine leiomyosarcoma
Uterine serous	Endometrial stromal sarcoma
Clear cell carcinoma	Undifferentiated endometrial sarcoma
Carcinosarcoma (mixed mullerian tumor)	Other rare tumors like adenosarcoma, rhabdomyosarcoma

Table 29.1 Bokhman suggested two pathogenic types[4]	
Type I	*Type II*
• Estrogen dependent endometrioid adenocarcinoma • Seen in women with obesity, hyperlipidemia and hyperestrogenism	• Estrogen independent nonendometrioid tumor i.e. Clear cell and papillary serous tumor
• Most common histologic type and accounts for more than three fourths of all cases	• Rare type
• Low grade, well differentiated, superficial myometrial invasion	• High grade, poorly differentiated, deep myometrial invasion
• Precursor lesion is endometrial intraepithelial neoplasia (also known as atypical endometrial hyperplasia)	• Significant risk of extrauterine disease
• Confined to the uterus	
• Good prognosis, 5-year survival is 85%	• Poor prognosis, 5-year survival 58%

Based on the FIGO grading system proposed in 1989, the differentiation is determined by architectural growth patterns and nuclear features and is expressed as three *Grades*:
- *Grade 1*: <5% of tumor has a solid growth pattern
- *Grade 2*: 6–50% has solid growth pattern
- *Grade 3*: >50% of the tumor has a solid growth pattern.

In cases with notable nuclear atypia inappropriate for the architectural growth pattern, increases the tumor grade by one. Serous and clear cell are considered high grade tumors.
- Most of the cases are of endometrial cancer are seen in sporadic manner.
- Genetic anomalies may be associated with type 1 endometrial carcinomas:
  - DNA mismatch repair genes mutation found in hereditary nonpolyposis colon cancer (HNPCC) or Lynch II syndrome. HNPCC is associated with a lifetime risk of 30–61% for endometrial cancer.[4]
  - Mutation of the PTEN tumor suppressor gene noted in 8.3% of cases with clear cell carcinoma.
  - PIK3CA mutation was also noted in some cases of endometrial cancer.
  - K-Ras and β-catenin gene mutations are found in carcinoma with squamous differentiation.
  - p53 mutations and chromosomal instability may be associated with a form of intraepithelial serous carcinoma, referred to as 'endometrial intraepithelial carcinoma' (EIC).

Risk Factors

- Infertility, nulliparity, early age of menarche and late age of menopause all are high risk factor for development of endometrial hyperplasia which may later develop endometrial carcinoma.
- History of type 2 diabetes, hypertension are also risk factor for endometrial carcinoma
- Prolonged unopposed estrogen exposure due to endogenous conditions like chronic anovulation seen in PCOS, obesity and estrogen secreting tumors. There is increased peripheral conversion of androgen into estrone in adipose tissues.
- Selective estrogen receptor modulators which act as estrogen agonist in endometrial tissues like tamoxifen is risk factor for endometrial carcinoma while tamoxifen significantly reduces the risk of breast cancer and breast cancer recurrence.
- Hormone replacement therapy (HRT) with estrogen is associated with an eightfold increased incidence, the risk is more with prolonged use but the addition of progestin decreases this risk to baseline levels.[5,6]
- Lynch syndrome (hereditary nonpolyposis colorectal cancer) is an autosomal dominant syndrome characterized by a germline mutation in one of the mismatch repair genes, typically MLH1, MSH2, PMS2, or MSH6. It is associated with increased risk of developing colon cancer, ovarian cancer and type I endometrial cancer.
- Cowden disease is a rare autosomal dominant familial cancer susceptibility syndrome characterized by germline *PTEN* mutations. It is associated with an increased risk of breast, thyroid and endometrial cancers.

Symptoms and Signs

Presenting symptoms and signs depends on the stage of the disease.

Symptoms	Signs
Abnormal uterine bleeding (most common symptoms)[5] • Irregular menstruation • Intermenstrual bleeding • Postmenopausal bleeding	• On bimanual examination uterus may be enlarged

Contd...

Contd...

Symptoms	Signs
Patients with advanced disease: • Abdominal or pelvic pain • Abdominal distention • Bloating • Change in bowel or bladder function	In more advanced disease: • Restricted mobility of uterus • Adnexal mass • Ascitis

INVESTIGATIONS

All basic investigations. Any vaginal bleeding in a postmenopausal woman requires assessment to exclude malignancy.

For Diagnosis

- Endometrial thickness of 5 mm or more on *ultrasonography* in postmenopausal women has a sensitivity of 90% and a specificity of about 53% for the detection of endometrial cancer[8]
- *Endometrial sampling* with Karman's cannula or a Pipelle's device is an outpatient procedure and reliable method for diagnosis of endometrial cancer. It is the *method of choice* for histologic evaluation of the endometrium[7]
- Sometimes rare cases of endometrial carcinoma (particularly type II) can present with an endometrial thickness of less than 3 mm, persistent or recurrent uterine bleeding is an indication for a histologic evaluation of the endometrium regardless of endometrial thickness.

If office endometrial sampling has already been performed and has demonstrated no evidence of hyperplasia or malignancy, *hysteroscopy with endometrial sampling* is recommended.[9-11]

Once the diagnosis of endometrial carcinoma is established a *metastatic workup should be done* which includes:
- A baseline hemogram with platelet count, liver and kidney function tests and chest X-ray should be done. Further pre-perative assessment of presence of metastatic disease with imaging (computed tomography [CT], magnetic resonance imaging [MRI], or positron emission tomography [PET]/CT), may be clinically important in the following situations:[12-14]
  - Patient is high risk for surgery because of associated medical co-morbidities
  - Symptoms are suggestive of possible metastasis to unusual sites, such as bones or the central nervous system
  - Preoperative histology report shows a high-grade carcinoma (including grade 3 endometrioid, papillary serous, clear cell, and carcinosarcoma)[15,16]
- Magnetic resonance imaging (MRI) is considered to be the best tool for assessment of cervical involvement.[17,18]

Role of Genetic Screening

- Mostly endometrial tumors are sporadic, but 5% of cases caused by genetic mutation[19]
- Endometrial tumors caused by genetic mutation occur 10–20 years earlier than sporadic tumors.
- Genetic counseling and screening should be done in patients:
  - With strong family history of endometrial and/or colorectal cancer
  - And in those who develop endometrial and/or colorectal cancer at early age, i.e. before 50 years.

STAGING OF ENDOMETRIAL CANCER

International Federation of Gynecology and Obstetrics' Surgical Staging System for Endometrial Cancer (2009)[20]	
Stage I*	Tumor confined to the corpus uteri
IA*	No or less than half myometrial invasion
IB*	Invasion equal to or more than half of the myometrium
Stage II*	Tumor invades cervical stroma, but does not extend beyond the uterus#

Contd...

Contd...

Stage III*	Local and/or regional spread of the tumor
IIIA*	Tumor invades the serosa of the corpus uteri and/or adnexae^
IIIB*	Vaginal and/or parametrial involvement^
IIIC*	Metastases to pelvic and/or para-aortic lymph nodes^
IIIC1*	Positive pelvic nodes
IIIC2*	Positive para-aortic lymph nodes with or without positive pelvic lymph nodes
Stage IV*	Tumor invades bladder and/or bowel mucosa, and/or distant metastases
IVA*	Tumor invasion of bladder and/or bowel mucosa
IVB*	Distant metastases, intra-abdominal metastases and/or inguinal lymph nodes

*Either grade 1, grade 2, or grade 3
#Endocervical glandular involvement only should be considered as stage I and no longer stage II
^Positive cytology has to be reported separately without changing the stage

MANAGEMENT[19]

Pure Endometrioid Carcinoma

Primary treatment for endometrial cancer confined to uterus and who are medically operable is peritoneal cytology (peritoneal washings), total hysterectomy (TH) with bilateral saplingo-oophorectomy (BSO) along with surgical staging. Further adjuvant treatment depends on the surgical stage. In patients not suitable for surgery tumor directed radio therapy (RT) or hormone therapy CT should be considered.

In patients where gross cervical involvement is suspected a cervical biopsy or MRI should be considered. For patients with cervical involvement and are operable, a radical hysterectomy is recommended along with BSO, peritoneal cytology and surgical staging. In patients not suitable for surgery tumor directed radio therapy (RT) with or without chemotherapy CT can be given followed by surgical resection.

Suspicion of extrauterine disease warrants further investigations which include CA-125, MRI/CT/PET. If there is evidence of intra-abdominal disease (ascites, omental, nodal, ovarian or peritoneal involvement) total hysterectomy with BSO, peritoneal cytology, pelvic and surgical staging or debulking procedure should be performed. The surgical goal is to have no measurable residual disease. The degree of surgical staging depends on the intraoperative findings. Preoperative chemotherapy and or hormone therapy may be considered in selective cases.

Patients with unresectable extrauterine pelvic disease (Vaginal, bladder, bowel/rectal or parametrial involvement) are treated with radiotherapy and brachytherapy followed by re-evaluation for surgery.

The *principles of surgery and staging* are:
- Visual evaluation of the peritoneal, diaphragmatic and serosal surfaces with biopsy of any suspicious lesion is important to exclude extrauterine disease.
- Although peritoneal cytology does not affect staging, FIGO and AJCC recommend that it should be obtained as positive cytology is an adverse risk factor.
- During surgery after peritoneal exploration is done, bilateral cornua should be occluded by long Kelly clamps or tied using a silk ligature to prevent spillage of tumor into the peritoneal cavity through fallopian tubes.
- During the hysterectomy while clamping the uterine artery and cardinal ligaments the clamp should not be rolled off the cervix.
- Endometrial carcinoma should be removed en bloc, morcellation should be avoided.
- Excision of suspicious or enlarged lymph nodes in the pelvic or paraaortic regions is important to rule out nodal metastasis.
- Pelvic nodal dissection can identify important prognostic information that may alter further treatment decisions.
- Paraaortic lymphadenectomy up to the renal vessels may be considered for selective high risk situations like deeply invasive lesions, high grade histology and in serous carcinoma, clear cell carcinoma or carcinosarcoma.

Pathological Evaluation
- Uterus
  - Ratio of myometrial/stromal invasion to myometrial thickness
  - Cervical gland/stromal involvement
  - Histological type and grade
  - Tumor size
  - Location of tumor, fundus or lower uterine segment/cervix
  - Lymphovascular space invasion
  - Consider screening with IHC and MSI for inherited mismatch repair gene mutation in patient <50 years and patients with significant family history of endometrial or colon and/or significant risk features to identify familial cancer syndromes, such as Lynch syndrome HNPCC
- Fallopian tube, ovaries
- Peritoneal cytology
- Nodes – pelvic, common iliac, para-aortic

Table 29.2 Adjunant therapy

	Grade 1	Grade 2	Grade 3
Stage IA without adverse risk factors	Observe	Observe or vaginal brachytherapy	Observe or vaginal brachytherapy
Stage IA with adverse risk factors	Observe or vaginal brachytherapy	Observe or vaginal brachytherapy and/or EBRT	Observe or vaginal brachytherapy and/or EBRT
Stage IB without adverse risk factors	Observe or vaginal brachytherapy	Observe or vaginal brachytherapy	Vaginal brachytherapy and/or EBRT or observe
Stage IB with adverse risk factors	Observe or vaginal brachytherapy and/or EBRT	Observe or vaginal brachytherapy and/or EBRT	EBRT and/or vaginal brachytherapy ± chemotherapy
Stage II	Vaginal brachytherapy and/or *EBRT	Vaginal brachytherapy and/or EBRT	EBRT and/or vaginal brachytherapy ± chemotherapy
Stage IIIA	Chemotherapy + RT Or Tumor directed RT ± chemotherapy Or EBRT ± vaginal brachytherapy	Chemotherapy + RT Or Tumor directed RT ± chemotherapy Or EBRT ± vaginal brachytherapy	Chemotherapy + RT Or Tumor directed RT ± chemotherapy Or EBRT ± vaginal brachytherapy
Stage IIIB	Chemotherapy and/or tumor directed RT	Chemotherapy and/or tumor directed RT	Chemotherapy and/or tumor directed RT
Stage IIIC$_1$ (positive pelvic LN)	Chemotherapy and/or tumor directed RT	Chemotherapy and/or tumor directed RT	Chemotherapy and/or tumor directed RT
Stage IIIC$_2$ (positive paraaortic LN with or without pelvic LN)	Chemotherapy and/or tumor directed RT	Chemotherapy and/or tumor directed RT	Chemotherapy and/or tumor directed RT
Stage IVA	Chemotherapy and/or RT	Chemotherapy and/or RT	Chemotherapy and/or RT
Stage IVB	Chemotherapy and/or RT	Chemotherapy and/or RT	Chemotherapy and/or RT

Abbreviation: *EBRT, external beam radiotherapy

After surgical staging patients are considered for adjuvant therapy. Apart from the stage the presence of certain *adverse risk factors* also determine if adjuvant therapy should be given.

These include:
- age >60 years
- Lymphovascular space invasion
- Tumor size >2 cm
- Depth of invasion> 50%
- Invasion of cervical gland/stromal involvement

Adjuvant therapy is required in higher grade or advance stage (Table 29.2).

ADJUVANT THERAPY

Serous or Clear Cell Carcinoma or Carcinosarcoma

Uterine serous, clear cell and carcinosarcomas are the more aggressive histologic variants of malignant epithelial tumors. These are considered as high grade tumors. These also have a higher incidence of extrauterine disease at presentation. Initial work up should also include imaging with MRI/CT/PET and CA 125 levels.

Primary treatment of patients with uterine papillary serous and clear cell carcinoma includes TH/BSO with surgical staging, peritoneal cytology, peritoneal biopsies, bilateral pelvic and paraaortic lymphadenectomy and omentectomy (as typically performed for ovarian cancer).

FERTILITY SPARING OPTIONS

The primary treatment of endometrial cancer is hysterectomy. Continuous progestin based therapy (Magestrol, medroxyprogesterone and levonorgestrel IUD) may be considered only for patients with stage IA, grade 1 endometrioid adenocarcinoma who wish to preserve their fertility. Counseling is extremely important in such cases as fertility sparing treatment is not the standard care for treatment of endometrial carcinoma.

The following criteria must be met before fertility sparing therapy can be considered:

- Well differentiated grade I endometrioid on D and C, confirmed by expert pathologists.
- Disease limited to endometrium on MRI (preferred) or TVS
- Absence of suspicious or metastatic disease on imaging
- No contraindications for medical therapy or pregnancy.

Continuous progestin based therapy is given and endometrial sampling is repeated every 3-6 months. If endometrial cancer is present even at 6-9 months TH/BSO with staging is done.

If the patient shows complete response by 6 months patient is encouraged for an early conception. Surveillance is continued every 3-6 months. After childbearing is complete or if there is progression of disease on endometrial sampling, surgery is done.

Role of sentinel lymph node (SLN) mapping:
- It is a useful technique to identify lymph nodes that are at high risk for metastasis. It can be considered in patients with tumor likely to be confined to uterus as suggested by imaging.
- Radiolabelled colloid most commonly injected is technetium-99m (^{99m}Tc), colored dye such as methylene blue 1%, isosulfan 1%, patent blue 2.5% sodium.
- Indocyanine green (ICG) has recently emerged as a dye that requires infrared camera for localization and provides very high SLN detection rate.
- Combination of superficial (1-3 mm) and deep (1-2 cm) injection of dye in cervix leads to dye delivery to the origin of lymphatic channels in cervix and corpus, namely superficial subserosal, intermediate stromal and deep submucosal.
- Dye from uterine cervix reaches the main uterine lymphatic trunks that condense into parametria and appear in the broad ligament leading to pelvic and occasionally para-aortic sentinel lymph node.
- Uterine body lymphatics commonly cross over the obliterated umbilical artery with most common location of SLN being medial to external iliac, ventral to hypogastric, or in superficial part of obturator region.

- Excision of all mapped SLN with ultra-staging performed. Any suspicious nodes must be removed regardless of mapping.

Surveillance of Endometrial Cancer

Physical examination every 3-6 months for 2-3 years then 6 monthly or annually. CA-125 helps in detection of extrauterine recurrences. Imaging (CT/MRI/PET) is done as clinically indicated. Patients should be educated regarding symptoms of potential recurrence, lifestyle, obesity, exercise, smoking cessation and nutrition counseling.

Management of Local Recurrence

In patients where recurrences in vagina or pelvis alone are detected, radiotherapy plus brachytherapy can be given in patients who have not received prior RT.

In patients who have received RT before recommended therapy includes: (1) surgery with intraoperative RT; (2) hormonal therapy or (3) chemotherapy.

Management of Metastasis Detected on Surveillance

Management outline is explained in Flow chart 29.1.

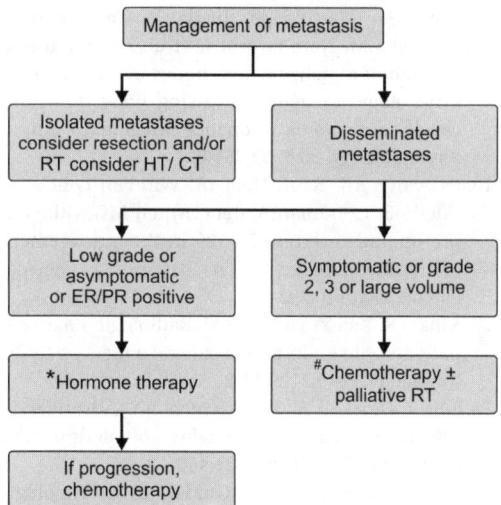

Flow chart 29.1 Outline of management of metastasis in endometrial cancer

Systematic therapy for recurrent, metastatic and high risk disease:
*Hormone therapy
Megestrol/tamoxifen
Progestational agents
Aromatase inhibitors
Tamoxifen

#*Chemotherapy regimens*
Multiagent chemotherapy regimen preferred if tolerated
Carboplatin/paclitaxel
Ifosfamide/paclitaxel
Carboplatin/docetaxel
Cisplatin/doxorubicin

Single agent
Cisplatin
Carboplatin
Doxorubicin
Topotecan
Ifosfamide

Survival Rates

Five year Survival rates based on National Cancer Data Base as published in the AJCC Staging Manual in 2010.

Stage	5-year survival rate
IA	88%
IB	75%
II	69%
IIIA	58%
IIIB	50%
IIIC	47%
IVA	17%
IVB	15%

REFERENCES

1. National cancer institute, surveillance, epidemiology, and end result program, http://seer.cancer.gov/statfacts/html/corp.html
2. National cancer institute. American Cancer Society. Cancer Facts & Figures 2016. Atlanta:

American Cancer Society; 2016, http://www.cancer.gov/types/common-cancers.
3. Balasubramaniam G, Sushama S. Hospital-based Study of Endometrial Cancer Survival in Mumbai, India. Asian Pacific J Cancer Prev. 14(2):977-80.
4. Di Saia, Creasman WT, Clinical Gynaecologic Oncology, 8th edition; 2012.pp.121-39.
5. Bergan L, Beilen MLR, Galee MPW, YHollera H, Benraade JK, Van leeuwen E. Risk & Prognosis of endometrial carcinoma after tamoxifen for breast carcinoma. The Lancet; 2000. pp. 356-881.
6. Weiderpass E, Adami HO, Baron JA, et al. Use of oral contraceptives and endometrial cancer risk (Sweden). Cancer Causes Control. 1999;10(4):277-84. (Pubmed Abstract).
7. The American College of Obstetricians and Gynecologists, practice bulletin, Number 149, April 2015.
8. Timmermans A, Opmeer BC, Khan KS, Bachmann LM, Epstein E, Clark TJ, et al. Endometrial thickness measurement for detecting endometrial cancer in women with postmenopausal bleeding: a systematic review and meta-analysis. Obstet Gynecol. 2010;116:160-7.
9. Epstein E. Management of postmenopausal bleeding in Sweden: a need for increased use of hydrosonography and hysteroscopy. Acta Obstet Gynecol Scand. 2004;83:89-95.
10. Ronghe R, Gaudoin M. Women with recurrent postmenopausal bleeding should be re-investigated but are not more likely to have endometrial cancer. Menopause Int. 2010;16:9-11.
11. Smith PP, O'Connor S, Gupta J, et al. Recurrent postmenopausal bleeding: a prospective cohort study. J Minim Invasive Gynecol. 2014;21:799-803.
12. Han SS, Lee SH, Kim DH, Kim JW, Park NH, Kang SB, et al. Evaluation of preoperative criteria used to predict lymph node metastasis in endometrial cancer. Acta Obstet Gynecol Scand. 2010;89:168-74.
13. Kitajima K, Murakami K, Yamasaki E, Fukasawa I, Inaba N, Kaji Y, et al. Accuracy of 18F-FDG PET/CT in detecting pelvic and paraaortic lymph node metastasis in patients with endometrial cancer. AJR Am J Roentgenol. 2008;190:1652-8.
14. Kitajima K, Murakami K, Yamasaki E, et al. Accuracy of integrated FDG-PET/contrast-enhanced CT in detecting pelvic and paraaortic lymph node metastasis in patients with uterine cancer. Eur Radiol. 2009;19:1529-36.
15. Nakai G, Matsuki M, Inada Y, Tatsugami F, Tanikake M, Narabayashi I, et al. Detection and evaluation of pelvic lymph nodes in patients with gynecologic malignancies using body diffusion-weighted magnetic resonance imaging. J Comput Assist Tomogr. 2008;32:764-8.
16. Olawaiye AB, Rauh-Hain JA, Withiam-Leitch M, Rueda B, Goodman A, del Carmen MG. Utility of pre-operative serum CA-125 in the management of uterine papillary serous carcinoma. Gynecol Oncol. 2008;110:293-8.
17. Kinkel K, Kaji Y, Yu KK, et al. Radiologic staging in patients with endometrial cancer: a meta analysis. Radiology. 1999;212:711-8.
18. Sala E, Rockall A, Kubik-Huch RA. Advances in magnetic resonance imaging of endometrial cancer. Eur Radiol. 2011;21:468-73.
19. NCCN Clinical Practice Guidelines in Oncology, Version 2. 2016.
20. Reprinted from Pecorelli S. Revised FIGO staging for carcinoma of the vulva, cervix, and endometrium [published erratum appears in Int J Gynaecol Obstet 2010;108:176]. Int J Gynaecol Obstet. 2009;105:103-4.

30

Ovarian Cancer

Latika Sahu

INTRODUCTION

Yearly throughout world 2,04,000 women are diagnosed to have ovarian cancer and 125,000 women die from this disease.[1] About 90–95% of all cases are epithelial ovarian carcinomas (EOCs). Three quarters of patients have advanced disease when they are diagnosed due to lack of good screening methods and few early symptoms.[2] Clinical remission, is achieved up to 80% of women by debulking surgery followed by chemotherapy. But usually there is relapse that leads to disease progression and death.[3] The median age of developing ovarian cancer is 63 years (6th and 7th decade of life) and the incidence increases with age.[2,4]

RISK FACTORS

For developing ovarian cancer, there are many reproductive and genetic risk factors. The risk of developing ovarian cancer increases in women with nulliparity and older age (>35 years) at first birth, pelvis inflammatory disease and women on hormone replacement therapy.[5] Use of ovulation induction drugs for *in vitro* fertilization increases the risk of low malignant potential (LMP) tumors of ovary.[6] The risk of ovarian cancer decreases by 30–60% in women with younger age at pregnancy or first birth ≤25 years of age, use of oral contraceptives and/or breastfeeding.[7] The lowest rates of ovarian cancer are found in developing countries and Japan.[8] This could be because of regional dietary habits—low fat and high fiber, carotene and vitamins are protective.

Early onset disease is found only in 15% of ovarian cancer patients.[7] Women who has family history of two or more first degree relative with ovarian cancer including *BRCA1* and *BRCA2* genotypes (Hereditary Breast Ovarian Cancer [HBOC] syndrome), or families affected by Lynch syndrome Hereditary nonpolyposis colorectal cancer (HNPCC) usually develop early onset ovarian cancer.[9]

CLINICAL PRESENTATION

Symtoms and Signs

Symptoms
• Often vague and nonspecific lower abdominal pain/discomfort
• Feeling bloated, anorexia, pain abdomen/pelvis
• Frequency/urgency of urination
• Ovarian cancer may found by chance during surgery for other cause or tests.
Signs: Cachexia
• Solid, irregular, fixed pelvic mass on abdominal/pelvic examination and/or ascites or abdominal distension
• Cul-de-sac nodules
• Edema of legs/varicose veins.

Investigations

Routine
- Complete blood count
- Urine analysis and culture
- Blood sugar (Fasting and postprandial)
- Liver function test
- Renal function test
- Occult blood in stool
- Chest X-ray PA view
- ECG
- Pap smear

Tumor markers

In epitheleal tumors
- Cancer antigen 125 (CA 125)
- Carcinoembryonic antigen (CEA)

In germ cell tumors
- Beta-HCG
- Alfa-fetoprotein
- Lactate dehydrogenase (LDH)

Imaging and other special investigations
- Ultrasound—to know the origin, size and nature of tumors, presence of free-fluid and metastases
- CT scan/MRI—if the origin of mass is doubtful and to assess spread, lymph nodes assessment,
- Gastrointestinal evaluation by endoscopy
- Biopsy—to plan management (if planned for neoadjuvant chemotherapy)
Endometrial aspiration and endocervical curettage, liver, bone and brain scan, if clinically indicated.

Malignancy Index

Risk malignancy index 1, RMI 1 index is calculated after multiplying ultrasonography (USG) parameter score, menopausal status and CA 125 level and malignancy suspected, if score is >250. There are no recommendations available for this.

Tissue Diagnosis

This is required, if the patient is to be planned for neoadjuvant chemotherapy in cases of advanced ovarian cancer.

Histology is preferred over cytology. Histology can be obtained by percutaneous image-guided biopsy. Laparoscopic biopsy should be done, if image-guided biopsy is not feasible. If histology not appropriate consider cytology.

EPITHELIAL OVARIAN CANCER SCREENING

For general population, routine screening for ovarian cancer is not recommended as most randomized controlled trials (RCTs) did not prove to detect ovarian cancer.[10] Annual pelvic examination screening in general population may detect ovarian cancer but in advanced stage.[3] In asymptomatic postmenopausal women with an average epithelial ovarian cancer (EOC) risk by evaluating the screening-related patient-relevant outcomes (EOC-specific mortality rates) the benefit and harms of transvaginal sonography (TVS) or serum CA125 or HE4 and multimodal testing, for ovarian cancer screening is now ongoing study in protocol stage and the results are awaited.[11] BRCA1 or BRCA2 mutation carriers who do not wish to undergo prophylactic oophorectomy should be offered at regular intervals thorough pelvic examination, transvaginal sonography (TVS) and CA125 testing.

Genetic Screening

Most of the inherited ovarian cancers (>90%) results from germline mutations in the *BRCA1* or *BRCA2* genes (autosomal dominant). Any women with personal history of both breast and ovarian cancer (HBOC), with ovarian cancer and close relative (1st/2nd/3rd degree) with breast cancer at <50 years of age or ovarian cancer at any age or women with breast cancer at ≤50 years of age and a close relative with ovarian cancer and women with 1st/2nd degree relative with a known *BRCA1/BRCA2* gene mutation are more than 20–25% chance of having genetic predisposition and should undergo genetic risk assessment.[3]

Prophylactic Salpingo-oophorectomy

It is the only way to prevent ovarian cancer. In carriers of *BRCA1* or *BRCA2* mutation, prophylactic bilateral salpingo-oophorectomy (BSO) may be performed either on completion of childbearing or at age 35 (90% effective in preventing ovarian cancer).[12] In women with

HNPCC, the prophylactic BSO is 100% effective in reducing risk of developing ovarian cancer.[13]

FIGO OVARIAN CANCER STAGING 2014[14]

Stage I tumor confined to ovaries	• 1A—tumor limited to one ovary, capsule intact, no tumor on surface, negative washings • 1B—tumor involved both ovaries, capsule intact, no tumor on surface, negative washings • 1C—tumor limited to one or both ovaries • 1C1—surgical spill • 1C2—capsule rupture before surgery or tumor on ovarian surface • 1C3—malignant cells in the ascites or peritoneal washings
Stage II	Tumor involves one or both ovaries with pelvic extension (below the pelvic brim) or primary peritoneal cancer. • IIA—extension and/or implants on uterus and/or fallopian tubes • IIB—extension to other pelvic intraperitoneal tissues
Stage III	Tumor involves one or both ovaries with cytologically or histologically confirmed spread to the peritoneum outside the pelvis and/or metastasis to the retroperitoneal lymph nodes • IIIA—positive retroperitoneal lymph nodes and/or microscopic metastasis beyond the pelvis • IIIA1—Positive retroperitoneal lymph nodes only • IIIA1(i)—metastases ≤10 mm • IIIA1(ii)—metastasis>10 mm • IIIA2—microscopic, extrapelvic (above the brim) peritoneal involvement ±positive retroperitoneal lymph nodes • IIIB—macroscopic, extrapelvic peritoneal metastasis ≤ 2 cm ± positive retroperitoneal lymph nodes Includes extensions to capsules of liver/spleen • IIIC—macroscopic, extrapelvic peritoneal metastasis >2 cm±positive retroperitoneal lymph nodes Includes extensions to capsules of liver/spleen
Stage IV	Distant metastasis excluding peritoneal metastasis. • IV A—pleural effusion with positive cytology • IVB—hepatic and/or splenic parenchymal metastasis, metastasis to extra-abdominal organs (including inguinal lymph node and lymph nodes outside the abdominal cavity)

Other Recommendations

- At staging histologic type including grading should be designated
- Primary site (ovary, fallopian tube or peritoneum) should be designated where possible
- Tumors that may otherwise qualify for stage I but involved with dense adhesions justify upgrading to stage II, if tumor cells are histologically proven to be present in the adhesions.

Information to be Given to Women Newly Diagnosed Ovarian Cancer

Any women diagnosed to have ovarian cancer should be informed about stage of the disease, treatment options available and prognosis, how to manage and treat the side effects of the disease in order to maximize wellbeing. She should be informed regarding sexuality and sexual activity, fertility and hormone treatment, symptoms and signs of disease recurrence, genetics including the chances of family members developing ovarian cancer, etc.

Role of Frozen Section of Suspicious Pelvic Masses

A review on role of frozen section of suspicious pelvic masses and to evaluate its accuracy and usefulness to diagnose histopathological ovarian cancer as verified by paraffin section of histopathological examination (ref standard). This review included 38 studies, in which 11,181 cases (3200 invasive cancer,1055 borderline tumors and 6926 benign tumors) were included. The authors concluded that there were no statistically significant differences between studies with pathologists of different levels of expertise. When a frozen section was used as a positive test to diagnose cancer (invasive cancer or a borderline tumor), then 280/1000 women would be diagnosed with cancer and 635 would be diagnosed without, 75 would be incorrectly diagnosed and in 10 women the diagnosis of cancer would be missed. In 94–99% of cases, the final HPE diagnosis would remain same, if frozen section report diagnose the mass as benign or malignant. There is 21% chance that final diagnosis would be a cancer, if the frozen section report is found as borderline tumor. In order to reduce the need for a second operation, if the final diagnosis turns out to be a cancer, in this group of women additional surgery may be performed at the time of initial surgery, if the surgeon decides.[15]

Primary Treatment[10]

Options

- Laparotomy and total abdominal hysterectomy (TAH), BSO with comprehensive staging or who desires fertility USO (unilateral salpingo-oophorectomy) for stage 1A, 1C, or all grade with comprehensive staging.
- Cytoreductive surgery for stage II, III, IV.
- Neoadjuvant chemotherapy (NACT) with interval debulking surgery (IDS) in case of poor surgical candidates due to comorbid conditions with bulky stage II/IV tumors.

Principles of Surgery

- Open laparotomy with midline incision.
- Intraoperative pathologic evaluation and frozen section, if necessary.
- For stage I, upon entering peritoneal cavity ascitic fluid should be aspirated, or if there is no ascites peritoneal lavage should be done. If metastasis found in the peritoneum, then excisional biopsy is taken otherwise random peritoneal biopsy taken from pelvis(POD), both right and left paracolic gutters and the undersurface of diaphragm (or scrapings from diaphragm).
- BSO/USO with every effort made to maintain the intact capsule during removal, and hysterectomy and omentectomy should be performed.
- Bilateral para-aortic lymph node dissection should be performed by removing the lymph node tissue stripped from vena cava and aorta to the level of inferior mesenteric artery and preferably to the level of renal vessels.
- Pelvic lymph nodes removed are bilateral common iliac, internal and external iliac and obturator nodes minimum anterior to the obturator nerve.

Debulking Surgery

Maximum cytoreduction should be done.
- Optimal cytoreduction—residual disease < 1 cm.
- Ascitic fluid aspiration should be performed and sent for cytology.
- If possible suspicious and/or enlarged nodes should be resected.
- Bilateral pelvic and para-aortic lymph node dissection should be done in patients with tumor nodules outside pelvis ≤ 2 cm (stage IIIB).
- Optimal cytoreduction procedure may include resection of bowel and/or appendectomy, stripping of the peritoneal surfaces of diaphragm and/or other sites, splenectomy, partial hepatectomy, partial cystectomy and/or ureteroneocystotomy, partial gastrectomy and/or distal pancreatectomy.

Risk Reducing Salpingo-oophorectomy (RRSO) (BRCA/HBOC) Protocol

Operative laparoscopy should be performed to visualize upper abdomen and pelvis. Biopsy should be taken from abnormal peritoneal sites. Pelvic washings of 50 mL normal saline aspirated. Total BSO to be performed with removal of 2 cm of proximal ovarian vasculature/Infundibulopelvic ligament, whole tube up to uterine cornua, and peritoneum surrounding the ovaries and tubes, especially peritoneum underlying areas of adhesion between tube and/or ovary and the pelvic side walls. There should be minimal handling with instrument of both ovaries and tubes should be done to avoid traumatic exfoliation of cells, and then placed in a endobag for retrieval from the pelvis. If occult malignancy found on histopathological examination, patient should be referred to a gynecologic-oncologist.

Mucinous Tumors

To rule out occult gastrointestinal (GI) primary with ovarian metastasis upper and lower GI tract should be evaluated and an appendectomy should be performed in all cases of mucinous ovarian neoplasm.

Low Malignant Potential Tumors

Lymphadenectomy need not be performed as it does not affect overall survival. However omentectomy and multiple biopsies of peritoneum should be done and that may upstage patients in approximately 30% of cases and thereby affect prognosis.

Secondary Cytoreduction

This surgery is performed in patients with recurrent ovarian cancer who recur >6-12 months after completion of initial chemotherapy, have an isolated/limited focus of disease amenable to complete resection and do not have ascites.

Palliative Surgical Procedures

In selected patients, these type of palliative surgical procedure can be done:
- Paracentesis/indwelling peritoneal catheter.
- Thoracentesis/pleurodesis/video assisted thoracoscopy/indwelling pleural catheter, ureteral stent/nephrostomy.
- Gastrostomy tube/intestinal stents/surgical relief of intestinal obstruction.

Primary Chemotherapy Regimens[10]

IP/IV Regimen

- Paclitaxel 135 mg/m^2 IV continuous infusion over 3 or 24 hour Day 1.
- Cisplatin 75-100 mg/m^2 IP Day 2 after IV Paclitaxel; Paclitaxel 60 mg/m^2 IP Day 8. Repeat every 3 weeks for 6 cycles.

IV Regimens

Paclitaxel 175 mg/m^2 IV over 3 hours followed by carboplatin AUC5-6 IV over 1 hour Day 1. Repeat every 3 weeks for 6 cycles.

Dose Dense Paclitaxel

- 80 mg/m^2 IV over 1 hour day 1, 8, 15 followed by carboplatin AUC 5-6 IV over 1 hour day 1. Repeat every 3 weeks for 6 cycles.
- Paclitaxel 60 mg/m^2 IV over 1 hour followed by carboplatin AUC 2 IV over 30 minutes, weekly for 18 weeks.

Docetaxel

60-75 mg/m^2 IV over 1 hr followed by carboplatin AUC5-6 IV over 1hr Day 1. Repeat every 3 weeks for 6 cycles.

Bevacizumab-containing Regimen

Paclitaxel 175 mg/m^2 IV over 3 hours followed by carboplatin AUC 5-6 IV over 1 hour and Bevacizumab 7.5 mg/kg IV over 30-90 minutes day-1 Repeat every 3 weeks for 5-6 cycles. Continue bevacizumab for up to additional 12 cycles.
or
Paclitaxel 175 mg/m^2 IV over 3 hours followed by carboplatin AUC5-6 IV over 1 hour Day 1. Repeat every 3 weeks for 6 cycles. Starting Day 1 of cycle 2, give bevacizumab 15 mg/kg IV over 30-90 minutes every 3 weeks for up to 22 cycles.

Treatment

Treatment options for newly diagnosed ovarian cancer
LMP tumors:
- Observation with follow-up tests
- Surgery to remove one ovary and its fallopian tubes + surgical staging
- Completion surgery ± chemotherapy next

Stage I
- USO (if cancer is only in one ovary) + surgical staging
- Hysterectomy with BSO + surgical staging

Stage II
- Hysterectomy with BSO and all cancer that can be seen + surgical staging.

Stage III and IV
- Hysterectomy with BSO and all cancer that can be seen + surgical staging
- NACT followed by surgery.

Treatment option for ovarian cancer found by prior surgery

Stage I
- No more surgery
- Surgical staging ± completion surgery

Stage II, III and IV
- No more surgery
- Completion surgery
- Chemo, then completion surgery

Treatment Options After Primary Treatment with Surgery[10]

Stage 1: Observation with follow-up tests or Chemotherapy for 3-6 cycles.

Role of systematic retroperitoneal lymphadenectomy: In stage I ovarian cancer lymph node assessment only to be done and avoid doing systematic retroperitoneal lymphadenectomy-enbloc dissection of retroperitoneal lymph node from pelvic sidewall up to renal vein level.[16]

Role of adjuvant systemic chemotherapy: Adjuvant platinum-based chemotherapy is effective in prolonging survival in women who have low risk (FIGO stage 1/IIa) epithelial ovarian cancer. Whether women with low and intermediate risk early stage disease (grade 1 or 2, stage 1a or 1b) will benefit as much from adjuvant chemotherapy as women having high-risk disease. Decision to use adjuvant chemotherapy in these women should be considering this uncertainty and the adverse events too. Treatment of women with lower risk disease should be individualized to take into account individual factors. In women with high-risk stage 1 disease (grade 3 or stage 1c), adjuvant chemotherapy with six cycles of carboplatin given. If a woman have had suboptimal surgical staging and appear to have stage I disease, the possible benefits and side effects of adjuvant chemotherapy should be explained to her.

The systematic review, includes five RCTs involving 1277 women with 10-year follow-up. This review showed an overall survival advantage with platinum based chemotherapy.[16]

Stage II, III, and IV: Aim of surgery should be complete resection of all macroscopic tissues.

If <1 cm of residual tumor after surgery for stage II/III—intraperitoneal chemotherapy (only clinical trial).

All patient after surgery—IV chemotherapy for 6-8 cycles.

Role of Intraperitoneal Chemotherapy for Advanced Ovarian Malignancy

Due to the chemosensitiveness of ovarian cancer and its confinement to the surface of the peritoneal cavity made it an obvious target for intraperitoneal (IP) chemotherapy. Which is given by infusion of chemotherapeutic agent directly into the peritoneal cavity. This might increase the anticancer effect and reduce the systemic adverse effects in comparison to IV therapy.

A systematic review included 9 RCTs studied 2119 women and compared the effectiveness of intravenous versus intraperitoneal chemotherapy for EOC of any FIGO stage following primary cytoreductive surgery. The authors concluded that intraperitoneal chemotherapy in advanced ovarian cancer cases increases overall survival and progression-free survival. But the disadvantages are related to peritoneal catheter including pain, catheter blockage, gastrointestinal effects and infection.[17]

Role of Interval Debulking Surgery in Advanced Ovarian Malignancy

A systematic review to assess effectiveness and complications of IDS for women with advanced stage ovarian cancer compared IDS, following NACT to primary debulking surgery followed by adjuvant chemotherapy included 3RCTs randomizing 853 women found inconclusive evidence weather IDS improves overall or progression-free survival (PFS) rates over primary debulking surgery. But IDS appeared to yield benefit only in women whose primary surgery was not performed by gynecologic-oncologists or was less extensive. Data on quality of life and adverse events were also inconclusive.[18]

Role of Maintenance Chemotherapy for Ovarian Cancer

In EOC the standard treatment of debulking surgery and six courses of platinum based chemotherapy results in complete clinical remission in up to 75% of cases. But 75% of the responders will relapse within a median time of 18 to 28 months and only 20–40% of women will survive beyond 5 years. A systematic review to assess the effectiveness and toxicity of maintenance chemotherapy for EOC and to evaluate the impact on quality of life, included 8 trials involving 1644 women and the authors concluded that there is no evidence to suggest that the use of platinum agents, doxorubicin or paclitaxel used as maintenance chemotherapy is more effective than observation alone.[19]

After Chemotherapy for Stage II, III/IV Ovarian Cancer

- *All signs and symptoms disappear:*
  - Clinical trial or
  - Observation with follow-up tests or
  - Maintenance treatment with paclitaxel or pazopanib.
- *Cancer shows some improvement/remain same/keep growing:* Clinical trial/recurrence treatment/supportive care alone or with treatment above.

Follow-up and Management of Recurrent Disease

Stage I, II, III, IV complete response

- Visit every 2–4 month for 2 year, then 3–6 month for 3 years, then annually after 5 years
- In each visit, physical examination including pelvic examination
- CA-125s or other tumor markers, if initially elevated
- Refer for genetic risk evaluation, if not previously done
- CBC and biochemistry profile as indicated
- Chest/abdominal/pelvic CT, MRI, PET-CT or PET as clinically indicated
- Chest X-ray as indicated.

- *Rising CA125 or clinical relapse without prior chemotherapy:*
  - Primary chemotherapy to be given after relevant investigations
- *Clinical relapse with prior chemotherapy:*
  - Treated as recurrence after relevant investigation
- *Rising CA125 with prior chemotherapy:*
  - Treatment is delayed till any clinical evidence of disease noticed (clinical relapse)
  - Follow up.

Treatment of Recurrence[10]

About 75% of women with advanced EOC will relapse following surgery and chemotherapy. Usually, the patients with relapse were treated with either platinum/non-platinum drugs depending on the platinum sensitivity and platinum-free interval. These drug regimens are generally well tolerated but have potential severe side effects. The available options are:

- No prior chemotherapy—surgical treatment with or without chemo.
- Relapse based on increase in CA 125 levels only—clinical trial/start recurrence treatment/wait till symptoms appear then treatment.
- Relapse <6 month after completion of chemotherapy—clinical trial/start recurrence treatment with different chemotherapy/supportive care with or without treatment.

- Relapse ≥6 month after end of chemotherapy- more surgery/clinical trial/platinum-based chemotherapy/different chemotherapy.

Surgical Cytoreduction for Recurrent Epithelial Ovarian Cancer

The standard treatment of women with recurrent ovarian cancer remains poorly defined. A review to evaluate the effectiveness and safety of optimal secondary cytoreductive surgery for women with recurrent epithelial ovarian cancer included 9 non-randomized studies involving 1194 women. The authors concluded that in women with platinum-sensitive recurrent ovarian cancer, ability to achieve surgery with complete cytoreduction (no visible residual disease) is associated with significant improvement in overall survival, however, the risks of major surgery need to be carefully balanced against potential benefits on a case-by-case basis.[20]

Chemotherapies for Recurrent Epithelial Ovarian Carcinomas

- Drugs for platinum sensitive disease are-carboplatin, carboplatin/docitaxel, carboplatin/gemcitabin, carboplatin/gemcitabin/bevacizumab, carboplatin/paclitaxel, Bevacizumab, Olaparib.
- For platinum-resistant disease—docitaxel, etoposide, gemcitabine, paclitaxel, bevacizumab, topotecan

Prognosis

Favorable prognostic factors[21]	Poor prognostic factors[10]
• Younger age • Good performance status • Cell type other than mucinous and clear cell, well-differentiated tumor, • Smaller disease volume prior to surgical debulking • Absence of ascites • Smaller residual tumor following primary cytoreductive surgery	• Patients who progress after 2 consecutive chemotherapy regimens without ever sustaining a clinical benefit (refractory) • For those whose disease recurs in <6 months (platinum-resistant)

NEWER THERAPY TRIALS

- *Poly (ADP-ribose) polymerase (PARP) inhibitors for the treatment of ovarian cancer*: PARP inhibitors are a novel medication that works by preventing cancer cells from repairing their DNA once they have been damaged by other chemotherapy agents. A review to determine the benefits and risks of PARP inhibitors for the treatment of epithelial ovarian cancer included 4 RCTs involving 599 women with epithelial ovarian cancer and concluded that they appear to improve PFS in women with recurrent platinum-sensitive disease.[22]
- *Luteinizing hormone releasing hormone (LHRH) agonists for the treatment of relapsed epithelial ovarian cancer*: A review included 2 studies involving 97 women, compared the effectiveness and safety of LHRH agonists with chemotherapeutic agents or placebo in relapsed EOC. The authors concluded that there is not enough evidence to comment on the safety and effectiveness of LHRH agonists in the treatment of platinum refractory and platinum resistant (relapsed) EOC.[23]
- *Interferon after surgery for women with advanced epithelial ovarian cancer*: A systematic review to assess the effectiveness and safety of interferon after surgery in the treatment of advanced (stage II-IV) EOC, included 5 trials involving 1476 participants (2 trials compared interferon with observation alone and 3 trials compared interferon plus chemotherapy with chemotherapy alone). The authors concluded that the addition of interferon to firstline chemotherapy did not alter the overall survival in postsurgical women with advanced EOC compared with chemotherapy alone. There is not enough evidence that interferon therapy alone alters overall survival or progression-free survival compared to observation alone in post-surgical women who have undergone 1st line chemotherapy.[24]

GERM CELL CANCER

Malignant germ cell tumor of ovary occurs in upto 0.07% of woman globally. This occurs in pediatrics population more than the adult population.

Any patient with pelvic mass should be investigated as for EOC but tumor markers to be tested are: CA125, inhibin, β-hCG, α-fetoprotein, lactate dehydrogenase (LDH) as clinically indicated.[10]

Treatment

Comprehensive surgical staging and fertility sparing surgery, if fertility desired, otherwise complete staging surgery should be done.[10]
- If the tumor found to be stage I dysgerminoma or stage I grade I immature teratoma then the patient should be kept under observation.
- Embryonal tumor or endodermal sinus tumor (yolk-sac tumor) of any stage or stage II-IV dysgerminoma or Stage I, grade 2/3 or stage II-IV immature teratoma should receive chemotherapy.

Primary Chemotherapy for Malignant Germ Cell Tumors

- Bleomycin, etoposide, cisplatin (BEP) Bleomycin 30 units per week, etoposide 100 mg/m^2 daily for day 1-5, cisplatin 20 mg/m^2 daily for Day 1-5. Repeat every 21 days for 3 cycles for good risk and 4 cycles for poor risk.
- *Etoposide/carboplatin*: For select patients with stage IB-III dysgerminoma for whom minimizing toxicity is critical, 3 courses of etoposide/carboplatin can be used. Carboplatin 400 mg/m^2 on day 1 plus etoposide 120 mg/m^2 on days 1, 2 and 3 every 4 weeks for 3 courses.

Follow-up

In germ cell tumor,
- Physical examination—in germ cell tumor every 2-4 month till 2 years, then annually.
- Serum tumor markers in germ cell tumor every 2-4 month till 2 years, then not indicated.
- Imaging studies as clinically indicated in germ cell tumors.

Recurrence therapy for malignant germ cell tumors: The chemotherapeutic agents can be used in case of recurrence are: Cisplatin/etoposide, Docetaxel/Carboplatin, Paclitaxel/ifosfamide, paclitaxel/carboplatin, Paclitaxel/gemcitabin, VIP (etoposide, ifosfamide, cisplatin), VeIP (vinblastin, ifosfamide, cisplatin), VAC (vincristine, dactinomycin, cyclophosphamide), TIP (paclitaxel, ifosfamide, cisplatin). Radiation therapy or supportive care.

Chemotherapy for malignant germ cell ovarian cancer in adult patients with early stage, advanced and recurrent disease.
A systematic review to evaluate the effectiveness and safety of chemotherapy in adult women with early stage, advanced and recurrent malignant germ cell ovarian cancers included one RCT and observational studies. The authors concluded that low quality evidence on the use of chemotherapy in malignant germ cell tumors of the ovaries.[25]

SEX CORD STROMAL TUMOR

They may be derived from female cells that secrete estrogen (granulose and theca cell) and male cells that secrete androgens (sertoli and leydig cells).

Treatment

Comprehensive surgical staging and fertility sparing surgery, if fertility desired, otherwise complete staging surgery should be done.[10]

Malignant sex chord stromal tumor-stage 1A/1C who desire fertility should be treated with fertility sparing surgery with complete staging. All other stage should undergo complete staging. Low-risk stage I patients can be observed and high-risk stage I, stage II-IV should receive chemotherapy. If there is relapse clinical trial/secondary cytoreductive surgery/recurrence therapy should be given.

Follow-up in Sex-cord Stromal Tumor

- *Physical examination*: In sexcord stromal tumor every 2-4 month for 2 years, then every 6 monthly.

- *Tumor markers*: In sexcord stromal tumor, every 2–4 month for 2 years, then every 6 monthly.
- *Imaging studies*: No supportive data for sex-cord stromal tumor.

Recurrence therapy for malignant sex cord stromal tumors: Aromatase inhibitors (anastrozole, letrozole), Bevacizumab, Leuprolide for granulose cell tumor. Docitaxel/Paclitaxel/ ifosfamide/carboplatin/Tamoxifen/VAC/ Radiation therapy.

Carcinosarcoma or malignant mixed mullerian tumor: It should have complete staging. Relapse is treated as EOC.

Low malignant potential (LMP) ovarian tumors: These tumors after diagnosis can be managed as follows:
- If previous surgical staging is comprehensive, then patient can only be observed. If staging is incomplete and there are invasive implants patient can be observed or treated as EOC. If there is residual disease after 1st procedure, complete surgery should be done, if fertility not desired or fertility sparing comprehensive surgery should be done.
- Follow-up should be done every 3–6 month for up to 5 years, then annually. In each visit, physical examination including pelvic examination should be done. If CA125 or other tumor marker elevated before should be done in each visit. Completion surgery should be performed after completion of childbearing in patients who underwent USO. Complete blood count (CBC), Biochem profile and ultrasound as indicated for patients with fertility—sparing surgery. If relapse occurs surgical evaluation and debulking surgery should be done.[10]

Ovarian Cancer During Pregnancy

Almost 5% of the adnexal masses found during pregnancy are malignant.[26] The incidence is 1/10,000 to 1/50,000 pregnancies. It is diagnosed by TVS, and if necessary MRI can be done after 1st trimester to confirm the features of malignancy. In most cases, it is possible to provide proper treatment to the mother without placing the fetus at serious risk. The investigation and management require a multidisciplinary approach with specialist in maternal-fetal medicine, gynecologic oncology and pediatrics as well as imaging and pathology as needed.[27]

In patients with USG suspected stage I malignant tumor, USO should be performed without rupture for stage IA and BSO for stage IB tumors associated with peritoneal cytology and complete abdominopelvic exploration in both cases (grade 2). Adjuvant chemotherapy, if indicated should be given as in nonpregnant patient. Treatment should start during or after pregnancy depending on prognosis, multidisciplinary decision and patient preference. The route of delivery should not be an issue. Postpartum secondary surgery should be considered according to multidisciplinary team decision and patient preference. For more advanced stage tumors (II to IV), preferable to consider termination of pregnancy before 24 weeks and perform routine treatment as non-pregnant. After 24 weeks, a biopsy may be taken USG-guided or by laparotomy/laparoscopic depending on the stage of tumor and the gestational age. Depending on the stage, NACT/ surgery can be performed. Dates for the last chemotherapy session and delivery for which a cesarean section is most frequently required should be choosen accordingly. Procedures should take place at a 4 week interval so cesarean section is not planned during a period of aplasia, harmful to both mother and child. It is reasonable to have preterm delivery between 32–36 weeks. Complete surgical treatment can be performed at cesarean section, if possible or after delivery.[27,28]

One study suggested, if chemotherapy is indicated that should be delayed until after delivery or at least after 20 weeks in order to minimize the potential fetal toxicity.[27]

KEY POINTS

- Most common ovarian malignancy is EOC.
- The risk of developing ovarian cancer increases in Nulliparous women and older

age at first birth, hormone therapy and pelvis inflammatory disease.
- Surgical staging followed by chemotherapy depending on histopathological studies is the primary treatment.
- NACT followed by IDS appeared to yield benefit only in women whose primary surgery was not performed by gynecologic-oncologists or was less extensive.
- Follow-up of the patient should be done according to protocol, and if recurrence diagnosed to be treated as per guideline.
- Younger age at diagnosis and complete debulking during primary surgery are the good prognostic indicators.
- Treatment of ovarian cancer during pregnancy should start during or after pregnancy depending on prognosis, multidisciplinary decision and patient preference.

REFERENCES

1. Sankarnarayanan R, Ferlay J. Worldwide burden of gynaecological cancer: the size of the problem. Best Pract Res Clin Obstet Gynecol. 2006;20:207.
2. Howlader N, Noone AM, Krapcho M, et al. SEER cancer statistics review, 1975-2012, based on November 2014 SEER Data submission, posted to the SEER website, April 2015. Bethesda.MD. National Cancer Institute; 2015. Available at *http://seer.cancer,gov/csr/1975, 2012/*.
3. Hoffman BL, Scorge JO, Schaffer JI, Halvorson LM, Bradshaw KD, Cunningham FG. Epithelial ovarian cancer, chapter-35. In: Williams Gynecology, 2nd edn, McGraw Hill Medical. New York; 2012.pp.853-78.
4. Jelovac D, Amstrong DK. Recent progress in the diagnosis and treatment of ovarian cancer. CA Cancer J Clin. 2011;61:183-203.
5. Morch LS, Lokkegaard E, Andreasen AH, et al. Hormone therapy and different ovarian cancers: a National Cohort study. Am J Epidemiol. 2012;175:1234-42.
6. Pearce CL, Templeman C, Rossing MA, et al. Association between endometriosis and risk of histological subtype of ovarian cancer: a pooled analysis of case-control studies. Lancet Oncol. 2012,13:385-94.
7. Flemming GF, Seidman J, Lengyel E. Epithelial ovarian cancer. In: Barakat RR, Markman N,Randll ME (Eds). Principles and practices of gynecologic oncology, 6th edn. Philadelphia: Lippinkott Williams & Wilkins; 2013.pp.757-847.
8. Jemal A,Bray F, Center MM, et al. Global cancer statistics. CA Cancer J Clin. 2011;61:69.
9. Lancaster JM, Powell CB, Chen LM, et al. Society of Gynecologic Oncology statement on risk assessment for inherited gynaecologic cancer predispositions. Gynecol Oncol. 2015;136:3-7.
10. NCCN Clinical Practice Guidelines in Oncology, Ovarian Cancer. 2015. available at *www.nccn.org*.
11. Mosch CG, Iaschinski T, Eikermann M. Impact of epithelial ovarian cancer screening on patient-relevant outcomes in average risk postmenopausal women, Cochrane Database of Systematic Reviews; 14 July 2014:*DOI:10,1002/14651858,CD11210*.
12. American College of Obstetricians and Gynecologists: Hereditary Breast and Ovarian cancer syndrome. Practice Bulletin No 103, April 2009.
13. Schmeler KM, Lynch HT, Chen LM, et al: prophylactic surgery to reduce the risk of gynecologic cancers in the Lynch syndrome. N Engl J Med. 2006;354:261.
14. Prat J, FIGO Committee on Gynecologic Oncology. Staging classification for cancer of the ovary, fallopian tube and peritoneum. Int J Gynecol Obstet. 2014;1244(1):1-5.
15. Ratnavelu ND, Brown AP, Mallett S, Scholten RJ, Patel A, Founta C, et al. Intraoperative frozen section analysis for the diagnosis of early stage ovarian cancer in suspicious pelvic masses. Cochrane Database of Systematic Reviews; 1st March 2016:DOI:10.1002/14651858,CD010360.
16. Theresa AL, Winter RBA, Heus P, Kitchener HC, adjuvant (postsurgery) chemotherapy for early stage epithelial ovarian cancer. Cochrane Database of Systematic Review.published online 17 Dec 2015. *DOI:10.1002/14651858 CD 004706.*
17. Iaaback K, Johnson N, Lawrie T A. Intraperitoneal chemotherapy for the initial management of primary epithelial ovarian cancer. Published 12 Jan 2016. Cochrane Database of Systematic Review. *DOI: 10.1002/14651858. CD005340.*
18. Tangiitgamol S, Manusirivithaya S, Laopaiboon M, Lumbiganon P, Bryant A. Interval debulking surgery for advanced epithelial ovarian cancer. Cochrane Database of systematic reviews. published 9th Jan 2016.*DOI:10,1002/14651858. CD006014.pub7.*
19. Mei L, Chen H, Wei DM, Fang F, Liu G, Xie H Y, et al. Maintenance chemotherapy for ovarian cancer. Cochrane Database of Systematic Reviews. 29 June 2013.*DOI:10.1002/14651858.CD007414.*

20. Rawahi TA, Lopes AD, Bristlow RE, Bryant A, Elattar A, Chattopadhyay S, et al. Surgical cytoreduction for recurrent epithelial ovarian cancer cochrane systematic Database Review. 28 Feb 2013;DOI:10.1002/14651858.CD008765,pub3.
21. National cancer institute: ovarian epithelial cancer treatment (PDQ) available at:*www.cancer.gov/ cancertropics/pdq/treatment/ovarian epithelial/ healthprofessional.Accessed May* 12.2011c.
22. Wiggans AJ, Cass GKS, Bryant A, Lawrie TA, Morrison J. Poly (ADP-ribose) polymerase (PARP) inhibitors for the treatment of ovarian cancer. Cochrane Database of Systematic Reviews, 20th May 2015.DOI:10.1002/14651858.CD007929.
23. Wuntakal R, Seshadri S, Montes A, Lane G. Luteinising hormone releasing hormone (LHRH) agonists for the treatment of relapsed epithelial ovarian cancer, Cochrane Database of Systematic Reviews; 29 June 2016. *DOI:10.1002/14651858. CD011322.pub2.*
24. Lawal AO, Musekiwa A, Grobler L. Interferon after surgery for women with advanced (stage II-IV) epithelial ovarian cancer; Cochrane Database of Systematic Reviews. 6 June 2013. *DOI:10.1002/14651858.CD009620.pub2.*
25. Razak ARA, Li L, Bryant A, Padilla I D. Chemotherapy for malignant germ cell ovarian cancer in adult patients with early stage, advanced and recurrent disease. Cochrane Database of Systematic Reviews, 16 March 2011;*DOI-10.1002/14651858.CD007584. pub2.*
26. Whitecar MP, Turner S, Higby MK. Adnexal masses in pregnancy: a review of 130 cases undergoing surgical management. Am J Obstet Gynecol. 1999; 181:19-24.
27. Marret H, Lhomme C, Lecuru F, Canis M, LevequeJ, Golfier F, et al. Guidelines for the management of ovarian cancer during pregnancy. Eur J Obstet Gynecol Reprod Biol. 2010;149(1):18-21.
28. Morice P, Lhomme C, Lecuru F, Canis MJ, Leveque J, Golfer F, et al. Guideline for the management of ovarian cancer during pregnancy. France, 16 Dec, 2008.

31

Borderline Ovarian Tumors

Devender Kumar, Savita Arora

INTRODUCTION

Borderline ovarian tumors (BOTs) are mostly epithelial ovarian tumors which are neither clearly cancers nor taken as benign. Significance of these tumors was recognized by Taylor, in 1929 as semimalignant.[1] These tumors were recognized as low malignant potential (LMP) tumors. Histologically these tumors have nuclear atypia but no stromal invasion so they have better prognosis.[1,2]

INCIDENCE

Borderline ovarian tumors mostly occur in women with age less than 40 years and limited to ovary (80% in Stage I) for long time. The common borderline ovarian tumors are mucinous or serous type. Incidence of these tumors is approximately 15–20% of all ovarian tumors.

Other low malignant potential tumors are as follows:
- Endometrioid tumors
- Clear cell tumors
- Transitional cell tumors.

CLASSIFICATION OF OVARIAN TUMORS[3-6]

Surface epithelial (65%), germ cell (15%), sex cord-stromal (10%), metastases (5%), miscellaneous (5%) are the gross classification of ovarian tumors. Epithelial ovarian tumors have sub-classification as borderline tumors under serous, mucinous, endometrioid and clear cell tumors depending on atypia.

CLINICAL PRESENTATION

Asymptomatic adnexal mass detected incidentally.

Lower abdominal pain/discomfort.

Rarely similar to malignant ovarian tumors as 20–25% of borderline ovarian tumors spread beyond ovary.[3,6] High suspicion of malignancy if irregular solid tumor, presence of ascites, papillary projections and irregular multilocular solid tumor ≥10 cm.

Patients with borderline ovarian tumors can be grouped in two categories:
1. No risk of recurrence if primary resected.
2. Risk of recurrence if primary resected.

The most important site of recurrence is preserved ovary.[6,7] Recurrence is not associated with following:
- Capsular status
- Presence of psammoma bodies
- Cribriform pattern
- Stratification
- Tumor size
- Surgical spillage.

Investigations

Patient with ovarian mass must be evaluated to rule out malignancy. All cases in young patients must have frozen section. Frozen section cannot rule out frank malignancy in BOT but helps in planning fertility sparing surgeries.[8]

They are worked in line with ovarian cancer so investigations are same as in ovarian tumor.

Routine Investigations

- Complete blood count
- Urine analysis and culture
- Blood sugar (Fasting and postprandial)
- Liver function test
- Renal function test
- Chest X-ray PA view
- ECG
- Pap smear.

Tumor Markers

- CA-125
- CEA.

Imaging and Other Special Investigations

- Ultrasound—to know the origin, size and nature of tumors, presence of free fluid and metastases
- CT scan/MRI—if the origin of mass is doubtful and to assess spread, lymph nodes assessment
- Gastrointestinal evaluation by endoscopy.

MALIGNANCY INDEX SCORE[9]

Risk of malignancy index (RMI) is calculated ultrasonography (USG) findings, menopausal status and serum CA-125 levels. Risk of malignancy index score = U × M × serum CA-125 concentration (U/mL), where U is USG findings (multilocularity, solid areas, bilateral masses, ascites, and evidence of metastases). U is 0 if none, 1 if one feature and 3 if two or more features observed. M is menopausal status. Value assigned is 1 if premenopausal and 3 if postmenopausal status.

Score of 200 or more is considered as malignant.

HISTOLOGY OF BORDERLINE OVARIAN TUMORS

Histology of these tumors have following characteristic:

- Epithelial multilayering of more than four cell layers
- Not more than four mitoses per 10 high power fields
- Mild nuclear atypia (slight pleomorphism, sometimes prominent nucleoli)
- Increased nuclear/cytoplasmic ratio
- Slight to complex branching or bridging of epithelial papillae and pseudopapillae
- Epithelial budding and cell detachment into the lumen
- No destructive stromal invasion.

The definite criteria to diagnose borderline ovarian tumors are:

- Epithelial proliferation with papillary formation and pseudostratification
- Nuclear atypia and increased mitotic activity
- Absence of true stromal invasion.

Differential Diagnosis

Adnexal masses always pose a diagnostic dilemma. The list of differential diagnosis of adnexal masses is extensive and is as follows:

- Ovarian tumors like dermoid, adenoma, etc.
- Endometrioma
- Benign lesions of the uterus like subserous fibroid
- Hydrosalpinx/pyosalpinx
- Ovarian cyst torsion
- Pelvic abscess
- Pelvic kidney
- Paraovarian or peritoneal cyst
- Uterine anomalies.

Management

Staging laparotomy is the standard surgical procedure but decision of conservative surgery is taken depending on age of patient, desire of fertility, preoperative clinical findings, biomarkers and intraoperative findings (including frozen section).[7,8,10] Laparoscopic staging is possible but chance of tumor rupture and incomplete staging is high.[7]

Majority of the patients are in stage I and reproductive age group so conservative treatment is choice, that is, cystectomy or oophorectomy or salpingo-oophorectomy but appropriate staging is must.[8,11] FIGO staging (2014) for ovarian cancer has incorporated TNM classification. T1 N0 M0 tumors without malignant cells on ovarian surface or in ascitic fluid are considered for conservative management and follow-up.[3,5]

Criteria for conservative surgery is as follows:[12,13]

Stage Ia grade I
- No ascites
- No dense adhesion
- No surface excrescence
- Unruptured
- Unilateral confined neoplasm.

If fertility is not desired then after collecting peritoneal washing for cytology (ascitic fluid if present) total abdominal hysterectomy with bilateral salpingo-oophorectomy with omentectomy is done (with appendicectomy in mucinous tumor). Para-aortic lymph nodes sampling is also performed with pelvic lymphadenectomy.[14]

Surgical staging is considered adequate if histology shows borderline tumor with no metastasis anywhere else like no evidence of malignancy in peritoneal lavage, resected omentum or lymph nodes. Other ovary and endometrium should also show no evidence of disease.

Postoperation chemo or radiotherapy (RT) is not indicated. Only follow-up of the case is sufficient. Cystectomy is advised in unilateral tumor confine to ovary alone. Though conservative surgery in serous and mucinous BOT is major cause of recurrence but conservative or radical surgery has similar impact on overall survival in stage I cases. In 2006, Marcickiewicz and Brännström published long-term consequences of fertility sparing surgeries in borderline ovarian tumors in reproductive age-group desiring fertility and recommended conservative approach to preserve fertility with no apparent risk of recurrence.[10] Damak et al in 2014, advised unilateral salpingo-oophorectomy with omentectomy and multiple peritoneal biopsies and washing, but once the fertility is not desired they recommended radical surgery as mandatory in stage I disease.[6]

In case of invasive disease or clinical progression (advance stage), primary cytoreductive surgery followed by chemotherapy is recommended. Regimens of postsurgery chemotherapy are Cisplatin and cyclophosphamide.[13,14] Most common complication of chemotherapy is leukemia. Chemotherapy have little value because tumor cells are very similar to normal epithelium in metabolic activities and only small fraction of cells are in susceptible phase of cell cycle, so adjuvant chemotherapy in early stages have no advantages over observation. Radiotherapy appeared to extend the disease free interval in advance stage.

Ziari et al. (2015) reported 7% and 21% recurrence in serous and mucinous BOT (stage I) respectively. In their retrospective review, they found 86% of patients in stage I of the disease and overall survival was 100% and 93% for serous and mucinous tumors respectively.[14]

Second look laparotomy is indicated if the initial evaluation was inadequate. Five-year survival is almost 100% is surgical staging was adequate in stage I.

Prognosis mainly depends on histology of tumor, stage of disease and residual disease after surgery.[8,11,14]

FOLLOW-UP

Cases are followed with history and clinical examination with pelvis sonography and CA-125 if initially elevated. Frequency is more and regular in cases with conservative management. Cases are followed once in 3 months up to 2 years, thereafter twice a year. Risk of recurrence beyond 5 years follow-up is 2–4% so annual follow-up is advised thereafter.[7]

KEY POINTS

- Histologically they have nuclear atypia and increased mitotic activity.
- The hallmark of these tumor is absence of true stromal invasion.
- Conservative management is advised in younger patients who desire fertility.
- Radical surgery must be performed once the family is complete in cases with stage more than Ia and grade 1.
- It is prudent to follow-up these cases religiously and sincerely.
- Survival and good quality of life is high if diagnosed in stage I and staging is done accurately.

REFERENCES

1. Serov SF, Scully RE, Sobin LH. International histological classification of tumors, no 9 Histological Typing of Ovarian Tumours. Geneva: World Health Organization; 1973.
2. Bostwick DG, Tazelaar HD, Ballon SC. Ovarian epithelial tumors of borderline malignancy: a clinical and pathologic study of 109 cases. Cancer. 1983;58:2052-64.
3. SB Edge, DR Byrd, CC Compton, et al. American Joint Committee on Cancer. Ovary and primary peritoneal carcinoma AJCC Cancer Staging Manual 7th edition (New York: Springer); 2010.pp.419-28.
4. Scully RE. Classification of human ovarian tumors. Environ Health Perspect. 1987;73:15-24.
5. Prat J. FIGO Committee on Gynecologic Oncology. Staging classification for cancer of the ovary, fallopian tube, and peritoneum. Int J Gynecol Obstet. 2014;124(1):1-5.
6. Damak T, Ben Hassouna J, Chargui R, Gamoudi A, Hechiche M, Dhieb T, et al. Borderline tumors of the ovary. Tunis Med. 2014;92(6):411-6.
7. D Fischerovaa, M Zikana, P Dundrb, et al. Diagnosis, Treatment, and Follow-Up of Borderline Ovarian Tumors. The Oncologist. 2012;17(12):1515-33.
8. Jones MB. Borderline ovarian tumors: current concepts for prognostic factors and clinical management. Clin Obstet Gynecol. 2006;49(3):517-25.
9. Jacobs I, Oram D, Fairbanks J, Turner J, Frost C, Grudzinskas JG. A risk of malignancy index incorporating CA-125, ultrasound and menopausal status for the accurate preoperative diagnosis of ovarian cancer. Br J Obstet Gynaecol. 1990;97:922-9.
10. Marcickiewicz J, Brännström M. Fertility preserving surgical treatment of borderline ovarian tumour: long-term consequence for fertility and recurrence. Acta Obstet Gynecol Scand. 2006;85(12):1496-500.
11. Morice P, Uzan C, Fauvet R. Borderline ovarian tumour: pathological diagnostic dilemma and risk factors for invasive or lethal recurrence. Lancet Oncol. 2012;13(3):e103-15.
12. Tropé C, Kaern J, Vergote IB. Are borderline tumors of the ovary overtreated both surgically and systemically? A review of four prospective randomized trials including 253 patients with borderline tumors. Gynecol Oncol. 1993;51:236-43.
13. Vasconcelos I, de Sousa Mendes M. Conservative surgery in ovarian borderline tumours: a meta-analysis with emphasis on recurrence risk. Eur J Cancer. 2015;51(5):620-31.
14. Ziari K, Soleymani E, Alizadeh K. Survival analysis and prognosis for patients with serous and mucinous borderline ovarian tumors: 14-year experience from a tertiary center in Iran. Acta Med Iran. 2015;53(4):199-203.

32
Introduction to Radiotherapy and Chemotherapy

Kishore Singh, Savita Arora, Arun Kumar Rathi

Radiation is being used in treatment of carcinoma since early 1900s. Dr Emile Grubbe treated a case of breast cancer using Roentgen rays in 1896 and is credited to be the first physician to clinically utilize radiation therapy.[1] Later in 1898, Madame curie discovered radium. The first case reported to be cured by radium was that of the uterine cervix and results were published in 1915.

The teletherapy machine consisting of radioisotope became popular with the advent of cobalt-60 (Co-60) source. The first cobalt machine was installed in August 1951 in Canada.[2] Within the last 100 years both radiotherapy treatment techniques as well as the equipment for treatment delivery have improved a lot leading to better conformity and sparing of the normal tissues.

RADIOTHERAPY

There are two methods of delivering radiotherapy:
1. External beam radiotherapy
2. Brachytherapy.

External Beam Radiotherapy

When the source of radiation is placed away from the tumor and treatment is carried out, it is called external beam radiotherapy. The EBRT is delivered either by Co-60 machine or linear accelerator. Nowadays, most of the centers are using linear accelerators for treatment delivery of EBRT. The linear accelerators are versatile equipment capable to treat tumor in any part of the body with precision.

Three types of EBRT techniques are commonly used:
1. Conventional technique (2D)
2. Three dimensional conformal radiotherapy (3-DCRT)
3. Intensity-modulated radiotherapy (IMRT).

Brachytherapy

Brachytherapy is derived from the Greek word "brachy" which means short range. Brachytherapy is the term used to describe the treatment of malignant diseases by the interstitial, intracavitary and surface application of sealed radioisotopes.

Three types of brachytherapy techniques are there depending upon the dose rate:
1. Low dose rate brachytherapy dose rate (0.4–2 Gy/hr)
2. Medium dose rate brachytherapy (2–12 Gy/hr)
3. High dose rate brachytherapy (>12 Gy/hr).

In case of low dose radiotherapy (LDR), applicator is kept in place for 48–72 hours but in case of HDR the procedure is completed within minutes. Nowadays, high dose radiotherapy (HDR), is becoming very popular throughout the world as it can be done on an outpatient basis. Due to availability of remote after loading technique, here is now no radiation exposure to the doctors and other healthcare personnels and the caregivers. The source of radiation used in brachytherapy are iridium-192, cesium-137, etc.

INTRACAVITARY RADIOTHERAPY

Treatment by placing radioactive sources inside natural body cavity is called as intracavitary radiotherapy (ICRT). Though various sites have been treated with this method, gynecological malignancies are the most important application of this method. This technique offers the advantage of homogeneous dose distribution to the tumor volume and spares the normal tissues and organs in the vicinity of tumor.

Interstitial Brachytherapy

In this form of brachytherapy, radioactive sources are implanted into the tumor and surrounding tissues and allowed to remain there for a definite period (temporary implants) or indefinitely (permanent). The sources can be in the form of needles or wires. In case of carcinoma cervix, it is generally used when there is bulky parametrial disease or distorted anatomy as in these cases, ICRT fails to provide optimal dose distribution. Currently, there are two different systems of interstitial implants are used: Martinez Universal Perineal Interstitial Template (MUPIT) and the Syed-Neblett applicator system.

CHEMOTHERAPY

Chemotherapy refers to the treatment that uses cytotoxic drugs to stop the growth of cancer cells, either by killing the cells or by stopping them from dividing. Nitrogen mustard was the first chemotherapeutic agent introduced in 1941 in the cancer treatment. Modern day chemotherapy came into existence about half a century back, now >100 chemotherapy drugs are in use.

Cell Cycle

Although some chemotherapeutic agents have activity in resting cells, most chemotherapy, in general, targets dividing cells at various points within the cell cycle.
- G_o *phase*: The resting phase, the most prolonged phase of cell cycle, lasting up to months.
- G_1 *phase*: The first gap phase; the most variable phase of cell cycle; can be briefed or prolonged. The late G_1 phase is associated with an increase in deoxyribonucleic acid (DNA) replicative enzymes.
- *S phase*: The DNA synthesis phase of the cell cycle; lasts 8–30 hours.
- G_2 *phase* is gap 2 phase before mitosis.
- *M phase*: Mitosis; usually lasts 30–90 minutes.

Anticancer Agents: Classification and Mechanism of Action

- *Alkylating agents*: Impair tumor cell function by binding covalently with DNA, ribonucleic acid (RNA) or proteins. These agents exert their major effect in the G_1 phase. This class includes agents like cyclophosphamide, ifosfamide and melphalan.
- *Antimetabolites*: Structural analogs of naturally occurring metabolites that exert their cytotoxic effect by competing with or substituting for key metabolites involved in DNA or RNA synthesis. Most antimetabolites are active when tumor cells are in S-phase of the cell cycle. Methotrexate, 5-flourouracil and gemcitabine belong to this group.
- *Platinum complexes*: Compound derived from plants, fungi, etc. that have been found to have cytotoxic effect through a variety of mechanisms, e.g. cisplatin and carboplatin.
- *Antimicrotubule agents*: Plant compounds that bind microtubules and inhibit mitotic spindle formation during the M-phase of cell cycle. Examples include paclitaxel and docetaxel.
- *Antitumor antibiotics*: Compounds derived from fungus, that mediate DNA damage through various mechanisms. Examples in the group include bleomycin and doxorubicin.

PRINCIPLES OF CHEMOTHERAPY[3]

Nitrogen mustard was the first chemotherapeutic agent introduced in 1941 for cancer treatment.

The field of chemotherapy has come a long way since then and an array of agents are available these days. Chemotherapy delivered as curative approach usually consists of a combination of agents.

Following are the principles for the combination chemotherapy:
- Only those agents with proven efficacy should be used.
- Each drug should have a different mechanism of action.
- Each drug should have a different toxicity profile.
- Sometime interval should be given between therapy cycles to allow for the recovery of normal tissue.

Chemotherapy can be used in a number of ways in the treatment of cancer.

Induction (Neoadjuvant) Chemotherapy

When chemotherapy is initiated as first-line therapy prior to main modality of treatment is known as induction or neoadjuvant chemotherapy.

Adjuvant Chemotherapy

It is given when a disease is localized and has been controlled primarily by another therapeutic modality either surgery or radiotherapy.

Concomitant Chemotherapy

The rationale of this approach is utilization of direct interaction of radiotherapy and chemotherapy. The drugs used in this approach have radiation enhancing properties.

Salvage Chemotherapy

Although objective tumor regression and cure is the objective of chemotherapy, a group of patients need chemotherapy with an attempt to salvage the recurrent disease. The salvage chemotherapy is generally attempted when patients have good performance status and there is reasonable expectancy of life.

The interdigitation of modalities of radiotherapy and chemotherapy in a logical sequence leads to excellent cure rates.

Drug Resistance

Resistance to drug is a major problem in systemic chemotherapy. The drug resistance may be primary, unresponsiveness from the start or secondary, where the tumor initially responds and later becomes resistant. Drug-resistant cells may be there because of genetic instability of that particular tumor.

The other factors associated with chemotherapy resistance are:
- Multiple drug resistance (MDR) phenotype
- Decreased drug uptake
- Increased drug inactivation.

Future Directions

Apart from dose intensive regimens and associated bone marrow transplant, the targeted drug therapies to target the drug solely towards the tumor site, specific receptor targets have been identified and continuous research in this field has led to the development of the "Targeted drug Therapy". The cytogenetic study of various neoplasms and research to identify the specific oncogenes has also helped in development of new treatment strategies.

REFERENCES

1. Hodges PC. The life and times of Emile H. Grubbe. University of Chicago; 1964.
2. Johns HE, Bates IM, Watson TA. 1000 curie cobalt units for radiation therapy. The Saskatchewan Cobalt-60 unit. Br J Radiol. 1952;25:296.
3. Devita VT Jr, Schien PS. The use of drugs in combination for the treatment of patients with cancer. Rationale and Results. N Eng J Med. 1973; 288:298.

33

Chemotherapy in Gestational Trophoblastic Neoplasia

Kishore Singh, Savita Arora, Arun Kumar Rathi

Gestational trophoblastic neoplasia is an uncommon, chemosensitive malignancy, which is curable in almost all the cases. Treatment is tailored according to International Federation of Gynecology and Obstetrics (FIGO) anatomic staging and FIGO 2000 risk factors (Table 33.1) (related to chances of developing relapse).[1]

The following model is a prognostic scoring system which has been developed to determine the appropriate chemotherapy regimens that helps in optimal management by reducing the risk of developing resistance to chemotherapy. Patients with low chances of relapse (score <7) are treated with single drug only whereas high relapse risk patients (score >7) are subjected to multidrug chemotherapy.

LOW-RISK

Majority of gestational trophoblastic (GTN) patients are low-risk (95%) with score of ≤6. Mostly single drug on outpatient basis is administered in this good prognosis group. There is not much difference between different protocols, eventually all will lead to cure with preservation of fertility. Most commonly methotrexate and folinic acid (Mtx FA) combination is used as first line, results in high cure rate with least toxicity. A second course is generally not required. Actinomycin D is the other regimen used, especially in the presence of hepatic dysfunction or failure of first line methotrexate.[2]

Table 33.1 FIGO 2000 risk scoring system based on prognostic factors

Prognostic factors	Score			
	0	1	2	4
Age (Years)	<40	>39	–	–
Antecedent pregnancy	Mole	Abortion	Term	–
Interval (months)	<4	>3, <7	>6, <13	>12
Pretreatment serum hCG (mIU/mL)	<10^3	10^3 to <10^4	10^4 to <10^5	>10^5
Largest tumor, including uterine (cm)	—	3 to <5	>4	—
Site of metastases	Lung spleen,	kidney	Gastrointestinal tract	Brain, liver
Number of metastases	—	1–4	5–8	>8
Prior failed chemotherapy	—	—	Single drug	Two drugs

DURATION OF CHEMOTHERAPY AND FOLLOW-UP

Generally, a single course of chemotherapy is required in low risk category. Remission in low risk group is achieved when the hCG level becomes undetectable for 3 consecutive weeks. At this point, the patient should be followed with monthly hCG for one year. During this time the contraception is mandatory.

Chemotherapy Regimens for Low-risk Patients

Mtx
Methotrexate (Mtx) 0.5 mg/ kg IV or IM daily for 5 days
Pulse Mtx weekly 50 mg/m² IM weekly
Mtx/FA
Methotrexate (Mtx) 50 mg by IM injection repeated every 48 hours for a total of four doses
Calcium folinate (Folinic acid) 15 mg orally/IV 30 h after each injection of methotrexate
Courses repeated every 2 weeks, i.e. days 1, 15, 29, etc.
Actinomycin D
1.25 mg/m² IV every 2 weeks

HIGH RISK GESTATIONAL TROPHOBLASTIC NEOPLASIA

These have score of ≥7, indicating high risk of developing drug resistance. Therefore such cases are treated with EMA/CO from the beginning. This is the preferred first line regimen, which results in 80–90% response rate. Treatment is generally well tolerated, in the event of neutropenia; G-CSF (Granulocyte colony stimulating factor) can be given.[3]

DURATION OF CHEMOTHERAPY AND FOLLOW-UP

Treatment is continued until hCG level becomes undetectable and remains undetectable for 3 consecutive weeks. Generally additional 3 cycles of chemotherapy is required after normalization of hCG, to ameliorate higher risk of relapse. After completion of chemotherapy patients with high risk disease should be followed for 24 months. Contraception is mandatory during this period. Those who conceive after this period, ultrasound is done at week 10 of gestation to confirm normal pregnancy. Six weeks after delivery, hCG is repeated again to rule out GTN.

Chemotherapy Regimens for High-risk Patients

EMA/CO
EMA
Day 1
Etoposide 100 mg/m² by IV infusion over 30 min
Folinic acid rescue (starting 24 hours after commencing the methotrexate infusion) 15 mg IV or orally every 12 h for four doses
Actinomycin D 0.5 mg IV bolus
Methotrexate 300 mg/m² by IV infusion over 12 h
Day 2
Etoposide 100 mg/m² by IV infusion over 30 min
Actinomycin D 0.5 mg IV bolus
Omit day 2 etoposide and actinomycin D in the event of myelosuppression
CO
Day 8
Vincristine 1 mg/m² IV bolus (maximum 2 mg)
Cyclophosphamide 600 mg/m² IV infusion over 30 min

ROLE OF SURGERY/RADIOTHERAPY

The use of radiation therapy in patients with GTN is limited to the treatment of brain metastasis. Solitary superficial cerebral lesion can be treated with surgery. Hysterectomy is considered in patients large, bulky intrauterine disease unresponsive to chemotherapy regardless of patient's parity.

RECURRENT/RESIDUAL LESION

There is a real possibility of this event in high risk lesions (stage IV/III). Three drug regimen consisting of paclitaxel, etoposide and cisplatin (TE/TP) achieved good response rate. actinomycin D and 5-fluorouracil combination has also shown effectiveness in this setting. Good cure rate of 80–90% is possible with modern combination chemotherapy in this condition, which otherwise carries poor prognosis (Table 33.2).

Placental Site Trophoblastic Tumors

They are managed similarly with surgery as first line choice in compared to chemotherapy. This is associated with survival of almost 100%.

CONCLUSION

Chemotherapy is highly effective in most patients with GTN. Despite the success of chemotherapy, the other modalities such as surgery and radiotherapy should be judiciously included when indicated. The best results are achieved when the patients are treated under the auspices of multidisciplinary team.

REFERENCES

1. FIGO Oncology Committee, FIGO staging for gestational trophoblastic neoplasia. International Journal of Gynecology & Obstetrics. 2000;77:285-7.
2. Seckl MJ, Sebire NJ, Berkowitz RS. Gestational trophoblastic disease. Lancet. 2010;376:717-29.
3. Seckl MJ, Sebire NJ, Fisher RA, et al. Gestational trophoblastic disease: ESMO Clinical Practice Guidelines for diagnosis, treatment and follow-up. ESMO Guidelines Working Group. Annals of Oncology. 2013;24(Suppl 6):vi39–vi50.

Table 33.2 Chemotherapy in relapsed GTN

Regimen	Schedule
Day 1	
Dexamethasone	20 mg oral (12 h pre-paclitaxel)
Dexamethasone	20 mg oral (6 h pre-paclitaxel)
Ranitidine	50 mg IV
Pheniramine	25 mg bolus IV
Paclitaxel	135 mg/m² in 250 mL NS (Glass bottle, infusion by codan set) over 3 h IV
Mannitol	10% in 500 mL over 1 h IV
Cisplatin	60 mg/m² in 1 L NS over 2 h IV
Post-hydration 1 L NS + KCl 20 mmol + 1 g MgSO$_4$ over 2 h IV	
Day 15	
Dexamethasone	20 mg oral (12 h pre-paclitaxel)
Dexamethasone	20 mg oral (6 h pre-paclitaxel)
Ranitidine	50 mg IV
Pheniramine	25 mg bolus IV
Paclitaxel	135 mg/m² in 250 mL NS (Glass bottle, infusion by codon set) over 3 h IV
Etoposide	150 mg/m² in 1 L NS over 1 h IV

34
Chemoradiotherapy in Carcinoma Vulva

Kishore Singh, Savita Arora, Arun Kumar Rathi

Vulvar cancer most commonly arises from the labia majora and labia minora. It shows lymphatic spread to the ipsilateral superficial inguinofemoral lymph nodes, followed by the deep inguinofemoral lymph nodes and then into the pelvis. Contralateral nodes or pelvic lymph nodes are usually uninvolved in the absence of ipsilateral nodes except in case of lesions approaching midline. Direct involvement of midline structures like urethra and vagina may have direct spread to the pelvic nodes.

Approximately, 30–40% of patients with clinically negative lymph nodes can have positive lymph nodes. Pathologic staging of the lymph nodes at risk is crucial, considering 30–40% chances of harboring microscopic metastases in clinically negative nodes. Therefore, ipsilateral nodes are assessed in all the patients. However, contralateral LN assessment is warranted in cases when tumor approaches midline; clinically enlarged nodes or metastases in ipsilateral lymph nodes.

Tumor thickness, lymphovascular invasion (LVI), age above 55 years, and poor differentiation are risk factors for nodal involvement.[1] The risk of contralateral nodal involvement increases with each additional risk factor.

ROLE OF SURGERY

Previously en bloc radical vulvectomy with bilateral (B/L) groin dissection with or without bilateral pelvic node dissection was the treatment of choice. However, it was associated with substantial acute and chronic postoperative morbidity like lower limb edema following radical lymphadenectomy, pelvic relaxation, organ prolapse, urinary incontinence, shortening of vaginal depth and associated psychological sequelae.[2-5]

Presently the focus of vulvar cancer management has moved towards decreasing the morbidity and mortality of extensive surgery, specifically in early stage and prognostically favorable tumors and improving results by integrated multimodality treatment including conservative surgery, radiotherapy and chemotherapy.[6]

For tumors with less than 2 cm diameter and 1 mm depth (Stage IA), lymphadenectomy may be omitted because the incidence of lymph node metastases in this subset of patients is almost zero.[7,8] Dissection of the groin nodes (unilateral or bilateral) should be performed when the depth of invasion is greater than 1 mm (FIGO stage Ib or worse) or the maximum diameter of the tumor is greater than 2 cm.[9] This surgery can often be undertaken through separate groin and vulval incisions (triple incision technique) to reduce morbidity. The incidence of skin bridge recurrence in early-stage disease is very low.[10]

Risk of local recurrence is inversely related to the width of tumor free resection margin. Multiple studies have shown substantial decrease in local recurrence in resection with tumor free margin of ≥8 mm.[11,12] Hence, in nonfixed state, tumor free margin of atleast 1–1.5 cm is desirable to achieve good local control. However, some clinicians endorse margins of 1.5–2 cm.

Published evidence suggests that macroscopic unifocal primary squamous vulval cancers measuring <4 cm in maximum dimension with no clinical or radiological evidence to suspect lymph node metastasis and no known safety issues for the use of Patent Blue dye and/or technetium-99, might safely be managed by excision of the sentinel lymph nodes identified in either groin.[13] Full-therapeutic groin dissection may be omitted in patients with discrete, unifocal vulvar tumors <4 cm in diameter because subsequent groin relapse in these patients will be as low as 2.3%, as shown in GROINSS-V study. If one or more sentinel nodes harbor tumor cells, surgery should generally be proceeded to complete therapeutic superficial and deep groin lymph nodes dissection.[14] GROINSS-V II study has shown that in unifocal squamous cell carcinoma of vulva that is <4 cm in diameter and less than 2 mm of sentinel lymph node metastases, further lymphadenectomy may be substituted by groin irradiation to 50 Gy of external beam radiotherapy (EBRT). Sentinel lymph node metastases more than 2 mm resulted in substantial in-field recurrence, if treated with groin irradiation alone.[15]

Extensive cross-over of lymphatic channels of the vulva may result in nodal involvement of the contralateral groins in addition to the ipsilateral groin nodes. Therefore, bilateral groin node dissection is usually required. A lateralized lesion is defined as one in which wide excision, at least 1 cm beyond the visible tumor edge, would not impinge upon a midline structure (clitoris, urethra, vagina, perineal body, anus). Lymphatic cross-over is less likely in lateral tumors; therefore, only an ipsilateral groin node dissection need initially be performed.[16] Contralateral lymph node assessment and dissection may be omitted in well-lateralized tumors, i.e. one which are ≥1.5 cm away from midline structures because of very less incidence of contralateral lymph node recurrence has been seen in these cases.

Radical vulvectomy is generally treatment of choice in multifocal invasive disease, invasive disease with extensive vulvar intraepithelial neoplasia and in patients with symptomatic vulvar dystrophy unresponsive to topical therapies.

ROLE OF RADIATION THERAPY

Adjuvant Postoperative Radiotherapy

Absolute indications for postoperative radiotherapy (RT) include (1) gross node metastases; (2) extracapsular extension; (3) microscopic metastases to two or more lymph nodes; and (4) close or positive margins. Depth of invasion more than 5 mm and presence of lymphovascular invasion are relative indications for adjuvant RT.

Gynecologic oncology group (GOG) conducted a randomized trial (GOG 37) to determine if pelvic RT improves survival over standard pelvic lymph node dissection. 114 patients of invasive squamous cell vulvar carcinoma and positive groin nodes after radical vulvectomy and bilateral groin lymphadenectomy were randomized to receive either RT or pelvic node resection. Fifty-three of the 59 patients were randomized to 45–50 Gy of external beam RT to bilateral groins and midplane of the pelvis, even if only unilateral positive groin nodes had been detected. However, no radiation was given to the central vulvar area. Fifty-three of the 55 patients were randomized to further pelvic node resection performed on the side containing positive groin nodes either unilaterally or bilaterally. Acute and chronic morbidity was similar for both regimens. The difference in survival for the 114 evaluable patients was significant, favoring the adjunctive RT group ($p = 0.03$). The estimated two-year survival rates were 68% for the RT group and 54% for pelvic node resection group. The most dramatic survival advantage for RT was in patients who had either gross node metastases, extracapsular extension or metastases to two or more lymph nodes. The major effect of RT was a reduction in groin failure from 24% (surgery only group) to 5% in irradiated group of patients. In this randomized prospective study, the addition of adjunctive groin and pelvic RT after radical vulvectomy and inguinal lymphadenectomy proved superior to pelvic node resection.[17] Observational study by Faul et al. showed that patients with <8 mm of surgical resection margin were benefited by addition of postoperative vulvar RT. Local recurrence occurred in 58% of observed patients and 16% or patients treated with adjuvant RT.[18] Role of adjuvant local RT to overcome the negative prognostic impact of depth of invasion and LVI is still to be explored.

LOCALLY ADVANCED VULVAR CANCER

Locally advanced vulvar cancer may be defined as nonmetastatic vulvar disease that is either beyond curative surgical resection or definitive curative surgery would be associated with considerable morbidity. Curative surgical treatment options usually involve pelvic exenteration in these patients, to obtain adequate surgical margins. The surgery is often followed by adjuvant radiotherapy (RT) or chemoradiotherapy depending on risk of disease recurrence. Such procedures are usually undesirable or inappropriate in view of high surgical mortality, complication rates, physical and psychological morbidity with permanent colostomy and/or urinary diversion. Presently there is no noninvasive imaging technique that can exclude the presence of lymph node metastasis with a sufficiently high negative predictive value.[19,20]

These patients are generally candidates for neoadjuvant therapies for down-staging of initial disease bulk to limit the morbidity associated with extensive surgery. However, subset of these patients may be considered for definitive chemoradiotherapy. Role of neoadjuvant therapies has been describing under various subheadings.

Neoadjuvant Radiotherapy Alone

The apparent advantages of this combined therapeutic approach over exenterative surgery include high probability of bladder and/or rectal preservation, low primary mortality, low treatment morbidity, and very good results in cancer control.

Boronow et al.[21] studied the role of neoadjuvant RT as a therapeutic alternative to exenteration for locally advanced vulvovaginal cancer. The purpose of the study was to alleviate the need of exenterative surgery. Authors reported 48 treated cases of vulvar carcinoma (37 primary cases and 11 cases of recurrent disease). With 48 patients treated, 48 bladders and 48 rectums were at risk for surgical removal had exenteration been employed. One patient had a total pelvic exenteration for local failure, and one had a posterior exenteration for local failure. One bladder and one rectum were lost to permanent diversion because of radiation injury. Thus, 5 of these major viscera were lost of the 96 total, and 91 (94.8%) were retained. No residual disease was identified in 42.5% of surgical specimens. The 5-year survival rates were 75.6% for the primary cases, 62.6% for the recurrent cases and an overall 72% for all 48 cases treated. Published FIGO survival for stage III is 32% and for stage IV is 10.5%.

Neoadjuvant Chemoradiotherapy

Studies have shown promising results with the use of neoadjuvant chemoradiation in patients of locally advanced vulvar carcinoma.

GOG 101[22] conducted a phase II study to determine the feasibility of using preoperative chemoradiotherapy to avert the need for more radical surgery for patients with T3 primary tumors, or the need for pelvic exenteration for patients with T4 primary tumors, not amenable to resection by standard radical vulvectomy. Seventy-three evaluable patients with clinical stage III–IV squamous cell vulvar carcinoma were enrolled in this prospective, multi-institutional trial. Treatment consisted of a planned split course of concurrent cisplatin/5-fluorouracil and radiation therapy followed by surgical excision of the residual primary tumor plus bilateral inguinal-femoral lymph node dissection. Radiation therapy was delivered to the primary tumor volume only, if the nodes were clinically negative. Patients with inoperable groin nodes received chemoradiation to the primary vulvar tumor, inguinal-femoral and lower pelvic lymph nodes. RT was given in a split-course, twice-daily regimen in 1.7 Gy fractions to a dose of 47.6 Gy, combined with cisplatin plus 5-fluorouracil chemotherapy. Following chemoradiotherapy, 33/71 (46.5%) patients had no visible vulvar cancer at the time of planned surgery and 38/71 (53.5%) had gross residual cancer at the time of operation. Using this strategy of preoperative, split-course, twice-daily radiation combined with cisplatin plus 5-fluorouracil chemotherapy, only 2/71 (2.8%) had residual unresectable disease. In only three patients it was not possible to preserve urinary and/or gastrointestinal continence. Toxicity was acceptable, with acute cutaneous reactions to chemoradiotherapy and surgical wound complications being the most common adverse effects. Study group concluded that preoperative chemoradiotherapy in advanced squamous cell carcinoma of the vulva is feasible, and may reduce the need for more radical surgery including primary pelvic exenteration.

The GOG 205[23] conducted a study to determine the efficacy and toxicity of radiation therapy and concurrent weekly cisplatin chemotherapy in achieving a complete clinical and pathologic response when used for the primary treatment of locally-advanced vulvar carcinoma. Patients with locally-advanced (T3 or T4 tumors not amenable to surgical resection via radical vulvectomy), previously untreated squamous cell carcinoma of the vulva were treated with radiation (1.8 Gy daily fraction to a total of 57.6 Gy) plus weekly cisplatin (40 mg/m²) followed by surgical resection of residual tumor (or biopsy to confirm complete clinical response). Among 58 evaluable patients, there were 40 (69%) who completed study treatment. 64% (37/58) patients had complete clinical response. Among these women 78% had complete pathological response as well. Common adverse effects included leukopenia, pain, radiation dermatitis, pain, or metabolic changes. Authors of this study concluded that the combination of radiation therapy plus weekly cisplatin successfully yielded high complete clinical and pathologic response rates with acceptable toxicity.

Neoadjuvant Chemotherapy

Preoperative neoadjuvant chemotherapy has been used in the treatment of locally advanced vulvar cancer.[24-27] Response rates have been quite variable and although complete clinical and pathologic response have been recorded, these are rare. This approach has not gained broad acceptance, presumably because response to combined chemoradiotherapy is predictable.

DEFINITIVE CHEMORADIOTHERAPY

High dose radiotherapy with or without concurrent chemoradiotherapy should or can replace radical surgery for vulvar cancer is still unclear and investigational. However, there is a trend to employ concurrent chemoradiotherapy for unresectable disease that is considered to extensive for conservatively functional surgery.[28-31]

Unfortunately, due to highly variable selection criteria, radiotherapy dose regimen, chemotherapeutic agent and small number of patients, optimal regimen has not been framed till present times. However, it seems that definitive chemoradiotherapy can emerge as a viable treatment option for medically inoperable and tumors that need extensive exenterative surgeries. The currently active GOG 279 protocol is studying the role of radiotherapy dose escalation to 64 Gy with addition of concurrent dual chemosensitizing agents, i.e. cisplatin and gemcitabine. Unlike former studies this study is employing intensity modulated radiotherapy, a technique of conformal radiation dose delivery system with expected minimal radiation toxicity.

Randomized trials may be difficult to perform because of the small number of patients with locally advanced vulvar cancer. However, results of trials in other types of cancer are encouraging: trials that demonstrated improved local control and survival when concurrent cisplatin-containing chemotherapy was added to radiation treatment of cervical cancers[32,33] and improved colostomy-free survival when mitomycin-C and 5-FU were added to radiation treatment of anal cancer.[34]

REFERENCES

1. Homesley HD, Bundy BN, Sedlis A, et al. Prognostic factors for groin node metastasis in squamous cell carcinoma of the vulva (a Gynecologic Oncology Group study). Gynecol Oncol. 1993;49(3): 279-83.
2. McKelvey JL, Adcock LL. Cancer of the vulva. Obstet Gynecol. 1965;26(4):455-66.
3. Andersen BL, Hacker NF. Psychosexual adjustment after vulvar surgery. Obstet Gynecol. 1983;62(4):457-62.
4. Green MS, et al. Sexual dysfunction following vulvectomy. Gynecol Oncol. 2000;77(1):73-7.
5. Stellman RE, et al. Psychological effects of vulvectomy. Psychosomatics. 1984;25(10):779-83.
6. Thomas GM, et al. Changing concepts in the management of vulvar cancer. Gynecol Oncol. 1991;42(1):9-21.
7. Magrina JF, et al. Stage I squamous cell cancer of the vulva. Am J Obstet Gynecol. 1979;134(4):453-9.
8. Kneale BLG, Elliott PM, McDonald IA. Microinvasive carcinoma of the vulva. Clinical features and management. In: Coppleson M (Ed) Gynecologic Oncology, Edinburgh, UK, Churchill Livingstone; 1981. p. 320.
9. Sedlis A, Homesley H, Bundy BN, Marshall R, Yordan E, Hacker N, et al. Positive groin lymph nodes in superficial squamous cell vulvar cancer. A Gynecologic Oncology Group Study. Am J Obstet Gynecol. 1987;156:1159-64.
10. Hacker NF, Leuchter RS, Berek JS, et al. Radical vulvectomy and bilateral inguinal lymphadenectomy through separate groin incisions. Obstet Gynecol. 1981;58:574-9.
11. De Hullu JA, et al. Vulvar carcinoma. The price of less radical surgery. Cancer. 2002;95(11):2331-8.
12. Chan JK, et al. Margin distance and other clinico-pathologic prognostic factors in vulvar carcinoma: A multivariate analysis. Gynecol Oncol. 2007;104(3):636-41.
13. Levenback CF, van der Zee AG, Rob L, Plante M, Covens A, Schneider A, et al. Sentinel lymph node biopsy in patients with gynecologic cancers: Expert panel statement from the International Sentinel Node Society Meeting, February 21, 2008. Gynecol Oncol. 2009;114:151-6.
14. Van der Zee AG, et al. Sentinel node dissection is safe in the treatment of early-stage vulvar cancer. J Clin Oncol. 2008;26(6):884-9.
15. Peters WA, 3rd, et al. Concurrent chemotherapy and pelvic radiation therapy compared with pelvic radiation therapy alone as adjuvant therapy after radical surgery in high-risk early-stage cancer of the cervix. J Clin Oncol. 2000;18(8): 1606-13.
16. Stehman FB, Bundy BN, Dvoretsky PM, et al. Early stage I carcinoma of the vulva treated with ipsilateral superficial inguinal lymphadenectomy and modified radical hemivulvectomy: a prospective study of the Gynecologic Oncology Group. Obstet Gynecol. 1992;79:490-7.
17. Homesley HD, Bundy BN, Sedlis A, et al. Radiation therapy versus pelvic node resection for carcinoma of the vulva with positive groin nodes. Obstet Gynecol. 1986;68(6):733-40.
18. Faul CM, et al. Adjuvant radiation for vulvar carcinoma: Improved local control. Int J Radiat Oncol Biol Phys. 1997;38(2):381-9.
19. Bipat S, Fransen GA, Spijkerboer AM, et al. Is there a role for magnetic resonance imaging in the evaluation of inguinal lymph node metastases in patients with vulva carcinoma? Gynecol Oncol. 2006;103(3):1001-6.
20. Oonk MH, Hollema H, de Hullu JA, et al. Prediction of lymph node metastases in vulvar cancer: a review. Int J Gynecol Cancer. 2006;16(3):963-71.
21. Boronow RC, Hickman BT, Reagan MT, et al. Combined therapy as an alternative to exenteration for locally advanced vulvovaginal cancer. II. Results, complications, and dosimetric and surgical considerations. Am J Clin Oncol. 1987;10(2): 171-81.
22. Moore DH, Thomas GM, Montana GS, Saxer A, Gallup DG, Olt G. Preoperative chemoradiation for advanced vulvar cancer: a phase II study of the Gynecologic Oncology Group. Int J Radiat Oncol Biol Phys. 1998;42(1):79-85.
23. Moore DH, Ali S, Koh WJ, Michael H, Barnes MN, McCourt CK, et al. A phase II trial of radiation therapy and weekly cisplatin chemotherapy for

the treatment of locally-advanced squamous cell carcinoma of the vulva: a gynecologic oncology group study. Gynecol Oncol. 2012;124(3): 529-33.
24. Benedetti-Panici PL, et al. The role of neoadjuvant chemotherapy followed by radical surgery in the treatment of locally advanced cervical cancer. Eur Gynaecol Oncol. 2003;24(6):467-70.
25. Geisler JP, Manahan KJ, Buller RE. Neoadjuvant chemotherapy in vulvar cancer: Avoiding primary exenteration. Gynecol Oncol. 2006;100(1):53-7.
26. Domingues AP, et al. Neoadjuvant chemotherapy in advanced vulvar cancer. Int J Gynecol Cancer. 2010;20(2):294-8.
27. Aragona AM, et al. Tailoring the treatment of locally advanced squamous cell carcinoma of the vulva: Neoadjuvant chemotherapy followed by radical surgery: Results from a multicenter study. Int J Gynecol Cancer. 2012;22(7):1258-63.
28. Iversen T. Irradiation and bleomycin in the treatment of inoperable vulval carcinoma. Acta Obstet Gynecol Scand. 1982;61(3):195-7.
29. Evans LS, et al. Concomitant 5-fluorouracil, mitomycin-C, and radiotherapy for advanced gynecologic malignancies. Int J Radiat Oncol Biol Phys. 1988;15(4):901-6.
30. Whitaker SJ, et al. A pilot study of chemo-radiotherapy in advanced carcinoma of the vulva. Br J Obstet Gynaecol. 1990;97(5):436-42.
31. Thomas G, et al. Concurrent radiation and chemotherapy in vulvar carcinoma. Gynecol Oncol. 1989;34(3):263-7.
32. Eifel PJ, Winter K, Morris M, et al. Pelvic irradiation with concurrent chemotherapy versus pelvic and para-aortic irradiation for high-risk cervical cancer: an update of Radiation Therapy Oncology Group trial (RTOG) 90-01. J Clin Oncol. 2004;22: 872-80.
33. Rose PG, Bundy BN, Watkins J, et al. Concurrent cisplatin-based chemotherapy and radiotherapy for locally advanced cervical cancer. N Engl J Med. 1999;340:1144-53.
34. Cummings B. Anal canal carcinomas. In: Meyer JL, Vaeth JM, (Eds). Frontiers in Radiation Oncology. Vol 26. Basel, Switzerland: Karger; 1992:131.

35
Chemoradiotherapy in Carcinoma Vagina

Kishore Singh, Savita Arora, Arun Kumar Rathi

According to International Federation of Gynecology and Obstetrics (FIGO) system, tumors that involve the cervix or vulva are not considered vaginal cancers and are classified as cervical or vulvar primaries.[1] Therefore, primary carcinoma of the vagina is a rare entity accounting for only 3% of all gynecologic cancers.

TREATMENT OPTIONS OVERVIEW

Roles of Radiation, Surgery and Chemotherapy

Due to rarity of primary vaginal cancer, treatment recommendations are usually based on retrospective, single institutional case series that may span a number of years. Further these recommendations are complicated by non-uniform staging approach, treatment modalities and radiotherapy techniques including the shift to high-energy accelerators and conformal- and intensity-modulated radiation.

Factors that are considered while treatment planning of patient with vaginal cancer includes stage and size of the lesion, proximity to radiosensitive organs or organs that preclude radical resection without unacceptable functional deficits (e.g. bladder, rectum, urethra), ability to retain a functional vagina, presence or absence of the uterus and whether there has been prior pelvic radiation therapy.

Early-stage vaginal cancer is defined as an invasive disease confined to the vaginal mucosa and/or paravaginal tissues (FIGO stages I–II). The treatment options include surgical resection or definitive radiotherapy. The advantages of surgery are the preservation of ovarian and sexual function and elimination of the risk of radiation-associated malignancy.[2] However, proximity of the vagina to the bladder and rectum limits surgical treatment options and increases short- and long-term surgical complications including functional deficits of these organs. For patients with stages III and IVA disease, radiation therapy is standard of care. The lymphatics may drain to pelvic or inguinal nodes or both, depending on tumor location, and consideration should be given to these areas in treatment planning. Radiation-induced toxicity using conventional techniques may include rectovaginal fistulas, vesicovaginal fistulas, rectal or vaginal strictures, cystitis, proctitis, premature menopause from ovarian damage, soft tissue or bone necrosis.

In an attempt to improve local control, concurrent chemoradiotherapy with 5-fluorouracil or cisplatin and radiation are sometimes advocated, again based solely on extrapolation from cervical cancer management strategies.[3-5] However, experience is limited to small case series and the incremental impact on survival and local control is not well-defined.

For patients with stage IVB or recurrent disease that cannot be managed with local treatments, current therapy recommendations are inadequate. Palliative chemotherapy is currently employed to these patients.

Management of the extremely rare vaginal clear cell carcinoma is generally similar to the management of squamous cell carcinoma, though techniques that preserve vaginal and ovarian function are recommended in treatment planning, given the young average age at diagnosis.[6]

STAGEWISE TREATMENT APPROACH

Vaginal Intraepithelial Neoplasia Including Squamous Cell Carcinoma In Situ

Vaginal intraepithelial neoplasia (VAIN) has been observed to be associated with human papillomavirus (HPV) infection; therefore, it seems to share similar etiology as cervical intraepithelial neoplasia (CIN).[7] It is further classified as VAIN 1, 2, and 3, denoting involvement of the upper one-third, two-thirds, and more than two-third of the epithelial thickness, respectively.

Women with VAIN 1 can usually be observed carefully without ablative or surgical treatment, since the lesions often regress spontaneously. The intermediate grade, VAIN 2, is variously managed by careful observation or initial treatment. VAIN 3 lesions are also denoted as carcinoma *in situ* (CIS). It is often multifocal and commonly occurs at the vaginal vault. VAIN 3 are felt to be at substantial risk of progression to invasive cancer and are treated immediately. The selection of treatment depends on patient factors, anatomic location, evidence of multifocality, and local expertise. Lesions with hyperkeratosis respond better to excision or laser vaporization than to fluorouracil. Standard treatment options include:

- *Laser therapy:*[8] The lesions should first be sampled adequately to rule out invasive components that could be missed with this treatment approach.
- Wide local excision with or without skin grafting.[9]
- Partial or total vaginectomy, with skin grafting for multifocal or extensive disease.[10]
- Intravaginal chemotherapy with 5% fluorouracil cream. This option may be useful in the setting of multifocal lesions.[11]
- Intracavitary radiation therapy.[12,13] This treatment is primarily used in the setting of multifocal or recurrent disease, or when the risk of surgery is high. The entire vaginal mucosa is usually treated.[14]
- Imiquimod cream 5%, an immune stimulant used to treat genital warts, is an additional topical therapy that has a reported complete clinical response rate of 50–86% in small case series of patients with multifocal high-grade HPV associated VAIN 2 and 3.[15] However, it is investigational, and it may have only short-lived efficacy.[16]

Stage I, II Vaginal Cancer

Standard treatment options include radiotherapy or surgery. Surgery[17] includes wide local excision or total vaginectomy with vaginal reconstruction, especially in lesions of the upper vagina. Bilateral pelvic lymph node dissection is usually required, given the extensive lymphatic network of the vagina and the risk of occult nodal spread. Surgical series have reported rates of pathologic nodal involvement that range from 6% to 14% for stage I disease and from 26% to 32% for stage II disease.[18,19] For distal vaginal lesions, the surgical approach involves total vaginectomy, or vulvovaginectomy, and inguinofemoral lymph node dissection. In cases with close or positive surgical margins, adjuvant radiation therapy is often added.[20] In cases with close or positive surgical margins, adjuvant radiation therapy is often given.[21] Combined local therapy may be used in selected cases which may include wide local excision, lymph node sampling, and interstitial therapy.[22]

These tumors may be amenable to intracavitary brachytherapy alone,[23] and/or external-beam radiation therapy (EBRT) to a total dose of at least 75 Gy to the primary tumor.[24,25] Pelvic failure rates following brachytherapy alone range from 14% to 33%.[26] In stage II (both squamous or adeno-histology), most centers prefer combination of brachytherapy and external-beam radiation therapy (EBRT) to deliver a combined dose of 70 Gy to 80 Gy to the primary tumor volume.[27,28] For lesions of the lower third of the vagina, elective radiation therapy of 45–50 Gy is given to the pelvic and/or inguinal lymph nodes.

Five-years survival rate is 90% for women with stage I disease treated with surgery alone, compared with 63% who receives definitive radiotherapy.[29] Survival outcomes for stage II disease shows nonstatistical difference with surgery and radiotherapy. However, patients with stage II disease are more likely to require total vaginectomy or an exenterative procedure to obtain negative surgical margins. Neoadjuvant chemotherapy (cisplatin and paclitaxel) has also been used as a downstaging method prior to radical surgery.[30]

Stage III and IVA Vaginal Cancer

Surgery is rarely employed in this setting. Standard treatment include external beam radiotherapy (EBRT) alone, or in combination with interstitial/intracavitary brachytherapy for a total tumor dose of 75–80 Gy and dose of up to 55–60 Gy to the lateral pelvic wall. Survival rates range from 23% to 59% for stage III disease and from 0% to 25% for stage IV disease. Corresponding pelvic control rates are 62–71% and 12–30%, respectively.

Use of neoadjuvant chemotherapy prior to radical surgery has been studied in randomized trials of patients with locally advanced cervical cancer, and no detectable survival advantage was found. Case reports and small series of neoadjuvant chemotherapy for locally advanced vaginal cancer have been published, although experience is limited and most patients relapsed and died.[31] Up front exenteration may also be considered for patients with resectable advanced-stage disease, an approach that may provide palliation in the setting of rectovaginal or vesicovaginal fistula in otherwise localized disease.

Stage IVB Vaginal Cancer

Current therapy is of unclear benefit for patients with stage IVB disease. No established anticancer drugs has proven clinical benefit, although patients are often treated with regimens used to treat cervical cancer. Radiation may be used for palliation of symptoms.

RECURRENT VAGINAL CANCER

Recurrence carries a grave prognosis. In a large series, only five of fifty patients with recurrence were salvaged by surgery or radiation therapy. All five of these salvaged patients originally presented with stage I or II disease and had tumor recurrence in the central pelvis. Most recurrences occur in the first 2 years after treatment. In centrally recurrent vaginal cancers, some patients may be candidates for pelvic exenteration or radiation therapy.

Follow-up

The standard follow-up for vaginal cancer involves a clinical examination every 3 months for 2 years, less frequent intervals thereafter. Based on the practice for locally advanced cervical cancer, consideration of post-treatment PET/CT surveillance is reasonable for patients with initial bulky disease.

REFERENCES

1. Edge SB, Byrd DR, Compton CC, et al. Vagina. AJCC Cancer Staging Manual, 7th edn. New York, NY: Springer; 2010.pp.387-9.
2. Cutillo G, Cignini P, Pizzi G, et al. Conservative treatment of reproductive and sexual function in young woman with squamous carcinoma of the vagina. Gynecol Oncol. 2006;103(1):234-7.
3. Grigsby PW. Vaginal cancer. Curr Treat Options Oncol. 2002;3(2):125-30.
4. Dalrymple JL, Russell AH, Lee SW, et al. Chemoradiation for primary invasive squamous carcinoma of the vagina. Int J Gynecol Cancer. 2004;14(1):110-7.

5. Samant R, Lau B, E C, et al. Primary vaginal cancer treated with concurrent chemoradiation using Cis-platinum. Int J Radiat Oncol Biol Phys. 2007;69(3):746-50.
6. Senekjian EK, Frey KW, Anderson D, et al. Local therapy in stage I clear cell adenocarcinoma of the vagina. Cancer. 1987;60(6):1319-24.
7. Smith JS, Backes DM, Hoots BE, et al. Human papillomavirus type-distribution in vulvar and vaginal cancers and their associated precursors. Obstet Gynecol. 2009;113(4):917-24.
8. Krebs HB. Treatment of vaginal intraepithelial neoplasia with laser and topical 5-fluorouracil. Obstet Gynecol. 1989;73(4):657-60.
9. Cheng D, Ng TY, Ngan HY, et al. Wide local excision (WLE) for vaginal intraepithelial neoplasia (VAIN). Acta Obstet Gynecol Scand. 1999;78(7):648-52.
10. Indermaur MD, Martino MA, Fiorica JV, et al. Upper vaginectomy for the treatment of vaginal intraepithelial neoplasia. Am J Obstet Gynecol. 2005;193:577-80.
11. Stefanon B, Pallucca A, Merola M, et al. Treatment with 5-fluorouracil of 35 patients with clinical or subclinical HPV infection of the vagina. Eur J Gynaecol Oncol. 1996;17(6):534.
12. Chyle V, Zagars GK, Wheeler JA, et al. Definitive radiotherapy for carcinoma of the vagina: outcome and prognostic factors. Int J Radiat Oncol Biol Phys. 1996;35(5):891-905.
13. Graham K, Wright K, Cadwallader B, et al. 20-year retrospective review of medium dose rate intracavitary brachytherapy in VAIN 3. Gynecol Oncol. 2007;106(1):105-11.
14. Perez CA, Garipagaoglu M. Vagina. In: Perez CA, Brady LW, (Eds): Principles and Practice of Radiation Oncology, 3rd edn. Philadelphia, PA: Lippincott-Raven Publishers. 1998.pp.1891-914.
15. Iavazzo C, Pitsouni E, Athanasiou S, et al. Imiquimod for treatment of vulvar and vaginal intraepithelial neoplasia. Int J Gynaecol Obstet. 2008;101(1):3-10.
16. Haidopoulos D, Diakomanolis E, Rodolakis A, et al. Can local application of imiquimod cream be an alternative mode of therapy for patients with high-grade intraepithelial lesions of the vagina? Int J Gynecol Cancer. 2005;15(5):898-902.
17. Tjalma WA, Monaghan JM, de Barros Lopes A, et al. The role of surgery in invasive squamous carcinoma of the vagina. Gynecol Oncol. 2001;81(3):360-5.
18. Al-Kurdi M, Monaghan JM. Thirty-two years experience in management of primary tumours of the vagina. Br J Obstet Gynaecol. 1981;88(11):1145-50.
19. Davis KP, Stanhope CR, Garton GR, Atkinson EJ, O'Brien PC. Invasive vaginal carcinoma: analysis of early- stage disease. Gynecol Oncol. 1991;42(2):131-6.
20. Stock RG, Chen AS, Seski J. A 30-year experience in the management of primary carcinoma of the vagina: analysis of prognostic factors and treatment modalities. Gynecol Oncol. 1995;56(1):45-52.
21. Rubin SC, Young J, Mikuta JJ. Squamous carcinoma of the vagina: treatment, complications, and long-term follow-up. Gynecol Oncol. 1985;20(3):346-53.
22. Senekjian EK, Frey KW, Anderson D, et al. Local therapy in stage I clear cell adenocarcinoma of the vagina. Cancer. 1987;60(6):1319-24.
23. Perez CA, Camel HM, Galakatos AE, et al. Definitive irradiation in carcinoma of the vagina: long-term evaluation of results. Int J Radiat Oncol Biol Phys. 1988;15(6):1283-90.
24. Frank SJ, Jhingran A, Levenback C, et al. Definitive radiation therapy for squamous cell carcinoma of the vagina. Int J Radiat Oncol Biol Phys. 2005;62(1):138-47.
25. Andersen ES. Primary carcinoma of the vagina: a study of 29 cases. Gynecol Oncol. 1989;33(3):317-20.
26. Perez CA, Grigsby PW, Garipagaoglu M, Mutch DG, Lockett MA. Factors affecting long-term outcome of irradiation in carcinoma of the vagina. Int J Radiat Oncol Biol Phys. 1999;44(1):37-45.
27. Tran PT, Su Z, Lee P, et al. Prognostic factors for outcomes and complications for primary squamous cell carcinoma of the vagina treated with radiation. Gynecol Oncol. 2007;105(3):641-9.
28. Lian J, Dundas G, Carlone M, et al. Twenty-year review of radiotherapy for vaginal cancer: an institutional experience. Gynecol Oncol. 2008;111(2):298-306.
29. Shah CA, Goff BA, Lowe K, Peters WA, 3rd, Li CI. Factors affecting risk of mortality in women with vaginal cancer. Obstet Gynecol. 2009;113(5):1038-45.
30. Benedetti Panici P, Bellati F, Plotti F, et al. Neoadjuvant chemotherapy followed by radical surgery in patients affected by vaginal carcinoma. Gynecol Oncol. 2008;111(2):307-11.
31. Taylor MB, Dugar N, Davidson SE, Carrington BM. Magnetic resonance imaging of primary vaginal carcinoma. Clin Radiol. 2007;62(6):549-55.

36
Chemoradiotherapy in Carcinoma Cervix

Kishore Singh, Savita Arora, Arun Kumar Rathi

Carcinoma cervix is the fourth common cancer in women worldwide, with 85% of cases occurring in developing countries, where cervical cancer is a leading cause of cancer death in women.[1] Persistent human papilloma virus infection is the most important factor in development of cervical cancer[2] the other epidemiological risk factors are smoking, parity, early age of onset of coitus, large number of sexual partners, history of sexually transmitted disease and chronic immunosuppression.

Squamous cell carcinoma account for approximately 80% of all cervical cancers and adenocarcinoma for approximately 20%. In developed countries, the decline in incidence is presumed to be result of effective screening and HPV vaccination.

DIAGNOSIS AND WORKUP

Early stage carcinoma of cervix may be asymptomatic or associated with a watery discharge and post-coital bleeding or intermittent bleeding.

Because of easy accessibility of uterine cervix, cervical cytology or Papanicolaou (Pap) smears and cervical biopsies can usually result in an accurate diagnosis.

The International Federation of Gynecology and Obstetrics (FIGO) evaluation procedures include biopsy, colposcopy, cystoscopy and proctosigmoidoscopy. Chest radiography, intravenous pyelogram (IVP) and barium enema are standard radiographic studies. Computed tomography (CT), magnetic resonance imaging (MRI) and positron emission tomography-computed tomography (PET-CT) are also used to guide treatment options.[3-4] Laboratory investigations include complete blood count along with liver and renal function profile.

PRIMARY MANAGEMENT

The primary treatment of early stage cervical cancer is either surgery or radiotherapy (Table 36.1). Surgery is typically reserved for early stage disease and smaller lesions, such as stage IA, IB1 and selected IIA1.[5] Chemoradiation is also recommended in early stage disease patients who are not candidates for surgery. The adenocarcinoma of cervix are treated in a similar manner to squamous cell carcinomas.

Stage IA1 Disease

Recommended options depend on the result of cone biopsy and whether patient,
- Wants to conserve fertility
- Lymphovascular space invasion (LVSI).

Fertility Sparing

Microinvasive disease, IA-1 with negative margin after cone biopsy and no LVSI, observation is an option if fertility preservation is desired.

Table 36.1 TNM and FIGO classifications for cervical cancer

TNM Categories	FIGO Stages	Surgical-Pathologic findings
Primary tumor (T)		
TX		Primary tumor cannot be assessed
T0		No evidence of primary tumor
Tis		Carcinoma in situ (preinvasive carcinoma)
T1	I	Cervical carcinoma confined to the cervix (disregard extension to the corpus)
T1a	IA	Invasive carcinoma diagnosed only by microscopy; stromal invasion with a maximum depth of 5.0 mm measured from the base of the epithelium and a horizontal spread of 7.0 mm or less; vascular space involvement, venous or lymphatic, does not affect classification
T1a1	IA1	Measured stromal invasion ≤ 3.0 mm in depth and ≤ 7.0 mm in horizontal spread
T1a2	IA2	Measured stromal invasion > 3.0 mm and ≤ 5.0 mm with a horizontal spread ≤ 7.0 mm
T1b	IB	Clinically visible lesion confined to the cervix or microscopic lesion greater than T1a/IA2
T1b1	IB1	Clinically visible lesion ≤ 4.0 cm in greatest dimension
T1b2	IB2	Clinically visible lesion > 4.0 cm in greatest dimension
T2	II	Cervical carcinoma invades beyond uterus but not to pelvic wall or to lower third of vagina
T2a	IIA	Tumor without parametrial invasion
T2a1	IIA1	Clinically visible lesion ≤ 4.0 cm in greatest dimension
T2a2	IIA2	Clinically visible lesion > 4.0 cm in greatest dimension
T2b	IIB	Tumor with parametrial invasion
T3	III	Tumor extends to pelvic wall and/or involves lower third of vagina and/or causes hydronephrosis or nonfunctional kidney
T3a	IIIA	Tumor involves lower third of vagina, no extension to pelvic wall
T3b	IIIB	Tumor extends to pelvic wall and/or causes hydronephrosis or nonfunctional kidney
T4	IV	Tumor invades mucosa of bladder or rectum and/or extends beyond true pelvis (bullous edema is not sufficient to classify a tumor as T4)
T4a	IVA	Tumor invades mucosa of bladder or rectum (bullous edema is not sufficient to classify a tumor as T4)
T4b	IVB	Tumor extends beyond true pelvis
Regional lymph nodes (N)		
NX		Regional lymph nodes cannot be assessed
N0		No regional lymph node metastasis
N1		Regional lymph node metastasis
Distant metastasis (M)		
M0		No distant metastasis
M1		Distant metastasis (including peritoneal spread; involvement of supraclavicular, mediastinal, or para-aortic lymph nodes; and lung, liver, or bone)

In IA-1 stage, patients with LVSI or positive margins after cone biopsy, radical trachelectomy in addition to pelvic lymphadenectomy is recommended.[6]

After childbearing is complete, hysterectomy is considered for patients who have persistent human papillomavirus (HPV) infections or persistent abnormal Pap smear.

Nonfertility Sparing

Simple hysterectomy is done in patients without LVSI and negative margins on cone biopsy, if they are medically operable.

Patients having positive margins or if LVSI is present, modified radical hysterectomy with lymph node dissection is recommended.

Stage IA2 Disease

Fertility Sparing

If margins are negative after cone biopsy, patients can be put on observation only. In case of positive margin, radical trachelectomy with pelvic lymph node dissection is recommended.

Nonfertility Sparing

For patients who do not wish to preserve fertility, the recommended surgical option is modified hysterectomy with bilateral lymph node dissection.

Pelvic radiation with brachytherapy (70–80 Gy to point A) is a treatment option for medically inoperable patients.[7]

Stage IB and IIA Disease

Depending on their stage and disease bulk, patients with stage IB or IIA tumors can be treated with surgery, RT or concurrent chemoradiation. Fertility sparing surgery radical trachelectomy with pelvic node dissection is only recommended for a select group of patients of stage IB1 where bulk of tumor is less than 2 cm.

Patients who do not wish to preserve fertility, radical hysterectomy with pelvic lymph node dissection is recommended especially for patients with stages IB1 or IIA1 disease while patients with stages IB2 or IIA2, pelvic RT and brachytherapy is another option. In this group of patients, who are treated with definitive RT concurrent Cisplatinum has been shown to improve survival.

Advanced Disease

Patients with stage IIB to IVA are included in this group. Concurrent chemoradiotherapy is the treatment of choice in this group.

For patients without nodal disease, treatment consists of pelvic RT and brachytherapy with concurrent cisplatin. However, patients with positive para-aortic or pelvic lymph nodes, require extended field radiotherapy.

Metastatic Disease

Cisplatinum containing multiagent chemotherapy is recommended. Individualized RT can be given to patients to palliate the symptoms of pain, bleeding, etc. in highly selected patients with isolated distant metastases; occasional long-term survival has been reported with surgery or local ablative therapies.

Post-hysterectomy Adjuvant Radiation Therapy

Following primary hysterectomy, the presence of one or more pathological risk factors, i.e. deep stromal invasion, vascular or lymphatic invasion and large tumor size (≥ 3 cm) may warrant the use of adjuvant radiotherapy.[8] A dose of 45–50 Gy in standard fractionation is usually recommended. In presence of high-risk in postoperative specimen, concurrent chemotherapy is indicated. The presence of high-risk features in which concurrent chemotherapy is given are positive pelvic lymph nodes, positive resection margins and parametrial involvement.[9]

Techniques of Radiotherapy and Radiotherapy Planning

The following are techniques of radiotherapy and its planning.

External Beam Radiotherapy

External beam radiotherapy is typically given prior to brachytherapy because for a proper brachytherapy application the normal anatomy should be maintained. MRI is the best imaging modality for determining soft tissue and parametrial involvement.

The radiation field covers the gross tumor as well as the regional draining lymph nodes. It includes the primary tumor, the parametrial or the vaginal extensions of the tumor and the pelvic group of lymph nodes. High energy photons (15 MV to 18 MV) are preferred for three dimensional conformal radiotherapy due to the skin sparing effect of the high energy radiotherapy.

Patient is usually treated in supine position with proper immobilization but in case of postoperative patients and in obese patients prone position is preferred as it removes the intestine away from the radiation field. In conventional technique using Co^{60} machine the upper border of the radiation field is placed at the L4–L5 vertebral junction to cover the common iliac lymph nodes, lower border must cover at least the obturator foramen and the lateral borders are taken 1.5–2 cm lateral to the pelvic brim. If the disease extends to lower 3rd of the vagina then the lower border of the field can be taken at the introitus to cover the entire primary tumor with adequate margin. In case of para-aortic node involvement, the field is extended to cover the para-aortic nodes. Coverage of microscopic nodal disease requires a dose of 45 Gy (in conventional fractionation of 1.8–2 Gy), and highly conformal boost of additional 10 Gy may be considered for gross unresected adenopathy.

In case of three-dimensional conformal radiothermal (3-DCRT) or intensity-modulated radiotherapy (IMRT), computerized treatment planning is done with help of contrast enhanced CT scans of abdomen and pelvis with the help of conformal techniques like 3-DCRT and IMRT the dose to the normal tissues can be grossly reduced with adequate dose of radiation to the tumor.

Brachytherapy

Brachytherapy was first used to treat cervical cancers in early 20th century and continues to play central role in the curative management of all patients with primary cervical cancer who are not candidates for surgery. Brachytherapy delivers a high dose to the central disease and the parametrium and spares the surrounding tissues. This sparing of the surrounding normal tissues occurs due to rapid dose fall off according to inverse square law.

Uterine cavity is an ideal site for intracavitary brachytherapy application. Most brachytherapy applicator system consists of an angled or curved intrauterine tandem with some form of intravaginal applicator. Intravaginal applicator may consist of two ovoids or colpostats or a ring intravaginal applicator. Various applicator system for intracavitary brachytherapy in carcinoma cervix include several modifications of Fletcher-Suit after loading colpostats, vaginal rings, French molds vaginal cylinders and others.

Vaginal packing is done to hold the applicator in place and to displace the bladder and rectum away from the source so that the bladder and rectum will get minimal radiation dose. Intrauterine tandem length is usually 6–8 cm. The longest tandem should always be used. The ovoids that are used are available in various diameters. The largest ovoid possible should be used. Brachytherapy is done in an operating room under general or spinal anesthesia. It can also be done under conscious sedation. Radiological confirmation of the proper placement of the applicator is done after the applicator insertion.

The dose in an intracavitary brachytherapy is prescribed to a single reference point referred to as point A representing a paracervical reference point. It is most widely used, validated and reproducible dosing parameter. Point A is defined as a point situated 2 cm superior to the tandem flange and 2 cm lateral from the center of tandem. Point B is a point situated 3 cm lateral to the point A and corresponds to the parametrium or the obturator nodes. Point B gets a dose approximately 1/3rd-1/4th of the dose to point A. Dose in low dose rate (LDR) technique is usually 15-20 Gy per fraction and total two fractions are given. The dose prescribed in high dose rate (HDR) technique is 6-7 Gy/fraction and total of 3-5 fractions are given.

CONCURRENT CHEMORADIOTHERAPY

At the end of the 1990s, number of studies provide evidence that adding chemotherapy to radiotherapy in treatment of carcinoma cervix leads to reduction in risk of local recurrence by as much as 50%. The chemotherapeutic agents that can be used concurrently with radiotherapy are cisplatin, carboplatin, 5 FU, taxanes, gemcitabine, etc. Most commonly used drug in carcinoma cervix with radiotherapy is cisplatin (40 mg/m^2 weekly). The rationale behind using chemotherapy with radiotherapy is that chemotherapeutic agents sensitize the tumor cells to the effect of radiation, they have a different toxicity profile than that of radiotherapy and also they can control both local as well as distant spread of the tumor.

There are five randomized landmark trials that proved the beneficial role of concurrent chemoradiotherapy in the treatment of carcinoma cervix, e.g. Rose et al. (GOG 120), Keys et al. (GOG 123), Whitney et al. (GOG 85), Peters et al. (INTERGROUP 0107/SWOG 87-97) and Pearcy et al. (NCIC Canada).[10-14]

A meta-analysis[15] in 2010, demonstrated the beneficial role of chemoradiation in locally advanced carcinoma cervix as compared to radiotherapy alone. The result showed that chemoradiation reduced the risk of death (HR- 0.69, 95% CI 0.61-0.77) which translated into a 10% absolute improvement in survival. The survival benefit associated with chemoradiation significantly decreased with increasing stage.

For women with stage IB to IIA, IIB, and III to IVA cervical cancer, the five-year survival benefit was 10%, 7%, and 3%, respectively (p = 0.017). Chemoradiation resulted in a reduction in the risk of recurrence (HR 0.66, 95% CI 0.59-0.73), which translated into a 13% absolute improvement in progression-free survival (PFS)but CTRT is associated with higher rates of serious (grade 3/4) adverse events, including gastrointestinal toxicity (OR 1.98, 95% CI 1.49-2.63).

DOSE OF RADIOTHERAPY

Definitive Radiation Therapy for an Intact Cervix

In patients with an intact cervix (i.e. who do not undergo surgery), the primary tumor and the regional lymphatics at risk are typically treated with definitive external beam radiotherapy (EBRT) of 45 Gy. The primary tumor is then boosted with brachytherapy with an additional 30-40 Gy to point A (in LDR equivalent dose), for a total dose of 80 gy to point A in small volume tumors or 85 Gy to larger volume disease.

Post-hysterectomy Adjuvant Radiation Therapy

Following primary hysterectomy, the presence of one or more pathological risk factors, i.e deep stromal invasion, vascular or lymphatic invasion and large tumor size (≥ 3 cm) may warrant the use of adjuvant radiotherapy. A dose of 45-50 Gy in standard fractionation is usually recommended. In presence of high-risk in postoperative specimen, concurrent chemotherapy is indicated. The presence of high-risk features in which concurrent chemotherapy is given are positive pelvic lymph nodes, positive resection margins and parametrial involvement.

Treatment Duration

Over all treatment time in carcinoma cervix patients should be as short as possible. Delay or interruption in treatment should be avoided.

Undue delay in overall treatment time adversely affects both local control as well as survival as detected by various studies (Lanciano et al., Chatani et al., Perez et al.). It was taken as a thumb rule that one day delay in treatment beyond 8 weeks leads to 1% treatment failure therefore we should always complete the total treatment including EBRT and brachytherapy within 8 weeks.

Toxicities during Radiotherapy

Mild toxicities are common during radiotherapy which are resolved spontaneously. Acute toxicities occur during and within 6 weeks of completion of radiotherapy. Acute toxicities include mild fatigue, mild to moderate diarrhea nausea, mild gastritis, cystitis, colitis, bone marrow suppression, permanent ovarian failure, dry or moist desquamation, pruritis, etc. Chronic toxicities include vaginal stenosis, ureteral stricture, vesicovaginal or rectovaginal fistula, intestinal obstruction or perforations, fracture of neck of femur, radiation induced proctitis leading to bleeding per rectum and hemorrhagic cystitis. Regular vaginal dilatation may be required to maintain vaginal vault size and sexual function.

Precautions to be Taken during Therapy

Hemoglobin level of the patient has a strong prognostic importance as studied in various trials. Therefore, the hemoglobin level should always be kept normal during the radiotherapy. Patients are strongly advised not to smoke during the treatment as smoking results in poorer outcome in patients of carcinoma cervix.

Drug Reactions

All the drugs used in cancer cervix have the potential to cause adverse reactions either during or after infusion. Mostly the reactions are mild but sometimes serious life-threatening anaphylaxis can happen. Patients who experience severe reaction should not receive the implicated agent again. If a mild reaction occurs, the precaution should be taken to desensitize the patient before next infusion.

RECENT ADVANCES

Screening of Cervical Cancer

Over the last few years, several randomized trials compared HPV based screening and cytology based screening tests. These trials showed HPV-based screening at 5 years intervals offered better protection than cytology alone at 3 years interval. In 2014, HPV test received FDA approval as the primary screening tool.[16]

New Agents

Nonplatinum combination chemotherapy has been proposed as a strategy to circumvent platinum resistance in carcinoma cervix. In this regard, Bevacizumab, a humanized vascular endothelial growth factor (VEGF) neutralizing monoclonal antibody has shown single agent activity in heavily pretreated recurrent carcinoma cervix.

In GOG-0240 (paclitaxel and cisplatin or Topotecan with or without bevacizumab in treating patients with stage IVB, recurrent or persistent carcinoma cervix), it improved survival by a significant 3.7 months.

REFERENCES

1. Parkin DM, Bray F, Ferlay J, Pisani P. Global cancer statistics,2002.CA Cancer J Clin. 2005;55:74-108.
2. Kjaer SK, Frederiksen K, Munk C, Iftener T. Long term absolute risk of cervical intraepithelial neoplasia grade 3 or worse following human papilloma virus infection: role of persistence. J Natl Cancer Inst. 2010;102:1478-88.
3. Amit A, Schink J, Reiss A, Lowenstein L. PET/CT in gynaecologic cancer: present applications and future prospects–a clinician's perspective. Obstet Gynaecol Clin North Am. 2011;38:1-21,vii.
4. Patel S, Liyange SH, Sahdev A, et al. Imaging of endometrial and cervical cancer. Insights imaging. 2010;1:309-28.
5. ACOG practice bulletin. Diagnosis and treatment of cervical carcinomas. Number 35, May 2002.

American College of Obstetricians and G. Gynaecologists. Int J Gynaecol Obstet. 2002;78: 79-91.
6. Abu Rustam NR, Sonoda Y. Fertility- sparing surgery in early-stage cervical cancer: indications and applications. J Natl Compr Canc Netw. 2010;8: 1435-8.
7. Small W Jr, Strauss JB, Jhingran A, et al. ACR appropriateness criteria (R) definitive therapy for early stage cervical cancer. Am J Clin Oncol. 2012;35:399-405.
8. Rotman M, Sedillis A, Piedmonte MR, et al. A phase III randomized trial of postoperative pelvic irradiation in stage IB cervical carcinoma with poor prognostic features: follow-up of a gynaecologic oncology group study. Int J Radiat Oncol Bio Phys. 2006;65:169-76.
9. Peters WA, Liu PY, Barrett RJ, et al. Concurrent chemotherapy and pelvic radiotherapy compared with pelvic radiation therapy alone as adjuvant therapy after radical surgery in high-risk early-stage cancer of cervix. J Cin Oncol. 2000;18:1606-13.
10. Rose PG, Bundy BN, Watkins EB, et al. Concurrent cisplatin-based radiotherapy and chemotherapy for locally advanced cervical cancer. N Engl J Med. 1999;340:1144-53.
11. Keys HM, Bundy BN, Stehman FB, et al. Cisplatin, radiation, and adjuvant hysterectomy compared with radiation and adjuvant hysterectomy for bulky stage IB cervical carcinoma. N Engl J Med. 1999;340:1154-61.
12. Whitney CW, Sause W, Bundy BN, et al. Randomized comparison of fluorouracil plus cisplatin versus hydroxyurea as an adjunct to radiation therapy in stage IIB-IVA carcinoma of the cervix with negative para-aortic lymph nodes: A Gynecologic Oncology Group and Southwest Oncology Group study. J Clin Oncol. 1999;17:1339-48.
13. Peters WA, Liu PY, Barrett RJ, et al. Concurrent chemotherapy and pelvic radiation therapy compared with pelvic radiation therapy alone as adjuvant therapy after radical surgery in high-risk early-stage cancer of the cervix. J Clin Oncol. 2000;18:1606-13.
14. Pearcey R, Brundage M, Drouin P, et al. Phase III trial comparing radical radiotherapy with and without cisplatin chemotherapy in patients with advanced squamous cell cancer of the cervix. J Clin Oncol. 2002;20:966-72.
15. Chemoradiotherapy for cervical cancer meta-analysis collaboration (CCCMAC). Reducing uncertainties about the effects of chemoradio-therapy for cervical cancer: individual patient data meta-analysis. Cochrane Database of Systematic Reviews 2010, Issue 1. Art. No.: CD008285. DOI: 10.1002/14651858.CD008285.
16. Society of Gynaecologic Oncology. Women's Cancer News. FDA panel approves HPV screening tool. Irving TX: Multibriefs; 2014.

37
Chemoradiotherapy in Carcinoma Endometrium

Kishore Singh, Savita Arora, Arun Kumar Rathi

INTRODUCTION

Adenocarcinoma of endometrium, also known as endometrial carcinoma or broadly as uterine carcinoma is the most common malignancy of female genital tract in United States, with a 2–3% lifetime risk of developing the disease.[1] The incidence of this disease is low in India, the highest being observed in Bengaluru.

More than 90% of cases occur in women more than 50 years of age with a median age of diagnosis of 63 years. The majority of patients (around 80%) are diagnosed early, with a 5-year survival rate of over 95%. Histopathologically, endometrial cancers are classified as malignant epithelial tumors or mesenchymal tumors. Epithelial tumors include pure endometrioid type, serous, clear cell carcinoma and carcinosarcoma. Mesenchymal tumors include uterine leiomyosarcoma, endometrial stromal sarcoma and undifferentiated endometrial sarcoma. The most common histopathological type is endometrioid adenocarcinoma.

RISK FACTORS

Increased levels of estrogen (caused by obesity, diabetes and high fat intake), early age at menarche, nulliparity, late age at menopause, Lynch syndrome and tamoxifen use are the main underlying risk factors for endometrial carcinoma.[2]

PROGNOSTIC VARIABLES IN ENDOMETRIAL CARCINOMA

The stages of disease are most significant risk factors and stage I patients have a 5-year survival of more than 90%. The adverse factors include lymphovascular space invasion (LVSI), advance age, clear and serous type of histology, higher grade of disease and more than one-third of myometrial invasion.

PRIMARY TREATMENT

The recommended treatment of endometrial carcinoma in a medically operable patient with disease clinically confined to uterus is total abdominal hysterectomy and bilateral salpingo-oophorectomy. The International Federation of Gynecology and Obstetrics (FIGO) recommends that peritoneal cytology should be collected and enlarged or suspicious lymph node should be excised to confirm or rule out metastatic disease.

If there is a suspected or gross cervical involvement, cervical biopsy or magnetic resonance imaging (MRI) should be considered prior to surgery. For operable patients with cervical involvement, radical hysterectomy along with bilateral sapingo-oophorectomy, peritoneal lavage and dissection of lymph node is recommended. Patients who are medically inoperable, tumor directed radiotherapy with or without chemotherapy can provide pelvic control and long-term progression free survival.

In patients with extra uterine disease and presenting with intra-abdominal disease (i.e. ascites, omental, peritoneal or nodal involvement), the treatment is total abdominal hysterectomy (TAH) with bilateral salpingo-oophorectomy (BSO) and peritoneal cytology, pelvic and para-aortic lymph node dissection and surgical debulking. Preoperative chemotherapy can be considered in these patients. Patients with unresectable extra uterine pelvic disease (rectal, bladder or parametrial), are typically treated with radiation therapy (RT) and brachytherapy with or without chemotherapy.

Table 37.1 summarizes the ESMO-EGO-ESTRO consensus guideline statement of 2015 on endometrial carcinoma.[3]

SYSTEMIC THERAPY IN ENDOMETRIAL CARCINOMA

The majority of patients with advanced or recurrent disease, require some form of systemic therapy during course of their disease. Systemic therapy consists of hormonal or cytotoxic chemotherapy.

Table 37.1 ESMO- EGO-ESTRO Consensus guidelines

Risk group	Description	Adjuvant therapy
Low	Stage I endometrioid, grade 1–2,<50% myometrial invasion, LVSI negative	Observation alone
Intermediate	Stage I endometrioid, grade 1–2, ≥ 50% myometrial invasion, LVSI negative	Vaginal brachytherapy, observation is an option in patients <60 years
High-intermediate risk	• Stage I endometrioid, grade 3, <50% myometrial invasion, regardless of LVSI status • Stage I endometrioid, grade 1–2, LVSI positive, regardless of depth of invasion	• Node negative—VBT • No nodal staging—pelvic EBRT for LVSI positive staging, VBT alone in LVSI negative cases
High risk	Stage I endometrioid, grade 3, >50% myometrial invasion, regardless of LVSI status	• Node negative—pelvic RT or vaginal brachytherapy • No nodal staging—pelvic RT and chemotherapy
	Stage II	• Node negative: Grade 1–2, LVSI negative—VBT Grade 3 or LVSI positive—pelvic RT and VBT • No nodal staging—pelvic RT and VBT • If grade 3 or LVSI positive—sequential adjuvant chemotherapy
	Stage III endometrioid, no residual disease	Pelvic RT and chemotherapy
	Nonendometrioid cancers	Stage IA, LVSI negative—VBT Stage IB or greater—pelvic RT and chemotherapy
Advanced	Stage III residual disease, stage IVA	Pelvic EBRT and chemotherapy

Abbreviations: VBT, vaginal brachytherapy; LVSI, lymphovascular space invasion; EBRT, external beam radiotherapy; RT, radiation therapy

Systemic Chemotherapy

Endometrial carcinoma is a chemosensitive disease. Response rates of 20–30% have been documented with single agent doxorubicin and cisplatin/carboplatin.[4] In a gynecologic oncology group (GOG) trial in patients with FIGO stage III–IV endometrial cancer, addition of paclitaxel to cisplatin and doxorubicin was associated with a higher progression free survival and response rate than cisplatin and doxorubicin alone (median PFS: 8.3 versus 5.3 months, respectively; P <0.01).

Miller et al. (GOG 209)[5] conducted a randomized trial on 1305 patients that compared the combination of paclitaxel 160 mg/m^2, cisplatin 60 mg/m^2 and doxorubicin 50 mg/m^2 (TAP) with paclitaxel 175 mg/m^2 and carboplatin AUC 6 (TC), both administered every 3 weeks. Both the regimes indicated a similar response rate (51.3% versus 51.2%) and progression free survival (PFS) (median 13.5 versus 13.3 months).

Agents like topotecan, liposomal doxorubicin and gemcitabine have been used as second line agents.

HORMONAL THERAPY

Hormonal therapy is preferred as systemic therapy in patients with hormone positive expression, low grade disease and with a long disease free interval. The progestogens, medroxyprogesterone acetate (MPA) are generally recommended. The reported response rates are in range of 15–20%. The 200 mg/day of MPA is the initial dose for treatment of advanced or recurrent endometrial cancer. If an objective response is achieved, the progestogens can be continued indefinitely. Side effects include weight gain, hypertension and thrombophlebitis.

RECENT ADVANCES

Angiogenesis inhibitors, bevacizumab and sunitinib are the new drugs showing promising result in pretreated patients with endometrial carcinoma. mTOR inhibitors temsirolimus and anti-EGFR agents like erlotinib are the new class of molecular targeted therapy. GOG -86P[6] is a three-arm trial which compared the addition of bevacizumab, temsirolimus or ixabepilone to first line TC in patients with advanced or recurrent endometrial carcinoma. Bevacizumab appeared superior when the median overall survival was compared with historical control data (34 versus 22.7 months).

REFERENCES

1. Jemal A, Seigel R, Xu J, Ward E. Cancer statistics, 2010. CA Cancer J Clin. 2010;60:277-300.
2. Van den Bosch T, Coosemans A, Mornia M, et al. Screening for uterine tumours. Best Pract Res Clin Obstet Gynaecol, 2011.
3. Colombo N, Creutberg C, Aman F, et al. ESMO_ESGO-ESTRO consensus conference on endometrial cancer: Diagnosis, treatment and follow up. Radiotherapy and Oncol. 2016;27(1):16-41.
4. Thigpen JT, Blessing JA, DiSaia PJ, et al. A randomized comparison of doxorubicin alone versus doxorubicin plus cyclophosphamide in the management of advanced or recurrent endometrial carcinoma: A Gynaecologic Oncology Group Study. J Clin Oncol. 1994;12:1408-14.
5. Miller D, Filaci V, Fleming G, et al. Randomized phase III non inferiority trial of first line chemotherapy for metastatic or recurrent endometrial carcinoma: a Gynaecologic Oncology Group Study. Gynaecol Oncol. 2012;125:771.
6. Aghajananian C, Filaci VL, Dizon DS. A randomized phase II study of paclitaxel/carboplatin/bevacizumab versus paclitaxel/carboplatin/temsirolimus and ixabepilone/carboplatin/bevacizumab as initial therapy for measurable III or IVA, stage IVB or recurrent endometrial cancer, GOG86P. J Clinic Oncol. 2015;33.

38

Chemotherapy in Ovarian Cancer

Kishore Singh, Savita Arora, Arun Kumar Rathi

Ovarian cancer is the fifth leading cause of cancer death among females. Primary malignant tumors of ovary include epithelial cell tumors, germ cell tumors and sex cord tumors. Epithelial ovarian tumors comprise the majority (about 90%) of malignant ovarian neoplasms.[1] Primary lymphoma, melanoma and sarcoma are rare. Ovarian low malignant tumors are noninvasive tumors confined to ovary.

Ovarian malignancy presenting symptoms are nonspecific and screening modalities are not effective. Early stage disease may get detected as an asymptomatic adnexal mass on routine examination. An adnexal mass in postmenopausal females is likely to be malignant.

DIAGNOSTIC WORKUP

The investigation plan of a pelvic mass should include a thorough history and full physical examination and pelvic examination. Ultrasound is the first noninvasive step for evaluation of a pelvic mass. Sonographic features of a malignant tumor include irregular borders; solid component; dense septa; enlarged nodes and presence of ascites. Other radiological studies include X-ray chest and computed tomography/magnetic resonance imaging (CT/MRI) scans of whole abdomen. CT/MRI are modalities to determine intra- and extra-abdominal extent of disease. Positron emission tomography (PET/CT) scan may be useful to assess indeterminate lesions.[2] Initial evaluation should include laboratory studies including complete blood counts, liver and kidney status.

Tumor markers including CA-125, (carbohydrate antigen) alpha-fetoprotein (AFP), beta-human chorionic gonadotropin, lactate dehydrogenase and total inhibin should be measured. Elevated CA-125 may reflect a greater burden of disease and a high grade serous histology. Increased level of AFP and beta-human chorionic gonadotropin (hCG) help in diagnosis of nonepithelial germ cell tumors. Appropriate evaluation of cardiac risk assessment should also be done. National Comprehensive Cancer Network (NCCN) guidelines now recommend that all patients of ovarian cancer should be referred for genetic risk evaluation.

Fine needle aspiration should be avoided for a suspected early stage ovarian cancer to prevent spilling of malignant cells into peritoneal cavity however, it can be safely performed in patients with bulky disease who are not candidates for surgical exploration.

Additional diagnostic studies including GI endoscopy are recommended in particular clinical situations only.

TREATMENT OF EPITHELIAL OVARIAN TUMORS

Epithelial ovarian cancer has four main histologic subtypes, i.e. serous, endometrioid, mucinous, and clear cell. Initial treatment is same for all the subtypes. Primary treatment for a presumed or histopathologically proven ovarian cancer is appropriate surgical staging and cytoreduction[3] followed by adjuvant treatment if indicated. It is the mainstay of diagnosis and initial treatment for ovarian and fallopian tube cancers. In early stage disease, it gives the accurate pathologic staging while in advanced disease, it helps in optimal debulking of tumor. It begins with an exploratory laparotomy including a total abdominal hysterectomy and bilateral salpingo-oophorectomy along with infracolic omentectomy and pelvic and para-aortic lymph nodes sampling when possible.

Peritoneal washings are taken for cytological examination. Surgical cytoreduction is optimal if residual tumor nodules are less than 1 cm.[4] Neoadjuvant therapy can be considered if goal of maximum cytoreduction cannot be achieved (3 or more cycles) however, the therapeutic benefit of this approach is still investigational and NCCN guidelines state that data is insufficient to recommend neoadjuvant chemotherapy (NACT) in potentially resectable patients and upfront debulking remains the treatment of choice. In a select stage 1 low grade young patients, unilateral salpingo-oophorectomy may be sufficient.

Prognostic Factors

Stage of disease and thoroughness of surgical staging determines the survival. Five years survival for early stage disease is nearly 80%, which is reduced to <30% for stage III and remains dismal at 5% for stage IV. Optimal cytoreduction improves median survival in advance stages. Among other factors pathologic grade, tumor volume, histologic subtype also influence survival. Mucinous and clear cell histopathology also indicate poor prognosis.

POSTOPERATIVE MANAGEMENT

Most patients with epithelial ovarian cancer receive postoperative systemic chemotherapy, which is known as adjuvant therapy.

Early Stage Disease

Women with early stage (FIGO stage 1A and 1B), grade 1 or 2 disease have low risk of relapse and > 90% of 5 years survival with surgical treatment alone.[5] In this subset of patients, no adjuvant treatment is required however, a complete surgical staging is mandatory.

Patients with stage 1, grade 3 tumors, and patients with clear cell histology require 3–6 cycles of postoperative adjuvant taxane and carboplatin.

All patients with disease beyond capsule, i.e. stage 1C, irrespective of grade are treated with 3–6 cycles of IV taxanes and carboplatin.[6]

Advance Stage Disease

In all patients with stage II to IV the recommendation is to give 6–8 cycles of intravenous taxane and carboplatin.

Chemotherapy Protocols for Epithelial Ovarian Tumors

Neoadjuvant/postoperative adjuvant therapy:
- Injection paclitaxel, 175 mg/m^2 over 3 hours intravenous infusion, followed by injection carboplatin, dosed at an area under the curve (AUC) of 5–6 intravenous over 1 hour on day 1 given every 3 weeks for 6 cycles.[7]
- Dose dense paclitaxel 80 mg/m^2 intravenous over 1 hour on days 1, 8 and 15 plus carboplatin AUC 5–6 intravenous over 1 hour on day 1 every 3 weeks for 6 cycles.
- Injection docetaxel 60–75 mg/m^2 as 1 hour infusion followed by carboplatin, at the dose of AUC of 5–6 intravenous over 1 hour on day 1, every 3 weeks for 6 cycles.

Old age patients, stage IV patients with comorbid conditions or poor performance may not tolerate above regimens. Single agent either paclitaxel or carboplatin may be given in such patients.

Intravenous versus Intraperitoneal Chemotherapy

Because of peritoneal dissemination of epithelial ovarian tumors, it is postulated that intraperitoneal administration of chemotherapeutic agents allows a several fold increase in drug concentration as compared to systemic therapy. NCCN guidelines recommend intraperitoneal chemotherapy for optimally debulked (<1 cm residual) stage-III tumors. Although recommended, this practice is not adopted much because of increased toxicity including leukopenia, renal toxicity and neurotoxicity along with catheter complications.

Monitoring of Patients on Chemotherapy

Patients planned for chemotherapy patients should have adequate organ functions (renal, hepatic and cardiac) and performance status.

Patients receiving above chemotherapy should get complete blood counts, renal functions and liver functions monitored before each cycle.

Regardless of which regimen is selected, patient should be re-evaluated after 2–3 cycles of chemotherapy to assess the response.

CA-125 levels should be checked prior to each cycle if initially raised.

Toxicity Profile

All drugs used in the protocols have the potential to cause infusion or allergic reactions.[8] Adverse reactions associated with taxanes (docetaxel, paclitaxel) tend to be infusion related and are due to cremophor in it.

Clinicians should be prepared to handle such reactions which can be life-threatening also. Adequate premedication with IV steroids, antihistaminic agents decreases the incidence of such episodes.

The potential side effects of above regimens include:
- Myelosuppression
- Renal toxicity
- Liver dysfunction
- Peripheral neuropathy (paclitaxel induced).

Follow-up Recommendations

Complete remission is defined as no objective evidence of disease, i.e. normal physical examination, normal CA-125 estimation and no disease evidence on CT scans.

Stage I–IV patients of epithelial ovarian carcinoma with complete clinical remission are followed-up 3–4 monthly initially for 2 years, then 6 monthly for 3 years and then annually after 5 years.

Each follow-up requires complete physical and pelvic examination and estimation of CA-125 levels if initially elevated. Pelvic/abdominal CT/MRI scan is done based on clinical indication.[9] PET-CT is routinely not recommended.

Recurrent Disease

Patients who experience an early recurrence, i.e. within 6 months of completion of initial chemotherapy or progress on chemotherapy are considered platinum resistant and are candidates of second-line chemotherapy. Treatment options include liposomal doxorubicin, gemcitabine, topotecan, nanoparticle albumin bound paclitaxel (nab paclitaxel), capecitabine or hormonal agents including leuprolide acetate and megestrol acetate. Response rate with these agents is in the range of 20–27%. Patients, who primarily progress on two different chemotherapy regimens without evidence of any clinical benefit, do not benefit from additional therapy.

Women with late recurrence, i.e. > 6 months after completion of chemotherapy are categorized as "platinum sensitive".[10] In this group, re-treatment with platinum-based chemotherapy is given.

In patients with rising CA-125 and no radiographic evidence of disease, the recommendation is the close observation only until clinical symptoms arise. Tamoxifen and other hormonal agents are recommended in this category of patients.

RADIOTHERAPY

Radiation therapy, known since 1912 to induce long-term remission in certain patients with ovarian cancer, has largely been excluded from routine use and is not currently used as a consolidative treatment although it may be used as salvage or palliative therapy in selective patients.

Whole-abdominal irradiation (WAI) was earlier a standard modality of postoperative treatment in completely resected ovarian cancer patients to treat all the peritoneal surface harboring the microscopic disease. Small fraction size, i.e. 100–125 cGy is given daily to the whole abdominal field. After delivering 25–27.5 Gy to the whole abdomen, a 20–22 Gy boost is given to pelvis. Organs at risk that are dose limiting include the kidneys, liver, small and large bowels and bone marrow.

Work continues on technique refinement, reduction, and management of long-term effects and patient selection. Presently, due to advancement in technology, the use of intensity modulated radiation therapy (IMRT) to deliver WAI has been proposed as a means to reduce dose to liver, kidney and bone marrow to decrease the incidence of myelotoxicity and renal damage.

Recent Advances

Serum Human Epididymis Protein (HE4) Measurement as Diagnostic Tool

Recently, HE4 measurement in serum has been proposed for improving the specificity of laboratory identification of ovarian carcinoma. Its serum levels measurement seems to be superior to CA-125 in terms of diagnostic performance for identification of ovarian carcinoma. Food and Drug Administrations (FDA) has approved use of HE4 and CA-125 for estimating risk of ovarian cancer in women with pelvic mass.

New Agents

Several modalities are now used to match individual patient's treatment requirement. Now, a variety of approaches can be used to predict therapeutic efficacy, including genetic panel testing, and molecular profiling. The genetic pathways involved in ovarian cancer are becoming clearer. For example, high-grade ovarian cancers (high grade serous carcinoma) almost always have a mutation in TP53, while borderline and low-grade ovarian cancers (endometrioid, transitional, low-grade serous) often have a mutation in BRAF or KRAS. Knowing which pathways are involved makes targeted therapies attractive. Targeting the VEGF pathway, i.e. antiangiogenesis agents with bevacizumab has led to improved progression-free survival in patients receiving up-front treatment or as maintenance therapy after completion of primary chemotherapy.[11] Several phase III trials have assessed the combination of bevacizumab with chemotherapy in platinum resistant, recurrent ovarian cancer.

One of the targeted drugs is the PARP (polyADP-ribose polymerase) inhibitors that exploits mutations in BRCA. The *BRCA* genes are a key component of homologous recombination. PARP proteins are crucial for DNA repair. PARP inhibitors act, in part, by providing a second hit to cells that are *BRCA*-deficient, blocking DNA repair via homologous recombination, thereby causing cell death. By targeting cells deficient in the *BRCA* gene, this treatment can more specifically target cancer cells, decreasing toxicity to the patient. There are a number of PARP (polyADP-ribose polymerase) inhibitor drugs including olaparib, (AZD2281), which received approval by the US Food and Drug Administration (FDA) in 2014 for the treatment of ovarian cancer (patients with BRCA1 and BRCA2 mutations have higher response rates than those who are BRCA patients negative) and who have earlier received treatment with 3 or more lines of chemotherapy. The PARP inhibitors show overall response up to 30% in patients with germline BRCA mutations. It is given as monotherapy in doses of 400 mg once daily.

Hyperthermic Intraperitoneal Chemotherapy

Hyperthermic Intraperitoneal Chemotherapy (HIPEC) refers to intraperitoneal administration of heated cytotoxic agents. The combination of heat and cytotoxic drugs frequently results in an increased cytotoxicity, beyond that predicted for an additive effect.[12] There is an abundance of experimental and clinical evidence that indicate that malignant cells are selectively destroyed by hyperthermia in the range of 41–43°C. HIPEC combines the pharmacokinetic advantage inherent to the intracavitary delivery of certain cytotoxic drugs, which results in regional dose intensification, with the direct cytotoxic effect of hyperthermia. Hyperthermia exhibits a selective cell-killing effect in malignant cells by itself, potentiates the cytotoxic effect of certain chemotherapy agents and enhances the tissue penetration of the administered drug effect. Delivery of HIPEC requires an apparatus that heats and circulates the chemotherapeutic solution so that a stable temperature is maintained in the peritoneal cavity during the procedure. Both an open abdomen (Coliseum) or closed abdomen technique are used, with no significant differences in efficacy proven. Different HIPEC drug regimens and dosages are currently in use. Concurrent intravenous chemotherapy administration (bidirectional chemotherapy, so-called "HIPEC plus") has been used in recent years, with the aim to further enhance the cytotoxic potential of HIPEC.

Criteria for Selection of Chemotherapeutic Agents

It is important for the agent to lack severe direct local toxicity after intraperitoneal administration. Moreover, the drug should have a well-established activity against the malignancy treated. Drugs that have to be metabolized systemically into their active form are inappropriate for intraperitoneal use. Agents like paclitaxel, cisplatin and mitomycin C have been used.

GERM CELL TUMORS

These tumors include dysgerminomas, immature teratomas, embryonal tumors and endodermal sinus (yolk sac tumors). They occur in younger age group and in contrast to epithelial tumors, they are diagnosed at an early stage. The work-up is identical to other ovarian tumors.

Estimation of beta-hCG and alpha-fetoprotein (AFP) is important in diagnosis and treatment.

Dysgerminomas are the most common of germ cell tumor, dysgerminoma presents as a bilateral tumor in 20% of cases. As an initial treatment, completion surgery with comprehensive staging is recommended in females who do not wish to maintain fertility. In a select group, (stage 1A dysgerminoma and early stage non-dysgerminoma) when patient wants to maintain fertility, a fertility sparing surgery with close follow-up is recommended.[13]

Postoperative Adjuvant Treatment

- *Stage-I dysgerminoma and stage-I grade-I immature teratoma*:
  - Observation only is recommended.
- *Stage-II to IV dysgerminoma*: 3–4 cycles of BEP regime are recommended.
- *Stage-I (grade-II to III) immature teratomas*: 3–4 cycles of BEP regime is the recommendation.
- *Stage-II to IV immature teratomas*: 3–4 cycles of BEP regime is recommended.

In all stages of embryonal or endodermal sinus tumors bleomycin, etoposide, cisplatin (BEP) regime is given as a postoperative adjuvant therapy.

Follow-up Recommendations

Patients who achieve complete response after chemotherapy should be followed-up clinically every 2–4 months. The assessment of tumor markers (AFP and β-hCG) is done on each visit for 2 years.

Sex Cord Stromal Tumor

This group includes granulosa cell tumors (most common), granulosa theca cell tumors and Sertoli-Leydig cell tumors. They all have good prognosis.

Patients diagnosed with stage–IA or IC sex cord stromal tumors, if desiring to preserve fertility should be treated with fertility sparing surgery.[14] For all other patients, comprehensive surgical staging is done. In high-risk stage-I tumors (tumor rupture or poorly differentiated histopathology), platinum-based chemotherapy can be considered. Adjuvant treatment is required in stage-II to IV tumors, 3–4 cycles of BEP regime are given postoperatively. Inhibin levels, if initially elevated, may be a useful marker in this group for follow-up.

Adjuvant BEP Regime

- Bleomycin 20 units/m^2 on day, intravenously
- Etoposide 100 mg/m^2 per day on day 1–5
- Cisplatin 20 mg/m^2 per day on day 1–5.
  The cycles are to be repeated every 3 weeks.

The 10-year survival for woman with stage-I disease is 90%, while in the advanced stages survival up to 50% is reported.

REFERENCES

1. Jelovac D, Armstrong DK. Recent progress in the diagnosis and treatment of ovarian cancer. CA Cancer J Clin. 2011;61:183-203.
2. American College of Obstetricians, Gynaeclogists. ACOG Practice Bulletin. Management of adenexal masses. Obstet Gynaecol. 2007;110:201-14.
3. Ledermann JA, Raja FA, Fotopoulou C, et al. Newly diagnosed and relapsed epithelial ovarian carcinoma. ESMO Clinical Practice Guidelines for diagnosis, treatment and follow up. Ann Onncol. 2013;(24 Suppl) 6:VI 24-32.
4. Fader AN, Rose PG, Role of surgery in ovarian carcinoma. J Clin Oncol. 2007;25:2873-83.
5. Young RC, Walton LA, Ellenburg SS, et al. Adjuvant therapy in stage I and stage II epithelial ovarian cancer. Results of two prospective randomized trials. N Engl J Med. 1990;322:1021-7.
6. Bell J, Brady MF, Young RC, et al. Randomized phase III trial of three versus six cycles of adjuvant carboplatin and paclitaxel in early stage epithelial ovarian carcinoma: a Gynaecologic Oncology Group study. Gynaecol Oncol. 2006;102:432-9.
7. Ozlos RF, Bundy BN, Greer BE, et al. Phase III trial of carboplatin and paclitaxel compared with cisplatin and paclitaxel in patients with optimally resected stage III ovarian cancer: a Gynaecologic Oncology Group Study. J Clin Oncol. 2003;21:3194-200.
8. Omano A, Torres MJ, Castells M, et al. Diagnosis and Management of drug hypersensitivity reactions. J Allergy Clin Immunol. 2011;127(3 Suppl):S67-73.
9. Fullham MJ, Carter J, Baldey A, et al. The impact of PET-CT in suspected recurrent ovarian cancer. A prospective multi-centre study as part of the Australian PET Data Collection Project. Gynaecol Oncol. 2009;112:462-8.
10. Fung-Kee-Fung M, Oliver T, Etill L, et al. Optimal chemotherapy treatment for women with recurrent ovarian cancer. Curr Oncol. 2007;14:195-208.
11. Hall M, Gourley C, McNeish I, et al. Targeted anti-vascular therapies for ovarian cancer. Br J Cancer. 2013;108:250-8.
12. Terence C Chua, Greg Robertson, Winston Liauw, et al. Intraoperative hyperthermic intraperitoneal chemotherapy after cytoreductive surgery in ovarian cancer peritoneal carcinomatosis: systematic review of current results. J of Cancer Research and Clinical Oncology. 2009;135:1637-45.
13. Lee Ih, Choi CH, Hong DG, et al. Clinicopathologic characteristics of granulose cell tumours of the ovary: a multicentre retrospective study. J Gynaecol Oncol. 2011;22:188-95.
14. Pectasides D, Pectasides E, Kassanos D. Germ cell tumours of the ovary. Cancer Treat Rev. 2008;34:427-41.

Index

Page numbers followed by *f* refer to figure and *t* refer to table.

A

Abdomen 168, 200, 332
  acute 260
  pain in
    lower 81
    upper right 81
  tenderness in lower 82
Abdominal cavity 30
Abdominal examination 164
Abdominal hysterectomy 115, 160
Abdominal mass 109
  large 34
  palpable 110
Abdominal radiograph 218
Abdominal wall sepsis 34
Abdominopelvic
  examination 216, 224
  exploration 306
  lump 109
Abortion
  medical 152
  spontaneous 45, 46, 109
  surgical 152
Abscess 23, 109
  diverticular 109
  fluctuant 83
Acanthosis nigricans 168
Acetic acid 39-42, 235, 286
  test 237*t*
Acetowhite epithelium 238
Ache, mild 81
Acid fast bacilli 89, 184
Acne 173
Acoustic shadows 22
Acquired immune deficiency
    syndrome 97
Actinomycin D 258
Activated partial thromboplastin
    time 192
Acyclical vaginal bleeding 255, 257
Adenocarcinoma 279
  in situ 248
  of endometrium 336
Adenoma malignum 279
Adenomyoma excision 135

Adenomyomectomy 26
Adenomyosis 21, 101, 106, 109, 123, 132, 133, 139, 141, 219
Adenomyotic
  deposits 135
  disease 135
  tissue 133
Adenosquamous carcinoma 279
Adherent adnexal masses 109
Adiana sterilization procedure 37
Adipocyte protein hormone 10
Adnexa 73, 153
  of ovaries 228
Adnexal cyst 218
Adnexal mass 82, 124, 216
  benign 216, 216*t*, 225
  complex 160
  complication of 227
  diagnosis of 219
  torsion of 24
Adnexal surgery 32
Adnexal tenderness 81, 82
Adnexal tumors 82
Adrenal androgen biosynthesis 180
Adrenal cortex 14
Adrenal hyperplasia, congenital 167
Adrenocorticotropic hormone 60, 179
Albicans species of Candida 75
Alcohol
  consumption 124, 266
  use of 184
Alendronate 63
Alkaline phosphatase 213
Allergy 46, 184
Alopecia 173
Alpha-fetoprotein 339
Alzheimer's disease 67
Amenorrhea 52, 103, 118, 163, 169, 170, 257
  management of secondary 168
  primary 163, 165
  prolonged 174
  secondary 163, 167, 169, 170
American Society for
    Reproductive Medicine 126

Amine test 73
Analgesia depends 39
Androgen 11, 191
  agonist 114
  biosynthesis 177
  excess, signs of 169
  insensitivity syndrome 164
  production 173
  receptors 10
  secreting tumor 167
  synthesis 178
Androgenic effect, low 52
Androstenedione 8*f*
Anemia 279
  signs of 110
Anesthesia 39
  adequate local 266
Anesthetic blocks 145
Anesthetic problems 37
Angiogenesis inhibitors 338
Angiotensin-converting enzyme 200
Anorectal angle, acute 196
Anorexia 165, 226, 297
  nervosa 163
Anovulation, chronic 173
Anovulatory bleeding 103
Anovulatory cycles 15, 185
Antenatal care 97
Antialdosterone 180
Antiandrogen 179, 180
Antiandrogenic compound 180
Antiandrogenic potential 174
Anticoagulation therapy. 34
Antimicrotubule agents 314
Anti-mullerian hormone 10, 60, 191
Antiovarian antibody 166
  testing 168
Antiprogestagenos 128
Antiprogestins 130
Antiretroviral therapy 97, 98
Antitubercular
  therapy 226
  treatment 90
Antitumor antibiotics 314
Antiviral therapy 93
Antral follicle count 184

Anus 32
Arcus tendineus
   fascia pelvis 197
   levator ani 197
Aromatase inhibitor 114
Ascites 22, 311
Ascitic fluid aspiration 300
Asherman's syndrome 34, 45, 102, 169, 183
Aspiration 84
   role of 223
Assisted reproductive techniques 152, 186, 187, 191
Atherogenic dyslipidemia 173
Atrophic endometrium 19
Atrophic stenosis of cervix 43
Atrophic vaginitis 74, 77
Ayre's spatula (wood/plastic) 40
Azithromycin 82

B

Back pain 81, 133
   low 143
Backache 279
Bacterial vaginosis 73, 77
Bacteroides 80
Baden-Walker classification 200
Baden-Walker halfway
   classification 202f
   system 201
Barium enema 280
Bartholin gland carcinoma 265
Basal cell carcinoma 265, 269
Bazedoxifene 62
   combination of 65
Beta-human chorionic
   gonadotropin 339
Bevacizumab-containing regimen 301
Biopsy 19, 75
   from pelvis, peritoneal 300
   local excision 250
   methods of 239
   wedge 239, 241
Bipolar electrosurgery 30
Bipolar electrosurgical device 32
Bipolar resectoscope
   electrosurgical system 36
Bisphosphonates 63
Bladder
   dysfunction 284
   endometriosis 124

function 205
hydrodistension 142
injury to 33, 84
mucosa 267
pillar 197
Bladder/bowel fistula 277
Bleeding 37, 43, 45, 102
   cycles 133
   irregular 257
   per vaginum
      excessive 260
      irregular 279
   prerectum 279
Bleomycin 305, 343
Blood 37
   count, complete 88, 110, 192, 228, 255, 298, 306, 310
   dyscrasias 155
   fresh 228
   in stool, occult 298
   in vagina 163
   loss myomectomy, reduction of 117
   loss, reduction of 53
   mixed discharge 279
   studies 145
   sugar 298, 310
   transfusions, multiple 284
   vessels 18
      injury to 33
Body mass index 164, 184
   low 124
Boggy uterus 133
Bone
   loss 62
   mineral density 63
   necrosis 325
Bony pelvis 196
Bowel
   abnormal 279
   disease, inflammatory 138
   dysfunction 284
   habits, regular 206
   injury 29, 284
      to small 84
   preparation 124
   syndrome, irritable 143
Brachytherapy 313, 332, 334
   delivers 332
   techniques, types of 313
Brain metastases 261
Breast 50, 67, 168
   cancer 65

disease, benign 61
examination 279
   clinical 58
feeding 155
tanner staging for 164
tenderness 180
ultrasound 60
Breath, shortness of 192
Brenner tumors 222
Bupivacaine 117
Butoconazole 76

C

Cachexia, signs 297
Calcium 64
Cancer 67
   alternate primary 219
   antigen 219
   cervix
      early 284
      new 286
      prevention of 286
   chemotherapy 182
   diagnose 300
   incidence of 67
   recurrent 284
   role in 37
   screening 44
Cancerous cells 39
Candida albicans 77
Candida glabrata 77
Candida species 73
Candida vaginitis 73
Candidiasis 78
Carbohydrate antigen 339
Carbon dioxide 28
   concentration, end-tidal 34
Carbonated drinks 143
Carcinoembryonic antigen 298
Carcinoma cervix 278, 286, 329
   stagewise treatment of 281t
   treatment of 333
   with pregnancy 285
Carcinoma *in situ* 326
Carcinoma vulva 265, 270
Cardiac arrest 33
Cardinal ligaments 197
Cardiometabolic abnormalities 173
Cardiopulmonary disease, severe 34
Cardiovascular disease 66
Catheter placement 208f
Cauliflower growth 279

Index

Ceftriaxone 82
Cell
- cycle 314
- keratinizing, large 279
- mediated immunity 88
- nonkeratinizing, large 279
- small 279
- theory, two 8
- tumors 309
  - clear 309

Cerebral metastases 258, 261
Cervical
- biopsy 39, 42
- canal 45, 160
- cancer 37, 40, 96, 96t, 236f, 237, 266, 278, 286, 334
  - classifications for 330t
- carcinoma 278, 280, 285
- conization 43
- consistency 279
- cytology 96
- fibroid 109
- glands 160
- hook 239
- infection 44
  - acute 44
- injury 45
- intraepithelial neoplasia 233, 247, 249, 252, 266, 275, 326
- laceration 46
- malignancy 39, 45
- motion tenderness 81
- polyp 106
- pregnancy 160
  - diagnosis of 160
- stenosis 37, 102, 183, 247, 282

Cervicitis 82, 245
Cervicopexy 27
Cervix 40, 41, 46, 67, 73, 123
- anatomy of 233, 234f
- barrel-shaped 160
- colposcopy of 239f, 267
- dilatation of 39, 43, 44
- growth in 42
- incompetent 282
- laceration of 43
- tear of 43
- ulcer in 42
- uteri 280
- visualized 44, 45, 46
- with swabs 42

Chemoradiation treatment 277
Chemoradiotherapy
- in carcinoma
  - cervix 329
  - vagina 325
  - vulva 319
- neoadjuvant 321

Chemosensitive malignancy 316
Chemotherapeutic agents 343
Chemotherapy 57, 184, 261, 273, 316
- complication of 311
- concomitant 315
- neoadjuvant 300, 322, 340
- prophylactic 260
- regimens
  - for high-risk patients 317
  - for low-risk patients 317
  - primary 301
- role of 272
- use of neoadjuvant 327

Chest 276
Childhood growth 164
Chlamydia 80, 183
- *trachomatis* 80, 81, 83, 142

Cholesterol 173, 177
Choriocarcinoma 257
Chromosomal abnormalities 163
Chromosome 10
Cigarette smoking 265, 266, 279
Cisplatin 305, 318, 334, 343
Clindamycin 77
Clitoris 320
Clomiphene citrate 175, 191
Clotrimazole 76
Clotting disorders 44
Coagulation test 103
Coccygeus 196, 197
Cochrane trial 128
Cognitive aging 66
Cogwheel appearance 24
Collagen 108
Colposcopic
- examination 41, 250
- of acetowhite cervix 238f
- of normal cervix 238f
- punctations 239f

Colposcopic-directed biopsy 239
Colposcopic-guided cervical biopsy 42
Colposcopy 39, 41, 75, 238, 275, 276, 280, 286
Columnar epithelium 41
Condyloma 40, 41

Condylomata lata 94
Cone biopsy 239, 241, 241f, 281, 282
- with cold knife 241f

Congenital adrenal hyperplasia 179
Conjugated equine estrogen 61, 63, 66
Constipation 109, 140, 227
- chronic 211

Contraception, recent advances in 49
Contraceptive
- gel 51
- newer emergency 55
- spray on 51, 51f
- use of barrier 84
- vaccines 56

Contralateral groin dissection 269
Contrast infusion sonography 111
Corpus luteum 9, 227, 228
- cysts 222

Corticotropin-releasing hormone 14
Cough
- breathlessness 255
- test 213

Cowden disease 290
Cribriform pattern 309
Cryotherapy 183, 245, 246
Cul-de-sac nodules 297
Culdocentesis fluid hematocrit 228
Cushing's syndrome 168
Cyclic leg pain 123
Cyclophosphamide 259
Cyproterone acetate 128, 179, 180
Cyst
- aspiration 26
- benign 228
- follicular 222
- functional 219, 228
- malignant 219
- simple 23, 217
- symptomatic 220

Cystectomy 26, 131
Cystic anechoic 21
Cystic spaces 21
Cystic teratoma, benign 220, 228
Cystourethroscopy 267
Cytokines, overproduction of 124
Cytomegalovirus 80
Cytoreductive surgery 304
Cytotrophoblast, clusters of 257

D

Dacron swabs 267
Danazol 147
Danazol-loaded intrauterine devices 135
Davydov vaginoplasty 166
Debulking surgery 300
Decidual cyst 153
Decubitus ulcer 200
    biopsy 206
Dehydroepiandrosterone 177
    sulfate 58, 60, 165, 174, 178
    supplementation 191
Delancey's biomechanical levels 199f
Delancey's classification 200
Denonvillier's fascia 197
Denosumab 64
Dense acetowhite epithelium 238
Dense adhesions 126, 126f, 311
Deoxyribonucleic acid 235, 265
Depot medroxyprogesterone acetate 62, 105
Depression 140, 173
    clozapine, treatment of 67
Dermal papilla, superficial 267
Dermoid cyst 22, 23, 30, 218, 220, 222, 223, 227, 228
Destructive stromal invasion 310
Dexamethasone 318
Diabetes mellitus 106, 175
Diarrhea 140, 227
Diffuse disease 132
Dihydrotestosterone 178
Discharge, nature of 73
Dispersive electrode 30
Disposable shielded trocars 30
Diverticulitis, acute 226
Docetaxel 301, 341
Dopamine agonists 169
Drug
    history 102
    reactions 334
    resistance 315
        phenotype, multiple 315
    resistant chemotherapy 260
    use of illicit 184
Dysmenorrhea 108, 110, 133, 140, 147, 224
    reduction of 53
Dyspareunia 108, 133, 140, 224, 272
Dysplasia 233
    mild 251
    moderate 252
    severe 251
Dysuria 140, 224

E

Eating disorder 164
Eccentric endometrial cavity 134
Echogenic endometrium, thick 24
Echogenic material 24
Echogenicity 19
Ectocervical lesion 245
Ectopic endometrial
    cells 124
    tissue 124
        hormonal dependence of 128
Ectopic mass 155
    size of 155
Ectopic pregnancy 24, 151, 152t, 153, 153t, 157, 158, 159
    classification of 151f
    linear salpingotomy 26
    nontubal 158
    previous 152
    sequelae of 152
Edema of
    legs 297
    lower limbs 279
Eflornithine 180
Ejaculation dysfunction 47
Electrical energy sources 30
Electrosurgical
    energy 32
    injury 31
    resources 30
Electrothermal injury 31
Embryo 185
    implantation 184
Embryonal tumor 305
Embryonic pharynx 5
Emotional disturbances 14
Endocervical
    brush device 40
    canal 282
    carcinoma 44
    curettage 42, 241, 248
    smear 75
    speculum 239
Endocervix 40
Endocrinological functions 14

Endocrinology
    of endometrium 11
    of menstruation 3
Endodermal sinus tumor 305
Endometria 18
Endometrial
    ablation 135
    adenocarcinoma 20
    biopsy 39, 44, 142, 169
        catheter 45
        specimens 88
    cancer 173, 289, 294, 295
        staging of 291
    carcinoma 37, 289, 290, 292, 336-338
        treatment of 336
    cavity 18, 35, 36, 37, 153
    cells 124
    curettage 154, 167
    dating 44
    factor 183
    glands 123, 140
    hyperplasia 19, 20, 44, 174, 290
    intraepithelial carcinoma 290
    layer 21
    polyp 19, 34, 109, 183, 185
    tissue 125
    tuberculosis 44
Endometrioid carcinoma, pure 292
Endometrioid tumors 309
Endometrioma 23, 30, 125, 141, 218, 223, 228, 310
    drainage 141
    surgical management of 130
Endometriosis 26, 32, 82, 108, 109, 123, 126, 131, 139-141, 183, 219
    associated pain 131
    component, deep 130
    diagnosis of deep 124
    fertility index 126
    medical management of 129t
    related pain, medical management of 128
    staging of 126
    surgery, prevention in 131
Endometriotic cells 124
Endometriotic lesion
    ablations 147
Endometrium 11, 18, 67, 108
    develops 18
    myometrium border 20
Endometroid 279

Endopelvic
  connective tissue, deep 196
  fascia, deep 197, 198f
Endosalpingiosis 139, 141
Endoscopic specimen 30
Endoscopy 26
  in gynecology 26
Endothelial cell 13
Enseal tissue sealing 31
Environmental hazards 184
Epinephrine 117
Epithelial tumors 298
Epithelium
  abnormal 266
  normal 266
Erythrocyte sedimentation rate 88
Essure sterilization procedure 36
Estradiol 4, 6, 8f, 11
  early intervention trial with 68
  late intervention trial with 68
Estrogen 4, 9
  breakthrough bleeding 13
  combined with estrogen
    agonist/antagonist 61
  deficiency 167
  dependent tumor 61
  increased production of 124
  levels of 103, 336
  receptor
    antagonist 114
    modulators 290
  therapy, local 65
  topical 277
  treatment, local 65
  vaginal cream 65
  withdrawal bleeding 13
Estrogen-progestin contraceptives 104
Ethambutol 90
Ethylene vinyl acetate 49
European Society of Human
    Reproduction and
    Embryology 123
Exfoliative cytology 267
Exogenous gonadotropins 175, 187
Extrafascial hysterectomy 282
Extraovarian masses, benign 24
Extraperitoneal
  insufflation of gas 33
  pelvic lymphadenectomy 269

F

Fallopian tube 28, 54f, 80, 124, 142, 158, 293, 302
  dilated 160
  diseased contralateral 158
Fascia lata 268
Fatty degenerations 109
Febrile illness 284
Fecal incontinence 272
Federation of Gynecology and
    Obstetrics 316
Female
  genital
    tract 86, 265, 275
    tuberculosis 90
  infertility 182
  reproductive system 80
  sterilization 54
Femoral
  hernia 272
  lymph nodes 267
  nerve injury 272
  node
    deep 268
    group 268
    metastases to 268
  vessels 268
Fertility
  cryopreservation 186
  desirous of 119
  prognosis 90
  sparing 329, 331
  surgery 282, 331
Fertilization, facilitate 46
Fetal cardiac activity 155
Fetal growth restriction 110
Fever 81
  low grade 226
Fibroid 19, 20, 109, 120, 183
  growth 109
  polyp 108
  presence of 61
  symptomatic 111, 116, 118
  types of 110
  uterus 108
    medical therapy of 113t
    signs of 109t
    symptoms of 109t
Fibromas 223

Fibromuscular portion of uterus, lower 233
Fibromyalgia 143
Fibronectin 108
Fibroplant 54
Fibrothecoma 23
Fluconazole 76, 78
Fluid management 193
Fluorouracil chemotherapy 322
Flutamide 179, 180
Folinic acid 258, 316
Follicle 227
  number criteria 22
  peripheral location of 23
Follicle-stimulating hormone 4, 5, 60, 103, 142, 173, 182, 187
Follicular stimulating hormone 165
Follistatin 10
Food and Drug Administration 61, 342
Fragility fracture 62
Fundal submucosal myoma, large 108

G

Gabapentin 62
Galactorrhea 103, 164, 168, 184
Gallbladder disease 61
Gardnerella vaginalis 80
Gas
  bubbles 37
  embolism 33, 34
Gaseous medium 35
Gastric 22
  surgery 27
Gastroesophageal reflux 33
Gastrointestinal
  causes 143
  evaluation 310
    by endoscopy 298
  tract 86
Gastrostomy tube 301
Gelatin-thrombin matrix 117
Genetic
  mutations 166
  screening 298
  role of 291
Genital symptoms, recurrent 93

Genital tract
    cancers 233
    infection, lower 46
    lower 257
    malignancy of 74
Genital tuberculosis 86, 88, 152, 219, 221, 226, 228
    endoscopy in 89, 90
Genital warts 94, 94t, 249
Genitourinary syndrome of menopause 64
Germ cell
    cancer 304
    ovarian cancer 305
    tumor 219, 298, 305, 343
        classification of 220t
        malignant 305
Gestational trophoblastic 316
    disease 254, 262
    neoplasia 254, 262, 316, 317
        chemotherapy in 316
        management of 254, 258
        persistent 256
        stages of 262t
Gestrinone 130
Glandular
    atypia 20
    cells 12
    epithelial cell 242
Glass echogenicity 124
Glucocorticoid 11
    receptors 10
Glucose tolerance, impaired 175
Glycine 35
Glycosylated hemoglobin 174
Gonadal biopsy 27
Gonadoblastoma 220
Gonadotropin 5, 11, 185, 187, 191
    high-dose 188
    levels 168
    regulation of 6
    releasing hormone 3, 141, 169, 187, 189f, 191, 193
        agonist protocol 188f
        stimulation protocol 189
Gonorrhoea 152
Gram-negative facultative bacteria 142
Granulosa cell 8
    interaction 8f
    tumors 344
Groin dissection, omission of 269
Groin lymphadenopathy 266
Groin nodes, multiple positive 269
Ground glass' appearance 24
Grounding pad 30
Growth hormone 14
Gynaefix 54
Gynecologic endoscopic 26
Gynecologic oncology group 320, 338
Gynecological
    cancer 65
    causes 140
    oncology 254
    symptoms 123
Gynecology, ultrasonography in 17
Gyrus plasma kinetic tissue management system 32

H

Haemophilus influenzae 80
Harmonic blade oscillates 31
Harmonic scalpel 31
Hasson technique 29
hCG vaccine 56
Headache 180, 255, 258
    symptoms of 164
Health service 98
Hearing loss, symptoms of 164
Hematocervix 221
Hematochezia 140
Hematocolpos 221
Hematogenous spread 86, 87, 267
Hematoma 118
Hematometra 221
    postsurgical 43
Hematosalpinx 217, 221
Hematuria 140
Hemivulvectomy
    anterior 268
    posterior 268
    with clitoral sparing, lateral 268
Hemodynamically unstable patient 34
Hemoglobin 205
    level 334
Hemogram 152
Hemogram-hemoglobin 102
Hemoperitoneum 255, 260
Hemoptysis 255
Hemorrhage 46, 108, 247, 280, 284
    post-partum 110, 120

Hemorrhagic corpus luteum cyst 23
Hemorrhagic cyst 22, 23, 222
Hemorrhagic ovarian cyst 217
Hemostasis 33
    system 31
Hepatic
    artery occlusion 261
    bleeding 261
    dysfunction 316
Hepatosplenomegaly 27
Herbal remedies 62
Hereditary nonpolyposis colon cancer 290
Herpes simplex virus 92
    in gynecology 93t
    specific glycoprotein 93
Heterogeneity 23
Heterogeneous 19, 23
    myometrium 21
Heterogenicity 20
Heterotopic
    endometrium 134
    pregnancy 25, 155
Hingorani sign 217
Hirsutism 169, 173, 174, 177, 184
    causes of 178, 178t
Homogeneous 19
    solid masses 23
Hormonal
    assays 179
    causes 183
    changes 58
    changes in menstrual cycle 7f
    injectable contraceptives 52
    methods 49
    sensors 10
    therapy 44, 338
        standard 61
    treatment 44
Hormone 14, 103
    analysis 60
    replacement therapy 165, 166, 214, 290
    secreted, levels of 170
    therapy 60, 67
Hot flashes, treatment of 67
Human chorionic gonadotropin 24, 102, 154, 187, 191
Human immunodeficiency virus 80, 97, 98
    infection 77
    positive patients 76

Human papilloma virus 94, 97, 235, 248, 265, 275, 278, 326, 331
　infection 235
　vaccines 286*t*
Human papillomavirus
　tests 96*t*
　types of 96*t*
Human placental lactogen 258
Human service 98
Hydatidiform mole 254, 257
　complete 25
Hydronephrosis 279
Hydroprotection 33
Hydrosalpinx 24, 217, 310
Hydroxy progesterone 179
Hydroxyethyl starch 193
Hygiene, poor perineal 278
Hymen
　imperforate 221
　on anterior wall 202*f*
　on posterior wall 203*f*
Hyperammonemia 35
Hyperandrogenic symptoms 168
Hyperandrogenism 172, 173, 175
　symptoms of 167
Hypercalcemia 109
Hyperechoic
　central stroma 23
　nodule 218
Hypergonadotropic hypogonadism 168
Hyperinsulinemia 173
Hyperkalemia 180
Hyperosmolar glucose 155
Hyperplasia 101, 109, 217
Hyperplastic
　myometrium 132
　reaction 21
　trophoblastic cells 257
Hyperprogestogenism 13
Hyperprolactenemia 15, 103, 169, 182
Hypertension, portal 27
Hyperthermic intraperitoneal chemotherapy 343
Hyperthyroidism 106
Hypoechoic inner functional layer 18
Hypoechoic mass 24, 218
Hypogonadotropic hypogonadism 165
Hyponatremia 34

Hypopituitarism 163
Hypotension cardiac arrhythmias 33
Hypothalamic
　amenorrhea 169
　disorder 183
　dysfunction 167
　hypogonadism 4
　production, absent 163
Hypothalamic-pituitary 6
　disease, symptoms of 167
　ovarian axis 10
Hypothalamus 3, 11, 14, 15, 182
　secretes 3
Hypothyroidism 15
Hypoventilation 33
Hysterectomy 108, 112, 136, 248, 294
　clamps 282
　emergency 260
　for endometriosis-associated pain 131
　number of 57
　primary 331
　total 292
Hysterography, abnormal 34
Hysteron-salpingogram 185
Hysteropexy 32
Hysterosalpingogram 36
Hysterosalpingography 89
Hysteroscopic morcellation systems 36
Hysteroscopic morcellator 36
Hysteroscopic myomectomy 115
Hysteroscopic sterilization 34, 36
Hysteroscopy 103
　diagnostic 34
　technique of 34

I

Iliac bifurcation, common 283
Iliac group, external 268, 283
Iliococcygeus 196
Immature squamous epithelium 40
Immune
　mechanism, defective 124
　status, low 278
Immunological deficiencies 142
In vitro fertilization 25, 47, 185, 187
Indocyanine green 294
Infection 37

Infertility 27, 47, 131, 133
　age-related 182
　care, seeking 182
　cases of 46
　causes of 182
　duration of 184
　evaluation for 44
　history of 152
　primary 183
　secondary 183
　treatment modalities for 185
　unexplained 34, 185
Infiltrative disease, deep 125
Inflammatory chemokines 12
Inflammatory masses 223, 225, 226
Infundibulopelvic ligament 142
Infusion pump 35
Inguinal ligament 268
Inguinal lymph node 268
　metastasis 268
Inguinofemoral lymph node 268, 270
　ulcerated 267
Inguinofemoral lymphadenectomy 270
　bilateral 268, 271
Inguinofemoral nodes 269
Injectable progestins 105
Insemination, artificial 46
Insulation failure 31
Insulin action, disordered 173
Insulin resistance, reduce 169
Insulin-like growth factor 14
Intensity-modulated
　radiation therapy 342
　radiotherapy 313, 332
Intercourse
　early 40
　pain during 81
　younger age at 278
Interferon gamma 88
　release assays 88
Intermenstrual bleeding 102
International Federation of Gynecology and Obstetrics 101, 280, 325, 329, 336
International ovarian tumor analysis 21
Interstitial brachytherapy 314
Interstitial cystitis 142
　prevalence of 142
Interstitial line sign 159
Interstitial portion 158

Interstitial pregnancy 158, 159
Interstitial therapy 277
Interval debulking surgery 300
Intestinal
　obstruction 83, 301
　stents 301
　vaginoplasty 166
Intestine, injury to 33
Intimate partner violence 144
Intra-abdominal pathology 117
Intracavitary brachytherapy
　application 332
Intracavitary radiation therapy 326
Intracavitary radiotherapeutic
　procedure 43
Intracavitary radiotherapy 314
Intracellular proteins 40
Intracranial pressure 255
Intramural, large 109
Intramuscular regimen 82
Intramuscular treatment 82
Intraperitoneal chemotherapy 340
Intrathecal methotrexate 261
Intrauterine
　adhesions 45
　contraceptive device 53, 159
　device 152
　disease 317
　growth 45
　insemination 39, 46, 185
　pregnancy 155, 157
　　advanced 34
Intravaginal chemotherapy 326
Intravaginal estradiol tablets 65
Intravenom pyelogram 75, 280, 329
Intravenous pyelography 267
Intrinsic sphincteric deficiency 211
Invasive cancer 41
Invasive carcinoma 40
　on cytology 41
Invasive disease 128
Ipsilateral nodal involvement 268
Ipsilateral salpingectomy 158
Ipsilateral superficial
　inguinofemoral lymph
　nodes 319
Ischemic heart disease 34
Isosulfan blue dye 270
Isotonic electrolyte 35
Itch-scratch cycle 265

J

Jadelle 52
Jeffcot's classification 200

K

Kallmann syndrome,
　cases of 164
Karman's cannula 291
Keyes punch 266f
Keyes punch biopsy 266
Kidney function test 192, 255
Kisspeptin 4
Koh smear 73

L

Labia 123
　majora 319
　minora 319
　　anterior 268
Labor 206
　preterm 110, 248
Lactate dehydrogenase 298, 305
Laparoscopic
　adhesiolysis 147
　appendectomy 147
　cannulas 30
　cystectomy 185, 221, 229
　endometriosis excision 147
　endoscopic single-site surgery 32
　grading of salpingitis 84
　hysterectomy 26, 115
　instruments 29
　lateral retroperitoneal 119
　myolysis 118
　myomectomy 116
　pelvic lymphadenectomy 282
　power morcellation 33
　salpingostomy 158
　surgery 28, 128
　　single incision 32
　trocar 30
　uterine
　　artery 119
　　nerve ablation 147
　uterosacral nerve ablation 27
　vaginoplasty 27
　Vecchietti procedure 166
Laparoscopic-assisted vaginal
　hysterectomy 26

Laparoscopy 26, 90
　indications of 26
　role of 84, 221, 226
　surgical technique of 27
Laser ablation 246
Laser energy 32
Laser energy source 30
Laser therapy 326
Leiomyoma 20, 101, 108, 224
Leiomyosarcomas 108, 120
Leptin 4, 10
Lesions
　atypical 125
　location of 250
　number of 250
　vulvoscopy for 267
Leukocyte count, total 205
Leukocytosis 227
Leukoplakia 40, 41
Leukorrhea 74, 78, 200
Leuprolide acetate 187
　microdose of 188
Leuprolide therapy 189
Levator ani 197
Levator plate 196
Levofloxacin 83
Levonorgestrel intrauterine
　device 129, 294
　system 147
Levonorgestrel releasing
　intrauterine device 128, 135, 175
Libido, loss of 180
Lichen sclerosus 265, 266
Life-threatening diseases 186
Ligament
　broad 43
　fibroid 109, 224
Lip
　anterior 46
　of cervix, anterior 44, 46
Lipoprotein
　high-density 173
　low-density 173
Liquid-based cytology 286
Lithotomy position 44
Liver
　acute 61
　cirrhosis 219
　disease, chronic 61
　dysfunction 341
　　transient 157

enlargement 255
function test 192, 298, 310
metastases 258, 261
Loop biopsy 239, 241
Loop electrosurgical excision procedure 246, 250
Lugol's iodine 41, 286
application of 42
visual inspection with 39, 235
Lugol's negative areas 41, 42
Lung 86
metastases 255, 261
Luteinizing hormone 4, 6, 58, 103, 131, 165, 173, 178
Luteinizing hormone-releasing hormone 3
Lymph node 86, 267, 270, 283, 284
assessment 310
detection, sentinel 284
dissection 270, 271
deep groin 320
enlarged 292
lateral group of 283
obturator chains of 283
positive inguinofemoral 271
procedure, sentinel 270
regional 330
sentinel 294
status 272
Lymphadenectomy 268, 269, 284, 319
unilateral 269
Lymphadenopathy 279
Lymphatic drainage 268
Lymphatic metastasis 267
Lymphatic spread 267
Lymphatics of vulva 268
Lymphedema, chronic 272
Lymphocyst formation 272, 284
Lymphoma 22, 279
Lymphoscintigraphy 270
Lymphovascular invasion 319
Lymphovascular space 268, 281, 282, 293, 329, 336
Lynch syndrome 290

M

Magestrol 294
Maintenance therapy 76
Malaise 226
Male contraceptive, newer 55
Malecot's catheter. 77
Malpas classification 200
Manchester repair 43
Mannitol 318
Mantoux test 88
Marriage, early 40
Masses, enlarging 220
Mastalgia 180
Matrix metalloproteinase 13
Mature teratoma 23
McCall culdoplasty 207
McIndoe vaginoplasty 166
Media delivering system 35
Medroxyprogesterone 66, 294
acetate 63, 105, 128, 129, 146, 338
Megavoltage radiotherapy 271
Meigs syndrome 222, 223
Melanoma, malignant 279
Menarche, early 124
Menopausal hormone therapy 60, 61, 63
Menopause 57
hormone therapy 68
late 124
Menstrual
abnormalities 97
bleeding 104t, 108, 133
abnormal 81
heavy 101, 102, 106
blood loss 135
cycle 11, 144
endocrine regulation of 5f
disorders 142
history 39, 102, 110, 184
irregularity 173, 180
cause of 167
parameters 14
periods, irregular 81
Menstruation 12, 18
factors affecting 14
reflux 124
Mesenchymal tumors 336
Metabolic activities 311
Metabolism in women 177
Metallic cannula 46
Metastasis in endometrial cancer, management of 295
Metastasis, management of 261
Metastasis, symptoms to 255
Metastatic disease 270, 331
Metastatic gestational trophoblastic neoplasi 258
management of high-risk 259
Metastatic lesion 255
Metastatic tumors to ovary 22
Methotrexate 26
dosage of 156
folinic acid 258
single dose 152
treatment protocol, multiple-dose 156t
Metronidazole 75-77, 78
gel, role of 75
Microcolpohysteroscope 37
Microinvasive disease 329
Midvaginal support 199
Migraine 61
Mirena 53, 53f
Mitochondrial disorders 186
Mitotic activity, increased 310
Molar evacuation 254
Molar pregnancy 25
Molecular testing 75
Molluscum contagiosum 94, 97, 97t
Monodermal teratoma 220
Monopolar electrical energy 30, 35
Mortality, low primary 321
Moxifloxacin 83
Mucinous cystadenoma 23, 218
Mucinous ovarian tumors 222
Mucinous tumor 301
Müllerian agenesis 163
Mullerian anomalies 27, 45
obstructive 219, 221
Mullerian fusion, anomalies of 183
Mullerian tumor, malignant mixed 306
Multidose methotrexate 152
Multidose regime better 76
Multilocular cysts 228
Muscle 196, 200
Musculoskeletal problems 143
Mycobacterium bovis 86
Mycobacterium tuberculosis 86, 88, 89
Mycoplasma genitalium 142
Mycoplasma hominis 80, 183
Myelosuppression 341
Myofascial pain 143
Myolysis 118
Myomectomy 32, 33, 108, 112, 115, 119, 185
abdominal 116
Myometrial reduction 135
Myometrium 18, 21, 25, 267

N

Nab paclitaxel 341
National Comprehensive Cancer Network 339
National Institute of Health 172
Natural orifice transluminal endoscopic surgery 32
Natural orifice transumbilical surgery 32
Nausea 81, 180, 258
Neisseria gonorrhoeae 75, 78, 80, 81, 83, 142, 183
Neoplasm
 benign 218
 malignant 275
Neoplastic cells 252
Neoplastic epithelial disorders 251
Nerve, injury to 284
Nerve-sparing radical hysterectomy 283
Neuroblastoma 219
Neuroendocrine 182
 carcinoma 279
Neurologic disorders 212
Neurological signs 255
Neurolytic therapy 146
Neuromatrix theory 139
Neuropathy, peripheral 341
Nitrous oxide 28
Nocturia 140
Node treatment, regional 276
Nodular lesions 279
Nonclotting blood, aspiration of 154
Noncontraceptive benefits 50
Noncyclical pelvic pain 123
Nonfertility sparing 331
Nonhormonal medications 62
Nonhormonal therapy 65
Noninfectious causes 183
Nonplatinum combination chemotherapy 334
Nonsteroidal androgen receptor antagonist 180
Nonsteroidal anti-inflammatory drug 105, 128, 141, 143, 146, 192
Norethindrone 54
 acetate 129
Norethisterone 128
 acetate 105
Norplant 51, 51*f*
Nuclear atypia 310
 mild 310
Nucleic-acid amplification testing 80
Nucleoproteins 40
Nulliparity 124
Nulliparous women 306
Nutrition
 improvement of 206
 poor 164
Nutritional deficiencies 279
NuvaRing 49*f*
Nystatin 76

O

Obesity 14, 173, 182, 206
 gross 34
Obstetric complication 109
Obstetric history infertility 110
Obstetrical bleeding, severe 167
Obstructive intestinal disease 34
Obstructive pulmonary disease, chronic 200
Ofloxacin 83
Oily sebaceous fluid 228
Oligomenorrhea 15, 169
Oocyte 185
 donation 166
 nuclear transfer 186
Oophorectomy 26, 142, 220
Open laparoscopy 29
Operative hysteroscope 35
Optical fibers 29
Oral
 agent 76
 antimicrobial therapy 82
 cancer 67
 contraceptive 128, 129, 146, 255
  combined 104
  pill 54, 102, 278
  pills, combined 113, 174, 179
 estrogen 66
 mebendazole 77
 progestins 129
  high dose 105
 regimens 82
  alternative 82
 temperature 81
 treatment 82
Organ prolapse 319
Organ sign, negative sliding 160, 161
Osteitis pubis 272
Osteopenia 63
Osteoporosis 63
 fracture 62
Outwardly convex borders 22

Ovarian biopsy 26, 166
Ovarian cancer 297, 298, 302-304
 advanced 298
 epithelial 304
 chemotherapy for 303, 339
 during pregnancy 306
 epithelial 297, 298, 304, 341
Ovarian cyst 139, 225
 adenofibroma 218
 aspiration of 223
 benign 22, 23
 functional 222, 227
 management of 226
 torsion 310
Ovarian cystectomies 57
Ovarian damage 277
Ovarian disease 167
Ovarian drilling 26, 57
Ovarian endometrioma 124
 diagnosis of 124
 in women, diagnosis of 124
Ovarian failure 118
Ovarian fibromas 23
Ovarian fibrothecoma 23
Ovarian hyperstimulation syndrome 187, 189, 191-193
Ovarian hyperthecosis 178
Ovarian insufficiency 182
Ovarian lesions on ultrasonography, malignant 22
Ovarian malignancy 306, 339
Ovarian mass 21, 225
 management of 223
Ovarian metastasis from breast 22
Ovarian pregnancy 159
 diagnosis of 159
Ovarian regulatory proteins 9, 9*f*
Ovarian remnant syndrome 139, 142
Ovarian reserve estimation 184
Ovarian steroid hormones 133
Ovarian steroidogenesis 174
Ovarian stimulation protocols 187
Ovarian surgery 26, 184
Ovarian tissue 159
Ovarian torsion 218
Ovarian tumor 109, 219, 221, 225, 228, 310
 benign 222
 borderline 309
 cases of 164
 classification of 309
 epithelial 340
 treatment of epithelial 339

Ovariotomy 26
Ovary 160
　bilateral enlarged 255
　mobilizing 130
　syndrome, residual 139, 142
Ovulatory dysfunction 101, 173, 182

P

Paclitaxel 318, 334, 341
Pain
　abdomen 297
　abdominal 155
　lower abdominal 297, 309
　pathway 140*f*
　perception, reduces 147
　reduction of 53
　relief with bowel movement 140
Painful induration 124
Painful urination 81
Painless vaginal 160
Palliative surgery 273
Palmer's point 27
Pancreatitis, acute 219
Panoramic 37
Pap smear 75, 103, 237, 267, 276, 286, 298, 310
　abnormal 184, 249
　conventional 286
Pap's test 39
　conventional 39
Papillary
　carcinoma 279
　structures 124
Para-aortic lymph node dissection 300
Para-aortic lymphadenectomy 292
Paracervical space 284
Paralytic ileus 34
Parametrial fibrosis 82
Parametrium 197
　excision of 284
Paraovarian cyst 24, 218, 224, 310
　excision of 26
Pararectal space 142
Parathyroid hormone 64, 109
Parenteral regimen, alternative 83
Parietal fascia 198*f*
　pelvic 196, 197
Pedunculated fibroids 23
Pelvic
　abscess 310
　　drainage of 83
　　midline 83
　　ruptured 83
　adhesiolysis 27
　adhesion 139, 183
　blood vessels 257
　bone 267
　cellulitis 43
　chemotherapy 57
　chronic 144
　congestion syndrome 139, 142
　discomfort 200
　examination 73, 145, 164, 213, 216, 255, 279
　　bimanual 44, 110, 276
　exenteration 271, 277, 284
　floor
　　anatomy 196
　　exercise 206
　　muscles 197*f*
　　musculature 144
　　myofascial syndrome 138
　infection 37
　　Chlamydia 152
　　chronic 139
　inflammatory disease 45, 80, 98, 102, 141, 182, 183, 184, 245
　　acute 44
　　complication of 217
　　prevention 84
　inflammatory disorder 80
　　acute 81
　　chronic 81
　irradiation 273
　kidney 109, 310
　lymph node 267, 283
　　removed 300
　lymphadenectomy 32, 282, 283
　　bilateral 277
　　routine 269
　lymphadenopathy 27
　mass
　　persistent 142
　　suspicious 299
　nerve pathways 131
　neuropathy 138
　nodal dissection 292
　node 268
　　bilateral 319
　　involvement 268
　　management of 269
　organ dysfunction 200
　organ prolapse 196, 198, 201, 207
　　causes of 199
　　classifications for 200
　organs 196*t*
　organs-hysterectomy 147
　pain 141, 142
　　acute 108
　　after hysterectomy 142
　　cause of chronic 139*t*
　　chronic 133, 138, 141, 146, 224, 279
　　cyclical 123
　　hormonal treatment of chronic 148
　　scale instructions 144*t*
　pathology 267
　peritoneum 123
　persistent 142
　pressure symptoms 109
　radiation 184
　　therapy 211
　　with brachytherapy 331
　recurrence, central 281
　relaxation 319
　surgery 131, 206, 211
　symptoms 123
　ultrasound 60, 103
　venography 142
　venous congestion 142
　wall 276
Pelvis 297
　frozen 224
　inflammatory disease 297
　sonography 311
Peptic ulcer disease, active 155
Percutaneous drainage 84
Percutaneous fluoroscopic 117
Perimenopausal
　period 175
　women, mildly symptomatic 119
Perimenopause 175
Perineal body 197, 320
Perineal fascia, deep 269
Peritoneal cavity 24, 27, 28, 30
Peritoneal cells, metaplasia of 124
Peritoneal cyst 310
Peritonitis 43, 260
Periumbilical adhesions 27
Periurethral surgery 211
Per-rectal examination 204
Per-speculum examination 276
Pheniramine 318

Phimotic fimbrial end,
 dilatation of 26
Phytoestrogens 67
Pinworms 77
Piriformis 197
Pituitary disease 167
Pituitary disorder 183
Pituitary gland 3, 5
 anterior 15
Pituitary hormones 3
Plasma kinetic energy 32
Platinum complexes 314
Platinum sensitive disease 304
Platinum-resistant disease 304
Pleural effusion 255
Plus doxycycline 82
Podophyllotoxin 95
Polycystic ovary 22, 169
 morphology 172-174
 syndrome 8, 103, 167, 169, 172, 172t, 173, 175, 178, 182, 185
Polycythemia 109
Polydipsia 164
Polyethylene fibers 36
 terephthalate 55
Polygenic disorder 173
Polyglutamates 26
Polymerase chain reaction 89, 93, 184
Polymeric sleeve 30
Polymorphonuclear leukocytes 142
Polypoid tumors 20
Polyuria 164
Postcoital bleeding 279
Postcoital test 184
Postexposure prophylaxis 98
Posthysterectomy pain 139
Postmenopausal 44, 266
 age group 225, 289
 bleeding 44, 279
 endometrium 19
 ovarian cysts 226
 vulvovaginal atrophy 64
 women 265
 causes in, causes in 225t
Postpartum
 and postabortal period 103
 intrauterine contraceptive device 55
Potassium chloride 26, 155
Potassium-titanyl-phosphate 32
Potential tumors, low malignant 301, 309

Pregnancy 37, 44-46, 109, 120, 211, 219, 242
 abdominal 160
 advice on future 261
 cervical 160
 chronic ectopic 224
 early termination of 43
 history 184
 loss 110
 might facilitate 133
 ovarian 159
 primary abdominal 160
 red degeneration in 108
 teenage 278
 test 192
 tubal ectopic 153
 unruptured tubal 155
Pregnant
 uterus, enlargement of 132
 women 77
Prehysterectomy 44
Preimplantation genetic testing 186
Premature menopause 277
Premature ovarian insufficiency 57, 60
Premenopausal 44, 266
 woman 124, 219
Premenstrual molimina 182
Prenatal diagnostic techniques 17
Prepubertal age group 219
Prepubertal girls 78
Presacral neurectomy 27
Pressure-sensor-equipped Veress needle 29
Primary cause, treatment of 103
Primary ovarian insufficiency 61
Primary screening test 96
Proctitis 277
Progesterone 4, 6, 11, 113, 179
 breakthrough bleeding 13
 challenge test 168
 receptor antagonist 114
 resistance to 124
 secretion 15
 vaginal ring 50f
 withdrawal bleeding 13
Progestin nestorone 51
Progestin-only contraceptive pills 175
Progestogen 66
Prolactin disorder 183
Proliferative phase, division of 12t
Prophylactic antibiotic 46

Prostaglandins 12
Proteoglycan 108
Prothrombin time 103
Psammoma bodies 309
Pseudogestational sac 153
Pseudo-Meigs syndrome 109
Psychological therapy 143
Psychosexual complications 272
Puberty, constitutional delay of 165
Pubic osteomyelitis 272
Pubocervical
 fascia 282
 ligaments 197
 septum 197
Puborectalis muscle 197f
Puerperium 206
Pulmonary
 arterial occlusion 255
 disease 155
 edema 35
 embolism 272, 284
 metastases 258, 261
 wedge resection 261
Punch biopsy 42, 239, 241, 266
 forceps 239
Purified protein derivative 88
Purplish red nodule 255
Pyometra with carcinoma cervix 285
Pyosalpinx 24, 217, 310
Pyrazinamide 90

Q

Quantiferon test 88
Quantiferon-TB gold in-tube test 88
Quiescent gestational trophoblastic disease 262

R

Radiation cystitis 277
Radiation therapy, role of 320
Radical hysterectomy 26, 32, 212, 282, 283
 complications of 284
Radical lymphadenectomy 319
Radical trachelectomy 282
Radical vulvectomy 268, 269, 271, 320
Ranitidine 318
Rectal examination 283
 bimanual 276

Rectal mucosa 267, 276
Rectal strictures 277
Rectovaginal, bidigital 204
Rectocele 272
Rectovaginal endometriosis 124
Rectovaginal fistula 272
Rectovaginal septum 197
Rectum 325
Rectus fascia 27
Reductase inhibitors 180
Reid colposcopy index 239
Renal
    failure 106, 279
    function test 298, 310
    toxicity 341
Reproductive age 18t, 221
    group, causes in 221t
    woman 101
Reproductive tract
    anomalies 124
    normal 165
Respiratory
    conditions, chronic 196
    discomfort 109
    distress 260
    pathogens 78
Retroperitoneal vessel injury 29
Rifampicin 90
Rising hematocrit 192
Robotic radical trachelectomy 282
Robotic surgery 32
Robotic-assisted laparoscopy 117
Robotic-assisted surgery 33

S

Sacrocolpopexy 32
Saline infusion
    sonography 103
    sonohysterography 21
Saline, normal 35
Salpingectomy 158
Salpingitis isthmica nodosa 183
Salpingo-oophorectomy 26
    bilateral 292, 298, 337
    prophylactic 298
    protocol 300
Salpingostomy 26, 158
Salvage chemotherapy 315
Sampson's transplantation
    theory 124
Saphenofemoral junction 269
Scar pregnancy, previous 161
Scar rupture 120

Second line drugs 104
Sensation 200
Sepsis 280
Septic shock 84
Serological tests 93
Serotonin reuptake inhibitor 143
Serous cystadenoma 23, 218, 222
Serous, low-grade 342
Sertoli-Leydig cell tumors 344
Serum
    creatinine 205
    dheas 179
    electrolytes 192
    estradiol 184
    human epididymis protein 342
    insulin measurement 169
    level 168
    plateauing of 257
    pooled prolactin levels 67
    progesterone 174, 184
        level 154
    prolactin 103
        level 179
    testosterone 103
    tumor markers 305
Sex cord stromal tumor 305, 344
Sex hormone-binding globulin
    173, 174, 178
Sex-cord stromal tumor 305
Sexual activity 250
    resumption of 277
Sexual assault
    past 144
    present 144
Sexual characteristics, poor 165
Sexual characters, secondary 164
Sexual dysfunction 47, 140, 184, 200
    persistent 182
Sexual exposure 164
Sexual intercourse, painful 81
Sexual partners, multiple 40, 278
Sexual trauma 140
Sexually transmitted
    diseases 81, 92, 278
    infections 80, 184
Shaw's classification 200, 201
Sheehan syndrome 170
Sim's speculum 205
Sinecatechins 95
Skeletal system 86
Skin 269
    disorders 74
Sleep apnea, obstructive 173

Sleep hygiene 14
Sling surgery 27
Smoking 14, 152, 206
    habits 40
Snow storm 255
Somatic type tumors 220
Spatial peak temporal average 25
Sperm
    antigens constitute 56
    under guidance 55
Spina bifida 212
Spinal anesthesia 34
Spine 200
Spiral arterioles 12
Spironolactone 179, 180
Splenic surgery 27
Spontaneous abortion, recurrent 34
Squamocolumnar junction 41,
    233, 234, 235f
Squamous cell cancer 265, 269, 276
Squamous cell carcinoma 94, 265,
    279, 322, 326, 329
Squamous epithelium 41, 42
Squamous hyperplasia 265, 266
Squamous intraepithelial lesion,
    low-grade 233, 241
Stellate ganglion block 62
Sterile draping done 44
Steroidal regulation 4
Stimulation protocol
    mild 191
    minimal 190
Stool examination 75
Stress 14
    physical 182
    urinary incontinence 208, 210, 213
Stromal endometrial layers 135
Stromal invasion 312
Stromal junction, epithelial 267
Stromal tissue 123
Strontium ranelate 64
Styrene maleic anhydride 55
Subcutaneous tissue 269
Subendometrial echogenic linear
    striations 21
Subfertility 124, 140
Submucosal fibroids 19, 20, 108
    large 118
Submucosal hemorrhage 142
Submucosal myoma 108
Submucosal pedunculated
    fibroids 118

Submucosal polyp 109
Submucous
  fibroid 183, 185
  leiomyomas 116
  myomas, classification of 19*t*
Subserosal edema 153
Subserosal fibroid 108, 109, 116
Subserous fibroid 310
Suburetheral nodule 255, 257
Subvaginal tissue 276
Suicidal ideation 140
Suppressive antiviral therapy 94
Systematic retroperitoneal
    lymphadenectomy 302
Systemic estrogen
  risks of 66
  therapy 65
Systemic illness 106
  severe 37
  signs of 168

T

Tamoxifen treatment 133
Tears, mapping of 205
Telerobotic arms 33
Tendon reflexes, deep 200
Tenesmus 109
Teratoma, benign 228
Terminal hair 177
Testosterone 4, 11, 174
  derivatives 114
Theca lutein cysts 25, 222
Therapeutic options 63
Thermal index 25
Thromboembolic complications 193
Thromboembolism 272
Thromboplastin time, activated
    partial 103
Thyroid
  disease 184
  disorder 182, 183
  function 166
    tests 179
  stimulating hormone 5, 103
Thyroid-releasing hormone 15
Tibolone 62, 63
Tinidazole 75, 77
Tissue 283
  connective 196
  diagnosis 298
  disorders, connective 196
  soft 325
  thermal destruction of 247

Tobacco, use of 184
Toxicities, mild 334
Toxicity 334
  profile 341
Tranexamic acid 105, 117
Transabdominal
  sonography 217
  ultrasound 17, 153
Transcervical endometrial
    coagulation 135
Transdermal contraception 50
Transdermal patch 50
Transperineal ultrasonography 25
Transuterine veress CO_2
    insufflation 28
Transvaginal
  color Doppler 153
  pelvic 17
  scan 25
  sonography 151, 159, 217, 298
    diagnostic 154
  ultrasonography 34, 124, 134,
    145, 188
  ultrasound 17, 124, 217, 228
Trichloroacetic acid 95
Trichomonal vaginitis 73, 75
Triphasic teratoma 220
Trocar insertion, direct 28
Trocars, placement of secondary 28
Trophectoderm cells 186
Trophoblastic
  cells 257
  disease, persistent 257
  sequelae 254
  tumor 257, 260, 262, 318
    epithelioid 258, 262
Tubal
  corrective surgery 152
  damage 152
  ectopics 155
  endometriosis 183
  factor 183
  hyperemia 81
  patency 27, 46
  polyp 183
  rupture 152
  spasm 183
  sterilization 26, 152
  surgery 26
Tuberculin skin testing 88
Tuberculosis 86
  in infertility patients 88
  of endometrium 87
  of Fallopian tubes 87
  of ovaries 87

Tubo-ovarian abscess 24, 43, 80,
    142, 224
Tubo-ovarian mass 109
  complex 217
  formation 126*f*
Tuboplasty 26
Tumor
  cells 311
  epithelial 222
  extent of 267
  invades bladder 276
  irregular solid 21
  malignant 257
  markers 219, 298, 306, 310
  of bowel 109
  of ovary, primary malignant
    339
  rupture 311
  size 309
  smooth multilocular 22
  thickness 268, 319
  well-lateralized 320
Turner's syndrome 165

U

Ultra low dose therapy 61
Ultraradical surgery 271
Ultraradical vulvectomy 269, 271
Ultrasonic cutting 31
Ultrasonic energy sources 30
Ultrasonography, indications of 17*t*
Umbilical surgery, one-port 32
Umbilicus 27, 29
Unifocal primary tumor 270
Unilateral oophorectomies 57
Unilocular cyst 22
Urea 205
Uremia 280
Ureteral injury 33, 284
Ureteral strictures 284
Ureteric involvement
    pyelonephritis 279
Urethra 320, 325
  causes of hypermobility of 211
  distal 269
  pipe stem 212
Urethral closure pressure,
    maximum 209
Urethral hypermobility 215
Urethral meatus, external 267
Urethral pressure 209
  maximum 209
  profile 209

Urethral support defect 211
Urinary
  catheter 272
  complaints 109
  frequency 224
  incontinence 210, 272, 319
    complaints of 205
    mixed 210, 214
    nonsurgical treatment of 214
  menotropins 188
  symptoms 200
  tract infection 82
Urination, urgency of 297
Urine
  analysis 298, 310
  culture 298, 310
  loss of 210
  pregnancy test 152
  retention of 221
  routine 205
  sediments 75
Urogenital diaphragm 269
Urological causes 142
Urticaria 180
Uteinized granulosa cells 10
Uterine 45
  anomalies 310
  artery 283
    embolization 117, 136
    intraoperatively 117
    ligation of 283
    occlusion, Doppler-guided 119
  bleeding
    abnormal 44, 45, 81, 101, 108, 205
    heavy 37
    in adolescents, treatment of abnormal 106
    irregular 102
  carcinoma 336
  cavity 36, 45, 46, 255, 267, 332
    empty 159, 160, 161
    removal of foreign body from 34
    visualization of 46
  cervix 329
  curettage 43, 255
  damage 37
  descent 201
  disease 167
  distension
    equipment for 35
    techniques for 35

echogenicity, decreased 134
enlargement 21
factor 183
fibroid 108, 185
  resection 34
  tumors 108
incision, anterior 117
infection, active 37
leiomyoma 219
lesion resistant to chemotherapy 260
ligaments 123
manipulators 30
musculature 257
perforation 37, 44-46, 255, 260
polyp 26
resectoscope 36
sarcoma 109
septum 183
  resection 34
size 279
smooth muscle cells 108
sounding 45
specimens 108
surgery 26, 133
tenderness 81
transplant 166
wall thickening 21
Utero-ovarian ligament 159 197
Uteroperitoneal fistula 160
Uterosacrals 197
Uterovesical fold 283
Uterus 3, 11, 18, 24, 73, 80
  bicornuate 183
  desirous of retaining 119
  distention of 116
  established 28
  fixed retroversion of 82
  large 118
  normal 109
  perforation of 43
  rupture 260
  sounding of 44

V

Vagina 32, 41, 73, 123, 320
  anterior 284
  bimanual examination of 276
  colposcopy of 267
  development of 275f
  palpation of 276
  posterior 284
    curve to 196

radiation necrosis of 277
satellite lesions in 246
upper 277
Vaginal approach 206
Vaginal areas 276
Vaginal bleeding
  abnormal 140
  irregular 52, 258
Vaginal cancer 275, 276, 326, 327
  early-stage 325
  primary 275
Vaginal contraceptive rings 49
Vaginal creams 40
Vaginal cuff 283
Vaginal delivery 211
Vaginal dilators 277
Vaginal discharge 73, 78, 82, 109, 110, 118, 226
  abnormal 81, 140
  causes of 74t
  purulent 258
  syndromic management of 78
Vaginal fibrosis 277
Vaginal fistulas 284
  rectal 284
  urinary 284
Vaginal fornix
  lesions in 277
  posterior 124
Vaginal hysterectomy 283
Vaginal infection 44
  acute 44
Vaginal inspection 275
Vaginal intraepithelial neoplasia 249, 275, 326
Vaginal length, total 204f
Vaginal moisturizers 66
Vaginal mucosa 168, 267, 284
Vaginal nodule 257
Vaginal packing 332
Vaginal ring 49
  combined 49
Vaginal septum, transverse 163, 164, 221
Vaginal speculum
  inserted 44-46
  posterior 43
Vaginal stenosis 334
Vaginal sulci, lateral 205
Vaginal support, distal 199
Vaginal tablet 76
Vaginal tube 30

Vaginal wall 205
　anterior 201, 255
　lesions, posterior 276
　posterior 201
Vaginectomy
　partial 250, 277, 326
　　upper 251
　total 250, 251, 326
Vaginitis 98, 245
Vague abdominopelvic pain 226
Varicose veins 297
Vascular endothelial growth factor 191, 334
Vascular obstruction 142
Vascular system 124
Vasomotor symptoms 61
Vasovagal reaction 46
Vein thrombosis, deep 284
Venetian blinds 21
Venlafaxine 62
Venous thromboembolism 61, 105, 174, 180
　disease 66
Venous thrombosis 66
Veress needle 29
　insertion 27
　　pneumoperitoneum 27
　modifications 29
Verrucous 265
　carcinoma 279
　tumor 269

Vesicovaginal fistula repair 32
Vesicovaginal septae 123
Vessel
　abnormal 239
　sealing devices 31
Villoglandular papillary adenocarcinoma 279
Viral infections in gynecology 92
Virological tests 93
Visceral pelvic fascia 196, 197
Visiport optical trocar 30
Visual disturbances, symptoms of 164
Visual problems 258
Vitamin 62
　D 64
Vomiting 81, 258
Vulva 73
　bimanual examination of 276
Vulval cancer 265, 267
　radiotherapy for 272
Vulval intraepithelial neoplasia 94
Vulval lesion, premalignant 266
Vulval varicosities 142
Vulvar cancer 265-267
　advanced 321, 323
　pathology of 265
Vulvar disease 251
Vulvar intraepithelial neoplasia 251, 251f, 265
　histopathology 252f

Vulvar pathology, classification of 251
Vulvar tissue, loss of 268
Vulvar wound 272
Vulvectomy 268
Vulvodynia 139
Vulvovaginal
　atrophy 64
　candidiasis 76
Vulvovaginitis, nonspecific 75

W

Wertheim hysterectomy 277
Whiff test 73
Whirlpool sign 227
White blood cell 81
Whole-abdominal irradiation 342
William's vulvovaginoplasty 166
Wilms' tumor 219
Women on hormone replacement therapy 297
Women, symptomatic 119
Women's health initiative 61, 66
World Health Organization 80, 138, 182
Wound breakdown 272

Y

Yolk sac tumors 343
Yttrium aluminum garnet 135